Huppert's Notes

Pathophysiology and Clinical Pearls for Internal Medicine

Huppert's Notes
Pathophysiology and Clinical Pearls for Internal Medicine

AUTHOR
Laura A. Huppert, MD
Clinical Fellow
Division of Hematology/Oncology
Department of Medicine
University of California, San Francisco

LEAD CONTRIBUTING EDITOR
Timothy G. Dyster, MD
Chief Resident
Department of Medicine
University of California, San Francisco

New York   Chicago   San Francisco   Lisbon   London   Madrid   Mexico City
New Delhi   San Juan   Seoul   Singapore   Sydney   Toronto

1 2 3 4 5 6 7 8 9   DSS   26 25 24 23 22 21

ISBN 978-1-260-47007-9
MHID 1-260-47007-5

This book was set in Proxima Nova by MPS Limited.
The editors were Kay Conerly and Christie Naglieri.
The production supervisor was Richard Ruzycka.
Project management was provided by Adwiti Pradhan.
The cover designer was W2 Design.
This book is printed on acid-free paper.

Library of Congress Cataloging-in-Publication Data

Names: Huppert, Laura A., author, editor. | Dyster, Timothy G., editor.
Title: Huppert's Notes : Pathophysiology and Clinical Pearls for Internal
Medicine / Editors, Laura A. Huppert, Timothy G. Dyster.
Other titles: Pathophysiology and clinical pearls for internal medicine
    Description: New York : McGraw Hill, [2021] | Includes bibliographical
    references and index. | Summary: "This text succinctly organizes the foundational
    science covered early in medical school and the clinical approaches
    encountered in clerkships and beyond. This marriage of pathophysiology
    and clinical medicine provides a framework for how to approach internal
    medicine concepts mechanistically, rather than through memorization.
    It is filled with concise descriptions of common medical conditions
    with diagnostic and management pearls, as well as high-yield
    diagrams and tables to emphasize key concepts."—Provided by publisher.
Identifiers: LCCN 2020044358 (print) | LCCN 2020044359 (ebook) | ISBN
    9781260470079 (softbound alk. paper) | ISBN 9781260470086 (ebook)
Subjects: MESH: Internal Medicine | Handbook
Classification: LCC RC46 (print) | LCC RC46 (ebook) | NLM WB 39 | DDC
    616—dc23
LC record available at https://lccn.loc.gov/2020044358
LC ebook record available at https://lccn.loc.gov/2020044359

McGraw Hill books are available at special quantity discounts to use as premiums and sales promotions, or for use in corporate training programs. To contact a representative please visit the Contact Us pages at www.mhprofessional.com

Contents

Contributors

Author
Laura A. Huppert, MD
Clinical Fellow, Division of Hematology/Oncology,
Department of Medicine,
University of California, San Francisco,
San Francisco, California

Lead Contributing Editor
Timothy G. Dyster, MD
Chief Resident, Internal Medicine Residency
Department of Medicine,
University of California, San Francisco,
San Francisco, California

CHAPTER 1: CARDIOLOGY

Contributing Author
Jacqueline T. DesJardin, MD
Clinical Fellow, Division of Cardiology,
Department of Medicine,
University of California, San Francisco,
San Francisco, California

Faculty Reviewer
Lucas S. Zier, MD, MS
Assistant Professor of Clinical Medicine,
Division of Cardiology,
Department of Medicine,
University of California, San Francisco,
San Francisco, California

CHAPTER 2: PULMONOLOGY

Contributing Author
Timothy G. Dyster, MD
Chief Resident, Internal Medicine Residency
Department of Medicine,
University of California, San Francisco,
San Francisco, California

Faculty Reviewer
Lekshmi Santhosh, MD, MAEd
Assistant Professor of Clinical Medicine and Associate
Program Director for Pulmonary & Critical Care Fellowship,
Division of Pulmonary, Critical Care,
Allergy and Sleep Medicine,
Department of Medicine,
University of California, San Francisco,
San Francisco, California

CHAPTER 3: CRITICAL CARE MEDICINE

Contributing Author
Michael Z. Root, MD, MBA
Resident Physician, Internal Medicine Residency
Department of Medicine,
University of California, San Francisco,
San Francisco, California

Faculty Reviewer
Brian L. Block, MD
Assistant Professor of Medicine,
Division of Pulmonary, Allergy,
Critical Care & Sleep Medicine,
Department of Medicine,
University of California, San Francisco,
San Francisco, California

CHAPTER 4: GASTROENTEROLOGY

Contributing Author
Lisa X. Deng, MD
Resident Physician, Internal Medicine Residency
Department of Medicine,
University of California, San Francisco,
San Francisco, California

Faculty Reviewer
Sara M. Lewin, MD
Assistant Professor of Medicine,
Department of Gastroenterology,
University of California, San Francisco,
San Francisco, California

CHAPTER 5: ENDOCRINOLOGY

Contributing Author
Saundra Nguyen, MD
Chief Resident, Internal Medicine Residency
Department of Medicine,
University of California, San Francisco,
San Francisco, California

Faculty Reviewer
Elizabeth Murphy, MD, PhD
Professor of Clinical Medicine,
Division of Endocrinology,
Department of Medicine,
University of California, San Francisco,
San Francisco, California

CHAPTER 6: NEPHROLOGY

Contributing Author
Jesse Ikeme, MD
Resident Physician, Internal Medicine Residency
Department of Medicine,
University of California, San Francisco,
San Francisco, California

Faculty Reviewer
Rafia Chaudry, MD
Assistant Professor of Clinical Medicine,
Division of Nephrology,
Department of Medicine,
University of California, San Francisco,
San Francisco, California

CHAPTER 7: HEMATOLOGY AND ONCOLOGY

Contributing Author
Kelsey H. Natsuhara, MD
Resident Physician, Internal Medicine Residency
Department of Medicine,
University of California, San Francisco,
San Francisco, California

Faculty Reviewer
Sam Brondfield, MD, MAEd
Assistant Professor of Clinical Medicine,
Division of Hematology & Oncology,
Department of Medicine,
University of California, San Francisco,
San Francisco, California

CHAPTER 8: INFECTIOUS DISEASES

Contributing Author
John C. Penner, MD
Resident Physician, Internal Medicine Residency
Department of Medicine,
University of California, San Francisco,
San Francisco, California

Faculty Reviewer
Jennifer M. Babik, MD, PhD
Associate Professor of Clinical Medicine,
Associate Program Director for the
Infectious Diseases Fellowship,
Associate Program Director for the Internal
Medicine Residency, Division of Infectious Diseases,
Department of Medicine,
University of California, San Francisco,
San Francisco, California

CHAPTER 9: RHEUMATOLOGY

Contributing Author
John P. Huizar, MD
Resident Physician, Internal Medicine Residency
Department of Medicine,
University of California, San Francisco,
San Francisco, California

Faculty Reviewer
Sarah Goglin, MD
Assistant Professor of Clinical Medicine,
Associate Program Director for the
Rheumatology Fellowship,
Assistant Program Director for the Internal Medicine
Residency, Division of Rheumatology,
Department of Medicine,
University of California, San Francisco,
San Francisco, California

CHAPTER 10: GENERAL MEDICINE

Contributing Author
Sarah J. Flynn, MD, MPhil
Resident Physician, Internal Medicine Residency
Department of Medicine,
University of California, San Francisco,
San Francisco, California

Faculty Reviewer
Molly Cooke, MD, MACP
Professor of Clinical Medicine,
Department of Medicine,
University of California, San Francisco,
San Francisco, California

CHAPTER 11: DERMATOLOGY

Contributing Author
Lowell Nicholson, MD
Resident Physician, Internal Medicine Residency
Department of Medicine,
University of California, San Francisco,
San Francisco, California

Faculty Reviewer
Ryan Y. Arakaki, MD
Assistant Professor of Dermatology,
Department of Dermatology,
University of California, San Francisco
San Francisco, California

CHAPTER 12: NEUROLOGY

Contributing Author
Lauren Patrick, MD
Clinical Fellow, Weill Institute for Neurosciences,
Department of Neurology,
University of California, San Francisco,
San Francisco, California

Faculty Reviewer
Megan Richie, MD
Assistant Professor of Neurology,
Weill Institute for Neurosciences,
Department of Neurology,
University of California, San Francisco,
San Francisco, California

CHAPTER 13: PSYCHIATRY

Contributing Author
Nicholas Rozón, MD
Chief Resident, Department of Psychiatry,
University of California, San Francisco,
San Francisco, California

Faculty Reviewer
Erick K. Hung, MD
Associate Professor of Clinical Psychiatry and
Residency Training Director,
Department of Psychiatry,
University of California, San Francisco,
San Francisco, California

ADDITIONAL CONTENT REVIEWER

Elizabeth Marshall, MD
General Internist, Wind River Cares Family and
Community Health Center,
Arapaho, Wyoming

Preface

Dear Reader,

Welcome to the first edition of *Huppert's Notes*! The story of these *Notes* begins when I was a third-year medical student at Harvard Medical School. I wanted a resource that distilled key concepts in internal medicine, bridging the pathophysiology that we learn in the beginning of medical school with the clinical concepts and approaches we learn on the wards. I perused a plethora of resources but never found a single resource that met this need. Therefore, I started creating my own set of notes – the earliest version of *Huppert's Notes* – compiling what I learned from articles, lectures, and clinical teaching. I printed and carried these *Notes* in my pocket, adding to them during each rotation. During internal medicine residency and chief residency at the University of California, San Francisco (UCSF), I further updated the *Notes* with diagnostic frameworks that I learned during morning reports and treatment approaches that I learned by caring for patients on the wards with my medicine team. Over time, the *Notes* became my comprehensive outline of internal medicine.

I originally wrote these *Notes* for myself, never intending to publish them. However, through a serendipitous series of events, an editor at McGraw Hill saw a copy of my *Notes* and introduced the prospect of publishing. I was excited to share this resource with a broader audience of trainees, and eager to use this opportunity to make them even more high-yield. Therefore, I recruited an amazing team of residents and faculty members, including individuals known to be the most dedicated and talented medical educators, to update and improve each chapter. The incredible work of the contributing authors transformed these *Notes* into the resource that you hold in your hands today. The book is titled "*Huppert's Notes*" in honor of its roots, but it now reflects the wisdom and expertise of all its contributing authors.

This book is designed to serve as a framework for your learning in internal medicine. In lectures or on the wards, use these *Notes* to frame your understanding and add your own notes in the designated space at the end of each chapter. Unless otherwise noted, every chapter is structured in the same way:

1. Anatomy and Physiology
2. Diagnostics
3. Approaches and Chief Complaints
4. Diseases and Pathophysiology
5. Key Medications and Interventions
6. Key Clinical Trials and Publications
7. Space for your personal notes

This book is primarily intended for medical trainees, from medical students to internal medicine interns and residents. Practicing physicians can also benefit from this reference – I still use these *Notes* in my own practice today! As an educational resource, this book is not intended to replace clinical or management guidelines; please use your clinical judgment and reference other resources as needed.

In closing, I hope that *Huppert's Notes* serves as a foundation for approaching internal medicine and sparks an enthusiasm for learning that is central to our profession. Enjoy!

Laura A. Huppert, MD

Acknowledgements

Huppert's Notes would not have been possible without an all-star team of residents and faculty that significantly contributed to this work. First, I am grateful to our incredible team of resident contributing authors and faculty content reviewers, who transformed this book into the incredible resource that it is today; I cannot imaging working with a more dedicated and talented group of colleagues who care so deeply about medical education. Second, I want to thank the lead contributing editor, Dr. Timothy Dyster, who co-reviewed the manuscript, contributed to multiple chapters, and whose passion, and talent for medical education was essential to the success of this project. Third, I want to thank my editor at McGraw Hill, Kay Conerly, who patiently and expertly guided us through the publishing process. I'm also grateful to the entire McGraw Hill team who worked on *Huppert's Notes* including Christie Naglieri, Libby Wagner, and Adwiti Pradhan. I also want to thank my family and friends who supported me throughout my medical training and the publishing process. Finally, I am grateful to those who taught me internal medicine over the last decade, including my peers and faculty mentors. These individuals shared their knowledge and passion for medicine with me, and in turn I hope that these *Notes* can help do the same for trainees in the future.

Cardiology

1

Cardiac Anatomy

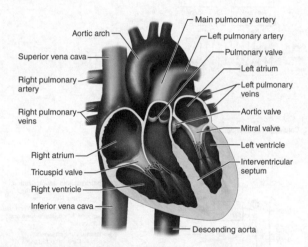

FIGURE 1.1: **Cardiac chambers, valves, and major vessels.**

Cardiac Electrophysiology

- Cardiac electrical conduction system: Sinoatrial (SA) node (1° pacemaker) → Atrioventricular (AV) node (stalls conduction; can also act as a backup pacemaker with rate of 40–60 bpm) → Bundle of His → Right/left bundle → Purkinje fibers → Ventricle
- Pacemaker cells (SA/AV node cells) automatically create electrical impulses that trigger myocyte cells (atrial/ventricular cells)
  - <u>Pacemaker action potential</u> is described using three phases (Phases 0, 3, and 4). It is automatic and initated by a slow inward Ca^{2+} current. The maximum diastolic potential (analogous to resting membrane potential) is ~−55 mV (Figure 1.2)
  - <u>Myocyte action potential</u> is described using five phases (Phases 0–4). It is automatic and triggered by a fast inward Na^+ current. The resting membrane potential is −90 mV, determined by K^+ conductance and equilibrium potential (Figure 1.3)

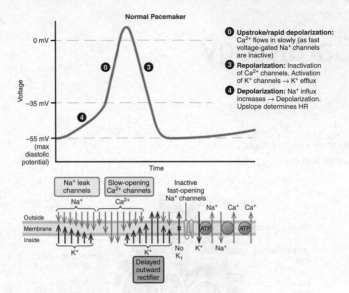

Normal Pacemaker

0 **Upstroke/rapid depolarization:** Ca^{2+} flows in slowly (as fast voltage-gated Na^+ channels are inactive)

3 **Repolarization:** Inactivation of Ca^{2+} channels. Activation of K^+ channels → K^+ efflux

4 **Depolarization:** Na^+ influx increases → Depolarization. Upslope determines HR

FIGURE 1.2: **Cardiac pacemaker cell action potential.**

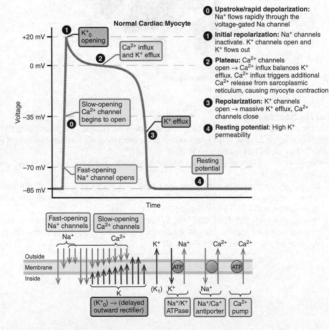

Normal Cardiac Myocyte

0 **Upstroke/rapid depolarization:** Na^+ flows rapidly through the voltage-gated Na channel

1 **Initial repolarization:** Na^+ channels inactivate. K^+ channels open and K^+ flows out

2 **Plateau:** Ca^{2+} channels open → Ca^{2+} influx balances K^+ efflux. Ca^{2+} influx triggers additional Ca^{2+} release from sarcoplasmic reticulum, causing myocyte contraction

3 **Repolarization:** K^+ channels open → massive K^+ efflux, Ca^{2+} channels close

4 **Resting potential:** High K^+ permeability

FIGURE 1.3: **Cardiac myocyte action potential.**

TABLE 1.1 · Hemodynamic Calculations Used Clinically

Volume Calculations
SV = EDV − ESV
SV = CO/HR
EF = SV/EDV = (EDV − ESV)/EDV. Normal 55–70%.

Pressure Calculations
MAP = (SBP + [2 × DBP])/3. Normal 65–100 mmHg.
MAP = CO × SVR
mPAP = (PASP + [2 × PADP])/3. Normal <20 mmHg.

Resistance Calculations
Ohm's Law: V = IR; R = V/I
SVR = (MAP − RAP) × 80/CO. Normal 800–1200 dynes × cm^{-5}.
PVR = (mPAP − PCWP)/CO. Normal <3 Wood units.

Flow Calculations
CO = HR × SV. Normal 4–8 L/min.
CO = VO$_2$/(Ca − Cv)
CO = VO$_2$/(Hgb × 13.6 × [PaO$_2$ − MvO$_2$]). Fick Principle.
CI = CO/BSA. Normal 2.4–4 L/min/m^2.

Abbreviations: Stroke volume (SV), End-diastolic volume (EDV), End-systolic volume (ESV), Cardiac output (CO), Heart rate (HR), Ejection fraction (EF), Mean arterial pressure (MAP), Systolic blood pressure (SBP), Diastolic blood pressure (DBP), Mean pulmonary artery pressure (mPAP), Pulmonary artery systolic pressure (PASP), Pulmonary artery diastolic pressure (PADP), Voltage (V), Current (I), Resistance (R), Right atrial pressure (RAP), Pulmonary vascular resistance (PVR), Pulmonary capillary wedge pressure (PCWP), Heart rate (HR), Stroke volume (SV), Oxygen consumption (VO$_2$), Arteriovenous oxygen difference (Ca − Cv), Hemoglobin (Hgb), Partial pressure of oxygen (PaO$_2$), Myocardial volume oxygen (MvO$_2$), Cardiac index (CI), Body surface area (BSA)

Determinants of Cardiac Function

- Preload: Myocardial stretch before contraction (i.e., the end-diastolic length of the cardiac fibers), which affects the force of contraction
  - Proxy: End-diastolic volume (EDV), end-diastolic pressure (EDP)
  - Frank-Starling curve: ↑Venous return → ↑SV + ↑CO
    - Increases preload: ↑Blood volume, exercise, sympathetic (reduced venous compliance), ↓HR (longer filling time)
- Afterload: Force to push against. Two types: Wall stress and vascular resistance
  - Proxy = systemic or pulmonary vascular resistance, ventricular wall stress
  - Wall stress = (pressure × radius) / (2 × wall thickness); ↑ Wall stress = ↑ O$_2$ demand
  - Systemic vascular resistance (SVR) (component of LV afterload) = (MAP − RAP) / CO
    - Increases LV afterload: Hypertension, aortic stenosis, systolic heart failure (↑ Wall stress)
  - Pulmonary vascular resistance (PVR) (component of RV afterload) = (mPAP − PAWP) / CO
    - Increases RV afterload: PE, pulmonary arterial hypertension
- Contractility: Inherent ability of the myocardium to contract independent of preload or afterload
  - Proxy: None (SV, CO, EF provide an impression; however, all are affected by preload/afterload)
    - Increases contractility: Sympathetic (catecholamine via β1 receptor), inotropic drugs (e.g., dobutamine via B1 receptor, digoxin via ↑intracellular Ca^{2+}), tachycardia (via Ca^{2+} buildup)
    - Decreases contractility: Parasympathetic (ACTH via M2 receptor), beta blocker/calcium channel blocker, CHF/MI, acidosis, hypoxia/hypercapnia

There are three ways to increase stroke volume (i.e., the area of a pressure-volume curve; Figure 1.4):
  - Increased preload → ↑SV (Frank-Starling)
  - Decreased afterload → ↑SV (increases linearly along the end-systolic pressure-volume relationship [ESPVR])
  - Increased contractility → ↑SV (increased slope of ESPVR line)

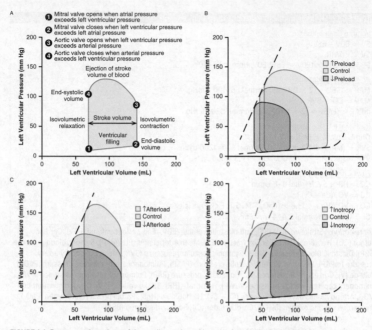

FIGURE 1.4: Pressure volume loop of the cardiac cycle and impact of preload, afterload, and inotropy.
A) Cardiac pressure-volume loop and key physiologic events. B) Interactions between preload and afterload at constant inotropy. C) Interdependent effects of changes in afterload. D) Interdependent effects of changes in inotropy.

Phases of the Cardiac Cycle
- Diastole:
  - Atrial pressure > ventricular pressure → Tricuspid and mitral valves open → Filling
  - Contraction: Atrial pressure < ventricular pressure → Tricuspid and mitral valves close → S1
    - Mitral valve snaps before the tricuspid valve because the LV contracts first (but normally heard as just one sound)
    - S1 is loudest at the apex (fifth intercostal space, mid-clavicular line)
- Systole:
  - ↑Ventricular pressure in isovolumetric contraction until ventricular pressure > pulmonary artery/aortic pressure → Pulmonic and aortic valves open → Ejection
  - End of ejection: Ventricular pressure falls → Pulmonic and aortic valves close → S2
    - Aortic sound occurs before the pulmonic sound because the aortic pressure is higher
    - S2 is loudest at the base (upper sternal border)
    - "Split S2": The close of the aortic valve (A_2) and the close of the pulmonary valve (P_2) are not synchronized and become wider during inspiration (i.e. widened A_2P_2) because ↓intrathoracic pressure → ↑Venous return → Longer RV emptying time → Pulmonic valve closes later → P_2 comes later

Extra Heart Sounds
- **S3** (Ventricular gallop): OVERLOAD; early diastolic sound, listen with the stethoscope's bell
  - Turbulent flow of blood hitting an overfilled ventricle
  - Differential diagnosis: Can be normal in patients age <35 yr or in pregnancy. Otherwise, specific sign of decompensated heart failure (92% specificity for LVEDP >15 mmHg and BNP >100 pg/mL)
- **S4** (Atrial gallop/kick): STIFF VENTRICLE; late diastolic sound, listen with the stethoscope's diaphragm
  - Atrium pushing blood against a stiff ventricle
  - Differential diagnosis: Always pathologic – ventricular hypertrophy (secondary to HTN), heart failure

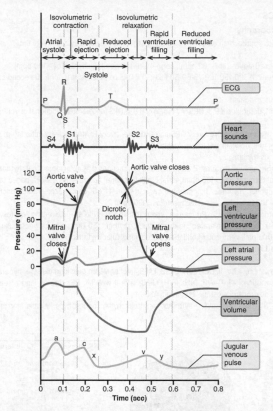

FIGURE 1.5: **The cardiac cycle.** This image depicts the relationship between various cardiac parameters over the course of a single cardiac cycle, including cardiac filling (black), ECG findings (dark green), heart sounds (purple), aortic pressure (light blue), left ventricular pressure (dark blue), left atrial pressure (green), ventricular volume (royal blue), and jugular venous pulse (lime).

Central Venous Pressure (CVP) Waveform / Jugular Venous Pulse (JVP)

- **a** wave: **a**trial contraction
- **c** wave: RV **c**ontraction (closed tricuspid valve bulging into the atrium)
- **x** descent: Atrial rela**x**ation and downward displacement of the closed tricuspid valve during ventricular contraction
- **v** wave: Increased RA pressure during systole because passive filling against a closed tricuspid **v**alve
- **y** descent: Tricuspid valve opens and empt**y**ing blood from RA fills RV

DIAGNOSTICS

Electrocardiography

It is important to approach an electrocardiogram (ECG) using the same system every time:

1. Rate
   - Definitions: Bradycardic (<60 bpm), normal (60–100 bpm), tachycardic (≥100 bpm)
   - Assessment: 1) 300-150-100-75-60-50 Rule; 2) # QRS complexes × 6 (for a 10-second strip)
2. Rhythm
   - Regular vs. irregular:
     - If not 1:1, determine if P > QRS (AV block) or if P < QRS (accelerated junctional or ventricular rhythm)
   - Sinus vs. nonsinus:
     - <u>Sinus rhythms</u>: P before every QRS and QRS after every P. Atrial activity initiating at sinus node: P upright in II, down in avR, sinusoidal in V1
     - <u>Nonsinus rhythms</u>:
       - Abnormal atrial rhythms: Premature atrial contractions (PACs), ectopic atrial rhythm (<100 bpm), atrial tachycardia (>100 bpm), atrial fibrillation, atrial flutter, AVNRT, AVRT, paced atrial rhythms
       - Junctional rhythms: Junctional escape rhythm (<60 bpm), accelerated junctional rhythm (60–100 bpm), junctional tachycardia (>100 bpm)
       - Ventricular rhythms: Premature ventricular beats (PVCs), idioventricular (escape) rhythm (<50 bpm), accelerated idioventricular rhythm (50–100 bpm), ventricular tachycardia (>100 bpm), ventricular fibrillation, paced ventricular rhythms
3. Axis (Figure 1.7)
   - Normal axis: +I, +II
   - L axis deviation: +I, −II. Ddx: LVH, LBBB, LAFB, inferior MI, chronic lung disease, hyperkalemia
   - R axis deviation: −I, +aVF. Ddx: RVH, LPFB, lateral wall MI, PE, chronic lung disease, arm lead reversal, dextrocardia, ostium secundum ASD
   - Extreme "NW" axis: −I, −aVF, +aVR. Ddx: Ventricular rhythm, pacing, hyperkalemia, lead misplacement

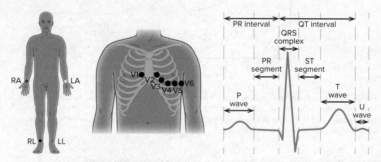

FIGURE 1.6: **Standard ECG lead placement and elements of a normal waveform.**

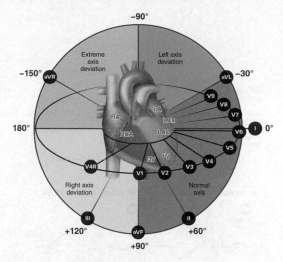

FIGURE 1.7: **ECG lead detection displayed in 360 degrees.**

4. Interval
- Measurement: Big box = 0.2 seconds, small box = 0.04 seconds
- Intervals:
  - **PR:** normal is 0.12–0.2 seconds (3-5 small boxes)
    - Ddx long PR: First-degree AV block, high vagal tone, conduction delay, AV nodal agents, hypokalemia
    - Ddx short PR: WPW, high catecholamine state
  - **QRS:** Normal is <0.12 seconds (<2.5 small boxes)
    - Ddx long QRS: 1) Ventricular rhythm; 2) Bundle branch block; 3) Intraventricular conduction delay (IVCD; slowing of both bundles, normal morphology but stretched QRS); 4) Medications (e.g., TCAs, antiarrhythmics); 5) WPW; 6) Paced rhythms
    - **Bundle branch blocks:** QRS may be narrow or wide; incomplete block = narrow QRS, complete block = wide QRS
      - **Fascicular blocks:** Typically narrow QRS (<0.12ms), then look at axis, I/avL, II/III/avF
        - LAFB: LAD (-45^0 to -90^0) with no other cause (diagnosis of exclusion), qR in I/avL, rS in II/III/avF
        - LPFB: RAD with no other cause (diagnosis of exclusion), rS in I/avL, qR in II/III/avF
      - **Unifascicular block:** QRS is wide; due to one slow conduction tract; can be normal (0.2% of normal population)
        - RBBB: V1 rSR' (QRS terminal forces POSITIVE), wide slurred S in lateral leads (I, avL, V5, V6)
      - **Bifascicular blocks:** QRS is wide; due to two unhealthy/slow conduction tracts; <u>always</u> abnormal and indicative of a diseased conduction system; should trigger workup for underlying heart disease (e.g., ischemia, infiltrative disease)
        - LBBB: V1 down (QRS terminal forces NEGATIVE), tall R in lateral leads, deep S in V1–V3 (Figure 1.8). New LBBB may suggest ischemia (see Table 1.2)
        - RBBB + LAFB (RBBB + LAD beyond −45 degrees)
        - RBBB + LPFB (RBBB + RAD beyond +120 degrees)
      - **Trifascicular block:** QRS is wide; due to three unhealthy/slow conduction tracts; always abnormal and indicative of a very diseased conduction system; should trigger workup for underlying heart disease and consideration of ambulatory ECG monitoring
        - Patients alternate between RBBB and LBBB
        - Any bifascicular block + AV block (especially second degree)
  - **QT:** Varies with HR. Ballpark QT less than half the RR interval is normal. Corrected QT (QTc): QTc = QT / $\sqrt{(R - R)}$: 0.33–0.47 seconds. If QT is prolonged, risk of torsades.
    - Ddx long QT: Hypocalcemia, hypomagnesemia, medications (e.g., antibiotics, ondansetron, certain psychiatric medications, methadone), long QT syndrome
    - Ddx short QT: Hypercalcemia, short QT syndrome, digoxin toxicity

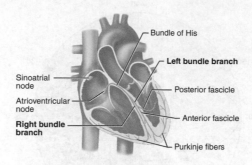

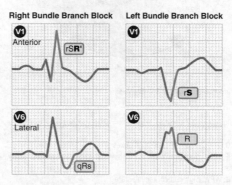

FIGURE 1.8: **Conducting system of the heart and ECG appearance of right and left bundle branch blocks.**

TABLE 1.2 · Identification of Ischemia in LBBB
• A LBBB does not always indicate a STEMI, but it may suggest ischemia and can make ST changes difficult to interpret
• Use modified Sgarbossa criteria (ANY of the following meets criteria for an acute MI):
1. Concordant ST elevation >1 mm
2. ST depression >1 mm V1-V3
3. ST elevation to S wave amplitude ratio >0.25 mm

5. Hypertrophy
   • Atrial abnormalities: Look at P waves (Figure 1.9)
     - <u>RA enlargement</u>: II- P tall and peaked >2.5 mm (*think **peaked** = **pulmonale***). V1–V2: Prominent initial positivity of P >1.5 mm
     - <u>LA enlargement</u>: II- P wide, double peaked >120 ms (*think of double humped "**m**" = **mitrale***). V1- More negative
   • Ventricular hypertrophy:
     - <u>RV hypertrophy (RVH)</u>: Right axis deviation required for RVH (unlike LVH); early R wave progression; V1 with tall R
     - <u>LV hypertrophy (LVH)</u>: Cannot call LVH in the setting of LBBB; there are multiple diagnostic criteria for patients >35 yr, but, no perfect diagnostic method:
       • Framingham: R in avL >11 mm in men or >9 mm in women (one of the quickest/easiest methods)
       • Sokolow Lyon criteria: S V1 + R V5 or V6 = 35 mm (fairly specific)
       • Cornell criteria: S in V3 + R avL >28 mm in men, >20 mm in women (65% sensitivity, 95% specificity)
       • Estes criteria: 1. Sokolow Lyon + LAA + repolarization changes (usually in I, avL, V4–6)

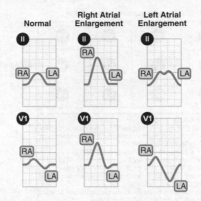

FIGURE 1.9: **ECG appearance of the p-wave in right and left atrial enlargement.** The p-wave is a complex wave that is influenced by both right and left atrial depolarization. When an atrium is abnormally enlarged, the duration of its depolarization increases, changing the p-wave's waveform. Abbreviations: RA = right atrium's contribution to the p-wave; LA = left atrium's contribution to the p-wave.

6. R wave progression
   - Normal R wave transition occurs V3–V4:
     - Ddx late R wave transition: Anterior MI, LVH, chronic lung disease, incorrect lead placement
     - Ddx early R wave transition: Posterior MI, RVH, RBBB, WPW, Duchenne's muscular dystrophy, incorrect placement
     - Ddx tall R wave in V1: Posterior MI, RVH, RBBB, WPW, Duchenne's muscular dystrophy, skeletal deformities, incorrect lead placement
7. Ischemia
   - Q waves:
     - Q waves tell you about the timing of the ischemic event. Pathologic if >25% R wave, 1 mm in width. Evidence of prior MI if ≥2 pathologic Q waves in contiguous leads.
     - S1Q3T3 pattern suggests RV strain (e.g., due to a pulmonary embolism)
   - ST segment:
     - **ST elevations:** Consider ischemia! Location of the ST elevations *can* help localize the lesion (Figure 1.10)
       - Infarct shortens the action potential
       - For ST elevation MI (STEMI): Requires new 1 mm ST elevation in two consecutive leads; in V1–V3 criteria is 1.5 mm ST elevation for women and 2 mm ST elevation for men. Measure from J point (beginning of ST segment). The criteria are different if LVH or LBBB is present (see Table 1.2).
       - Ddx for ST Elevation: STEMI should be at the top of the differential diagnosis! Other things to consider include normal early repolarization, LV aneurysm, pericarditis, hyperkalemia, Brugada syndrome
     - **ST depressions:** Consider ischemia! Location of ST depressions *cannot* help localize the lesion
       - For non-ST elevation MI (NSTEMI): Typically >0.5 mm downsloping or horizontal ST depressions
       - Ddx for ST depressions: NSTEMI, LVH, drugs, severe hypokalemia, rate-related
     - **T waves:** Evaluate for T wave inversions, peaking, flattening
       - Ddx for T wave inversions: Can be nonspecific, ischemia/infarction (especially if >2 mm, symmetric, and across precordium), hypokalemia, RV strain (S1Q3T3), LV strain, juvenile pattern, cardiomyopathy, myocarditis, intracerebral hemorrhage; normal in BBB (T wave should be opposite the terminal forces of the QRS)
     - **Evolution of ECG changes:** After an ischemic event, ECG changes will occur in a predictable pattern over time, with persistence of the Q wave (Figure 1.11)

CARDIOLOGY

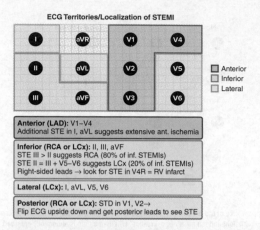

ECG Territories/Localization of STEMI

Anterior
Inferior
Lateral

Anterior (LAD): V1–V4
Additional STE in I, aVL suggests extensive ant. ischemia

Inferior (RCA or LCx): II, III, aVF
STE III > II suggests RCA (80% of inf. STEMIs)
STE II = III + V5–V6 suggests LCx (20% of inf. STEMIs)
Right-sided leads → look for STE in V4R = RV infarct

Lateral (LCx): I, aVL, V5, V6

Posterior (RCA or LCx): STD in V1, V2→
Flip ECG upside down and get posterior leads to see STE

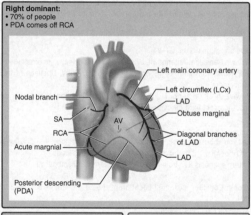

Right dominant:
• 70% of people
• PDA comes off RCA

Left dominant:
• PDA comes off LCx

Co-dominant:
• RCA and LCx both supply PDA and posterior lateral system

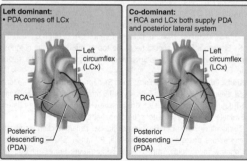

FIGURE 1.10: **Coronary anatomy and ECG territories.** Abbreviations: Left anterior descending artery (LAD), right coronary artery (RCA), left circumflex artery (LCx), posterior descending (PDA), right coronary artery (RCA), sinoatrial node (SA), atrioventricular node (AV), ST elevation (STE), ST depression (STD), ST elevation MI (STEMI), anterior (ant.), inferior (inf.)

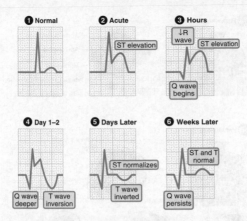

FIGURE 1.11: **Progression of myocardial infarction on ECG.** After an ischemic event, ECG changes will occur in a predictable pattern over time, with persistence of the Q wave.

Echocardiography

Transthoracic echocardiography (TTE)
- Definition: Most common type of echocardiogram. The ultrasound transducer is placed on the chest or abdomen of the patient to get various views of the heart to provide a noninvasive assessment of cardiac function, including an assessment of the heart valves and degree of cardiac contraction.

Transesophageal echocardiography (TEE)
- Definition: Echocardiogram performed using a transducer that is passed into the patient's esophagus, thus allowing better visualization of cardiac structures compared to a TTE.
- Indications: Evaluating for a cardiac source of embolism, endocarditis, prosthetic heart valve dysfunction, native valvular disease, and aortic dissection or aneurysm

Point-of-care (POC) echocardiography
- Definition: A bedside echocardiogram that can be done to assess for gross abnormalities. Bedside assessment is highly dependent upon user skill, so it is important to practice with a skilled point-of-care ultrasound (POCUS) provider. See Figure 1.12.
- Indications: A bedside echocardiogram can be performed to identify different causes of acute cardiac failure or hemodynamic instability. The size and ability to compress the inferior vena cava (IVC) can be used to estimate the right atrial (RA) pressure:
  - IVC >2.1 cm and <50% collapsible: Right atrial pressure approximately 15 mmHg
  - IVC <2.1 cm and <50% collapsible: Right atrial pressure approximately 8 mmHg
  - IVC >2.1 cm and >50% collapsible: Right atrial pressure approximately 8 mmHg
  - IVC <2.1 cm and >50% collapsible: Right atrial pressure approximately 3 mmHg

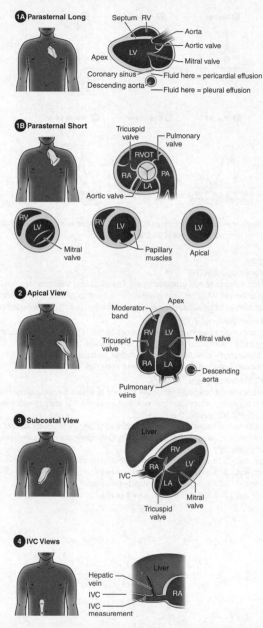

FIGURE 1.12: **Views in Cardiac Point of Care Ultrasound (POCUS).** This figure depicts four common views utilized in cardiac POCUS. For each view, the figure at left shows the position of the transducer on the patient's chest/abdomen. The figure at right shows a depiction of the cardiac structures visible using that view. Of note, POCUS is highly user-dependent so clinical findings should be confirmed with a formal TTE if indicated. Abbreviations: Right atrium (RA), Right ventricle (RV), Left atrium (LA), Left ventricle (LV), Inferior vena cava (IVC).

Cardiac Stress Testing

- Indications:
  - Assessment for a new diagnosis of coronary artery disease (CAD) in patients with chest pain who have been ruled out for acute coronary syndrome (ACS)
    - Helpful in patients who have INTERMEDIATE pre-test probability of CAD (Table 1.3)
      - If low pre-test probability of CAD, stress testing is not specific enough (positive results are often *false* positives)
      - If high pre-test probability of CAD, stress testing is not sensitive enough (negative results are often *false* negatives); instead proceed to coronary angiogram, which is more sensitive/specific
    - Chest pain quality and age together determine the probability of underlying CAD (Table 1.3)
      - Features of chest pain concerning for CAD:
        - Substernal location
        - Provoked by exertion or emotion
        - Improved by rest or with nitroglycerin
      - All features = Typical angina; 2–3 features = atypical angina; 0–1 features = nonanginal
    - Also adjust assessment of CAD risk using the Atherosclerotic Cardiovascular Disease (ASCVD) Risk Calculator and additional factors:
      - Very high risk: History of MI, stroke, TIA, peripheral arterial disease
      - High risk: Familial hypercholesterolemia, prior CABG or PCI, DM, HTN, CKD (eGFR 15–59), current smoker, LDL-C persistently ≥100 mg/dL despite treatment, heart failure
      - Other risk enhancers: Low HDL, LDL >160 mg/dL, family history of premature ASCVD (<55 yr in male first degree relative; <65 yr in female first degree relative), metabolic syndrome (TG >150 mg/dL, HTN, DM, low HDL-C, increased weight circumference), inflammatory conditions (especially RA, psoriasis, HIV), menopause before 40 yr, pregnancy complications (e.g., pre-eclampsia), high-risk ethnicity (e.g., South Asian)
- Contraindications: Recent MI or active ACS, decompensated heart failure, uncontrolled arrhythmias; severe hypertension may preclude testing or affect the validity of the results
- Pre-stress test patient instructions:
  - Instruct patients to take all medications as usual with the exception of beta blockers
  - Patients are allowed to eat, but cannot consume caffeine prior to vasodilator testing
- Types of stress tests: Can vary the combination of stressor and detector (Table 1.4)
  - Possible stressors:
    - Exercise – Treadmill or bike
    - Pharmacologic – Coronary vasodilators (adenosine derivatives, e.g., regadenoson) or β1 agonist (dobutamine)
  - Possible detectors:
    - ECG
    - ECHO
    - Nuclear (PET vs. SPECT such as 99m Tc-sestamibi)
    - Cardiac MR (new technology, only available in select centers)

TABLE 1.3 • Pre-Test Probability of CAD Based on Age and Features of Chest Pain				
Age (yr)	Typical Angina	Atypical Angina	Nonanginal Chest Pain	Asymptomatic
30–39	Intermediate	Very low	Very low	Stress testing is generally not indicated for asymptomatic patients
40–49	Intermediate	Low	Very low	
50–59	Intermediate	Intermediate	Low	
60–69	High	Intermediate	Intermediate	
>70	High	Intermediate	Intermediate	

Reference: Genders et al. Eur Heart J 2011;32(11):1316–30.

TABLE 1.4 · Types of Cardiac Stress Tests			
		Stressor	
	Exercise Pros: Can assess exercise tolerance Cons: Must be able to exercise	**Vasodilator (regadenoson)** Contraindications: WPW, COPD (risk of bronchospasm), sinus node dysfunction or high-degree AV block without pacemaker (risk of worsening conduction disease), baseline hypotension (risk of worsening) No caffeine within 24–48 hours	**Beta-1 agonist (dobutamine)** Contraindications: Frequent ventricular arrhythmias, afib with RVR, hemodynamically significant LV outflow tract obstruction, severe hypertension (SBP>180 mmHg) Consider holding beta blockers prior to test
Detector	**ECG only** Contraindications: Baseline abnormal ECG (e.g., paced, LBBB, LVH, ST depressions at rest, WPW, digoxin) Cons: Cannot localize ischemia, no hemodynamic assessment for valvular disease, not helpful in the setting of prior revascularization	Exercise ECG (frequently used pairing)	Not performed	Not performed
	Echo (+ ECG) Pros: Localize ischemia, assess valvular disease and hemodynamics, highest specificity Cons: Views may be limited in obesity or if poor echo windows	Exercise Echo	Vasodilator Echo (pairing not used in the US)	Dobutamine Echo (frequently used pairing)
	Nuclear (+ ECG) Pros: Localize ischemia, highest sensitivity Cons: Radiation exposure	Exercise NM	Vasodilator NM (frequently used pairing)	Dobutamine NM (pairing not used in the US)

Note: All stress tests include an ECG component.

Myocardial Viability Study
- Indications: Identifies "hibernating" myocardium that could regain function after revascularization
- Methods: MRI, FDG-PET

Coronary CT Angiography (CCTA)
- Indications: Direct anatomic assessment of the coronary anatomy (less sensitive than invasive coronary angiography); CT can increasingly provide physiologic assessment with FFR (fractional flow reserve, a measure of pressure/flow across a coronary lesion); CT-FFR allows clinicians to estimate the hemodynamic significance of coronary lesions noninvasively.
- Methods: Noninvasive ECG-gated CT during which contrast is timed to fill the coronary arteries. Heart rate must be low (e.g., <70 bpm) during testing.
- Utility: CCTA is increasingly being used in place of stress testing. In patients with stable angina, CCTA allows clinicians to rule out significant left main CAD (which benefits from revascularization, see Coronary Artery Disease section later), and thus start empiric medical therapy without invasive testing.

Left Heart Catheterization/Coronary Angiogram
- Procedure: A thin catheter is placed in an artery (usually radial, sometimes femoral), advanced to the ascending aorta, and then contrast is injected to visualize the coronary arteries from their origin off of the aorta (diagnostic). Can cross the aortic valve, but this is not always performed. In addition to getting diagnostic information, it is also possible to intervene upon blockages (i.e., percutaneous coronary intervention [PCI]).
- Indications:
  - CAD: Both diagnostic (can identify culprit lesion and directly measure FFR) and therapeutic (can place stent to open a blockage). Diagnose CAD in patients with symptoms, ACS, HF, VT, post-arrest.
  - Aortic stenosis: Determine the severity of AS (cross the aortic valve and measure the pressure gradient)
- Percutaneous coronary interventions (PCI):
  - Bare metal stents (BMS): Rarely done in current day. Largely replaced by drug-eluting stents (DES).
  - Drug eluting stents (DES): Standard of care. Lower rates of restenosis compared to BMS; current generation ("3rd") has better safety profile than first generation. Requires lifelong aspirin. Also need dual antiplatelet therapy (DAPT) × 6 months (or for 1 yr if DES is placed in the setting of ACS).
- Post-catheterization complications:
  - Immediately post-catheterization:
    - Stroke (risk ~0.05% at 30 days)
    - Vascular access complication (~4% risk femoral; <2% risk radial): Hematoma, retroperitoneal bleeding (get STAT CT abd/pelvis, transfuse empirically), vessel damage requiring intervention (e.g., pseudoaneurysm, dissection)
    - Renal injury: Risk of contrast-associated AKI in patients with CKD and high-volume contrast (>350 mL); newer low-osmolality contrast agents have reduced risk; Cr typically peaks within 3–5 days
    - Coronary artery dissection, procedure-related myocardial infarction
    - In-stent thrombosis: Typically presents as a STEMI that occurs minutes to months after PCI. Can occur due to a mechanical problem with the stent or discontinuation of antiplatelet therapy
  - Longer-term post-catheterization:
    - In-stent restenosis: Typically presents as gradual onset anginal symptoms that occur months to years after PCI

Right Heart Catheterization
- Procedure: Insertion of a catheter into the right heart and pulmonary arteries usually via the IJ or brachial vein in order to measure the RA, RV, PA, and wedge pressures as well as cardiac output.
- Indications: Diagnosis of pulmonary hypertension, assessment of hemodynamics in heart failure (specifically: pre-heart transplant, if unable to wean from inotropes, severe symptoms of hypotension despite medical therapy).

APPROACHES AND CHIEF COMPLAINTS

Chest Pain

Approach to chest pain

- Take a focused history: Ask about the character and quality of pain, provoking and relieving factors, duration and frequency.
- Perform a targeted exam: Vitals (including BP in both arms and legs), cardiac and chest wall exam, pulmonary exam, abdominal exam.
- Differential diagnosis:
  - Think about the five "cannot-miss" causes of chest pain: 1) ACS; 2) PE; 3) Aortic dissection; 4) Tension pneumothorax; 5) Esophageal rupture.
  - Then can consider a broader differential diagnosis by organ system (Table 1.5)
- Initial diagnostics:
  - ECG: Look for ST changes (ACS, pericarditis, demand), RV strain (PE), Q waves (evidence of prior ischemia)
  - CXR: Look for pneumonia, rib fractures, pneumothorax, widened mediastinum (can occur due to aortic dissection)
  - D-dimer: Use age-adjusted cutoff for patients >50 yr (age × 10 = upper limit cutoff); normal d-dimer can:
    - Rule out PE in low to intermediate clinical probability situations
    - Rule out aortic dissection in low risk patients (i.e., no connective tissue disease; no new murmur; no chest, abdominal, or back pain that is abrupt, severe, or ripping)
- CT scan: Timing of contrast differs slightly depending on whether the imaging focuses on the systemic or pulmonary arteries
  - CTA (CT angiography with arterial contrast) is used if most concerned for aortic dissection
  - CTPA (CT pulmonary angiography) is used if most concerned for PE

TABLE 1.5 • Etiologies of Chest Pain by System	
System	**Etiologies of Chest Pain**
Cardiac	**Angina:** Pain due to myocardial tissue ischemia (aka supply/demand mismatch) • Examples: ACS (STEMI, NSTEMI, unstable angina), stable angina, demand ischemia, vasospasm, spontaneous coronary artery dissection (SCAD), myocardial infarction with non-obstructive coronary arteries (MINOCA) • Characteristics: Especially concerning if "typical" features (i.e., substernal, exertional, improves with rest/nitroglycerin)
	Pericarditis: Pleuritic, sharp, retrosternal, relieved with sitting forward, +friction rub throughout the cardiac cycle
	Advanced heart failure or pulmonary hypertension (PAH): Pressure, often exertional dyspnea, syncope (with advanced PAH)
Vascular	**Aortic dissection:** Sudden onset tearing pain, radiates to the back, unequal pulses and discordant blood pressures in arms and/or legs, often occurs in the setting of hypertension or connective tissue disorders
	Pulmonary embolism (PE): Sudden onset, pleuritic, often associated with dyspnea
Pulmonary	**Pneumonia/pleuritis:** Lateral to midline, brief, often associated with dyspnea, cough, sputum production, fever
	Tracheobronchitis: Midline, burning discomfort, associated with coughing
	Pneumothorax: Sudden, pleuritic pain, dyspnea, decreased breath sounds. Spontaneous or associated with instrumentation (e.g., central line placement)
GI	**Peptic ulcer disease:** Burning, epigastric, relieved with food or antacids
	GERD: Burning, epigastric, worsened when lying flat after a meal
	Esophageal spasm: Pressure, tightness, retrosternal, mimics angina, often relieved by nitroglycerin (likely due to relaxant effect of nitrites on smooth muscle with resultant change in esophageal motility)
	Biliary disease: RUQ pain, may occur after meals
	Pancreatitis: Prolonged/intense epigastric/back pain, presence of certain risk factors (e.g., heavy alcohol use)
Neuromuscular	**Costochondritis:** Rare and often over diagnosed; sudden onset, intense/fleeting pain, may be reproduced with palpation
	Rib fracture: Reproducible on exam, associated with injury, localized, worse with movement, crepitus may be present
	Herpes zoster: Vesicular rash in area of discomfort, dermatomal distribution, burning
Psychological	**Panic disorder:** Chest tightness, palpitations, can have "typical" features, often associated with dyspnea

Syncope

- Definition: Transient loss of consciousness due to low blood pressure to the brain
- Rule out syncope mimickers: Stroke, seizure, TIA, atypical migraine, mechanical fall (e.g., due to dementia, gait abnormality, normal-pressure hydrocephalus, vision problems, neuropathy), weakness (e.g., due to anemia, metabolic derrangements, thyroid disorders, infection)
- Types:
  - Cardiogenic: No prodrome (i.e., sudden syncope without preceding symptoms). Get ECG, telemetry monitoring. Ddx:
    - Outflow obstruction (e.g., aortic stenosis, hypertrophic obstructive cardiomyopathy with exertion)
    - Arrhythmia (e.g., bradyarrhythmias or tachyarrhythmias)
  - Neurocardiac: Typically 3Ps: **P**rodrome, **P**ositional, **P**rovocation. Perform tilt-table test if possible. Ddx:
    - Vasovagal: Dizziness, weakness, nausea, diaphoresis, often identifiable trigger
    - Situational: Neurocardiogenic reflex that can occur with defecation, micturition, coughing, eating
    - Carotid sinus hypersensitivity: Stimulation of the carotid sinus can cause syncope
  - Orthostatic: Change in position triggers syncope. Get orthostatic vitals, which are abnormal if supine → standing ↓SBP ≥20 mmHg or ↓DBP >10 mmHg. Ddx:
    - Decreased volume (e.g., due to diarrhea, poor PO intake, hemorrhage)
    - Autonomic insufficiency: Medications (e.g., diuretics, nitrates, alpha-adrenergic blockers); neurogenic (e.g., neuropathy from diabetes or alcohol use, multiple sclerosis); elderly patients with decreased baroreceptor response
    - Adrenal insufficiency
- Workup:
  - Initial evaluation:
    - Take a thorough history
    - Perform orthostatic vital signs (e.g., check blood pressure with the patient lying, seated, and standing)
    - Physical exam: In particular, perform a careful cardiac exam (e.g., listen for murmurs), neurologic exam, and assess for volume status
    - ECG: Look for 1) Arrhythmias; 2) Conduction disease; 3) WPW – short PR, delta wave; 4) Long QT; 5) Brugada (V1: RSR', downsloping ST elevation)
  - If concerned for cardiac etiology, pursue further cardiac workup:
    - Continuous telemetry during the admission and consider discharging the patient with ambulatory cardiac monitoring
    - TTE: Determine whether the patient has a structurally normal or abnormal heart
      - Differential diagnosis of cardiogenic syncope with a structurally <u>normal</u> heart:
        - Channelopathies: Long QT, short QT, Brugada (V1: RSR', downsloping ST elevation)
        - Conduction system abnormalities: Sinus or AV node dysfunction, WPW
        - Ventricular tachycardia or fibrillation (e.g., catecholaminergic polymorphic VT)
        - Electrolyte disturbances
      - Differential diagnosis of cardiogenic syncope with a structurally <u>abnormal</u> heart:
        - Hypertrophic cardiomyopathy (HCM)
        - Arrhythmogenic right ventricular dysplasia (ARVD)
        - Arrhythmias related to cardiomyopathies or infiltrative disease (e.g., sarcoid, amyloid)
        - Congenital heart conditions
        - Valvular pathology (e.g., mitral or aortic stenosis)
        - Severe pulmonary arterial hypertension with RV dysfunction

DISEASES AND PATHOPHYSIOLOGY

Ischemic Heart Disease

Stable coronary artery disease (CAD)

- **Types:** Asymptomatic CAD or stable angina (angina that occurs reliably with exertion and emotional stress, relived with rest or nitroglycerin; due to fixed atherosclerosis)
- **Diagnosis:** Stress testing; computed tomography angiography (CCTA) vs. invasive coronary angiogram to assess anatomy
- **Workup:** HgA1c, lipid panel, ECG, TTE to assess LV function
- **Treatment:**
  - Address risk factors and disease pathology:
    - Smoking cessation
    - Exercise/weight loss/diet
    - Control hypertension (goal at least <140/90 mmHg), ACEi (or ARB if intolerant of ACEi)
    - Treat DM (preferably with SGLT2 inhibitors or GLP-1 agonists)
    - Treat HLD, start statin (e.g., atorvastatin, rosuvastatin; goal LDL <70 mg/dL)
      - Consider addition of ezetimibe if LDL not at goal (IMPROVE-IT 2015)
      - Consider addition of PCSK9 inhibitor if LDL still not at goal and/or family history (FOURIER 2018)
      - Consider addition of icosapent ethyl if fasting triglycerides >135 mg/dL in patients with known CAD or DM (REDUCE-IT 2019)
    - **Aspirin** (particularly if prior ACS event)
    - **Beta blocker (BB)** (particularly if prior ACS event)
  - Address symptoms (antianginal therapy for stable angina):
    - **Beta blocker (BB):** Increases coronary blood supply ($\downarrow$HR → $\uparrow$coronary diastolic filling time → $\uparrow$blood supply) and decreases myocardial demand ($\downarrow$contractility → $\downarrow$wall stress/O_2 demand)
    - **Calcium channel blocker (CCB):** If second agent required; similar mechanism as BB
    - **Nitrates:** Vasodilation of coronary arteries; venodilation → $\downarrow$preload → $\downarrow$wall stress/O_2 demand
      - Nitroglycerin (sublingual/ transdermal/ spray; taken as needed)
      - Isosorbide dinitrate (oral; taken BID or TID)
      - Isosorbide 5-mononitrate (oral; taken daily or BID)
    - **Ranolazine:** Inhibits late inward sodium current in ischemic myocytes (Phase 0) → $\downarrow$$Ca^{2+}$ overload → $\downarrow$wall stress/O_2 demand and $\uparrow$coronary blood flow.
    - **Revascularization:** Consider in patients who are symptomatic despite optimal medical therapy; only revascularize physiologically significant lesions as identified by stress testing or fractional flow reserve (FAME 2 2012; ISCHEMIA 2020).
      - EXCEPTIONS: Revascularization has mortality benefit in:
        - Significant left main disease (i.e., >50% stenosis LAD): All patients should be revascularized; CABG vs. PCI depends on anatomic complexity and surgical candidacy; decision should be made after multidisciplinary review.
        - Significant 3-vessel CAD (i.e., >70% stenosis in 3 vessels): All patients should be revascularized; CABG preferred to PCI in patients who are good surgical candidates (SYNTAX 2009), especially in patients with diabetes (FREEDOM 2012).
        - HFrEF: Consider revascularization, especially if severe CAD or viable myocardium (limited data, though may have long-term benefit).

Myocardial infarction

- Type I MI: Spontaneous MI (aka acute coronary syndrome from thrombus in a coronary artery) (Figure 1.13)
  - **ACS without ST elevation (NSTEMI)**
    - **NSTEMI:** *Subendocardial* ischemia
      - Criteria: Rise and/or fall in troponin (Table 1.6) AND at least one of the following:
        - Symptoms of acute myocardial ischemia
        - New ischemic ECG changes (e.g., significant ST-T changes or LBBB)
        - Development of pathologic Q waves
        - Imaging evidence of loss of myocardial function (e.g., new wall motion abnormality)
        - Coronary thrombus on angiography
    - Unstable angina: Angina at rest without troponin elevation or ECG changes; concept was developed in the era before sensitive biomarkers; becoming less clinically relevant and not included in the current guideline definition of MI; however, patients with worsening anginal symptoms often merit expedited evaluation with stress testing or coronary angiogram.
  - **ACS with ST elevation (STEMI):** *Transmural* ischemia

- Type II MI: MI due to ischemic imbalance (aka demand ischemia) (Figure 1.13)
  - Frequent cause of elevated troponin in patients with hemodynamic stressors (e.g., sepsis, severe hypertension), especially in patients with underlying stable CAD.
  - Treat the underlying hemodynamic cause.
- Coronary vasospasm:
  - Etiology: Transient coronary vasospasm that causes angina at rest.
  - Clinical: Classically chest pain that occurs at night in young women who smoke cigarettes and have migraines or Raynaud's; often co-occurs with CAD; can occur in patients on vasopressors.
  - Diagnosis: ECG with transient ST elevation that occurs during an episode of chest pain. Can mimic STEMI. Provocation testing: Hyperventilation, intracoronary acetylcholine.
  - Treatment: Smoking cessation, CCB, long-acting nitrate to prevent attacks, PRN nitrate to abolish attacks. Avoid nonselective beta blockers.

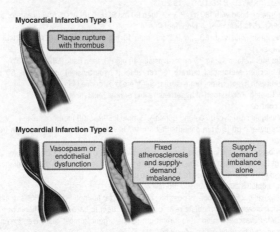

Myocardial Infarction Type 1

Plaque rupture with thrombus

Myocardial Infarction Type 2

Vasospasm or endothelial dysfunction

Fixed atherosclerosis and supply-demand imbalance

Supply-demand imbalance alone

FIGURE 1.13: **Pathophysiology of type 1 and type 2 myocardial infarction.**

TABLE 1.6 · Troponins: Definition and Assays
Definition: Troponins are proteins involved in cardiac contraction, which are detectable in the blood as biomarkers of myocardial injury and infarction.
Troponin assays: - <u>Conventional troponin assay</u>: Rises 3–5 hr after myocardial injury, peaks 24–48 hr, normalizes 5–14 d; trend q4–6 hours; risk of false negative when checked immediately after myocardial injury - <u>High-sensitivity troponin assay</u>: Use based on local algorithms, helpful in quickly ruling out myocardial infarction, increasingly preferred over conventional troponin assay

Acute coronary syndrome (ACS)
- Diagnosis: Diagnosis should be suspected based on a combination of history, ECG, and troponin; confirmed by invasive coronary angiography
- Initial medical therapy:
  - **Aspirin (ASA):** 325 mg PO ×1 chewed (VA Cooperative Study 1983; ISIS-2 1988), then 81 mg daily
  - **Anticoagulation:** Enoxaparin 1 mg/kg SQ q12h has the strongest evidence (ESSENCE 1997; ExTRACT-TIMI 25 2006), although heparin gtt often used because fast on/off if going to the cath lab so it can be held for arterial access; ensure SBP <180 mmHg and DBP <110 mmHg prior to administration of the anticoagulant
  - **PGY12 inhibitor:**
    - Clopidogrel (Plavix): Load with 600 mg ×1, then 75 mg daily (CURE 2001). Consider decreasing load to 300 mg if age >75 yr. If a patient is already on Plavix, reload in the setting of an acute ACS event (ARMYDA-8 RELOAD-ACS 2013).
    - Ticagrelor: Load with 180 mg PO ×1, then 90 mg PO BID (PLATO 2009 ticagrelor > clopidogrel; TREAT 2019 ticagrelor = clopidogrel)
    - Prasugrel: Load with 60 mg PO ×1, then 10 mg PO daily (ISR-REACT5 2019 prasugrel > ticagrelor)
  - **Statin:** Atorvastatin 80mg PO or rosuvastatin 40 mg PO, then daily (MIRACL 2001)
  - **Beta blocker:** Metoprolol tartrate (or carvedilol if hypertensive) to goal HR<60 bpm. Hold in patients with hypotension, bradycardia, or if there is evidence of heart failure
  - **ACEi:** Captopril or lisinopril if hypertensive and normal renal function
  - **Pain control:**
    - Sublingual nitroglycerin 0.4 mg q5min × 3, hold if SBP <100 mmHg, caution if RV infarct
    - Nitroglycerin gtt (start in patients that are still having pain after they have been treated with SL nitro ×3)
    - Ongoing chest pain indicates ongoing ischemia, so it is critical to use the above medications to try to get patients chest pain free. If chest pain cannot be resolved with medical management, then the patient should be taken to the cath lab urgently
    - Avoid opioids due to increased mortality
- Revascularization: PCI as soon as possible; can administer fibrinolytics/tPA if PCI is unavailable
  - **STEMI:** Indication for immediate revascularization; "door to balloon time" should be <90 min
  - **NSTEMI:** Revascularization is important but not as urgent in most cases (see exceptions below); generally can be done within 24–48 hr
    - Indications for immediate revascularization:
      - Acute heart failure or cardiogenic shock
      - Sustained ventricular arrhythmias
      - Mechanical complications (e.g., acute MR, VSD)
      - Refractory chest pain despite medication therapy
    - Urgent (within 24 hours) catheterization if intermediate to high risk (e.g., TIMI >3)
      Risk scores: 1) TIMI (Antman et al. 2000); 2) GRACE; 3) Killip. These scores can help determine the urgency of cardiac cath for NSTEMIs.
- Possible peri-MI complications:
  - Pump failure: Flash pulmonary edema, heart failure, cardiogenic shock
  - Thrombus and stroke (in setting of akinetic heart)
  - Recurrent infarction (hours–days)
  - Arrhythmias: Ischemic VT/VF
  - Mechanical complications:
    - Free wall rupture (hours–2 weeks): Pericardial tamponade with sudden hypotension, distant heart sounds; can cause PEA arrest and death
    - Interventricular septal rupture (hours–2 weeks): New VSD with holosystolic murmur with thrill, hypotension, respiratory distress
    - Papillary muscle rupture (2 days to 1 week): New MR with holosystolic murmur that radiates to the axilla, pulmonary edema, respiratory distress
    - Ventricular aneurysm: (weeks–months): ECG demonstrates persistent ST elevation; risk of clot/embolism, arrhythmias, angina, heart failure
  - Pericarditis:
    - Post-infarction pericarditis ([PIP], within days): Pleuritic, positional. Diffuse ST elevations, PR depressions. Treatment: Pain relief; continue ASA
    - Post-cardiac injury syndrome ([PCIS], also called Dressler's, weeks–months): Pericarditis due to an immune reaction; positional chest pain, friction rub, fever. Treatment: ASA +/− colchicine

- Post-MI management:
  - Aspirin 81 mg PO daily for life
  - Atorvastatin 80 mg PO daily for life (or another high-intensity statin); LDL goal <70 mg/dL (can add ezetimibe, PCSK9 inhibitor as needed)
  - PGY12 inhibitor (clopidogrel, ticagrelor, or prasugrel) for 1 yr post-MI (maybe longer if high ischemic risk and low bleeding risk)
  - Beta blocker
  - ACEi/ARB
  - Spironolactone/eplerenone if EF <40% and either DM or heart failure symptoms
  - TTE to assess LV function
  - Lifestyle modification: Smoking cessation, weight loss, exercise, diet
  - Diabetes control (ideally with SGLT2 inhibitors or GLP1 agonists)
  - Cardiac rehabilitation
  - Implantable cardioverter-defibrillator (ICD): Indicated if post-MI EF<35% despite medical therapy ×40 days or sustained VT/VF >2 days post-MI not due to reversible ischemia

Bradycardia
Approach to Bradycardia (HR <60 bpm)
- UNSTABLE:
  - Prepare for transcutaneous pacing (e.g., put pacing pads on the patient)
  - Atropine 0.5 mg IV q3–5 min, max 3 mg
  - Transcutaneous pacing
  - Dopamine 5–10 μg/kg/min or epinephrine 2–10 μg/min if pacing is not effective
  - Transvenous pacing
- STABLE: Observe, get ECG to rule out high-degree AV block, management depending on the etiology

Bradycardic Rhythms
Sinus bradycardia
- ECG: See Figure 1.14
- Physiologic causes: (Vast majority) Increased vagal tone or decreased sympathetic tone:
  - Sleep (HR can fall to 35–40 bpm normally, especially in young patients and those with OSA)
  - Well-conditioned athletes
  - Vasovagal episodes (e.g., vomiting, Valsalva)
  - Cushing's reflex due to increased intracranial pressure
  - Reflex bradycardia from severe hypertension
- Pathologic or extrinsic causes:
  - Medications (e.g., beta blockers, calcium channel blockers, clonidine, digoxin, amiodarone, timolol eye drops)
  - Ischemia (especially inferior MI)
  - Infiltrative diseases (e.g., sarcoid, amyloid)
  - Hypothermia, hypothyroidism, hypokalemia, hypoxia (if severe, prolonged)
- Treatment:
  - Asymptomatic or transient: No treatment required (majority of cases)
  - Symptomatic: Dizziness, hypotension, altered mental status
    - If unstable, give atropine and consider pacing as discussed above. Treat underlying problem. If beta blocker overdose, give glucagon. If calcium channel blocker overdose, give $CaCl_2$. Rarely, consider pacemaker placement.

Sinus arrhythmia
- Definition: Phasic variation in the sinus cycle; respiratory (variation with breathing) or nonrespiratory (variation not associated with breathing)
- Epidemiology: Most frequent arrhythmia; normal and common in young patients or those with high vagal tone

Sick sinus syndrome
- Definition: Nonspecific term referring to any or multiple of the following:
  - Persistent pathologic/symptomatic sinus bradycardia
  - Sinus arrest
  - SA exit block
  - Combinations of sinus and AV conduction disorders
  - Tachy-brady syndrome: Patients who alternate between any bradycardic rhythm and tachycardic rhythm (e.g., alternating paroxysmal Afib with RVR and symptomatic sinus bradycardia)
- Treatment: Consider pacemaker placement if symptomatic or associated with high-degree AV block

AV blocks
- First degree: Delayed conduction at the AV node. Prolonged PR (>200 ms), all atrial impulses conducted (1:1). Patients are usually asymptomatic and no treatment is necessary. Caution with use of beta blockers, calcium channel blockers.
- Second degree: Intermittent failure of conduction between the atria and ventricles (Figure 1.14).
    - Mobitz Type I (Wenckebach): Lengthening of PR until impulse not conducted and "dropped" beat (compare first/last). Usually a *nodal block* due to problems with the AV node itself (e.g., AV node damage due to ischemia/inflammation) or due to increased vagal tone (e.g., with sleep, drugs). Improves with atropine/exercise, worsens with carotid massage. No treatment needed unless symptomatic. Consider atropine and stop AV nodal blockers.
    - Mobitz Type II: No change in PR length but then sudden dropped beat. Usually an *infranodal block*, meaning that the issue is in the His-Purkinje system beneath the AV node (e.g., due to age, ischemia, aortic valve surgery). Improves with carotid massage, worsens with atropine/exercise. Can progress to third-degree block. Treatment: Pacemaker (Table 1.7).
- Third degree (complete): No AV conduction; no relationship between P and QRS (Figure 1.14). Escape, if present, is narrow (junctional) or wide (ventricular). Differential diagnosis: Ischemia, aging, lyme disease. Treatment: Pacemaker (Table 1.7).

TABLE 1.7 · Pacemakers: Indications and Types
• <u>General principle</u>: Pacemakers are implanted devices used to treat slow cardiac rhythms
• <u>Examples of indications for pacemaker placement</u>:
- Complete heart block with documented asystole >3 seconds in an awake patient, escape rates <40 bpm, escape rhythm with wide QRS
- Symptomatic second or third degree heart block
- Symptomatic bradycardia without reversible cause
• <u>Types of pacemakers</u>:
- RV pacemaker: 1 lead in apex of RV
- RV/RA pacemaker: 2 leads ("Dual"), sequential pacing
- Cardiac resynchronization therapy (CRT) pacemaker: 3 leads ("BiV," RA, RV, LV) pump synchronously, indicated if LBBB and HFrEF

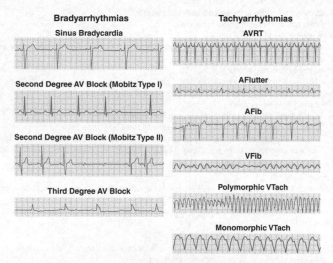

FIGURE 1.14: ECG examples of common bradyarrhythmias and tachyarrhythmias.

Tachycardia

Tachycardia is defined as having a heart rate >100 bpm. When approaching tachycardia, consider the following features: 1) Rate; 2) Wide (>0.12 s) or narrow (<0.12 s) QRS complex; 3) Regular or irregular

Narrow QRS Complex Tachycardia
Approach to Narrow QRS Complex Tachycardia

- UNSTABLE: If sinus tachycardia, treat the underlying cause if present (e.g., treat sepsis). If the tachycardia is due to a tachyarrhythmia, perform synchronized cardioversion.
- STABLE: Try to identify the rhythm (see rhythm abbreviations on the next few pages). Some clues:
  - Regular vs. irregular
  - Onset: Abrupt onset/offset suggests reentrant circuit (SANRT, AVNRT, AVRT)
  - Atrial rate:
    - Sinus tachycardia: typically 100–150 bpm (max rate = 220 − age)
    - Atrial tachycardia: typically 150–250 bpm
    - Atrial flutter: Atrial rate can be up to 300 bpm (ventricular rate often 150 bpm for 2:1 block)
    - Atrial fibrillation: Atrial rate can be 350+ bpm
  - P-wave morphology:
    - ST, SANRT: Sinus P waves
    - AVNRT: No P waves or distorts QRS (pseudo RSR' in V1)
    - AVRT: Retrograde or buried P waves
    - MAT: ≥3 P-wave morphologies before the QRS
    - Atrial fibrillation: No P waves
    - Atrial flutter: Flutter waves
  - RP intervals: See Figure 1.15
    - Short RP: P wave closer to the preceding R wave than the following R wave (i.e., first half of RR)
      - Ddx short RP: Typical AVNRT, antidromic/orthodromic AVRT, junctional tachycardia, atrial tachycardia with marked PR prolongation
    - Long RP: P wave closer to the following R wave than the preceding R wave
      - Ddx long RP: Sinus tachycardia, atypical AVNRT, orthodromic AVRT, atrial tachycardia
  - Response to vagal stimulation or adenosine (can be both diagnostic and therapeutic, see Table 1.8)
    - AVNRT, AVRT: Terminates arrhythmia, classically with P wave after the last QRS
    - ST, AT, MAT, atrial flutter: Slows ventricular rate enough to reveal an underlying atrial rhythm, but it doesn't usually terminate it (Exception: AT sometimes terminates with adenosine)

TABLE 1.8 · Adenosine Administration

- Indications: Used for diagnosis/treatment of narrow complex supraventricular tachycardias; DO NOT give for irregular wide complex tachycardias or if variable QRS morphology
- Administration: Warn the patient that they may feel flushing or palpitations but that it will be brief. Run the ECG strip while giving, push and flush 6 mg adenosine quickly, have external defibrillator available
- Dosing: Start with 6 mg, increase dose if no response: 6 mg → 12 mg → 18 mg (peripherally); 6 mg → 6 mg → 12 mg (centrally)

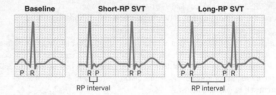

| Baseline | Short-RP SVT | Long-RP SVT |

FIGURE 1.15: **Interpretation of the RP interval.**

TABLE 1.9 · Wolff-Parkinson-White (WPW) and WPW Syndrome

WPW: Presence of an accessory pathway, recognized by preexcitation
- ECG features of preexcitation: 1) PR<0.12 seconds; 2) QRS>0.12 seconds due to delta waves (slow initial rise of QRS); 3) ST-T discordant changes (usually opposite vector from delta/QRS direction)
- Most patients with WPW pattern on ECG are asymptomatic, do not experience tachyarrhythmias, and require no treatment

WPW Syndrome: Patients with accessory pathways AND tachyarrhythmias
- AVRT: Most common; accessory pathway propagates the arrhythmia
- SVT with bystander accessory pathway:
  - When another atrial tachyarrhythmias (e.g., Afib, Aflut, Atach) occurs in a patient with WPW syndrome, the accessory pathway is a bystander (i.e., not the cause of the tachyarrhythmia), HOWEVER it can be very dangerous because the fast atrial rates can be transmitted directly to the ventricles via the accessory pathway and degenerate into ventricular fibrillation.
  - Recognize atrial fibrillation in WPW syndrome by an irregularly irregular wide QRS with changing morphologies; do not administer beta blockers/CCB/adenosine (they selectively inhibit AVN and promote rapid accessory pathway conduction to ventricles with risk of VF). Give procainamide instead.
- Treatment: Catheter ablation, occasionally antiarrhythmics

Regular Atrial Rhythms

Sinus tachycardia (ST)
- Etiologies: Infection, hypovolemia/hemorrhage, hypoxia, anemia, anxiety, PE, alcohol withdrawal, hyperthyroidism. In the outpatient setting in a patient with chronic sinus tachycardia without an underlying cause consider: 1) Chronic inappropriate sinus tachycardia or 2) Postural orthostatic tachycardia syndrome (POTS)
- Treatment: Treat underlying etiology

SA node reentrant tachycardia (SANRT)
- Description: Reentrant loop in the SA node; hard to discern from sinus tachycardia except rapid on/off. Relatively rare rhythm.

AV nodal reentrant tachycardia (AVNRT)
- Description: Reentrant circuit using fast and slow circuits within the AV node.
- ECG: Regular, narrow QRS with rate usually 120–220 bpm, no P waves (buried, occasionally can see pseudo-R' in V1, pseudo-S in inferior leads; only recognizable when comparing to the patient's normal QRS), short RP interval.
- Treatment: Acute: 1) Vagal maneuvers and 2) IV adenosine (breaks) (Table 1.8). Chronic: Ablation vs. nodal blocking agents.

AV reentrant tachycardia (AVRT)
- Description: Reentrant circuit using the AV node and accessory pathway; frequently occurs in patients with Wolf-Parkinson White (WPW) syndrome (Table 1.9)
- Subtypes:
  - Orthodromic (85%): Impulse travels down through the AV node and up through an accessory pathway. Narrow QRS, regular, rate often >200 bpm (Figure 1.14).
  - Antidromic (15%): Impulse travels down through an accessory pathway and up through the AV node. Wide QRS, regular (can look like VT), rate often >200 bpm.
- Treatment: 1) Vagal maneuvers, 2) IV adenosine (breaks), 3) Nodal agents

Atrial tachycardia (AT)
- Description: Impulse generated at a focus of enhanced automaticity in the atria other than the SA node. Associated with CAD, COPD, alcohol use, digoxin use; can occur in the absence of heart disease.
- ECG: P wave often looks different than a sinus P wave; atrial rate usually 110–250 bpm, ventricular rate can be regular or irregular (if variable block); narrow QRS, long RP interval; frequently occurs in recurrent self-terminating bouts.
- Treatment: Short-term use of BB or CCB. Long-term: BB, CCB, ablation.

Atrial flutter (Aflutter)
- Description: Irritable focus in the atria with reentrant circuit around the tricuspid annulus. Associated with mitral valve/tricuspid valve stenosis or regurgitation, or due to aging. Can occur in the absence of heart disease.
- ECG: Saw-toothed flutter waves best seen in leads II, III, aVF, or V1; atrial rate typically ~300 bpm; ventricular rate slower and can be regular (most common) or irregular (if variable AV nodal block); atrial to ventricular conduction usually in even ratio (e.g., 2:1 = 150 bpm, 4:1 = 75 bpm) (Figure 1.14).
  - Counterclockwise flutter (most common) = inverted flutter waves in the inferior leads
  - Clockwise flutter = upright flutter waves in the inferior leads

- Treatment: Similar to treatment of Afib.
  - Acutely: Rate control with metoprolol, diltiazem, but note that flutter is usually more difficult to rate control than Afib. If unable to rate control, consider TEE/cardioversion.
  - Chronically: Consider anticoagulation (by same criteria as Afib), ablation (success rate >90% in ablating flutter).

Irregular Atrial Rhythms

Premature atrial complexes (PACs)
- Description: Most common cause of irregular pulse and palpitations; benign, increased frequency with age, illness, tobacco/alcohol/caffeine
- ECG: Extra P waves, often with different morphology, and can be followed by a pause
- Treatment: None required unless symptomatic

Multifocal atrial tachycardia (MAT)
- Description: Increased automaticity at multiple sites in the atria. Associated with COPD, HF, hypokalemia, hypomagnesemia.
- ECG: ≥3 P waves with differing morphologies, atrial rates usually 100–130 bpm
- Treatment: CCB or BB if tolerated; treat underlying disease process

Atrial flutter with variable block
- Description: Atrial flutter with alternating block (e.g., 2:1 then 3:1). See Atrial flutter on prior page.

Atrial fibrillation (Afib)
- Description: Low-amplitude atrial activity that often originates in the pulmonary veins and oscillates at a rate of ~300–600 bpm; atrial activity is transmitted irregularly through the AV node, resulting in an irregular (often fast) ventricular rate
- Predisposing factors: Heart disease (e.g., CAD, MI, HTN, valve), older age, obesity, OSA
- Episodic/reversible triggers: Infection, heart surgery, VTE/PE, hyperthyroidism, alcohol, stress
- Symptoms: Fatigue, dyspnea, palpitations, irregular pulse, thrombi, stroke
- ECG: Irregularly irregular ventricular rhythm (e.g., irregular RR intervals, tiny erratic spikes), no P waves (Figure 1.14)
- Workup of new Afib: TSH, BMP, LFTs, TTE; calculate CHA_2DS_2-VASc and HAS-BLED scores (online calculators) to help determine need for anticoagulation, ambulatory ECG monitor (assess rate control), +/− sleep study
- Classifications:
  - Paroxysmal (<7 days) vs. persistent (>7 days) vs. long-standing persistent (>1 yr) vs. permanent (refractory to cardioversion)
  - Valvular vs. nonvalvular
  - Lone Afib (age <60 yr, without hypertension or structural heart disease)
  - Symptomatic (~75%) vs. asymptomatic (~25%)
- Treatment of Afib with rapid ventricular response (RVR):
  - Assess patient stability: Heart rate, blood pressure, mental status
    - UNSTABLE: Emergent synchronized cardioversion
    - STABLE: Manage as follows:
      - Identify and treat the triggering condition (e.g., infection, drugs, subarachnoid hemorrhage, medication noncompliance)
      - Rate control: Options for rate control agents include the following, in order of preference:
        - Beta blocker (careful in decompensated HF)
        - Calcium channel blocker (contraindicated in HF)
        - Amiodarone (also used for rhythm control so may result in cardioversion)
        - Digoxin (longterm use associated with increased mortality)
      - Consider cardioversion:
        - Types: Pharmacological (amiodarone) or electrical (direct current cardioversion [DCCV])
        - Obtain TEE before cardioversion in most patients, especially if not reliably anticoagulated for >4 weeks or Afib duration >48 hours (unless emergent)
        - Contraindication to cardioversion: Presence of left heart thrombus
        - Post-cardioversion: All patients require 4 weeks of anticoagulation due to increased stroke risk from cardiac stunning (although most will require lifelong anticoagulation due to an elevated CHA_2DS_2-VASc score)

- Treatment of chronic Afib:
  - **Treat reversible causes and triggers** (e.g., OSA, obesity, hyperthyroidism, heart failure)
  - **Reduce stroke risk:**
    - Anticoagulation:
      - Valvular Afib: e.g., Afib from mitral stenosis. Anticoagulate with warfarin (INR goal 2–3)
      - Nonvalvular Afib: Anticoagulate if history of TIA/stroke or CHA_2DS_2-VASc $\geq$2 (~2% annual stroke risk). Consider for CHA_2DS_2-VASc score of 1 (<1% annual stroke risk). Reconsider anticoagulation if HAS-BLED $\geq$5 ($\geq$12% annual major bleeding risk with warfarin). Choice of warfarin or direct oral anticoagulant (DOAC) (e.g., apixaban 5 mg BID, rivaroxaban 20 mg daily with food, or dabigatran 150 mg BID). If patient on DAPT for CAD and Afib, discontinue the second antiplatelet and only use dual therapy (RE-DUAL 2017).
      - Post-op Afib: Patients with new Afib after <u>cardiac</u> surgery usually don't need chronic anticoagulation; anticoagulate for 2–3 months, then discontinue if confirmed sinus on ambulatory ECG monitoring.
    - Procedures:
      - Left atrial appendage closure: Patients may be able to discontinue anticoagulation if success of closure confirmed by TEE; can be done surgically or percutaneously (WATCHMAN procedure).
  - **Manage the arrhythmia:**
    - Rate control:
      - Rate control is noninferior to rhythm control in asymptomatic patients >65 yr (AFFIRM 2002), although rhythm control is still preferred for certain patients
      - Types of rate control therapies:
        - Medications: BB or CCB to achieve goal HR <110 bpm with activity (RACE II 2010)
        - Procedures (less commonly used strategy): AV node ablation and pacemaker placement
    - Rhythm control:
      - Consider for:
        - Symptomatic patients
        - Young patients (generally recommend at least one DC cardioversion [DCCV] attempt)
        - HFrEF (catheter ablation may have improved outcomes, CASTLE-AF 2018)
      - Types of rhythm control therapies:
        - Cardioversion:
          - Indicated to restore sinus rhythm at least once in patients with persistent Afib who are <65 yr or $\geq$65 yr and symptomatic despite rate control
          - Duration of sustained sinus rhythm following cardioversion is variable, and early reversion to Afib occurs frequently in patients with a history of long-standing persistent Afib or LA diameter >5 cm
        - Antiarrhythmic drugs:
          - Scheduled medications: Goal to suppress Afib episodes to ~1×/year; rarely completely eliminates Afib. Options: Class IA (quinidine, procainamide), class IC (flecainide, propafenone), class III (sotalol, dofetilide); amiodarone (used for select patients given long-term side effects)
          - PRN dosing: Flecainide or propafenone "pill-in-pocket" strategy; appropriate in paroxysmal symptomatic Afib with CHA_2DS_2-VASc 0 in "lone Afib"
        - Procedures:
          - Cryoballoon ablation: Percutaneous; circumferential ablation around the pulmonary vein (PV) antrum for PV isolation; risk of phrenic nerve injury and PV stenosis; typically requires less technical skill and time than radiofrequency ablation
          - Radiofrequency catheter ablation: Percutaneous; mapping with directed ablation for PV isolation; similar efficacy to cryoballoon with possibly fewer complications
          - MAZE procedure: Surgical; intraoperative ablation to isolate PVs, most often performed in patients getting cardiac surgery for another indication or those who failed catheter ablation

TABLE 1.10 · Indications for Implantable Cardioverter Defibrillators (ICDs)

- General principle: ICDs are devices that are implanted into the body and can perform cardioversion, defibrillation, and pacing of the heart. Therefore, they can correct most life-threatening cardiac arrhythmias (i.e., fast rhythms)
- Examples of indications for ICD placement:
  - Secondary prevention: History of VT/VF arrest
  - Primary prevention: No history of VT/VF
    - Heart failure: EF <35% after optimal medical therapy for 3–6 months
    - Hypertrophic cardiomyopathy: Family history of sudden cardiac death, septal thickness >3 cm, unexplained syncope

Wide QRS Complex Tachycardia

Ventricular tachycardia (VT)

- Etiology: VT can be due to active ischemia, chronic ischemic heart disease (e.g., scar forms reentrant circuit), cardiomyopathy (e.g., congestive, hypertrophic, arrhythmogenic RV), inherited syndromes, congenital heart disease (e.g., tetralogy of Fallot), idiopathic
- Common artifact: It is common for telemetry artifact to look like VT. Get 12-lead ECG to evaluate.
- Diagnosis of VT:
  - Stable or unstable?
    - UNSTABLE: If the patient is hypotensive, non-responsive, or has chest pain, assume that it is VT and proceed with DCCV or ACLS
    - STABLE: If the patient is stable, you have more time to proceed to the next steps and try to differentiiate VT vs. SVT with aberrancy.
  - Does the patient have any risk factors for VT? (e.g., prior MI, prior cardiac surgery, known scars)? If so, it is safest to assume that it is VT.
  - Does the patient have a prior ECG with an old LBBB or RBBB? If the patient is stable AND has an old bundle branch block, it is more likely to be SVT with aberrancy, especially if the QRS morphology of their tachycardia looks like their baseline BBB.
  - Check for capture or fusion beats: If either of these is present, high positive predictive value for VT.
  - Check for A-V dissociation: Clear A-V dissociation confirms VT.
  - Check for concordance: Concordant QRS morphology in leads V1–V6 (i.e., all negative or all positive) suggests VT.
  - R wave in aVR? NW axis (aka up in aVR) is highly suggestive of VT.
  - Check the Brugada criteria. If any of the Brugada criteria are satisfied, it is likely VT. If none are satisfied, it is likely SVT. BUT no perfect criteria, which is why there are so many (e.g., Kindwall, Wellens, Brugada, Miller).
- Types of VT:
  - Monomorphic
    - ECG: Single QRS morphology
    - Etiology: Chronic ischemic heart disease (scar forms reentrant circuit), cardiomyopathy (e.g., congestive, hypertrophic, arrhythmogenic RV), inherited syndromes, congenital heart disease (e.g., tetralogy of Fallot), idiopathic
  - Polymorphic
    - ECG: QRS morphology varies from beat to beat
    - Etiology: Active ischemia (most common cause), long QT (torsades), catecholaminergic
    - Torsades de pointes: VT with varying QRS amplitude which occurs in the setting of long QTc (usually >500 ms) especially when bradycardic. Can be congenital or due to acquired causes (e.g., medications, hypokalemia, hypomagnesemia, bradycardia). Treatment: Magnesium 4 g IV, replete K to 4.5 mmol/L, keep HR >100 bpm (e.g., isoproterenol, epi, or pacing), lidocaine, stop QT-prolonging medications, defibrillation if unstable
- Treatment of VT:
  - Nonsustained (<30 seconds) or PVCs: Check electrolytes, evaluate for underlying heart disease; use beta blocker if symptomatic.
  - Sustained (>30 seconds): IV amiodarone (especially for monomorphic VT), lidocaine (especially for VT due to ischemia). Prepare for synchronized cardioversion. Look for underlying causes such as active ischemia, hypotension, hypo/hyperK, hypoMg.
  - Long-term management: ICD for secondary prevention after unstable VT or VT/VF arrest; pacemaker WITH antitachycardic pacing (PM senses VT then paces patient quickly to override the rhythm), antiarrhythmics (Class III e.g., sotalol; amiodarone), ablation.

SVT with aberrancy
- Description: A supraventricular tachycardia (Afib, Aflutter, Atach, orthodromic AVRT, AVNRT), which conducts through the AV node and down a slow conduction system (e.g., baseline RBBB or LBBB) causing the QRS to appear wide.
- Treatment: Adenosine, SVT treatment

Antidromic AVRT
- Description: AVRT that conducts down an accessory pathway and then up through the AV node causing the QRS to appear wide.
- Treatment: Adenosine

SVT with bystander accessory pathway
- Description: An SVT (other than AVRT or AVNRT) occurring in a patient with WPW syndrome, recognized by changing QRS morphologies.
- Treatment: Procainamide, amiodarone

Ventricular fibrillation (Vfib)
- Definition: Multiple foci in the ventricles fire rapidly, which can occur due to ischemia, drugs, rapid Afib with a bystander pathway, short-QT syndrome, Brugada syndrome (which is a Na^+ channelopathy; look for pseudo-RBBB with ST elevations in V1–V3 on resting ECG).
- ECG: Irregular, wide QRS (Figure 1.14)
- Treatment: Nonsynchronized defibrillation followed by amiodarone. If not associated with an MI, recurrence rate is 30% so ICD placement is indicated.

Heart Failure (HF)
- Etiology:
  - Left-sided HF: Ischemic vs. nonischemic (e.g., arrhythmia or tachycardia-mediated; valvular disease; hypertension; drugs/toxins [chemotherapy, alcohol, stimulants]; infiltrative diseases [sarcoid, amyloid, hemochromatosis])
  - Right-sided HF: Most often due to L-sided heart failure. Other causes: cor pulmonale (e.g., due to OSA, COPD, pulmonary arterial hypertension)
- Symptoms: Dyspnea, decreased exercise capacity, orthopnea, PND, nocturnal cough, fatigue, edema, abdominal bloating, early satiety
- Physical exam:
  - Signs of congestion: S3, pulmonary crackles, Cheyne-Stokes respirations (deep/fast breathing cycling with apnea), jugular venous distention, hepatojugular reflex, hepatomegaly, pulsatile liver, lower extremity or sacral edema, IVC >2.1 cm and <50% collapsible on POCUS, B-lines on lung POCUS (Table 1.11)
  - Signs of low cardiac output: Cool extremities, narrow pulse pressure, weak pulse, low SBP, altered mental status, reduced urine output (Table 1.11)
  - Other notable findings: Irregular rhythm, tachycardia, displaced point of maximal impulse (PMI), murmurs (e.g., MR, AS, TR), S4, reduced EF on POCUS
- Classification:
  - American College of Cardiology (ACC)/American Heart Association (AHA) stages and New York Heart Association (NYHA) functional classes:
    - **A** – At risk of HF but no diagnosis
    - **B** – Structural heart disease but without symptoms of HF
      - NYHA I – No limitations on physical activity
    - **C** – Structural heart disease with symptoms of HF
      - NYHA II – Slight limitation on physical activity, ordinary activity does not cause symptoms
      - NYHA III – Marked limitation on physical activity, ordinary activity causes symptoms
    - **D** – Refractory HF requiring advanced therapies
      - NYHA IV – Symptoms at rest and inability to participate in physical activity

TABLE 1.11 · Heart Failure: Signs of Congestion and Low Cardiac Output			
		Signs of Congestion	
		NO	YES
Signs of Low Cardiac Output	NO	"Warm and dry" (well compensated) Tx: Chronic HF management	"Warm and wet" Tx: Diuresis
	YES	"Cool and dry" Tx: Inotropes	"Cold and wet" Tx: Inotropes + diuresis

TABLE 1.12 · Diuretics				
Diuretic	Bioavailability	Equivalent Dose	Onset of Action (min)	Time to Peak (min)
Furosemide (Lasix)	50% PO	40 mg	30–60	60–120
	100% IV	20 mg	5	30
Bumetanide (Bumex)	90% PO	1 mg	30–60	60–120
	100% IV	1 mg	2–3	15–30
Torsemide (Demadex)	80% PO (no IV)	20 mg	60	60–120
Ethacrynic Acid (Edecrin)	100% PO	50 mg	30	120
	100% IV	50 mg	5	30

Add thiazide for sequential nephron blockade: Chlorothiazide 250–500 mg IV, Metolazone 2.5–5 mg PO.

- Diagnosis and work-up of heart failure:
  - TTE: Do when euvolemic
    - EF <40%: HF with reduced EF (HFrEF)
    - EF >50% with diastolic dysfunction: HF with preserved EF (HFpEF)
    - EF 40–50%: HF with mid-range EF (HFmrEF)
  - CXR: Kerley B-lines, pleural effusions, prominent interstitial markings and alveolar opacities ("butterfly" pattern)
  - Natriuretic peptides: Peptides released from the ventricles in response to stretch; elevated in acute and chronic HF but also increase with age, valvular disease, pulmonary hypertension, atrial arrhythmias (e.g., Afib), sepsis, CKD; false negative in obesity; useful to trend when patient's baseline is known; has prognostic value in HF
    - B-type natriuretic peptide (BNP): Uninterpretable in patients on sacubitril/valsartan (Entresto)
      - Can be used to exclude diagnosis of HF ("Breathing Not Properly" Study 2003)
        - <20 pg/mL = Rule out HF in asymptomatic outpatient with 96% NPV
        - <40 pg/mL = Rule out HF in symptomatic outpatient with 96% NPV
        - <50 pg/mL = Rule out Acute Decompensated HF (ADHF) in ED patient with 96% NPV
        - <100 pg/mL = Rule out ADHF in ED with 90% NPV
      - Can be used to identify HF:
        - >400 pg/mL = Identify ADHF in ED with 86% PPV
    - NT-proBNP: Useful in patients on sacubitril/valsartan (Entresto), <300 pg/mL useful to rule out ADHF in ED with 99% NPV (PRIDE study 2005)
  - ECG: Look for signs of the cause of HF such as LVH, atrial arrhythmias, tachycardia, Q waves, active ischemia, pacing spikes; low voltage ECG with LVH on ECHO suggests infiltrative disease
  - Troponin: Rule out active ischemia/ACS
  - Sodium: Hyponatremia may occur due to volume retention, diuretic use, increased neurohumoral activation; Na^+ <135 mEq/L associated with increased mortality in HF
  - Assess severity of advanced heart failure: BUN/Cr, LFTs, lactate
  - Assess for co-occurring conditions: HgA1c, lipid panel, TSH, iron studies
  - Assess heart failure etiology: Stress test or coronary angiogram (depending on pre-test probability of CAD), HIV, Utox, Upreg; sometimes: SPEP/SFLC, cardiac MRI, endomyocardial biopsy
- Goals of hospitalization for ADHF:
  - Decongestion: IV diuretics (see Table 1.12; typically start by doubling the patient's home diuretic dose, ensure urination within 30 min), BID electrolytes (repletion of K >4 mmol/L and Mg >2 mg/dL), strict I/Os (goal negative >2 L daily or more if tolerated), diurese fully to euvolemia (i.e., no JVD, no crackles, IVC<2.1 cm and >50% collapsible), establish dry weight, trial on PO diuretics prior to discharge
  - Define and reverse triggers: **FAILURES** mnemonic
    - **F**orgetting (i.e., not taking heart failure medications)
    - **A**rrhythmia (especially Afib)
    - **I**schemia
    - **L**ifestyle (e.g., fluids, alcohol, salt, drugs)
    - **U**p-regulation (e.g., in pregnancy, hyperthyroidism)
    - **R**enal failure
    - **E**mbolism
    - **S**tenosis (e.g., aortic stenosis, renal artery stenosis)
  - Establish HF etiology: Reassess the reason that the patient has HF, determine if additional workup is required to define the etiology

- Initiate and up-titrate guideline-directed medical therapy (GDMT): Prior to discharge, try to get patients on the maximum tolerated ACEi/ARB/ARNI, BB, MRA, SGLT2 inhibitor as indicated (see later)
- Prevent rehospitalization: Schedule outpatient follow-up within 2 weeks to reassess volume exam, weight, labs, and medication tolerance
- Additional measures for severe ADHF:
  - Noninvasive ventilation (NIV): Respiratory support for cardiogenic pulmonary edema (CPAP preferred, may trial bilevel NIV if hypercapnia present)
  - Inotropes: Dobutamine or milrinone
  - Pulmonary artery catheter (Swann-Ganz catheter): Continuously measures cardiac and pulmonary pressures and can calculate cardiac output; has not been shown to improve outcomes in ADHF (ESCAPE 2005), but has a role in some patients, particularly those with cardiogenic shock, mixed shock, RV failure due to pulmonary hypertension, or those with a challenging clinical assessment
- Treatment: Depends on the type of heart failure, as described below

HFrEF (EF <40%): Heart failure with reduced ejection fraction
- Lifestyle: Sodium restriction (<4 g/day), weight loss, smoking cessation, restrict alcohol, daily weights
- Symptomatic relief: Diuretics. Common recommendation for patients: If weight increases 3–5 lb, double diuretic and K^+ repletion and call provider.
- Guideline-directed medical therapy for HFrEF: Medications with mortality benefit
  - **ACE inhibitor (ACEi)** (SAVE 1992, SOLVD 1991)
    - ~20% mortality reduction
    - Recommended for EF <40%, NYHA I–IV
    - Medications: Lisinopril (initial = 2.5–5 mg qD; goal = 40 mg qD). Alternatively, can use short-acting captopril (initial = 6.25 mg TID; goal = 50 mg TID) for easier titration inpatient then convert to once-daily lisinopril prior to discharge. Ratio captopril:lisinopril is 5:1 (captopril 50 mg TID = lisinopril 30 mg qD). Other options: benazepril, enalapril, ramipril
    - Side effects: Hypotension, hyperkalemia, cough; careful in CKD, bilateral renal artery stenosis. Teratogen
  - **Angiotensin receptor blockers (ARBs)** (Val-HeFT 2001; HEAAL 2009)
    - ~15% mortality reduction
    - Recommended for EF <40%, NYHA II–IV
    - Medications: Losartan (initial = 12.5–25 mg; goal = 50 mg daily). Alternative for patients who do not tolerate ACEi (usually due to cough). Other options: valsartan, candesartan
    - Side effects: Hypotension, hyperkalemia. Cough less common with ARBs than ACEi, but can occur. Teratogen
  - **Angiotensin receptor neprilysin inhibitor (ARNI) + ARB (sacubitril/valsartan [Entresto])** (PARADIGM-HF 2014)
    - Up to ~15% mortality reduction (over ACEi)
    - Recommended for EF ≤35% and BNP ≥150 pg/mL *or* NT-proBNP ≥600 pg/mL *or* hospitalization
    - Medications: Sacubitril/valsartan (initial = 24/26 mg BID; goal = 97/103 mg BID)
    - Side effects: Hyperkalemia, angioedema. Do not combine with ACEi due to risk of angioedema
  - **Beta blockers** (MERIT-HF 1999)
    - ~35% mortality reduction
    - Recommended for EF <40%, NYHA I–IV
    - Medications: Carvedilol if hypertensive (initial 3.125 mg BID; goal = 25 mg BID) or metoprolol succinate if normotensive (initial = 12.5–25 mg qD; goal = 200 mg qD). When up-titrating can start with metoprolol tartrate q6h and then convert total daily dose 1:1 to metoprolol succinate at discharge
    - Side effects: Hypotension, bradycardia
    - Note: OK to continue home BB in stable patient with ADHF but do not start new BB until nearing euvolemia
  - **Mineralocorticoid receptor antagonists (MRAs)** (RALES 1999, EMPHASIS-HF 2011)
    - ~30% mortality reduction
    - Recommended for EF ≤35%, NYHA II–IV
    - Medications: Spironolactone (initial 12.5–25 mg qD; goal = 50 mg qD) or eplerenone (initial 25 mg qD; goal 50 mg qD, less gynecomastia)
    - Side effects: Hyperkalemia. Do not use in CKD (Cr >2.5)

- **SGLT2 inhibitors** (DAPA-HF 2019)
  - ~20% mortality reduction (over standard guideline-directed medical therapy [GDMT])
  - Recommended for EF ≤40%, especially in patients with diabetes
  - Medications: Dapagliflozin, canagliflozin, empagliflozin
- Less frequently used:
  - **Hydralazine-isosorbide dinitrate** (A = HeFT 2004)
    - Mortality reduction in persons who self-identified as Black (defined as of African descent). Beneficial if hypertensive and/or symptomatic despite GDMT, especially in African American patients
    - Medications: Hydralazine 37.5–75 mg/Isordil 20–40 mg TID
  - **Ivabradine** (SHIFT 2010)
    - No mortality reduction
    - SA node (funny current) blocker. Consider if HR<70 bpm after on maximum dose beta blocker
  - **Tolvaptan**
    - No mortality reduction
    - Consider if severe hyponatremia (e.g., Na^+ <120 mEq/L) despite fluid restriction. Initiated inpatient only with close sodium monitoring.
    - Do not use for >30 days. Do not use in liver disease.
  - **Digoxin**
    - Unclear mortality benefit and potential for harm. Consider rarely if a patient is symptomatic despite GDMT.
    - Dose 0.125 mg daily and maintain serum digoxin level <1 ng/mL
    - Side effects: Dizziness, diarrhea, rash, confusion
- Procedures:
  - **Implantable cardioverter defibrillator (ICD):** Consider if EF <35% after 3–6 months on medical therapy, for prevention of sudden cardiac death.
  - **Cardiac resynchronization therapy (CRT):** Cardiac resynchronization (placement of a pacemaker with RV and LV leads to synchronize RV/ LV contraction). Consider if EF <35%, NYHA II–IV, wide QRS (at least >120 ms; particularly with LBBB) after optimal medical therapy for 3–6 months.
  - **CardioMEMS:** Implantable device that monitors changes in pulmonary artery pressure to allow clinicians to remotely titrate diuretics. Consider in patients with frequent hospitalizations, difficult to manage volume status.
- Advanced therapies: Consider in ACC/AHA Stage D/NYHA IV despite guideline-directed medical therapy:
  - **LVAD (Left Ventricular Assist Device):** For bridge to transplant or destination therapy
  - **Heart transplant**
  - **IV inotropic therapy:** For symptom benefit/quality of life often as a bridge to transplant
  - **Palliative care:** For symptom benefit/quality of life

HFmrEF (EF 40–50%): Heart failure with mid-range ejection fraction

- Definition: Between HFrEF and HFpEF. Recognized by most as a subcategory of HFreF
- Treatment: Unclear how exactly to manage given limited clinical trials directed at this population, but generally treated like HFrEF

HFrecEF (EF <40% that improves to >50%): Heart failure with recovered ejection fraction

- Definition: HFrEF that recovers over time with treatment
- Treatment: Unclear exactly how to manage but should NOT stop HFrEF therapies

HFpEF (EF >50% + clinical symptoms of HF): Heart failure with preserved ejection fraction

- Treatment: Data less clear; unclear if standard HFrEF medications help this population, but trials have largely not shown benefit
- Mainstays of treatment:
  - Management of hypertension
  - Diuretics, lifestyle changes, consideration of remote hemodynamic monitoring (e.g., CardioMEMs) when difficult to control
  - MRAs: Spironolactone decreases hospitalizations (TOPCAT 2014; controversial study due to differences in subgroup analysis by region)
  - SGLT-2 inhibitors may have benefit (trials on-going)

Pulmonary Hypertension

- Diagnosis: Mean pulmonary artery (mPA) >20 mmHg on RHC; suspect when PASP or RVSP >35 mmHg on TTE
- WHO Classification: A mnemonic that is useful: **AVRT-other**
  - Group 1: **A**rterial: Primary PAH, connective tissue disease, toxins (e.g., methamphetamines) HIV
    - Pre-capillary (PVR >3 Wood units; PAWP <15 mmHg); arterial remodeling
    - Treatment: Pulmonary vasodilators (e.g., PD5 inhibitors, endothelin antagonists, prostanoids)
  - Group 2: **V**enous: Backup from left heart due to LV failure (HFrEF or HFpEF)
    - Post-capillary (PAWP >15 mmHg); venous congestion
    - Treatment: Treat underlying heart failure
  - Group III: **R**espiratory, due to pulmonary disease: ILD, OSA, COPD, chronic hypoxia
    - Usually pre-capillary (PVR >3 Wood units, PAWP <15 mmHg); capillary destruction
    - Treatment: Treat underlying lung disease, supplemental oxygen, lung transplantation, sometimes treprostinil
  - Group IV: **T**hromboembolic disease: Chronic thromboembolic pulmonary hypertension (CTEPH)
    - Usually pre-capillary (PVR >3 Wood units, PAWP <15 mmHg); arterial obstruction
    - Treatment: Anticoagulation, pulmonary artery thromboendarectomy or angioplasty
  - Group V: **O**ther: Sarcoid, sickle cell, hemolytic anemia, metabolic disease
    - Variable or mixed
    - Treatment: Directed at underlying disease, occasionally pulmonary vasodilators

Valvular Heart Disease

Aortic stenosis (AS)

S1 S2

- Etiology: 1) Age-related calcific degeneration of a normal valve (generally age >70 yr) or a bicuspid aortic valve (generally age 40–60 yr); 2) Rheumatic disease
- Clinical presentation: Angina, syncope, heart failure. Parvus et tardus: Diminished carotid upstroke, weak pulse
- Heart sound: Harsh crescendo-decrescendo systolic murmur (see depiction at right), best heard at the second right intercostal with radiation to the carotid. The more severe the stenosis, the longer duration of the murmur and the more likely it peaks later in systole.
- Staging:
  - <u>Mild to moderate AS</u>: Repeat TTE q1–5 yr depending on severity
  - <u>Severe AS</u>: "1-4-40" on TTE: AV area <1 cm², max velocity ≥4 m/s, or mean gradient ≥40 mmHg. Repeat TTE q6mo to 1 yr and consider treatment with valve replacement
- Treatment: SAVR (surgical) vs. TAVR (transcatheter) for severe AS
  - TAVR increasingly preferred to SAVR (**PARTNER trials**); SAVR preferred when there are other indications for cardiac surgery
  - Bioprosthetic AV: Placed by TAVR or SAVR, no anticoagulation, requires ASA, lasts ~10 yr
  - Mechanical AV: Placed by SAVR, requires warfarin (INR 2–3) and ASA; lasts >20 yr (often indefinitely)

Aortic regurgitation (AR)

S1 S2

- Etiology: 1) Aortic root problems (e.g., dilation due to age-related degeneration, hypertension, ankylosing spondylitis, syphilis, dissection, Marfan's syndrome); 2) Valve problems (e.g., bicuspid aortic valve, endocarditis, rheumatic)
- Clinical presentation: Dyspnea, PND, orthopnea, palpitations when lying down, wide pulse pressure, bounding pulse
- Heart sound: Diastolic blowing decrescendo murmur (see depiction at right), best heard at the apex/ left sternal border
- Treatment: Surgical AVR +/– aortic root replacement; consider when symptomatic, EF<50%, or severe LV dilation. Asymptomatic: Can consider initiation of ACEi

Mitral stenosis (MS)
- Etiology: Rheumatic fever, mitral annular calcification (e.g., in the setting of CKD), congenital
- Clinical presentation: Dyspnea, hemoptysis, Afib, risk of emboli. Dilated LA can compress the recurrent laryngeal nerve and cause hoarseness
- Heart sound: Opening snap, low-pitched diastolic rumble, and loud S1 (see depiction at right), best heard at the apex when the patient is in the left lateral decubitus position
- Treatment:
  - Chronic medical management of mitral stenosis:
    - Symptoms: Diuretics
    - Valvular atrial fibrillation:
      - Rate control: BB, CCB, digoxin (control HR to increase ventricular filling time)
      - Anticoagulation: warfarin (goal INR 2.0–3.0)
  - Procedural:
    - Indicated for moderate to severe symptoms or if pulmonary hypertension occurs to provide definitive management
    - Options: Percutaneous balloon valvuloplasty, surgical mitral valve replacement, percutaneous mitral valve replacement

Mitral regurgitation (MR)
- Etiology:
  - Acute: Endocarditis, MI with papillary muscle rupture, chordae tendineae rupture
  - Chronic: 1) Primary problem with valve: mitral valve prolapse (MVP, i.e. prolapse due to myxomatous degeneration), rheumatic carditis, prior endocarditis, Marfan's syndrome, carcinoid (rare); 2) Secondary to dilation of MV annulus (e.g., dilated cardiomyopathy)
- Clinical presentation: Acutely, may cause flash pulmonary edema. Chronically, may cause pulmonary edema (DOE, PND, orthopnea), right heart failure
- Heart sound: Holosystolic murmur (see depiction at right), best heard at the apex radiating to the axilla, back, or clavicle
- Treatment:
  - Acute MR: Decrease afterload (e.g., give ACEi nitroprusside, IABP); surgical repair
  - Chronic primary MR: Consider treatment if symptomatic or EF ≤60%
    - Surgical repair: Preferred if possible
      - Bioprosthetic MV: Surgical, requires 3–6 months warfarin then ASA monotherapy, last ~10 yr
      - Mechanical MVR: Surgical, requires warfarin (INR 2.5–3.5) and ASA, last >20 yr
    - MitraClip: Transcatheter mitral repair that is <u>only</u> used in patients with high surgical risk; surgery always preferred if possible
  - Chronic secondary MR: Consider MitraClip (MITRA-FR 2018 [negative trial]; COAPT 2018 [positive trial])

Tricuspid regurgitation (TR)
- Etiology: Either due to 1) Primary valve problem (e.g., rheumatic, Ebstein anomaly, carcinoid, endocarditis or 2) Secondary to elevated RV pressures (e.g., pulmonary hypertension, LV failure, restrictive cardiomyopathy)
- Clinical presentation: Murmur similar to MR but louder with <u>inspiration</u>
- Treatment: Often none, consider bioprosthetic TV +/– annuloplasty, off-label MitraClip

Pearls about heart murmurs:
- Provocative maneuvers and how they affect heart sounds:
  - Inspiration: Louder **R** heart murmur
  - Expiration: Louder **L** heart murmur
  - Standing/Valsalva: Increases murmur associated with mitral valve prolapse (MVP), hypertrophic cardiomyopathy (HCM)
  - Hand grip (increased SVR): Increases murmur associated with AR, MR, VSD; decreases murmur associated with HCM
- Systolic murmurs can be benign; diastolic murmurs are always pathologic

Cardiac Valve Infection and Inflammation

Rheumatic fever

- Etiology: Complication of inflammatory reaction to group A *strep* spp. Jones criteria: Strep infection and two major criteria OR one major criteria and two minor criteria:
  - <u>Major criteria</u>: Migratory polyarthritis, erythema marginatum, cardiac problems (pericarditis, CHF, valve), chorea, subcutaneous nodules
  - <u>Minor criteria</u>: Fever, ESR $\geq$60 mm/hr or CRP $\geq$3 mg/L, polyarthralgias, prolonged PR interval on ECG
- Treatment: Treat strep pharyngitis with penicillin; NSAIDs or steroids. Consider penicillin prophylaxis to prevent recurrence.

Endocarditis

- Infective endocarditis: See Infectious Diseases Chapter 8
- Nonbacterial thrombotic endocarditis (marantic endocarditis): Rarely, malignancy can cause sterile depositions of fibrin/platelets that attach to the cardiac valves. Treatment: Anticoagulation.
- Nonbacterial verrucous endocarditis (Libman-Sacks endocarditis): Noninfectious endocarditis that occurs in the setting of systemic lupus erythematosus, typically with vegetations on both sides of the valve. Treatment: Anticoagulation, treat lupus or underlying condition.

Congenital Heart Diseases

Congenital Heart Disease with Late Cyanosis (L $\rightarrow$ R shunt)

Atrial septal defect (ASD)

- Etiology: Defect in the middle (ostum secundum, most common) or lower (ostum primum, which occurs in Down syndrome) part of atrial septum
- Clinical presentation: Small defects are often asymptomatic. Large ASDs are typically detected/closed in childhood; if not patients may become symptomatic by middle age, causing exercise intolerance, dyspnea, fatigue
- Complication: Pulmonary hypertension, Eisenmenger syndrome, right heart failure, Afib, stroke with paradoxical emboli
- Heart sound: Loud S1, wide fixed split S2. More pulmonic flow = mild systolic ejection murmur, diastolic rumble across the tricuspid valve
- Treatment: Most do not require closure. When pulmonary to systemic flow is high (Qp/Qs >1.5) or RV overload, consider closure. Closure contraindicated after right to left shunt develops.

Patent foramen ovale (PFO)

- Etiology: The foramen ovale is an atrial opening that usually closes at birth, PFO = persistent opening (25% of the population)
- Clinical presentation: Common and usually benign. May cause cryptogenic strokes and select patients may benefit from closure (CLOSE, RESPECT, REDUCE trials)

Ventricular septal defect (VSD)

- Etiology: Defect in the muscular or membranous portion of the ventricular septum
- Associations: Fetal alcohol syndrome, Down syndrome
- Clinical presentation: Most large VSDs are detected and closed in childhood; if not patients may become symptomatic with eventual pulmonary hypertension and right to left shunting
- Heart sound: Harsh blowing holosystolic murmur with thrill, loudest at the left third intercostal space with handgrip (smaller defect = louder murmur)
- Treatment: Consider closure if large, but contraindicated after right to left shunt develops

Patent ductus arteriosus (PDA)

- Etiology: Persistent communication between the aorta and pulmonary artery. Associated with congenital rubella, prematurity.
- Clinical presentation: Depends on the size; small PDAs are usually asymptomatic; moderate PDAs cause Eisenmenger syndrome if not diagnosed; large PDAs cause infantile heart failure.
- Heart sound: Machine-like murmur, best heard at the left second intercostal space; wide pulse pressure and bounding peripheral pulses.
- Treatment: Consider closure; options include pharmacologic therapy (e.g., indomethacin; used exclusively in premature infants), surgical ligation, percutaneous catheter occlusion.

Coarctation of the aorta (CoA)

- Etiology:
  - Infantile: Lower extremity cyanosis with weak pulses; associated with Turner's syndrome
  - Adult: Can also be acquired due to inflammation of the aorta (e.g., Takayasu's)
- Clinical presentation: Upper extremity hypertension, low/unobtainable lower extremity blood pressure, and diminished/delayed femoral pulse; CXR can reveal "notched ribs" after age 4–12 yr due to erosion by collateral arteries; in adulthood, if previously undetected, likely to present with hypertension
- Treatment: Indicated for CoA gradient >20 mmHg, radiologic evidence of significant collaterals, hypertension due to CoA, or HF due to CoA; options include balloon angioplasty, stenting, or surgery

Congenital Heart Disease with Early Cyanosis (R → L shunt)

Tetralogy of Fallot

- Etiology: Associated with Down syndrome; includes four anatomic components: 1) VSD; 2) Right ventricular hypertrophy; 3) Pulmonary stenosis; 4) Overriding aorta
- Clinical presentation: Progressive hypoxemia in childhood
- Heart sound: Harsh crescendo-decrescendo systolic ejection murmur best heard at the left upper sternal border (due to RVOT obstruction), single S2 (because pulmonic component rarely audible).
- CXR: Boot-shaped heart
- Treatment: Early surgical repair

Transposition of the great vessels

- Etiology: Congenital defect involving the abnormal spatial rearrangement of any of the great vessels (SVC, IVC, pulmonary artery, pulmonary vein). If involving only the pulmonary artery and aorta, belongs to a subtype called transposition of the great arteries (TGA) which is the most common congenital heart condition. Causes are largely unknown (some association with genetics, viral illness in pregnancy, advanced maternal age)
- Clinical presentation: Cyanotic newborn, tachypnea; requires shunt (e.g., VSD, PDA, PFO) to allow mixing of blood
- Treatment: Surgical repair

Persistent truncus arteriosus

- Etiology: Congenital defect where there is a single vessel leaving the heart rather than both the pulmonary artery and aorta; typically occurs spontaneously
- Clinical presentation: Cyanosis at birth, heart failure may occur within weeks

Tricuspid atresia

- Etiology: Congenital defect where there is complete absence of the tricuspid valve. Therefore, there is no right atrioventricular connection and it requires ASD and VSD for viability. Causes unknown
- Clinical presentation: Congenital cyanosis
- Treatment: Administer PGE to maintain patent ductus arteriosus and surgical repair

Myocardial Diseases

Myocarditis

- Etiology: Inflammation of the myocardium due to a viral infection (e.g., adenovirus, coxsackievirus parvovirus B19, HIV, HHV6), parasitic infection, bacterial infection, autoimmune condition (e.g., SLE, sarcoidosis, poly/dermatomyositis), medications (e.g., sulfonamides, doxorubicin, cocaine), idiopathic
- Symptoms: May have preceding symptoms depending on the etiology (e.g., URI prior to viral myocarditis). May be asymptomatic or can cause fever, fatigue, chest pain, pericarditis, heart failure, arrhythmias. Often ↑ESR, CRP
- Treatment: Supportive care

Hypertrophic cardiomyopathy (HCM)

- Etiology: Hypertrophied and stiff LV due to sarcomere protein abnormality, sometimes due to inherited autosomal dominant mutations
- Problems:
  - Structural: Septal hypertrophy obstructs LVOT
  - Hemodynamic: Flow acceleration sucks anterior MV leaflet into the left ventricular outflow tract (LVOT) by the Venturi effect, worsening obstruction and causing MVR
  - Ischemic: Supply/demand mismatch given thick/highly contractile heart
  - Arrhythmias
- Symptoms: Dyspnea on exertion, angina, syncope after exertion/Valsalva, sudden death
- Heart sound: Sustained PMI, loud S4, rapid carotid upstroke, crescendo-decrescendo systolic ejection murmur louder with Valsalva/standing and softer with hand grip
- Diagnosis: Requires 1) Appropriate clinical symptoms; 2) Wall thickness >15 mm visualized anywhere in the ventricle; 3) Absence of secondary cause of LVH (e.g., hypertension, aortic stenosis, infiltrative diseases) **or** if LVH is out of proportion to the stressor
- Suggestive features: Helpful but not required for diagnosis: Septal hypertrophy with or without obstruction (LVOT gradient >30 mmHg at rest); genetic testing
- Treatment:
  - Decrease LVOT obstruction and improve symptoms; avoid anything that increases contractility or impairs filling (e.g., avoid dehydration, diuretics, isometric exercise, nitrates, dobutamine); give BB or CCB, disopyramide; consider procedures (e.g., myectomy, catheter-based alcohol septal ablation).
  - Prevent sudden death: ICD indicated for secondary prevention, or if family history of sudden death, LV wall >30 mm, and/or unexplained syncope.

Restrictive cardiomyopathy
- Etiology: Infiltrative diseases (e.g., amyloid, sarcoid, hemochromatosis), lysosomal storage diseases (e.g., Fabry disease), endomyocardial damage (e.g., XRT, fibrosis), scleroderma, carcinoid
- Symptoms: Stiff poorly filling ventricles may cause diastolic dysfunction. Right heart failure is common (because right heart is thin walled, and thus more sensitive to change).
- Diagnosis: ECG: Low voltages; PYP scan for ATTR amyloid; often need cardiac biopsy to diagnose other etiologies
- Treatment: Treat underlying disorder; e.g., hemochromatosis (phlebotomy, deferoxamine), sarcoid (steroids), amyloid (chemotherapy for AL amyloid; tafamidis for ATTR amyloid)

Pericardial Disease
Acute pericarditis
- Etiology: Inflammation of the pericardial sac
  - Infectious:
    - Viral: Preceded by URI or coxsackievirus, EBV, influenza, HIV, hepatitis A/B
    - Bacterial: *Staphylococcus, Pneumococcus, Streptococcus* (rheumatic pancarditis), *Haemophilus, Mycoplasma, Mtb*
    - Fungal: *Histoplasma, Aspergillus, Blastomyces, Coccidioides, Candida*
    - Parasitic: *Echinococcus*, amebic, *Toxoplasma*
  - Post-MI: Immediate (PIP) or weeks later (PCIS; "Dressler's")
  - Autoimmune (e.g., SLE, RA, SSc)
  - Neoplasm (metastatic: Hodgkin's, lung, breast; primary; paraneoplastic)
  - Uremic (especially BUN >60 mg/dL)
  - Iatrogenic (e.g., trauma, XRT, drug-induced lupus from procainamide, hydralazine)
- Symptoms: **P**ericardial **P**ain is **P**leuritic (sharp worse with inspiration unlike MI) and **P**ositional (better leaning forward); patients may also develop fever
- Diagnosis: Chest pain with pericardial features, pericardial friction rub, ECG with diffuse ST elevations and/or PR depression in avR, pericardial effusion, may have leukocytosis
- Treatment: Aspirin, NSAIDs, colchicine. Do not give NSAIDs for post-MI pericarditis

Constrictive pericarditis
- Description: Fibrous scarring of the pericardium and loss of elasticity of the pericardial sac
- Etiology: Idiopathic or viral (>50%), post-cardiac surgery, prior XRT, post-infectious, connective tissue diseases, uremia
- Symptoms: Fluid overload, diminished cardiac output (with fatigue, DOE), elevated JVP with Kussmaul's sign (i.e., increase during inspiration rather than decrease), pericardial knock (mid-frequency heart sound occurring slightly earlier than an S3), pericardial calcification (highly specific, but uncommon)
- Diagnosis: Based on typical symptoms/signs and typical features on TTE (e.g., increased pericardial thickness, abnormal septal motion/bounce, pronounced respiratory variation in ventricular filling, biatrial enlargement).
- Treatment: Diuretics for fluid overload, NSAIDS/colchicine for inflammation. Pericardectomy indicated if no improvement in 2–3 months or if presenting with late disease.

Pericardial effusion and cardiac tamponade
- Definitions:
  - Pericardial effusion: Accumulation of extra fluid in the pericardial space around the heart
  - Cardiac tamponade: Accumulation of pericardial fluid causes resulting compression of the heart
- Etiology:
  - Idiopathic, malignancy, infection (e.g., HIV, lyme, coxsackievirus, TB), cardiac (Post-MI, Dressler's, post-cardiac surgery), metabolic (uremia, hypothyroidism), other: SLE, trauma, drugs (e.g., doxorubicin, minoxidil, phenytoin, hydralazine, procainamide via drug-induced SLE)
- Clinical presentation:
  - Pericardial effusion: The patient may be asymptomatic if small effusion, or can develop progressive shortness of breath, chest pain
  - Cardiac tamponade: Beck's triad: 1) Hypotension; 2) Elevated JVP; 3) Muffled heart sounds. More specific: Pulsus paradoxus (>10 mmHg decrease in SBP during inspiration)
- Diagnosis: TTE (+/− RV collapse), CXR ("water bottle" shaped heart if large/chronic effusion); ECG (low voltage or electrical alternans [i.e., varied QRS height])
- Workup: Consider differential diagnosis and work-up based on the clinical scenario; review medication list, CBC, BMP, TFTs (myxedema), rheumatologic work-up, HIV, serologic lyme testing, PPD, albumin/urine protein (nephrotic syndrome), consider evaluation for malignancy (e.g., breast cancer, lung cancer)
- Treatment:
  - Stable pericardial effusion: Monitor, serial TTEs, treat underlying condition
  - Cardiac tamponade: Give IVF (fill the collapsing RV), consult cardiology, and perform urgent pericardiocentesis

Diseases of the Vasculature

Hypertensive emergency
- Definitions: Elevated SBP with end-organ damage
- Etiology: See etiologies for hypertension in General Medicine Chapter 10; in particular consider medication noncompliance, stimulant use (e.g., cocaine, methamphetamines), hyperaldosteronism, pheochromocytoma, Cushing's, preeclampsia, vasculitis, renal artery stenosis
- Symptoms: CNS symptoms (e.g., mental status changes, visual changes, papilledema, encephalopathy), renal injury (e.g., hematuria, AKI), cardiac injury (e.g., ACS, ADHF), pulmonary edema
- Treatment: Reduce mean arterial pressure (MAP) by 25% in 1–2 hours (then slower after). IV medications: Nitroprusside or nicardipine gtt

Aortic dissection
- Definitions:
  - Type A: Dissection of the ascending aorta
  - Type B: Dissection of the descending aorta
- Etiology: Risk factors: Hypertension (most common), stimulant use (e.g., cocaine, methamphetamines), connective tissue disease, bicuspid aortic valve
- Clinical presentation: 1) Abrupt onset tearing pain in the chest or back; 2) Pulse and/or BP asymmetry in each arm or between the arms and the legs
- Diagnosis: CT Angiogram. On CXR, see widened mediastinum. Sometimes need TEE to confirm the diagnosis.
- Treatment:
  - Type A: Emergent surgery, in meantime medical management
  - Type B: Medical management: IV BB to lower HR, then IV nitroprusside to lower BP (goal SBP 100–120 mmHg within 20 minutes)

Abdominal aortic aneurysm (AAA)
- Etiology: Atherosclerosis, hypertension, smoking, syphilis, connective tissue disorders
- Clinical: Pulsatile abdominal mass (rarely detect clinically); instead usually diagnosed on screening imaging or incidentally on abdominal imaging obtained for another purpose
- Screening: Ultrasound: One-time screening ultrasound indicated in men age 65–75 yr who have ever smoked. Insufficient evidence for screening ultrasounds in women
- Treatment: Open vs. endovascular repair
  - Repair if 1) AAA >5.5 cm in men or AAA >5 cm in women; 2) Rapid rate of expansion, >0.5 cm in 6 months or >1 cm in 1 yr; 3) Symptoms due to the AAA
  - Rupture: Triad of 1) Abdominal pain; 2) Hypotension; 3) Palpable pulsatile abdominal mass Treatment: Open repair

Peripheral artery disease (PAD)
- Etiology: Abnormal narrowing of the arteries, most commonly affecting the legs. Risk factors = atherosclerotic risk factors. Common vessels affected include the superficial femoral artery, popliteal artery (causes calf pain), aortoiliac artery (causes butt/hip pain)
- Clinical presentation: Claudication, leg pain at rest (especially at night, hanging foot over the bed often relieves the pain). Signs: Diminished pulses, less hair over legs/feet, ulcers
- Diagnosis: Ankle-brachial index (ABI): ABI <1.0 is diagnostic of PAD. Claudication typically develops if ABI <0.7 and rest pain if <0.4. If vessel calcification is present (ABI >1.4) then non-interpretable and get toe-brachial index
- Treatment: Smoking cessation, exercise, aspirin, (phosphodiesterase-3 inhibitor (e.g., cilostazol, contraindicated in heart failure). Percutaneous intervention (e.g., balloon angioplasty, stenting), surgery (i.e., bypass grafting).

Acute arterial occlusion
- Etiology: Native arterial thrombosis, arterial (or paradoxical) embolism, arterial injury
- Clinical: Six Ps: Pain (acute), Pallor, Poikilothermic (cold), Paralysis, Paresthesia, Pulselessness
- Diagnosis: CTA to determine the site of occlusion
- Treatment: Immediate IV heparin gtt and vascular procedure/surgery; Use anticoagulation with caution for suspected cholesterol emboli

KEY MEDICATIONS AND INTERVENTIONS

TABLE 1.13 · Common Medications used in Cardiology

Class	Examples	Mechanism	Typical Uses	Side Effects
Diuretics	See Nephrology Chapter 6			
Calcium channel blockers (CCB)	Dihydropyridine: • amlodipine • clevidipine • nicardipine • nifedipine • nimodipine	Block voltage-dependent L-type Ca^{2+} channels → muscle contractility; acts on vascular smooth muscle	• Hypertension • Angina (including Prinzmetal) • Raynauds • Nimodipine: Prophylaxis against vasospasm in SAH	• Peripheral edema • Flushing • Dizziness
	Non-DHP: • diliazem • verapamil	Block voltage-dependent L-type Ca^{2+} channels → muscle contractility; acts on heart	• Hypertension • Angina • Afib/flutter	• Cardiac depression • AV block • Hyperprolactinemia • Constipation • Gingival hyperplasia
ACE-inhibitors (ACEi)	• captopril • enalapril • lisinopril • ramipril	Inhibition of ACE lowers angiotensin II, with reduction in GFR due to relaxation of efferent arteriole; prevents inactivation of bradykinin (i.e., a vasodilator)	• Hypertension • Heart failure • LV hypertrophy • Diabetic nephropathy	• Cough • Hyperkalemia • Angioedema • Teratogen (contraindicated in pregnancy)
Angiotensin receptor blockers (ARB)	• losartan • candesartan • valsartan	Blocks binding of angiotensin II; does not increase bradykinin levels	• Same as ACEi above • Often used second line if the patient develops cough with ACEi	• As with ACE inhibitor, but cough/angioedema much more rare
Vasodilator	• hydralazine	Relaxes smooth muscle via cGMP; arteriole dilatation > venodilation	• Acute severe hypertension • Combination therapy with organic nitrates for hypertension	• Compensatory tachycardia (contraindicated in CAD) • Headache • SLE-like syndrome
Nitrodilators	• nitroprusside	Vasodilation via direct action; arteriole dilatation > venodilation	• Hypertensive emergency • ADHF (afterload reduction)	• Cyanide toxicity • Careful in renal failure
	Organic nitrates: • nitroglycerin • isosorbide dinitrate • isosorbine mononitrate	Vasodilation via increased nitrous oxide; venodilation >> arteriole dilatation	• Angina • ACS	• Contraindication: Right ventricular MI • Reflex tachycardia, hypotension • Flushing, headache
Ranolazine	—	Inhibits late phase Na^+ current particularly in ischemic cardiomyocytes; thereby decreases wall tension and O_2 consumption	• Refractory angina	• Dizziness, headache • Nausea • QT prolongation

(Continued)

TABLE 1.13 · Common Medications used in Cardiology (*Continued*)				
Class	**Examples**	**Mechanism**	**Typical Uses**	**Side Effects**
Milrinone	—	Selective PDE-3 inhibitor; increases inotropy/chronotropy via Ca^{2+} influx to cardiomyocytes; also relaxes vascular smooth muscle	• Acute, decompensated HF	• Hypotension • Arrhythmia
Glycosides	Digoxin	Inhibits Na^+/K^+ ATPase, which indirectly inhibits Na^+/Ca^{2+} exchanger, resulting in increased inotropy; also slows HR via vagal nerve stimulation	• Heart failure • Afib	• Cholinergic effects • Hyperkalemia • Toxicity, particularly in renal failure
Class I antiarrhythmic (Na^+ channel blockers)	A: quinidine procainamide disopyramide B: lidocaine mexiletine C: flecainide propafenone	Slows or blocks phase 0 conduction, particularly for depolarized cells	A: Atrial/ventricular arrhythmia B: Post-MI ventricular arrhythmia, digitalis-induced Arrhythmia C: SVT, including Afib	A: QT prolongation, SEL-like syndrome (procainamide) B: CNS effects C: Proarrhythmic, particularly post-MI
Class II antiarrhythmic (β blockers)	• metoprolol • propranolol • esmolol • atenolol • timolol • carvedilol	Decreases SA <AV nodal activity; decreases slope 4 of abnormal pacemaker cells	• Rate control for Afib/flutter or other SVTs	• Bradycardia • Masked signs of hypoglycemia • Impotence • Dyslipidemia (metoprolol)
Class III antiarrhythmic (K^+ channel blockers)	• amiodarone (I-IV) • ibutilide • dofetilide • sotalol	Increased duration of action potential/effective refractory period	• Afib/flutter • VT (amiodarone, sotalol)	• Prolong QT • Amiodarone: pulmonary, hepatic, and thyroid toxicity
Class IV antiarrhythmic (Ca^{2+} channel blockers)	• verapamil • diltiazem	Decrease conduction velocity and increase effective refractory period	• Rate control in Afib, SVTs conducted by the AV node	• Edema • Constipation • Flushing • Bradycardia, AV block

Procedural/Surgical Interventions

Many procedures are done by cardiologists or cardiac surgeons. Some examples include:

- Percutaneous coronary intervention (PCI): Coronary catheterization can be both diagnostic to identify coronary abnormalities and therapeutic if a stent is placed to allow better coronary perfusion.
- Coronary artery bypass graft (CABG): The main indications for CABG are the presence of triple-vessel coronary disease, severe left main artery stenosis, or severe stenosis of the proximal left anterior descending artery (LAD) with concurrent stenosis of the proximal circumflex artery or EF <50%.
- Valve replacement: E.g., surgical aortic valve replacement (SAVR) or transcatheter aortic valve replacement (TAVR) in patients with aortic stenosis.
- Radiofrequency ablation: Used to disrupt electrical signals that are causing arrhythmia.
- Heart transplantation: The most common indications for heart transplantation are nonischemic cardiomyopathy (~59%) and ischemic cardiomyopathy (~40%).

KEY CLINICAL TRIALS AND PUBLICATIONS

Cardiovascular Disease Risk Prevention

- **FOURIER.** *N Engl J Med* 2017;376(18):1713-1722.
  - Randomized, double-blind, placebo-controlled trial that included 27,564 patients with atherosclerotic cardiovascular disease and LDL cholesterol levels of 70 mg/dL or higher who were receiving statin therapy. Patients were randomly assigned to receive evolocumab (PCSK9 inhibitor, either 140 mg every 2 weeks or 420 mg monthly) or placebo. The primary efficacy end point was the composite of cardiovascular death, myocardial infarction, stroke, hospitalization for unstable angina, or coronary revascularization. Relative to placebo, evolocumab treatment significantly reduced the risk of the composite primary end point (1344 patients [9.8%] vs. 1563 patients [11.3%]).

Coronary Artery Disease (CAD)

- **FAME-2.** *N Engl J Med* 2012;367(11):991–1001.
  - In this trial, 888 patients with stable CAD for whom PCI was being considered underwent, fractional flow reserve (FFR) testing to measure the percentage of functionally significant stenosis. Patients with at least one functionally significant lesion were randomly assigned to FFR-guided PCI plus best medical therapy vs. best medical therapy alone. This trial demonstrated that FFR-guided PCI reduced the composite endpoint of death, nonfatal MI, and urgent recatheterization in patients with stable CAD compared to best medical therapy alone.
- **SYNTAX.** *N Engl J Med* 2009;360:961–972.
  - This trial randomized 1800 patients with previously untreated three-vessel or left main coronary artery disease (or both) to undergo coronary artery bypass graft (CABG) vs. PCI. In this trial, rates of major adverse cardiac or cerebrovascular events at 12 months were significantly higher in the PCI group (17.8%, vs. 12.4% for CABG; P = 0.002). Therefore, CABG remains the standard of care for patients with three-vessel or left main coronary artery disease.
- **ISCHEMIA.** *N Engl J Med* 2020;382:1395–1407.
  - This trial randomized 5179 patients with moderate to severe stable coronary disease to conservative strategy (medical management) vs. early interventional strategy (revascularization). There was no significant difference in ischemic cardiovascular events or death over a median of 3.2 yr.
- **ORBITA.** *The Lancet* 2017;391:31–40.
  - This trial randomized 230 patients with stable coronary artery disease and ischemic symptoms to revascularization of flow-limiting lesions vs. a placebo procedure. There was no difference in exercise time or symptom scores at 6 weeks follow up.

Acute Coronary Syndrome (ACS) and Post-ACS Care

- **CAPRICORN.** *The Lancet* 2001;357(9266):1385–1390.
  - This trial randomized 1959 patients who had had a hemodynamically stable MI with reduced LVEF of ≤40% who were already on an ACE inhibitor (unless proven intolerance) to receive carvedilol or placebo. Treatment with carvedilol was associated with decreased all-cause mortality (12% vs. 15% in placebo group).
- **MIRACL.** *JAMA* 2001;285(13):1711–1718.
  - This trial randomized 3086 patients who were hospitalized for unstable angina/NSTEMI to receive either atorvastatin 80 mg or placebo daily. The early initiation of atorvastatin reduced the combined endpoint of death, nonfatal MI, cardiac arrest, and ACS requiring hospitalization at 16 weeks.
- **IMPROVE-IT.** *N Engl J Med* 2015;375(25):2387–2397.
  - This trial randomized 18,144 patients with recent ACS to simvastatin 40 mg daily plus ezetimibe 10 mg daily vs. simvastatin 40 mg alone. The combination of ezetimibe and simvastatin reduced CV events (CV mortality, major CV event, or nonfatal stroke) when compared to statin therapy alone.

Atrial Fibrillation

- **AFFIRM.** *N Engl J Med* 2002;347(23):1825–1833.
  - This trial randomized 4060 patients with nonvalvular atrial fibrillation and a high risk of stroke or death to rate-control (using beta blocker, calcium channel blocker, and/or digoxin) vs. rhythm-control strategies. There was no survival benefit between the two strategies, but patients who underwent rhythm control trended toward increased mortality.
- **RACE-II.** *N Engl J Med* 2010;362(15):1363–1373.
  - This trial randomized 614 patients with permanent atrial fibrillation to a lenient rate control strategy (resting HR <110 bpm) vs. a strict rate control strategy (resting HR <80 bpm). A lenient rate control strategy was noninferior to a strict rate control strategy in preventing CV events (composite outcome of CV death, CHF hospitalization, stroke, systemic embolism, bleeding, and life-threatening arrhythmic events) over 3 yr.

Heart Failure with Reduced Ejection Fraction (HFrEF)

- **PARADIGM-HF.** *N Engl J Med* 2014;371(11):993-1004.
  - This trial randomized 8399 patients with HFrEF (LVEF ≤40%) and NYHA class II–IV symptoms to an angiotensin receptor–neprilysin inhibitor sacubitril + valsartan combination (Entresto) 200 mg PO BID vs. enalapril 10 mg PO BID. Treatment with Entresto reduced CV mortality and HF hospitalizations compared to enalapril and was also associated with reduced all-cause mortality.
- **DAPA-HF.** *N Engl J Med* 2019;381(21):1995–2008.
  - This trial randomized 4744 patients with HFrEF (EF ≤40%) and NYHA II-IV symptoms, with or without diabetes, to receive the SGLT-2 inhibitor dapagliflozin or placebo. The addition of dapagliflozin decreased rates of CV death or worsening HF and all-cause mortality.

Heart Failure with Preserved Ejection Fraction (HFpEF)

- **TOPCAT.** *N Engl J Med* 2014;370(15):1383–1392.
  - This trial randomized 3445 patients with HFpEF (LVEF >45%, findings or HF, and either a HF hospitalization or elevated BNP) to receive spironolactone or placebo. Spironolactone did not reduce the composite endpoint of CV mortality, aborted cardiac arrest, or HF hospitalizations compared to placebo, but it was associated with a small reduction in HF hospitalizations. Of note, this is a controversial study due to differences in subgroup analysis by region.

Aortic Stenosis

- **PARTNER A**. *N Engl J Med* 2011;364(23):2187–2198; **PARTNER B**. *N Engl J Med* 2010;363(17):1597–1607.
  - These studies demonstrated that transcatheter aortic valve replacement (TAVR) is equivalent (and in some cases superior) to surgical aortic valve replacement (SAVR) at decreasing death, stroke, and rehospitalization in severe aortic stenosis.

NOTES

Pulmonology

ANATOMY AND PHYSIOLOGY

Anatomy of the Lungs

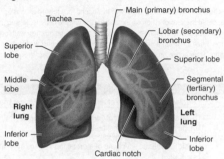

FIGURE 2.1: **Anatomy of the lungs.** Shown are the five lobes of the lung and the anatomy of the tracheobronchial tree.

Overview

- Mechanics:
  - **Statics** refer to forces acting on the lung that affect volumes and elastic behavior
    - Lungs = collapsing forces; chest wall (CW) = expanding forces (Figure 2.2)
  - **Dynamics** refer to the forces moving air, including flow patterns and resistance
- Gas exchange: Handling of O_2/CO_2

Statics: Volumes/Capacities, Compliance, and Surface Tension

- Volumes and Capacities:
  - Definitions (Table 2.1)
  - Changes in pathologic states (Figure 2.3)
    - **Obstructive lung disease** (e.g., asthma, emphysema): ↑TLC, FRC, RV; ↓↓FEV₁, ↓FVC, FEV₁/FVC < 0.7
    - **Restrictive lung disease** (e.g., fibrosis): ↓TLC, FRC, RV; ↓FEV₁, ↓↓FVC, ↑ or normal FEV₁/FVC
- Compliance: $C = \Delta V/\Delta P$

  $V = volume, P = pressure$
  - Compliance = Filling term; ability of lungs to stretch
  - Elastance = Expiration term; ability of lungs to collapse from stretched position
  - Obstructive diseases = ↑Compliance, ↓Elastance; **Restrictive diseases** = ↓**Compliance**, ↑Elastance
- Surface tension: $P = 2T/r$

  $P = pressure, T = surface\ tension, r = radius$
  - **Law of Laplace:** Large alveoli remain open due to high radius, and small alveoli collapse, causing atelectasis
  - **Surfactant:**
    - Increases surface tension → Decreases pressure → Increases compliance and reduces alveolar collapse
    - Produced by Type II alveolar cells: Choline + diacylglycerol → dipalmitoylphosphatidylcholine (DPPC)
    - Surfactant contains lecithin; if lecithin:sphingomyelin ratio ≥ 2:1 in amniotic fluid = lung maturity
  - **Hysteresis:** Compliance (i.e., the slope of a pressure/volume curve) changes with inspiration and expiration; compliance is lower during expiration and at extreme volumes (i.e., very full lungs or very empty lungs)

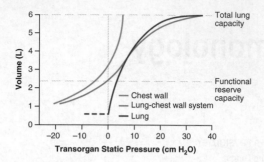

FIGURE 2.2: The lung–chest wall system. The chest wall has a tendency toward expansion, while the lungs have a tendency toward collapse. At the end of a normal exhalation, the volume of air remaining in the lungs is the functional reserve capacity. While at the functional reserve capacity, the expanding chest wall forces and the collapsing lung forces are in balance. Since initiating a new breath requires the lung–chest wall system to shift away from this equilibrium point, inhalation is an active process that requires the use of the respiratory muscles.

TABLE 2.1 · Volumes and Capacities		
Volumes	TV	Tidal volume – Volume of air taken with normal, quiet breath
	E/IRV	Expiratory / inspiratory reserve volume – Volume of air that can be expired/inspired beyond a normal breath
	RV	Residual volume – Volume of air retained in lungs even after maximal expiration
Capacities	TLC	Total lung capacity – Volume in lungs after maximal inspiration
	FRC	Functional residual capacity – Volume in lungs after normal expiration (i.e., resting state)
	VC	Vital capacity – Volume that can be expired following maximal inspiration
	IC	Inspiratory capacity – Volume that can be inspired after a normal, quiet expiration

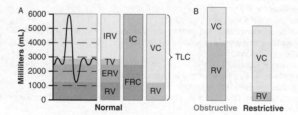

FIGURE 2.3: Lung volumes and capacities in health and disease. A) The four components of volume in the lung: Tidal volume (TV), expiratory reserve volume (ERV), inspiratory reserve volume (IRV), and residual volume (RV), as well as capacities which are measurements of two or more volumes. Functional residual capacity (FRC) = ERV + RV. Inspiratory capacity (IC) = TV + IRV. Vital capacity (VC) = ERV + TV + IRV. TLC (total lung capacity) is the volume of the lungs at maximal inflation. **B)** The changes in residual volume (RV), vital capacity (VC), and total lung capacity (TLC) in obstructive and restrictive lung diseases.

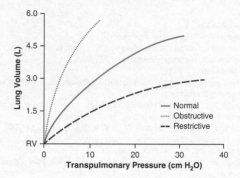

FIGURE 2.4: Transpulmonary pressures by lung volume in health and disease. Transpulmonary pressure is the pressure across the lung that produces pulmonary ventilation. It is equal to the difference between pleural and alveolar pressure. At a given lung volume, transpulmonary pressures are higher in restrictive disease and lower in obstructive disease.

PULMONOLOGY

Dynamics: Flow, Resistance, and V/Q Matching

- Flow:
  - **Ohm's Law ($\Delta P = Q \times R$)**
    $P = pressure, Q = flow, R = resistance$
    - Laminar flow: ΔQ proportional to ΔP (peripheral airway). Reynold's # < 2000.
    - Turbulent flow: ΔQ proportional to $\sqrt{\Delta P}$ (central airway). Reynold's # >2000.
    - Reduce density of gas $\rightarrow$ favors turbulent over laminar flow $\rightarrow$ decrease work of breathing
  - **Breathing cycle**
    - At rest: Lung collapsing forces = Chest wall expanding forces; Intra-alveolar pressure = 0 cm H_2O (i.e., equal to atmospheric pressure); pleural pressure negative (-5 cm H_2O); Transmural pressure positive ($+5$ cm H_2O); Lung volume = FRC.
    - Inspiration: Inspiratory muscles contract $\rightarrow$ Thoracic volume increases $\rightarrow$ Intra-alveolar pressure <0 cm H_2O (i.e., becomes lower than atmospheric pressure) $\rightarrow$ Air flows in $\rightarrow$ Intrapleural pressure becomes more negative; Lung volume = FRC + TV.
    - Expiration (passive): Elastic forces of lungs compress greater volume of air in alveoli $\rightarrow$ Alveolar pressure > atmospheric pressure $\rightarrow$ Air flows out $\rightarrow$ Intrapleural pressure returns to baseline (-5 cm H_2O)
    - Forced expiration: Similar to passive expiration, except use of musculature (abdominal wall, internal intercostals) results in even _more_ positive intrapleural pressure, which rapidly forces air out of the lungs
- Resistance/Poiseuille's Law: **$R = 8\eta l/\pi r^4$**
  $R = Resistance\ to\ flow, \eta = viscosity\ of\ gas, l = length\ of\ airway, r = radius\ of\ airway$
  - Medium-sized airways = Highest resistance (small-sized bronchi exist in parallel, so less resistance)
  - Resistance influenced by:
    - Modification of airway radius via bronchial smooth muscle
      - Sympathetic stimulation: $\beta 2$ receptors $\rightarrow$ smooth muscle relaxation $\rightarrow$ airway dilation $\rightarrow$ decreased resistance (e.g., $\beta 2$-agonist inhalers)
      - Parasympathetic stimulation: Smooth muscle contraction $\rightarrow$ airway constriction $\rightarrow$ increased resistance (e.g., anticholinergic toxicity)
    - Modification of airway radius by lung volume
      - High volume = more traction holding airways open, thus decreased resistance (and vice versa)

- V/Q Matching:
  - **Calculating ventilation**
    - Minute ventilation = Tidal volume × breaths/min
    - Alveolar ventilation = (Tidal volume − dead space) × breaths/min
  - **Dead space:** Ventilation but no perfusion (Figure 2.5)
    - Types of dead space:
      - <u>Anatomic dead space</u>: Volume of the conducting airways (i.e., areas that move air but do not participate in gas exchange; ~150 mL)
      - <u>Physiologic dead space</u>: Functional measurement of the volume of the lungs that does not participate in gas exchange
        - Calculating physiologic dead space: $\mathbf{V_D = V_T \times (P_ACO_2 - P_ECO_2)/(P_ACO_2)}$
          - V_D = Physiologic dead space, V_T = Tidal volume, P_ACO_2 = PCO_2 of arterial blood = PCO_2 of alveolar gas, P_ECO_2 = PCO_2 expired air
    - If physiologic dead space > predicted anatomic dead space, then pathology is present that increases dead space
      - E.g., pulmonary embolism – clot disrupts blood flow (i.e., Q = 0) → V/Q = infinity; 100% O_2 will help
  - **Shunt:** Perfusion but no ventilation (Figure 2.5)
    - E.g., airway obstruction (i.e., V = 0) → V/Q = 0; 100% O_2 does <u>NOT</u> help
  - **V/Q mismatch is more likely to cause <u>hypoxemia</u> than hypercapnia**
    - O_2 has a sigmoidal hemoglobin binding curve and thus is generally saturated in the alveolar–capillary bed (i.e., exchange only increases with increased blood flow) → hyperventilating does not help
    - CO_2 has a linear hemoglobin binding curve, and increased ventilation can increase removal from blood → hyperventilating can help/compensate for mismatch

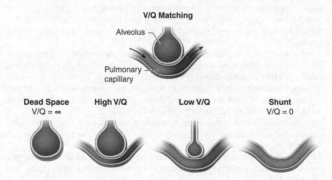

FIGURE 2.5: Dead space and shunt. Dead space refers to areas that are ventilated but not perfused, whereas shunt refers to areas that are perfused but not ventilated. V = ventilation; Q = blood flow.

Gas exchange

- Oxygen:
  - Oxygen is transported in two forms: 1) Dissolved in blood; 2) Bound to Hgb (most important/majority)
    - Hemoglobin: $2\alpha2\beta$ subunits; heme moiety with iron-containing porphyrin
    - O_2 capacity refers to the maximum amount of O_2 that can be bound to Hgb
      - Upper limit of how much O_2 can be carried by the blood
      - Must be measured at 100% saturation
    - O_2 content refers to the total O_2 carried in blood = Hgb-bound O_2 + dissolved O_2 = (1.34 × [Hgb] × % Sat) + (0.0031 + PaO_2)
  - Oxygen–Hgb dissociation curve is SIGMOIDAL (Figure 2.6)
    - **Shift L:** Increased O_2 affinity = ↓ PCO_2, ↓ 2,3 DPG, ↓Exercise, ↓Temperature, ↓H^+, Fetal Hb, CO
    - **Shift R:** Lower O_2 affinity = ↑ **P**CO_2, **A**ltitude, ↑ 2,3 **D**PG, **E**xercise, ↑ **T**emperature, (**CADET**), ↑H^+
- Carbon dioxide:
  - Carbon dioxide transport: 1) HCO_3 formed by carbonic anhydrase (~90% of CO_2), 2) Dissolved CO_2, 3) Carbaminohemoglobin (i.e., Hgb-CO_2)
  - Hgb–CO_2 dissociation curve is LINEAR
    - In lungs, Hgb is oxygenated → Hgb–CO_2 dissociation curve shifts right + down → CO_2 unloads (Haldane effect)
- Variations/disruptions in Hgb function:
  - **Methemoglobinemia** (Met-Hgb): Involves iron in Hgb converting from ferrous [Fe^{2+}] to ferric [Fe^{3+}] form, making it unable to bind oxygen. Medication culprits include dapsone, nitrates. Tx: Methylene blue.
  - **Carboxyhemoglobin** (CO-Hgb): Product of reaction between carbon monoxide and hemoglobin; CO releases more slowly than CO_2 from Hgb. Symptoms: Tiredness, dizziness, unconsciousness, death. Tx: Nonrebreather, hyperbaric chamber. Involve toxicology.

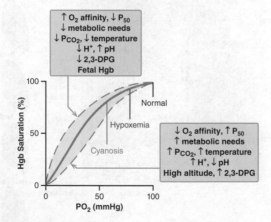

FIGURE 2.6: Oxygen–hemoglobin dissociation curve. "Right shifts" in the curve allow oxygen to be released from hemoglobin more easily, whereas "left shifts" cause oxygen to bind hemoglobin more tightly. O_2 = oxygen; P_{50} = oxygen tension at which hemoglobin is 50% saturated; PCO_2 = partial pressure of carbon dioxide; H^+ = hydrogen ions; 2,3-DPG = 2,3-diphosphoglyceric acid

DIAGNOSTICS

Chest x-ray (CXR)

- Types of CXR:
  - <u>PA and lateral CXR</u>: Method: Radiation *posterior → anterior*; obtained with lateral images. Indications: Most common modality used for lung imaging.
  - <u>AP portable CXR</u>: Method: Radiation *anterior → posterior*. Indications: Does not provide as much information as a PA CXR, but used for unstable or hospitalized patients since it is portable. Subject to issues with patient rotation. No lateral images and enlarges the cardiac silhouette.
  - <u>Lateral decubitus CXR</u>: Method: Patient placed in the lateral decubitus position (on side) for CXR. Indications: Assessment of free-flowing vs. loculated pleural fluid. Increasingly replaced by point of care ultrasound (POCUS), especially for assessment of effusions.
- Approach to interpretation of CXR:
  - Verify patient name and date
  - Identify CXR type
  - Evaluate quality:
    - **R**otation: Clavicular symmetry, trachea midline
    - **I**nspiration: Count for 8.5–11 rib spaces above the diaphragm
    - **P**enetration: If thoracic spine seen through heart, film is overexposed
  - Read systematically:
    - **A**irway (i.e., trachea)
    - **B**ronchoalveolar markings (Figure 2.7)
    - **C**ardiac silhouette (and assessment of mediastinum)
    - **D**iaphragm
    - **E**xtras/**E**verything Else (i.e., lung parenchyma, MSK, lines/tubes)

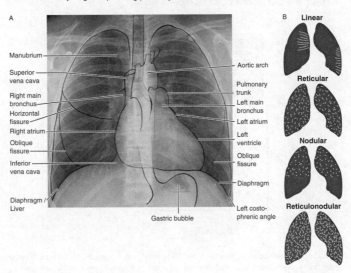

FIGURE 2.7: Normal CXR and depiction of CXR findings. A) Normal CXR with anatomy labeled. B) Patterns on a CXR can be described as linear, reticular, nodular, or reticulonodular.

Chest CT

- Types of Chest CT:
  - <u>Standard</u>: Images may be obtained with or without contrast. Indications for use of contrast include malignancy workup and evaluation for infection of chest wall/mediastinum
  - <u>High resolution</u>: Very thin cuts with outstanding spatial resolution that helps to detect interstitial lung disease (particularly honeycombing, which can be missed on standard chest CT). Expiratory views are useful to detect air trapping, which helps with diagnosis of certain interstitial lung diseases (e.g., hypersensitivity pneumonitis)
  - <u>CT angiography</u>: Image with contrast; timing of image attainment can be optimized for detection of specific diagnoses, such as pulmonary emboli
  - <u>Low radiation dose CT (LDCT)</u>: Screening for lung cancer (National Lung Cancer Screening Trial, *New Engl J Med* 2011)
- Interpreting chest CT images:
  - **Images provide information about density:** Dense = bright/white
    - Air: Black
    - Fluid/Soft tissue: Gray
    - Blood: White
    - Bone/Contrast: Dense white
  - **Windows adjust what densities are displayed in the image** (can aid interpretation)
    - Lung window: Lung, airways, lung parenchyma
    - Soft tissue window: Mediastinal structures, heart, thyroid, muscles, lymph nodes
    - Bone window: Bone
- Approach to interpretation of chest CT:
  - Verify patient name and date
  - Identify chest CT type, including whether contrast was administered
  - Select appropriate window (*often start with lung, then use soft tissue*)
  - Read systematically:
    - **A**ir: Airway, lung parenchyma
    - **B**one: Evaluate for fractures, metastases
    - **C**ardiac/vessels: Assess for anatomy, clots, false lumen
    - **D**igestive: Evaluate esophagus patency
    - **E**xtras: Tubes, foreign bodies
    - **S**oft tissue: Muscles, fat
  - The radiographic finding(s) can be used to help create a differential diagnosis (Table 2.2)

Pulmonary Function Testing (PFTs)

- Approach to interpreting PFTs:
  - Key questions:
    - Is there obstruction?
    - Is there restriction?
    - Is there pathology disruptive to the alveolar–capillary membrane?
  - Approach: See Figures 2.8 and 2.9
    - **Assess flow–volume loop**, if available (curvilinear = obstructive; steep/vertical = restrictive)
    - **Evaluate FEV_1/FVC** (<0.7 = obstructive)
      - If obstructive, assess reversibility and DLCO to determine etiology
    - **Evaluate TLC** ($<80\%$ predicted = restrictive)
      - If restrictive, assess DLCO to determine etiology
    - **Evaluate DLCO**
      - Consider methacholine challenge, as asthma may have baseline normal FEV_1/FVC, TLC, DLCO

TABLE 2.2 · Differential Diagnoses of Pulmonary Processeses Based on Radiographic Findings	
Finding	**Differential Diagnosis**
Segmental/Lobar Consolidation	• Common bacterial pathogens (including *Legionella*) • Less common: TB, *Nocardia*, fungal

Solitary nodule	• Benign (>99%)
	  - Infectious: Endemic fungi (histoplasmosis, coccidioidomycosis), mycobacteria (TB, NTM); less commonly, abscess-forming bacteria (e.g., *S. aureus*)
	  - Tumor: Hamartoma
	  - Pulmonary AV malformation
	  - Other: Inflammatory lesions (e.g., RA, GPA, sarcoidosis, amyloidosis), rounded atelectasis
	• Malignancy (<1%)
	  - Primary lung cancer
	  - Metastatic cancer, especially melanoma, sarcoma, or carcinoma of bronchus, colon, breast, kidney, or testicle

Multiple nodules	• Centrilobular:
	  - Most common: Infection and aspiration; infection can be bacterial, fungal, mycobacterial, or nontuberculous mycobacteria (NTM)
	  - Less common: Hypersensitivity pneumonitis (HP), respiratory bronchiolitis (RB), endobronchial tumor
	• Perilymphatic:
	  - Inflammatory: Sarcoidosis, pneumoconiosis, lymphocytic interstitial pneumonia (LIP)
	  - Malignancy: Lymphangitic carcinomatosis, leukemia/lymphoma
	  - Amyloidosis
	• Random distribution:
	  - Hematogenous infection: Septic emboli, disseminated fungal, miliary TB
	  - Hematogenous malignancy, Langerhans cell histiocytosis (LCH, accompanied by cysts)

Cavitation	• Lung abscess and necrotizing pneumonia
	  - Bacteria: Anaerobes (most common), MRSA, less commonly *Pseudomonas*
	  - Atypicals: TB/NTM (including MAC), *Nocardia*
	  - Fungal
	    • Yeasts: *Cryptococcus*
	    • Dimorphic (endemics): *Histoplasma, Coccidioides*
	    • Molds: *Aspergillus*, Zygomycetes
	• Septic emboli
	• Malignancy: Primary lung cancers (e.g., bronchogenic carcinomas), lymphoma, Kaposi's sarcoma, or metastatic disease
	• Rheumatologic: Granulomatosis with polyangiitis; less commonly rheumatoid arthritis and sarcoidosis
	• Pulmonary embolism
	• Other: Bronchiolitis obliterans with organizing pneumonia, Langerhans cell histiocytosis, and amyloidosis

Ground Glass Opacities (GGOs; "*pus, water, blood*")	• Most common: Edema (cardiogenic or noncardiogenic) • Infectious: Viral – respiratory viruses (e.g., influenza, RSV) or CMV • Atypicals (rarely *Mycoplasma, Chlamydia*, Q fever, leptospirosis) • Pneumocystis pneumonia (PCP) • Parasitic and fungal, including *Toxoplasma* and *Strongyloides* • Hemorrhage, including diffuse alveolar hemorrhage (DAH) • Others: Drug-induced acute lung injury (ALI)
Cystic	• Lymphangioleiomyomatosis (LAM) • Langerhans cell histiocytosis (LCH, accompanied by nodules) • Lymphocytic interstitial pneumonia (LIP)
Fibrotic	• Diffuse parenchymal lung disease (DPLD) due to a known cause (e.g., associated with rheumatologic disease, secondary to medication) • Idiopathic DPLD (e.g., idiopathic pulmonary fibrosis [IPF]) • Granulomatous DPLP (e.g., sarcoidosis) • Other DPLD

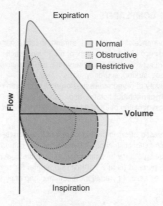

FIGURE 2.8: PFT Flow–volume loops in health and disease. In obstructive disease, the flow–volume loop becomes curvilinear, whereas in restrictive disease the flow–volume loop becomes steep/vertical.

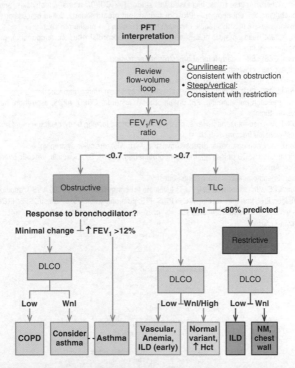

FIGURE 2.9: An approach to PFT interpretation. Abbreviations: PFT = Pulmonary function test; FEV$_1$ = forced expiratory volume in one second; FVC = forced vital capacity; DLCO = diffusion capacity for carbon monoxide; Wnl = within normal limits; ILD = interstitial lung disease; NM = neuromuscular disorder; Hct = hematocrit

APPROACHES AND CHIEF COMPLAINTS

Key Terms and Definitions

- Dyspnea: Subjective experience of breathing discomfort, must be self-reported
- Respiratory distress: Presence of increased work of breathing, which signals approaching respiratory collapse; physical exam may reveal high respiratory rate, use of accessory muscles, evidence of acute obstruction (e.g., wheezing, stridor), and/or cyanosis
- Hypoxia: Insufficient delivery of oxygen to tissues/organs, which can result from anemia, hypoxemia, circulatory dysfunction, hypermetabolic states, and/or the presence of histotoxins (e.g., cyanide)
- Hypoxemia: Insufficient oxygenation of arterial blood; directly measured by blood gas

Dyspnea

- Pathophysiology: 1) Increased effort in setting of respiratory muscle fatigue. 2) Acute hypercapnia > acute hypoxemia. 3) Bronchoconstriction. 4) Dynamic airway compression. 5) Afferent mismatch.
- Differential diagnosis: Etiologies may be pulmonary, cardiac, metabolic, hematologic, acid–base, and psychiatric; the dyspnea pyramid (Figure 2.10) can be helpful for remembering how common each etiology is for dyspnea (i.e., base of pyramid most common, top of pyramid least common)
- Physical exam:
  - Vital signs: HR, RR, SpO_2
  - General: Distress, mental status
  - HEENT: Airway exam
  - Volume: JVD, rales, edema, S3 ($\rightarrow$ CHF)
  - Pulm: Wheeze, pursed lips, increased I/E, stridor ($\rightarrow$ COPD/asthma, anaphylaxis, angioedema), rhonchi/crackles, egophony ($\rightarrow$ PNA), distant/absent breath sounds, dull to percussion ($\rightarrow$ pleural effusion), absent breath sounds, resonant to percussion ($\rightarrow$ pneumothorax)
  - CV: Distant heart sounds, pulsus paradoxus ($\rightarrow$ pericardial effusion, tamponade), palpitations/irregular rhythm
  - Neuro: GCS <8 ($\rightarrow$ early intubation), strength/sensation
  - Abd: Ascites or distention
- Differential diagnosis by system: (Figure 2.10)
  - Cardiac: ACS, CHF, cardiomyopathy, valvular disease, arrhythmia, tamponade
  - Pulm: Infection (pneumonia), PE, pneumothorax, asthma, COPD, ARDS, aspiration, hemorrhage, effusion, tumor
  - HEENT: Angioedema, anaphylaxis, pharyngeal infection, foreign body, neck trauma
  - Chest wall: Rib fracture, flail chest
  - Neuro: CVA, neuromuscular disease (myasthenia gravis, muscular dystrophy)
  - Toxic/metabolic: CO poisoning, methemoglobinemia, sepsis, DKA, anemia, narcotic overdose
  - Psych: Anxiety
  - Other: Pneumomediastinum, ascites, obesity
- Workup: CBC with differential, BMP, LFTs (evaluate for congestion), CXR, ECG, A/VBG; additional testing to consider: BNP, troponin, cardiac/IVC POCUS, TTE; pulmonary POCUS; CT chest/CT-PE/HRCT chest
- Management: If "**respiratory distress**" is present, see next section; otherwise, treat suspected underlying cause

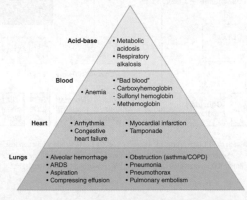

FIGURE 2.10: The dyspnea pyramid. The etiologies of dyspnea are listed here, with more common causes of dyspnea on the bottom of the pyramid and less common causes at the top.

Respiratory Distress
- Ask for help: Call your team and consider rapid response
- Confirm code status
- Provide respiratory support: Oxygen via nasal canula, non-rebreather, or high-flow nasal canula. Consider non-invasive positive pressure ventilation (NIPPV) if not contraindicated or intubation if needed.
- Perform physical exam: See physical exam under dyspnea above
- First-pass diagnostics: STAT ABG, CBC with differential, CXR, ECG. Consider BMP, BNP, troponin, VBG with lactate, cardiac and/or pulmonary POCUS, CT chest/CTPE (based on stability)
- Differential diagnosis: Consider differential diagnosis based on patient characteristics (Table 2.3)
- Use ABG to further characterize the respiratory failure:
  - Calculating the A-a gradient
    - $A\text{-a}DO_2 = PAO_2 - PaO_2$
      $PAO_2 =$ partial pressure of O_2 in alveolar gas, $PaO_2 =$ partial pressure of O_2 in arterial blood
    - PaO_2 is measured directly on ABG
    - PAO_2 must be calculated:
      - $PAO_2 = [(P_{atm} - PH_2O) * FiO_2] - (PaCO_2/R) = (760 - 47)(0.21) - (PaCO_2/0.8) = 150 - 1.25(PaCO_2)$
  - Interpreting the A-a gradient
    - There are multiple rules of thumb to age-adjust the A-a gradient normal value
      - Normal A-a gradient $= (Age/4) + 4$
      - Normal A-a gradient $= 0.3 * Age$

PULMONOLOGY

TABLE 2.3 · Differential Diagnosis for Causes of Acute or Emergent Respiratory Distress		
Suspected Condition	**Potential Intervention**	**Considerations**
Tension pneumothorax	Needle thoracostomy (5th ICS, mid-axillary)	Consider tension physiology with acute hypotension, tachycardia, hypoxemia; consider checking POCUS for lung slide
Pulmonary embolism	Empiric heparin gtt/TPA	Consider whether the patient is on oral anticoagulation, evidence of active bleed, prior bleeding history, contraindications to anticoagulation
Pleural effusion	Thoracentesis	Check INR, platelet count. Correct coagulopathy or thrombocytopenia
COPD	Nebulizer, non-invasive positive pressure ventilation (NIPPV), methylprednisolone 125 mg IV	Steroids can worsen cardiogenic pulmonary edema
Anaphylaxis	Epi (1:1000) 0.3 mg IM, methylprednisolone 125 mg IV, diphenhydramine, famotidine	Epi acutely raises blood pressure and is pro-arrhythmogenic
Congestive heart failure	IV diuresis, NIPPV	Trial of NIPPV requires prompt reassessment for improvement. if no improvement, consider intubation
Acute coronary syndrome	Aspirin 325 mg, atorvastatin 80 mg, heparin gtt. See Cardiology Chapter 1	Discuss patient with cardiology early (even NSTEMI is indication for urgent cath if new-onset HF present)
Opiate overdose	0.4–2 mg q3min PRN IV/IM naloxone (Narcan)	Narcan has a short half-life; consider ICU admission for Narcan drip if leading diagnosis
Pneumonia	IV antibiotics	CXR or lung imaging would show consolidation

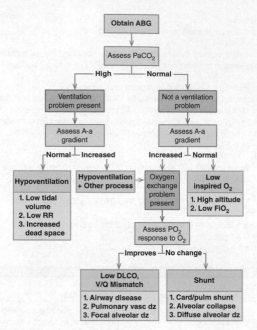

FIGURE 2.11: **An approach to interpreting arterial blood gas (ABG) using the A-a gradient.** Abbreviations: TdV = tidal volume; RR = respiratory rate; PO_2 = partial pressure of oxygen; O_2 = oxygen; DLCO = diffusing capacity for carbon monoxide; FiO_2 = fraction of inspired oxygen; dz = disease

Hypoxemic Respiratory Failure

- Definition: PaO_2 <60 mmHg, P/F <300, *or* PaO_2 decrease from baseline of 10 mmHg
- Pathophysiology: Hypoxemia has five major mechanisms:
  - Hypoventilation (↑$PaCO_2$, Normal $AaDO_2$): See "hypercarbic respiratory failure" in next section
  - Low inspired FiO_2 (Normal $PaCO_2$, Normal $AaDO_2$): High altitude
  - Low DLCO/diffusion impairment (Normal $PaCO_2$, ↑$AaDO_2$, Response to O_2)
    - In normal states, O_2 is a perfusion-limited gas (i.e., O_2 exchange at alveolar–capillary bed limited by blood flow since O_2 in the blood and alveolus equilibrates early along the capillary). Therefore, issues with O_2 diffusion requires significant diffusion impairment
    - In physiologic stress (e.g., intense exercise) or pathologic states, O_2 becomes a diffusion-limited gas; examples include pulmonary fibrosis (due to alveolar membrane thickening) and emphysema (due to destruction of lung → decreased surface area for diffusion)
  - V/Q mismatch (Normal $PaCO_2$, ↑$AaDO_2$, Response to supplemental O_2)
    - Normal V/Q = 0.8 (highest at apices, lowest at bases)
    - Occurs with focal alveolar processes (e.g., pneumonia, pulmonary edema, aspiration/mucus plugging, ILD)
  - Shunt (Normal $PaCO_2$, ↑$AaDO_2$, No response to supplemental O_2)
    - Perfused (Q > 0) but not ventilated (V = 0; therefore, V/Q = 0). Supplemental O_2 does not help.
    - Both pulmonary and cardiac etiologies exist
      - Pulmonary shunting: Physiologic (pulmonary edema, ARDS, DAH, atelectasis), AVM, hepatopulmonary syndrome
      - Intracardiac shunting (assess using TTE with bubble):
        - R→L shunt: Blood from the right heart enters circulation without going through the lungs (tetralogy of Fallot). Reduced PaO_2
        - L→R shunt: More common because left pressure higher (patent ductus arteriosus, trauma). Does NOT reduce PaO_2. Over time, can get reversal of shunt to R→L causing hypoxemia (Eisenmenger's syndrome)
- Physical Exam: See physical exam under dyspnea above

- Workup:
  - ABG: PaO_2 measures gas exchange; $PaCO_2$ measures ventilation. A-a gradient: PaO_2-PaO_2, normal (age+4)/4
  - EKG: Evaluate for ischemia, evidence of right heart strain to support PE (S1Q3T3, RAD, RBBB)
  - Labs: CBC, BMP, troponin, BNP
  - CXR: Evaluate for infiltrate or lobar collapse, pneumothorax, pulmonary edema, hyperinflation, or for no evidence of abnormality (Pearl: CXR often looks normal for PE, COPD, early aspiration)
- Treatment: Supplemental O_2, airway clearance (i.e., suction secretions), consider furosemide, albuterol, antibiotics, NIPPV, intubation and/or escalation of care (i.e., transfer to ICU)

Hypercarbic Respiratory Failure

- Definition: Respiratory failure due to alveolar hypoventilation → ineffective carbon dioxide elimination
- Pathophysiology: 1) Impaired respiratory drive (i.e., CNS cause) 2) Impaired neuromuscular strength 3) Increased load on respiratory system
- Differential diagnosis by mechanism:
  - **Impaired respiratory drive**
    - Brainstem injuries
    - Drug overdose (e.g., opiates, sedatives)
    - Severe hypothyroidism
  - **Impaired neuromuscular strength**
    - Neuromuscular diseases (e.g., myasthenia gravis, amyotrophic lateral sclerosis, Guillain-Barré syndrome, multiple sclerosis)
    - Weakness of respiratory muscles (e.g., myopathy, fatigue from increased work of breathing, severe electrolyte derangement)
  - **Increased load**
    - Increased resistive load: Bronchospasm (e.g., COPD, asthma)
    - Decreased compliance:
      - Lung: Restrictive disease, auto-PEEP
      - Chest wall: Chest wall skeletal disorder, obesity, pleural effusion, ascites/distension
    - Increased required minute ventilation: DKA, sepsis, pulmonary embolism
- Physiologic response:
  - Hyperventilate to increase alveolar ventilation and blow off more CO_2
  - Vicious cycle: $\uparrow PaCO_2$ → decline in mental status → reduction in ventilator drive → further $\uparrow PaCO_2$
- Physical exam: See physical exam under dyspnea above
- Work-up:
  - ABG or VBG, CBC, CMP, consider troponin, BNP
  - CXR, ECG, cardiac and pulmonary point of care ultrasound (POCUS), consider Chest CT or CT-PE
  - Consider PFTs, testing maximum inspiratory pressure (MIP) and maximum expiratory pressure (MEP), other testing based on clinical suspicion
- Treatment:
  - Identify and treat underlying cause
  - Consider NIPPV if not contraindicated; best evidence for use in COPD exacerbations

PULMONOLOGY

Chronic Cough (>8 wk) in Immunocompetent Adults

- Evaluate for red flags: Evaluate for red flags and consider CXR. If red flags present or concerning findings on CXR, proceed with a more urgent workup
- Etiology and diagnosis: Consider common causes of subacute to chronic cough: See Table 2.4
- Refractory chronic cough:
  - If symptoms continue despite evaluation/empiric treatment for common causes, consider less common causes of chronic cough. Differential diagnosis:
    - Infectious: *Mycobacterium tuberculosis*, Nontuberculous mycobacterium (including *Mycobacterium avium complex* (MAC), *Mycobacterium kansasii*, and *Mycobacterium abscessus*), endemic fungal infections
    - Cardiac: LV failure, dilated left atrium, mitral stenosis
    - Other: Post-infectious cough, chronic aspiration, sarcoidosis, laryngeal spasm, non-asthmatic eosinophilic bronchitis, allergic bronchopulmonary aspergillosis (ABPA), psychogenic cough
  - Workup may include: Labs (including CBC with differential to evaluate for eosinophilia), repeat CXR, advanced imaging, sputum cultures, PFTs, sleep apnea testing, TTE, referral to pulmonary/ENT/ID, bronchoscopy

Hemoptysis

- Evaluate for massive hemoptysis:
  - Defined as >**500 cc blood in 24 hr or >100 cc/hr**
    - If massive, call airway team for intubation and contact procedural consultants (e.g., interventional radiology, interventional pulmonology) due to concern for arterial bleeding
    - If not massive, consider differential diagnosis in Table 2.5
- Rule out hemoptysis mimics: Hematemesis, nasopharyngeal bleeding
- Work-up: Order first pass work-up and consider additional testing based on differential diagnosis
  - First-pass work-up: CBC, coags, sputum cx, UA, CXR. Also consider CT chest, AFB/airborne isolation if concern for MTB
  - Differential diagnosis by categories of disease process:
    - Hemorrhage, including diffuse alveolar hemorrhage (DAH)
    - Infection: TB, bronchiectasis, lung abscesses
    - Malignancy: Lung cancer, metastatic disease
    - Rheum: Capillaritis
    - Pulm: PE
    - Cardiac: Heart failure, mitral stenosis, congenital heart disease
    - Coagulation diseases: Severe thrombocytopenia, uremia, anticoagulation medications
    - Other: Airway trauma (iatrogenic postprocedure or post-traumatic), foreign body

TABLE 2.4 · Differential Diagnosis for Causes of Subacute to Chronic Cough	
Diagnosis	**Notes**
ACE inhibitor	Classically causes a dry cough; can switch to ARB; however, 3% of patients develop ARB-associated cough
GERD	Assess for classic features (heartburn, metallic taste, worse at night/with recumbence), trial PPI for 4 weeks. Laryngopharyngeal reflux (LPR) can cause hoarseness, globus sensation
Upper airway cough syndrome (UACS)	Formerly "postnasal drip." Assess for classic features (rhinorrhea, sensation of dripping), then trial intranasal glucocorticoids (e.g., fluticasone, mometasone)
Cough-variant asthma or COPD	Diagnosis requires PFT; if already on therapy, assess whether escalation of treatment is needed
Smoking/environmental	Counsel on lifestyle modification

DISEASES AND PATHOPHYSIOLOGY

Alveolar Hemorrhage

- Definition: Bleeding into the alveolar space due to disruption of the alveolar–capillary basement membrane
- Etiologies: See Table 2.5
- Clinical presentation:
  - Cough, fever, hemoptysis, or diffuse GGOs + other concerning features (e.g., extrapulmonary signs of vasculitis, known condition associated with DAH, declining hemoglobin without clear reason)
  - Pearl: Hemoptysis is only present in 50% of cases and absence does not predict hemorrhage severity
  - Also consider alveolar hemorrhage in a patient with GGOs who is failing to progress as expected (e.g., patient with suspected cardiogenic pulmonary edema who is not improving with diuresis)
- Diagnostics:
  - Labs: CBC, BUN/Cr, UA, ESR, CRP. Consider rheumatologic w/u, which may include ANA, dsDNA, RNP, C3, C4, RF, CCP, ANCA, MPO, PR3, cryoglobulins, anti-GBM, RVVT, cardiolipin, B2-glycoprotein Ab
  - Imaging: Noncontrast chest CT (consider contrast if suspect other causes of hemoptysis): Imaging shows patchy or diffuse GGOs
  - Bronchoscopy: 1) Serial lavage – gets progressively more hemorrhagic; 2) Rule out infection; 3) Check CBC with differential to evaluate for eosinophilia
- Management:
  - **Capillaritis**: Immunosuppression
    - For ANCA-associated vasculitis, typically give pulse-dose steroids first and then adjunctive therapies like cyclophosphamide, rituximab, etc. if lack of response
  - **Bland hemorrhage** or **diffuse alveolar damage**:
    - Treat underlying cause, supportive care

TABLE 2.5 · Etiologies of Alveolar Hemorrhage Based on Mechanism		
Mechanism	**Pathophysiology**	**Differential diagnosis**

Capillaritis	PMNs infiltrate lung interstitum → necrosis of alveolar septa → RBCs leak into the alveolar space	• ANCA-associated small vessel vasculitis
		  - GPA: Granulomatosis with polyangiitis, formerly Wegener's: Sinus, lungs, kidneys. Most common. c-ANCA, anti-PR3
		  - EGPA: Eosinophilic granulomatosis with polyangiitis, formerly Churg-Strauss: Asthma, eosinophilia, p-ANCA, anti-MPO
		  - MPA: Microscopic polyangiitis: Lungs and kidneys. p-ANCA, anti-MPO
		• Pulmonary renal syndromes, ANCA negative
		  - Anti-GBM
		  - IgA nephropathy
		• Other connective tissue disease associated/immune-complex mediated processes
		  - SLE
		  - Anti-phospholipid antibody syndrome (APLS)
		  - Cryoglobulinemia

Bland hemorrhage	RBCs leak into the alveolar space without associated inflammation or alveolar destruction	• Elevated LVEDP: Left sided heart failure, mitral stenosis • Drugs: Complication of anticoagulation, drug-induced thrombocytopenia • Thrombocytopenia or bleeding disorders • Uremia
Diffuse alveolar damage	Pattern seen in ARDS with edema in the alveolar septa and hyaline deposition in the membranes	• Infections: Infection related to ARDS, viral infection, opportunitic infection • Drug toxicity (e.g., cocaine, amiodarone, nitrofurantoin) • Connective tissue diseases: SLE, polymyositis • Other: Noninfectious causes of ARDS, pulmonary infarct, tuberous sclerosis

PULMONOLOGY

Obstructive Lung Diseases

- Obstructive = ↑compliance, ↓elastance → problem emptying the lung.
  - ↑TLC, ↑RV, problem pushing air out → air trapping
  - ↓↓FEV$_1$ ↓FVC = FEV$_1$/FVC ratio <0.7

Chronic obstructive pulmonary disease (COPD)

- Epidemiology: Most common in former smokers (although can affect persons in cities with air pollution, women may develop with less significant smoking history). Typical onset age >40 yr
- Definitions:
  - **COPD:** Persistent airflow limitation resulting from the consequences of chronic inflammation from smoking. Classic subtypes were chronic bronchitis and emphysema, although these are not included in the current definition
    - Chronic bronchitis: Clinical diagnosis of chronic productive cough for 3 mo/yr for >2 yr. Normal DLCO.
    - Emphysema: Pathologic diagnosis that describes permanent enlargement of the airspaces and destruction of the alveoli, which causes loss of diffusing capacity and reduced elastic recoil. ↓DLCO.
      - Centrilobular: Tobacco activates PMNs, inhibits α1-antitrypsin, ↑oxidative stress. Upper lung predominant.
      - Panlobular: Alpha-1 antitrypsin deficiency. Lung bases with bilateral basilar bullae and can also have liver disease (PAS+).
    - Small airway disease: Third characteristic feature of COPD. Small bronchioles are narrowed and reduced in number. Small airway destruction is a hallmark of advanced COPD.
  - **Asthma–COPD overlap syndrome** (some reversibility with bronchodilators)
- Pathogenesis:
  - Airways: Chronic inflammation, increased numbers of goblet cells and mucous glands; airway collapse due to the loss of tethering caused by alveolar wall destruction
  - Lung parenchyma: Affects structures distal to the terminal bronchiole
  - Pulmonary vasculature: Smooth muscle hypertrophy → chronic hypoxic vasoconstriction of the small pulmonary arteries
- Clinical presentation: Dyspnea, chronic cough, sputum production
- Physical exam:
  - Early in disease: Normal or only prolonged expiration or wheezing on forced exhalation
  - Increasing severity: Hyperinflation (increased resonance to percussion), decreased breath sounds, wheezes/crackles
  - Pearl: Clubbing is NOT typical in COPD; suggests comorbidities such as lung cancer, ILD, or bronchiectasis
- Diagnosis:
  - CXR may be normal, as evidence of hyperinflation often not present; CXR is only 50% sensitive for detection of COPD
  - PFTs: ↓FEV$_1$, FEV$_1$/FEC <0.70, ↑TLC,↑RV
  - Consider testing for alpha-1 antitrypsin deficiency in young patients (<45 yr) or non/minimal smokers. Patients with alpha-1 antitrypsin deficiency may also have liver disease
  - Rule out other causes of subacute/chronic dyspnea (e.g., consider BNP, TTE, chest imaging including CT-PE)
- Characterization:
  - Characterize symptom burden and risk of exacerbation using the **GOLD Group A-D** classification system
    - Based on exacerbation history (# exacerbations per year and # resulting in hospital admission) and symptom burden (measured by questionnaires such as mMRC, CAT)
- Chronic treatment:
  - Three things improve survival: 1) Smoking cessation; 2) Home supplemental oxygen (if PaO$_2$ <55 mmHg, cor pulmonale); 3) Lung volume reduction surgery
  - Initial treatment regimen: Here is a general approach, which much be tailored for each patient:
    - Start by prescribing a short-acting beta agonist (SABA) or short-acting muscarinic antagonist (SAMA) to be used as needed
    - Add a long-acting muscarinic antagonist (LAMA) (e.g., Spiriva)
    - Add a long-acting beta agonist (LABA)
    - Add an inhaled corticosteroid (ICS)
  - Treatment of refractory COPD:
    - Consider adjuvant therapies like a PDE4 inhibitor (roflumilast) if inflammation is a significant factor or chronic azithromycin to prevent recurrent exacerbations
    - If failing triple therapy (LAMA/LABA/ICS) and eosinophilia is present, consider targeted therapies for eosinophilic lung disease
    - For select patients with apical predominant refractory disease, surgery may be an option
    - Recommend pulmonary rehabilitation as evidence demonstrates substantial impact on quality of life

- Treatment of acute COPD exacerbation:
  - History of prior exacerbations is the best predictor of recurrent exacerbation (ECLIPSE trial, *New Engl J Med* 2010)
  - Cardinal symptoms: Increased dyspnea, sputum quality, sputum purulence
  - Etiology: Viral/bacterial infection (70%), inhaler nonadherence, pollution/poor air quality, forest fires, pulmonary embolism, idiopathic
  - Management:
    - Bronchodilator β2-agonist (albuterol) and anticholinergic (ipratropium)
    - Systemic corticosteroids
      - Improve FEV_1/SpO_2, shorten recovery time/length of stay
      - PO as effective as IV, benefit may be greatest if peripheral eosinophilia is present
      - Prednisone 40 mg PO × 5 days (noninferior for preventing re-exacerbation compared to 14-day course, REDUCE trial, *JAMA* 2013)
    - Supplemental O_2 (SpO_2 goal 88–92%), avoid hyperoxia
    - Ventilatory support
      - Indicated for acute hypercapnic respiratory failure
      - Benefit demonstrated for non-invasive positive pressure ventilation
      - Reassess in 1–2 hours; if not improving, consider intubation
    - Antibiotics
      - Consider use of antibiotics if 3/3 cardinal symptoms present, 2/3 with one being sputum purulence, or if the patient requires non-invasive mechanical ventilation
      - Total antibiotic course typically 5–7 days
      - Drug choice based on local antimicrobial resistance. Commonly used: doxycycline, azithromycin
- Prevention:
  - Influenza vaccine annually
  - Pneumonia vaccines: PCV13 (if not previously given) followed by PPSV23 $\geq$8 weeks later, then PPSV23 q5yr
- Complications:
  - Compensatory polycythemia (Hct >55% men, >47% women)
  - Pulmonary hypertension
  - Compensatory metabolic alkalosis: Check BMP to assess for elevated HCO_3

Asthma
- Pathogenesis: Triad: 1) Airway inflammation, 2) Airway hyper-responsiveness, 3) Reversible airflow obstruction
- Clinical presentation: Shortness of breath, wheezing
- Asthma syndromes: There are many asthma syndromes/variants:
  - **Allergic asthma:** +IgE
  - **Cough-variant asthma**
  - **Exercise-induced bronchospasm**
  - **Occupational asthma:** Farmers, factory workers, and other exposures.
  - **Aspirin-exacerbated respiratory disease:** "Samter's triad": Asthma, sinus inflammation with nasal polyps, and sensitivity to aspirin/NSAID. Avoid aspirin/NSAIDS or consider aspirin desensitization.
  - **Reactive airways dysfunction syndrome:** Syndrome of acute airway hyperreactivity in response to an inhaled irritant; NOT to be confused with the sometimes nonspecifically used term "reactive airways" or "airway reactivity" to describe transient wheezing.
  - **Allergic bronchopulmonary aspergillosis (ABPA):** Chronic hypersensitivity in response to colonization with *Aspergillus*, typically in patients with asthma or cystic fibrosis. Clinical features: Recurrent exacerbation of asthma, peripheral eosinophilia, high IgE titers, +*Aspergillus* IgG/IgE, radiographic findings (classically central bronchiectasis, upper lobe parenchymal opacities). Tx: Steroids, consider antifungals in some cases.
- Differential diagnosis:
  - **Virus-induced bronchospasm**
  - **Chronic eosinophilic pneumonia (CEP):** Idiopathic disorder with accumulation of eosinophils in the interstitium/alveoli. Median age of onset 30–40 yr. Clinical features: Fever, dyspnea, productive cough, weight loss, wheezes or crackles, peripheral eosinophilia. Classic CXR = bilateral peripheral/pleural-based opacities. Tx: Steroids.

- **Eosinophilic granulomatosis with polyangiitis (EGPA, formerly *Churg-Strauss*):** Clinical features: Chronic rhinosinusitis, asthma, and pronounced peripheral eosinophilia. +pANCA. Tx: Steroids. If refractory, consider cyclophosphamide and/or other adjuvant therapies
- **Vocal cord dysfunction:** Consider if the patient is diagnosed with "asthma" but does not improve with treatment or if the patient dramatically improves immediately with intubation. In some cases worsened by stress or can be induced by patient "on command." Diagnosed by direct laryngoscopy or characteristic flow – volume loop on PFT.
- Common comorbidities: GERD, sinus disease, OSA, obesity. Management of these comorbidities may improve asthma symptoms
- Diagnosis: PFTs; spirometry before and after albuterol administration (increase in $FEV_1 \geq 12\%$ = "reversibility"); bronchoprovocation test (i.e., methacholine, a synthetic choline ester)
- Classification: Asthma severity is characterized by impairment from symptoms and risk of exacerbation requiring oral steroids (Table 2.6)
- Chonic treatment:
  - Initial controller therapy is based on classification (Figure 2.12)
  - Step-up therapy is based on the principles of Assess, Adjust, and Review Response (GINA Guidelines 2020)
    - Assess: Patient's symptom burden, goals, and inhaler technique
    - Adjust: Treat modifiable risk factors, review nonpharmacological strategies, provide education about inhaler use, escalate asthma medications
    - Review Response: Symptom burden, exacerbations, side effects, lung function, patient satisfaction
- Treatment of acute asthma exacerbation:
  - Clinical features: Dyspnea, wheezing, increased home inhaler use; abnormal peak flow by peak flow meter (in general, <200 L/min consistent with severe obstruction); hypoxia
  - Etiology: May be triggered by viruses, allergens, occupational exposures, environmental pollution, aspirin/NSAIDs, exercise, inadequate chronic asthma treatment, or medication non-compliance
  - Management:
    - Assess severity: HR, RR, O_2 saturation, pulsus paradoxus, use of accessory muscles, inability to speak in full sentences
    - Evaluate for major risk factors for fatality: 1) Recent history of poorly controlled asthma, 2) Prior history of near-fatal asthma. Minor risk factors = allergies, aspirin-associated asthma
    - Provide therapies:
      - Supplemental O_2 to maintain SpO_2 >92%
      - Short-acting beta2 agonists (e.g., albuterol nebulizers every 4 hr)
      - Ipratropium bromide
      - Oral corticosteroids (if used, total duration 5–7 days)
      - If severe, consider IV steroids, IV magnesium, and high-dose inhaled corticosteroids

TABLE 2.6 • Classifications of Asthma: Clinical Features and Recommended Treatments					
Classification	**Symptoms/ SABA Use**	**Nighttime Awakening**	**Interference with Activity**	**Exacerbations Requiring Steroids**	**Initial Treatment (see *Figure 2.12*)**
Intermittent	<2 days/ week	<2×/month	None	0–1/year	Step 1
Mild persistent	>2 days/ week, but not daily	3–4×/month	Minor	≥2/year	Step 2
Moderate persistent	Daily	>1×/week, but not nightly	Some	≥2/year	Step 3 + PO steroid course
Severe persistent	Throughout the day	Often nightly	Extreme	≥2/year	Step 4/5 + PO steroid course

| ❶ Assessment | • Confirm diagnosis of asthma (e.g., PFTs, rule out other diagnoses)
• Address modifiable risk factors (e.g., smoking cessation)
• Address co-morbidities (e.g., obesity)
• Review inhaler techniques/adherence
• Assess patient goals and preferences | | |

❷ Management	Frequency of symptoms	Preferred controller	Preferred reliever
	<2 times per month	As needed low dose ICS-formoterol	• As needed low-dose ICS-formoterol OR • PRN short-acting beta2-agonist
	2+ times per month but less than daily	Daily low dose ICS OR as-needed low dose ICS-formoterol	
	Symptoms most days - mild	Low-dose ICS-LABA	
	Symptoms most days - moderate	Medium dose ICS-LABA	

	Symptoms most days - severe	• High dose ICS-LABA
		• Consider additional therapies:
		  • Tiotropium
		  • Anti-IgE
		  • Anti-IL5/5R
		  • Anti-IL4R
		• Severely uncontrolled: may need short course oral corticosteroids	

FIGURE 2.12: **Selecting Initial Controller Treatment in Adults with Asthma.** Abbreviations: PFT = pulmonary function test, ICS = inhaled corticosteroid, PRN = pro re nata, a.k.a. as needed; LABA = long-acting beta agonist

Asthma–COPD overlap syndrome
- Background:
  - Asthma/COPD are increasingly recognized as heterogeneous and at times overlapping conditions (Postma et al., *New Engl J Med* 2015)
    - Prototypical versions of each diagnosis differ on several features (e.g., typical age of onset, presence of atopy, smoking history/pack years, reversibility)
  - Historical approaches to research have reinforced the asthma and COPD prototypes
    - COPD studies excluded nonsmokers or patients with bronchodilator reversibility
    - Asthma studies excluded smokers and patients without bronchodilator reversibility
- Treatment: Sporadic trials with various definitions; may be increasingly described in the future, and thus may at some point become an important clinical entity

Bronchiectasis
- Etiology: Irreversible pathologic dilation of the bronchi or bronchioles due to an infectious process occurring in the context of airway obstruction (e.g., tumor, TB, COPD), impaired drainage (e.g., cystic fibrosis, ciliary dysfunction), or abnormality in host antimicrobial defense (e.g., CVID); however, approximately 50% cases ultimately deemed idiopathic
- Clinical presentation: Productive cough (excessive sputum), recurrent pneumonia
- Diagnosis: PFTs with mild moderate obstruction. High resolution chest CT can be used to definitively diagnose
- Treatment: Airway clearance, antibiotic therapy for exacerbations, pulmonary rehabilitation

Cystic fibrosis (CF)
- Etiology: Autosomal recessive mutation in CF transmembrane conductance regulator (*CFTR*) gene
- Diagnosis: Typically diagnosed in children; occasionally diagnose atypical/delayed presentation in adults. Diagnose by genetic testing (*CFTR* mutation present) or biochemical testing (sweat test)
- Comorbidities: Diabetes, infertility, osteoporosis, liver disease
- Treatment: Airway clearance, antibiotic therapy, nutritional support including pancreatic enzyme replacement, diabetes management, psychosocial support
- Complications: Bronchiectasis, ABPA, NTM, *Burkholderia cepacia infection*, sinusitis, male infertility, pancreatitis, intestinal intussusception

PULMONOLOGY

Restrictive Lung Diseases

- Restrictive = ↓Compliance, ↑Elastance→ Problem getting air in.
  - ↓DLCO in ILD. Normal DLCO in neuromuscular disorders. ↑DLCO in obesity
  - ↓TLC, ↓RV. Increase in radial traction, so tethered more strongly and airways remain open
  - FEV₁↓, FVC↓↓ → FEV₁/FVC ratio normal or increased

Extrapulmonary Restrictive Disease (Normal DLCO)

- Neuromuscular diseases: Guillain-Barré, myasthenia gravis, poliomyelitis, post-polio, ALS. These disorders may cause weakening of the respiratory muscles.
- Diaphragmatic disease
- Conditions affecting the chest wall: Kyphoscoliosis; obesity hypoventilation syndrome; "Pickwickian syndrome," BMI >50, hypoventilation due to ↓central drive to breathe. Tx: Weight loss and noninvasive positive pressure ventilation. Consider "last resort" treatment with respiratory stimulants, such as progestin or acetazolamide.

Overview of Interstitial Lung Disease (ILD) (↓DLCO)

- Definitions: Large group of diagnoses, most of which cause progressive scarring/fibrosis of the lung, with resultant restrictive physiology
- Clinical presentation: Chronic progressive dyspnea with associated dry cough. "Velcro-like crackles," wheezing, clubbing. May also present with symptoms or signs of an underlying pathology (e.g., clinical features of connective tissue disease). PFTs reveal restrictive physiology with low DLCO.
- Etiologies/classification: See Figure 2.13
- Imaging/pathology pattern correlates:
  - **Usual interstitial pneumonia (UIP)** on high-resolution chest CT (honeycombing with or without traction bronchiectasis, reticular abnormalities, distributed in a subpleural, basilar predominant pattern) = UIP on path → often idiopathic pulmonary fibrosis (IPF) if other exposures are excluded
  - **Nonspecific interstitial pneumonia (NSIP)** on high-resolution chest CT (symmetric bilateral ground glass opacities, fine reticulations, traction bronchiectasis, immediate subpleural sparing) = NSIP on path → Ddx: autoimmune, drug, XRT
- Clinical history:
  - Hypersensitivity pneumonitis (HP) exposures (e.g., birds, down comforter/pillows, molds, sauna/indoor hot tub), occupational exposures (e.g., hard metals, coal, silica), smoking history
  - Medications (nitrofurantoin, amiodarone), radiation
  - Extra-pulmonary symptoms of connective tissue diseases (e.g., Raynaud's, rash, arthritis)
  - Family history of ILD, early graying of hair

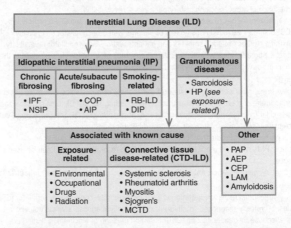

FIGURE 2.13: **Classification of interstitial lung diseases.** Abbreviations defined in the chapter text.

- Diagnosis:
  - PFTs: Restrictive pattern, low DLCO
  - High-resolution chest CT (HRCT)
  - Autoimmune serologies: Start with ANA, Jo1, SSA/SSB, RF, CCP $+/-$ ANCA
    - If positive, consider: MCTD (U1RNP) SLE (SM, dsDNA), scleroderma (Topo-1, RNA polymerase III)
    - If negative, consider myositis panel if concern for myositis
- Treatment:
  - Supplemental O_2, pulmonary rehab, transplant referral if indicated
  - IPF: Nintedanib vs. pirfenidone
  - Most others: Immunosuppression

Additional Details About Specific ILD Diagnoses
- Idiopathic interstitial pneumonias (IIPs):
  - Definition: A broad classification within ILDs of unknown cause. These are noninfectious interstitial lung diseases. Most common among them is idiopathic pulmonary fibrosis (IPF).
    - Idiopathic pulmonary fibrosis (IPF)
      - Etiology: Unknown. May be due to mucin gene mutation or related to telomere length. Older adults (typical age >60 yr), former smoker, absence of an underlying cause.
      - Diagnostics: HRCT: UIP pattern (usual interstitial pneumonitis). Fibrosis worst at the bases (basilar predominant) and peripherally distributed. Honeycombing with traction bronchiectasis. Lack of air trapping (which would suggest HP). Pathology: UIP pattern (can forego obtaining pathology in certain classic populations, typically elderly white men).
        - Ddx: Rule out 1) hypersensitivity pneumonitis (ask about exposures) and 2) connective tissue disease (ask about rheumatology ROS)
      - Treatment: Two options: nintedanib or pirfenidone (both slow progression and may reduce risk of ILD flare but do not improve function or halt progression). Immunosuppression is harmful (PANTHER trial, *New Engl J Med* 2012). Avoid intubation if possible.
        - Nintedanib (BID, side effect: nausea, GI side effects. Contraindication: CAD or anticoagulation)
        - Pirfenidone (TID, side effect: photosensitivity)
    - Nonspecific interstitial pneumonia (NSIP): Can be idiopathic, overlap with other IIP, or be associated with HIV, connective tissue diseases, drugs, and hypersensitivity pneumonitis. Idiopathic NSIP predominantly affects never-smoker, middle-aged women. Imaging: HRCT findings are basilar predominant and include reticular markings, subpleural sparing, and ground glass opacities. Classic finding: Basilar GGO with subpleural sparing. Tx: Mild disease may be self-limited; otherwise, initial treatment is steroids or other immunosuppressive adjuncts.
    - Cryptogenic organizing pneumonia (COP, formerly BOOP): Rare form of ILD in which the bronchioles and alveoli become inflamed. Most common in patients 40–50 yr. Clinically mimics pnumonia. Chest imaging often with recurrent, "migratory," peripheral-predominant opacities. Tx: Steroids. High risk of recurrence.
    - Acute interstitial pneumonia (AIP, Hamman-Rich syndrome): Acute onset, rapidly progressive course (unlike other IIPs). Median age ~50 yr. Presents with fever, cough, progressive dyspnea over 7–14 days. Imaging findings mimic ARDS (bilateral opacification, often symmetric on CT chest). Tx: Supportive care, steroids. Prognosis: 50% mortality.
    - Desquamative interstitial pneumonia (DIP): Most common in patients with heavy smoking history (>90%). Median age 30–40 yr. Imaging: CXR may be normal (20%). HRCT reveals GGO/centrilobular nodules; no peripheral reticulation (i.e., which helps distinguish from UIP pattern). Tx: Smoking cessation, ?steroids.
    - Respiratory bronchiolitis-associated ILD (RB-ILD): On a clinical spectrum with DIP. Median age 30–40 yr, typically smokers, M:F = 2:1. Imaging: Similar to DIP. Tx: Smoking cessation, ?steroids.
    - Lymphoid interstitial pneumonia (LIP): Usually associated with rheumatic disease, immunodeficiency, or infection (such as EBV), less commonly idiopathic (<20%). Imaging: Similar to NSIP; HRCT findings are basilar predominant and include GGO, centrilobular nodules, and interstitial thickening. Cysts are common (>60%), and not seen in NSIP. Tx: Depends on underlying cause. Complications: May progress to lymphoma (5%).
    - Pleuroparenchymal fibroelastosis (PPFE): Rare. Idiopathic or associated with chemotherapy. Imaging: HRCT reveals upper lobe predominant pleural and subpleural lung parenchymal fibrosis.

PULMONOLOGY

- Exposure-related:
  - **Environmental/occupational:**
    - Hypersensitivity pneumonitis (HP, also called "extrinsic allergic alveolitis"): Results from exposure to a causative agent, such as bird feathers or mold. Presentation is variable, ranging from acute (i.e., 4–6 hours after exposure and self-limited with exposure removal) to chronic (insidious onset of cough with constitutional symptoms and fibrosis). For chronic HP, HRCT demonstrates small centrilobular nodules, ground-glass attenuation, and lobular areas of decreased attenuation and vascularity; rarely HRCT shows UIP but with air trapping, which is suggestive of HP. Tx: Detailed history and removal of all potential exposures. Partial lung function may return.
    - Pneumoconiosis: Requires an exposure, such as silica, asbestos, coal, talc, beryllium, or hard metal. Imaging findings differ based on causative agent.
  - **Drug/radiation-induced:** Nitrofurantoin, amiodarone, chemo, XRT, immunotherapy (e.g., PD-1 inhibitors or other immunotherapy)
  - **Smoking-related:** See DIP, RB-ILD under IIP
- Connective tissue disease (CTD-ILD): Systemic sclerosis, RA, myositis, Sjogren's, MCTD
- Granulomatous:
  - Sarcoidosis:
    - Epidemiology: Young to middle-age adults; more common in black individuals
    - Etiology: The exact etiology and pathogenesis of sarcoidosis remain unknown
    - Clinical features: Three classic features: 1) Bilateral hilar adenopathy; 2) Pulmonary reticular opacities; and 3) Skin, joint, and/or eye lesions. Other features include elevated ESR/CRP, hypercalciuria, and serum ACE level elevations, which are suggestive but of variable clinical utility in making the diagnosis
    - Diagnostics: No single definitive test; diagnosis relies on compatible clinical/radiographic features, exclusion of other differential diagnoses (e.g., mycobacterial infection, fungal infection, other ILD), and noncaseating granulomas on pathology
    - Treatment: Steroids as first-line
- Other:
  - Acute eosinophilic pneumonia (AEP): Rare, cause unknown. Age varies, most commonly 20–40 yr. M:F = 2:1. Nonproductive cough, dyspnea, and fever are present in nearly all patients. Usually symptoms for less than 1 week, occasionally as long as 1 month. Leukocytosis initially neutrophilic, but may become eosinophilic. ESR/CRP, IgE elevated. Imaging: CXR: Subtle reticular or GGO, later diffuse GGO. HRCT not necessary, but helpful to select an area for BAL (BAL cell count shows eos >25%). Tx: Steroids.
  - Chronic eosinophilic pneumonia (CEP): Rare, cause unknown. Age varies, most commonly 30–50 yr. M:F = 1:2. Association with asthma/atopy. Chronic onset of dyspnea, weight loss, fever, and productive cough. Imaging: Bilateral peripheral or pleural-based consolidations ("photographic negative" of pulmonary edema). BAL cell count shows eosinophils >25%. Tx: Steroids.
  - Pulmonary alveolar proteinosis (PAP): Diffuse lung disease characterized by the accumulation of amorphous, PAS-positive material (mostly surfactant and apoproteins) in the distal airspaces. Can be primary (due to impaired surfactant clearance, excess surfactant production) or secondary (due to high-level dust exposure, hematologic dyscrasia, post-hematopoietic stem cell transplant). Age 40–50 yr, M:F=2:1, affects smokers disproportionately. Patients present with dyspnea on exertion, cough, fatigue, weight loss, fever over weeks to months, and rarely expectoration of "chunky" gelatinous material. Imaging: CXR reveals alveolar opacities in "bat wing" pattern, HRCT reveals GGO in homogenous distribution with or without "crazy paving" pattern on CT.
  - Lymphangioleiomyomatosis (LAM): Rare, multisystem disease due to mTOR pathway activation that mostly affects young women. May be primary or associated with tuberous sclerosis complex (TSC-LAM). Classic feature is diffuse cystic lung disease due to infiltration of smooth muscle cells into the pulmonary parenchyma. Common symptoms include progressive dyspnea, spontaneous pneumothorax, pleural effusion, and fatigue, associated with chylothorax, chyloperitoneum, and benign masses of the kidneys, retroperitoneum/pelvis, and uterus. Imaging: CXR nonspecific, HRCT reveals hallmark thin-walled cysts. Tx: Sirolimus, everolimus (mTOR kinase inhibitors).
  - Amyloidosis: May cause ILD, although more common pulmonary manifestations are tracheobronchial infiltration, persistent pleural effusions, parenchymal nodules (amyloidomas).

Diseases of the Pleura

- Pleural Effusion:
  - Thoracentesis should be performed for new effusion to calculate Light's criteria
  - Light's criteria: Must have at least one to be considered exudative:
    - Pleural **P**rotein/serum protein >0.5 (think **P** for **P**entagon [five-sided])
    - Pleural LDH/serum LDH >0.6 (think **H** for **H**exagon [six-sided])
    - LDH >2/3 upper limit of normal
- Transudative: Increased hydrostatic pressure (CHF), decreased oncotic pressure (cirrhosis, nephrotic, other hypoalbuminemia). pH 7.4–7.55
- Exudative: Increased permeability or decreased lymphatic drainage (infection, malignancy, connective tissue disease, CABG, PE). pH 7.3–7.45; <7.2 typical for empyema
  - Other useful features: High amylase (pancreatitis, malignancy), milky fluid (chylothorax, lymphatic), bloody fluid (malignancy; may need multiple thoracenteses to increase yield of cytology if malignancy expected), lymphocytic predominance and/or ADA elevation (TB)
- Treatment:
  - Transudative: Diuretics, sodium restriction
  - Exudative: Treat underlying process. If complicated, involve pulmonology to discuss therapies like indwelling pleural catheters, chest tubes, etc. See Empyema in Infectious Diseases Chapter 8.

Pneumothorax

- Spontaneous:
  - Primary: Typically occurs in tall lean men when a dilated alveolar bleb ruptures.
  - Secondary: Complication of lung disease, resulting in more severe symptoms
- Traumatic: Iatrogenic (e.g., central line, thoracentesis – always check post-procedure CXR). Mediastinum shifts TOWARD pneumothorax.
- Tension: Accumulation of air with one-way valve collapses ipsilateral lung and mediastinum shifts AWAY from the pneumothorax. Causes: Mechanical ventilation, CPR, trauma. Medical emergency! Perform immediate needle thoracostomy (large-bore needle; fifth intercostal space, mid-axillary), followed by chest tube placement.

Diseases involving the Vasculature

Pulmonary Embolism (PE)

- Etiology: Virchow's triad: 1) Endothelial injury, 2) Venous stasis, 3) Hypercoagulability.
- Risk factors: Older age, malignancy, prior VTE, hypercoagulable state (factor V Leiden mutation, protein C/S deficiency), prolonged bed rest, CHF, obesity, orthopedic surgery, trauma, pregnancy, oral contraceptive pills (OCPs)
- Diagnosis:
  - EKG: Classic findings: S1Q3T3, RV strain, new incomplete RBBB. Most common finding: Sinus tachycardia
  - CXR: Classic findings (rare): Hampton's hump, Westermark's sign. Most common finding: Normal
  - Well's criteria (most commonly used, but subjective), Geneva Score (objective), **PESI score** (objective)
    - LOW pre-test probability → D-dimer. D-dimer has high sensitivity (95%), but low specificity (50%) (Christopher study, *JAMA* 2006)
    - HIGH pretest probability (or +D-dimer) → CT-PE (Stein et al., *New Engl J Med* 2006)
- Approach:
  - Assess hemodynamic stability
    - If unstable, manage emergently
    - If stable, assess PE risk (i.e., low risk, intermediate-low risk, or intermediate-high risk)
- Comment on PE management:
  - Management approach for PE depends on risk stratification, features of individual patients, access to advanced therapies, and local practice
  - Treatment modalities include tPA, catheter-directed thrombolysis, and systemic anticoagulation alone
  - One possible approach stratified by risk classification is described on the next page

PULMONOLOGY

- Classifications and management:
  - **Massive PE** (high-risk PE)
    - Key features: SBP <90 mmHg, SBP drop >40 mmHg, or shock for >15 minutes despite IVF
    - Treatment: Fibrinolytic (catheter-directed or reduced-dose systemic thrombolysis)
      - Absolute contraindications to tPA: History of hemorrhagic stroke or stroke of unknown origin; ischemic stroke in previous 6 months; central nervous system neoplasm; major trauma, surgery, or head injury in previous 3 weeks; bleeding diathesis; active bleeding
  - **Nonmassive PE**
    - **Intermediate-high risk PE**
      - Key features: Acute PE without hypotension but with evidence of abnormal RV function by echocardiography (or a clearly dilated right ventricle by CT pulmonary angiography), plus an elevated troponin and/or brain natriuretic peptide (BNP) level; BOVA score >4 may also be suggestive
      - Treatment: Anticoagulation, plus multidisciplinary discussion about role for fibrinolytics (systemic vs. catheter-directed)
    - **Intermediate-low-risk PE**
      - Key features: Acute PE without hypotension or evidence of abnormal RV function, but sPESI screen is positive (i.e., at least one of the following: Age >80 yr, cancer, cardiopulmonary disease, HR >110 bpm, SBP <100 mmHg, SpO$_2$ <90%)
      - Treatment: Anticoagulation
    - **Low-risk PE**
      - Key features: Acute PE with negative sPESI screen (i.e., all of the following: Age <80 yr, no cancer, no cardiopulmonary disease, HR <110 bpm, SBP >100 mmHg, SpO$_2$ >90%)
      - Treatment: Consider outpatient management with direct oral anticoagulants (DOAC); admission may be appropriate based on safety of discharge plan, likelihood of follow-up, etc.

Pulmonary Hypertension (PH)

- Note: See Cardiology Chapter 1 for additional details
- Classifications of PH: Mneumonic = **AVRT O**ther
  - **Group 1: A**rterial- Primary PAH. SLE, scleroderma, toxins (methamphetamine, cocaine), HIV
    - Dx: Utox, ANA, RF, TTE, HIV, hepatitis serologies, LFTs
    - Tx: PDE5 inhibitor (first line, e.g., sildenafil), endothelin receptor antagonists (second line), prostacyclins (third line, e.g., Flolan), and treat underlying cause. Consider lung transplant referral.
  - **Group 2: V**enous- Back up from left heart due to cardiac disease (valve disease, cardiomyopathy)
    - Dx: Right heart cath, TTE
    - Tx: Diuresis
  - **Group 3: R**espiratory, due to pulmonary disease- OSA, COPD
    - Dx: High-resolution chest CT, sleep study, PFTs
    - Tx: Supplemental oxygen, treat underlying disease
  - **Group 4: T**hromboembolic disease (i.e., chronic PEs)
    - Dx: VQ scan (preferred over CT-PE to diagnose chronic PEs)
    - Tx: Anticoagulation
  - **Group 5: O**ther: Sarcoid, sickle cell, hemolytic anemia, metabolic disease

KEY MEDICATIONS AND INTERVENTIONS

Respiratory Support

See Critical Care Chapter 3.

Thoracentesis

- Indications: 1) Diagnostic for pleural effusion of unknown cause; 2) Therapeutic for respiratory symptoms due to large effusions
- Tests to consider:
  - Pleural fluid protein and LDH (for Light's criteria)
  - Cell count and differential (PMN predominance suggests an acute process such as a parapneumonic effusion or PE; mononuclear predominance suggests cancer or TB)
  - Gram stain and culture
  - Hct (1–20% suggests cancer, PE, trauma; >50% suggests hemothorax)
  - Glucose (<60 mg/dL suggests parapneumonic effusion or empyema, cancer, or possibly TB, RA, SLE, or esophageal rupture)
  - Cytology
  - pH (can be helpful to diagnose parapneumonic effusion or empyema since pH <7.2 in most cases)
  - Triglycerides (>100 mg/dL suggests chylothorax)
  - Amylase (level may be elevated if pleural effusion due to pancreatic disease, esophageal rupture)
- Relative contraindications: 1) Coagulopathy/thrombocytopenia (especially DIC), 2) Overlying cellulitis, 3) Inability to tolerate a potential complication (e.g., if patient only has one functional lung at the time)
- Complications:
  - **Pneumothorax**: Rare. Even when present, rarely requires the placement of a chest tube. Obtain post-procedure CXR if air was aspirated during the procedure, if the patient develops chest pain, dyspnea, or hypoxia, if there were multiple needle passes during the procedure, or if the patient is critically ill and/or receiving mechanical ventilation.
  - **Other:** Minor: Pain, coughing, localized infection. Severe: Hemothorax, intraabdominal organ injury, air embolism, and postexpansion pulmonary edema (although this is rare, increasingly controversial, and can probably be avoided by limiting therapeutic aspirations to <1500 mL).

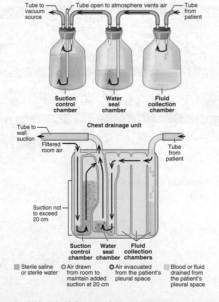

FIGURE 2.14: The chest tube: A "three-bottle" system. A chest tube uses a three bottle system for fluid collection, forming a water seal, and controlling suction.

PULMONOLOGY

Chest Tubes

- Description: Flexible plastic tube placed into the pleural space (or mediastinum) through the chest wall for drainage of air, fluid, or pus
- Indications:
  - Air (tension pneumothorax)
  - Fluid (hemothorax, persistent effusion; do NOT put in for hepatohydrothorax)
  - Pus (empyema)
- Components: Three-bottle system (Figure 2.14)
  - Collection trap – Tubes on right side
  - Water seal (gradient to flow out) – Look for air leak in form of bubbles
  - Suction to wall (with suction regulator) – Normal to see bubbles
- Parameters to report on rounds:
  - Suction: Is the tube on water seal or suction? If on suction, at what pressure (measured in cm H_2O)?
  - Volume: How much has the chest tube drained? What is the rate of drainage and is it increasing/decreasing?
  - Quality: What color is the fluid that has drained?
  - Air leak: Is there an air leak?

Inhaler Glossary

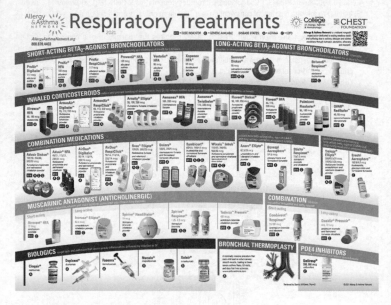

FIGURE 2.15: Respiratory treatments by inhaler class.

Source: Allergy & Asthma Network.

KEY CLINICAL TRIALS AND PUBLICATIONS

Asthma

- **Comparison of a beta 2-agonist, terbutaline, with an inhaled corticosteroid, budesonide, in newly detected asthma.** *New Engl J Med* 1991; 325:388–92.
  - Randomized, blinded trial comparing terbutaline and budesonide, which provided early evidence useful for establishing inhaled corticosteroids as a first-line treatment in asthma management.
- **The Salmeterol Multicenter Asthma Research Trial (SMART).** *Chest* 2006;129(1):15–26.
  - Randomized, double-blinded, placebo-controlled trial of salmeterol BID for asthma in patients >12 yr old. Demonstrated a small but statistically significant increase in respiratory- and asthma-related deaths for the population receiving salmeterol, particularly for African Americans who were enrolled in the trial.
- **As-needed budesonide-formoterol versus maintenance budesonide in mild asthma.** *N Engl J Med* 2018;378(20):1877–1887.
  - Randomized, double-blinded, placebo-controlled trial that demonstrated budesonide–formoterol PRN was noninferior to budesonide BID with respect to the rate of severe asthma exacerbations and resulted in approximately one-quarter of the inhaled glucocorticoid exposure. However, symptom control was inferior in the budesonide–formoterol PRN group.

COPD

- **Antibiotic therapy in exacerbations of COPD.** *Ann Intern Med* 1987;106:196–204.
  - Randomized, double-blinded, placebo-controlled study assessing antibiotic use when all three cardinal symptoms of an acute exacerbation of COPD were present (i.e., increased dyspnea, increased sputum production, increased sputum purulence). Results demonstrated less failure with use of antibiotics; however, this improvement was not significant after controlling for use of oral steroids.
- **Antibiotics in addition to systemic corticosteroids for acute exacerbations of chronic obstructive pulmonary disease.** *Am J Respir Crit Care Med* 2010;181:150–157.
  - Randomized, placebo-controlled study to evaluate the effect of adding doxycycline to prednisone for patients presenting with dyspnea and increased sputum volume; patients with fever or chest radiograph consistent with pneumonia were excluded. The results demonstrated no significant improvement in 30-day clinical response with antibiotics, although clinical cure/clinical success at day 10 were improved in the antibiotic arm.

Interstitial Lung Disease

- **A phase 3 trial of pirfenidone in patients with idiopathic pulmonary fibrosis.** *N Engl J Med* 2014;370:2083–2092.
  - Randomized, placebo-controlled trial which demonstrated that pirfenidone slowed the rate of decline in FVC (23% vs. 9.7% placebo for no decline; 17% vs. 32% placebo for >10% decline).
- **Efficacy and safety of nintedanib in idiopathic pulmonary fibrosis.** *N Engl J Med* 2014;370:2071–2082.
  - Randomized, placebo-controlled trial which demonstrated that nintedanib slowed the rate of decline in FVC (−115 mL vs. −240 mL for placebo over 1 yr).

Cystic Fibrosis

- **A CFTR potentiator in patients with cystic fibrosis and the G551D mutation.** *N Engl J Med* 2011;365:1663–1672.
  - Seminal study that demonstrated a considerable benefit from a therapy that targeted cystic fibrosis's underlying genetic cause. In this study, patients with at least one G551D-CFTR mutation who received the CFTR potentiator ivacaftor showed an absolute increase in predicted FEV_1 of 10% compared to a small FEV_1 decline for the placebo group.

Pulmonary Embolism

- **Age-adjusted D-dimer cutoff levels to rule out pulmonary embolism: The ADJUST-PE study.** *JAMA* 2014;311:1117–11124.
  - Prospective study that evaluated the reliability of a modified D-dimer level cut-off for patients age >50 yr who had low clinical probability of PE (age-adjusted D-dimer level = patient age × 10). Among the patients for whom D-dimer was greater than the standard cutoff but below the age-adjusted cut off (n = 337), 0.3% had a DVT or PE in the following 3 months.

PULMONOLOGY

NOTES

Critical Care Medicine

3

INTRODUCTION

Goals of Intensive Care Unit (ICU) Care

- Stabilize, diagnose, and treat patients with acute life-, limb-, or organ-threatening conditions
- Monitor patients who are at high risk of developing acute life-, limb, or organ-threatening conditions
- Prevent complications associated with care for the critically ill patient
- Provide compassionate care for patients at the end of life

Common ICU Indications

- Need for mechanical ventilation or noninvasive ventilation
- Need for vasoactive medications such as vasopressors, inotropes, or vasodilators
- Monitoring or nursing needs beyond the capabilities of the floor or other units
- Persistent abnormal vital signs: Often sufficient to warrant intensive care

ANATOMY, PHYSIOLOGY, AND DIAGNOSTICS

Please see Chapters 1 and 2 for cardiac and pulmonary anatomy/physiology, respectively. In this chapter, we combine anatomy, physiology, and diagnostics into a single section, which reflects the use of diagnostics in critical care medicine to characterize altered physiology in critically ill patients.

Assessment of Fluid Responsiveness

- Hypotension is a common problem in the ICU
- Various methods exist to determine whether a patient with hypotension is likely to be "fluid responsive," which is defined as an increase in cardiac stroke volume with a fluid bolus
- Each of the following methods can help inform this decision, but no single measure is perfect: 1) Assessment of pulse pressure variation (PPV); 2) Central venous pressure (CVP); 3) Dynamic measurement of the inferior vena cava (IVC using POCUS); and 4) Passive leg raise
- Please note that these measures were validated in specific settings and may not be valid in alternative clinical scenarios

Arterial Line and Pulse Pressure Variation (PPV)

- Indications for arterial line placement:
  - Invasive hemodynamic monitoring
  - Frequent laboratory draws, often arterial blood gases (ABGs)
- Interpretation of the arterial line tracing:
  - Waveform shows systolic peak pressure, dicrotic notch, and end-diastolic pressure (Figure 3.1)
  - Mean arterial pressure (MAP) is calculated and shown on the monitor
  - Position of the transducer will affect the blood pressure readings
    - Device should be zeroed at the level of the heart
    - When the transducer is ABOVE the patient, then the measured pressure will be LOWER than actual
    - When the transducer is BELOW the patient, then the measured pressure will be HIGHER than actual
- Measuring PPV using the arterial line: See Figure 3.2
  - PPV is a predictor of fluid responsiveness in mechanically ventilated patients
    - PPV >13% suggests that the patient is fluid responsive
    - PPV 9–13% is indeterminate
    - PPV <9% suggests that the patient is not fluid responsive
  - Pulse Pressure (PP) = (Systolic Pressure − Diastolic Pressure)
    - PP maximum occurs during inspiration; PP minimum occurs during expiration
    - PPV is calculated with the following formula:

$$\text{Pulse Pressure Variation (PPV)} = \frac{(PP_{max} - PP_{min})}{PP_{mean}}$$

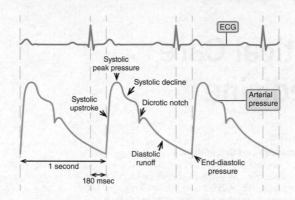

FIGURE 3.1: Arterial Line waveform. The arterial pulse waveform includes a systolic phase, the dicrotic notch, and a diastolic phase. The systolic phase corresponds to left ventricular ejection, the dicrotic notch represents closure of the aortic valve, and the diastolic phase represents runoff into the peripheral circulation.

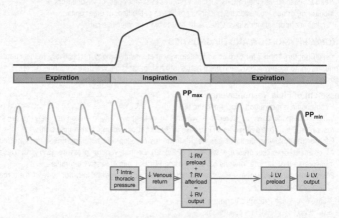

FIGURE 3.2: Physiologic mechanism of pulse pressure variation. Pulse pressure variation (PPV) allows bedside assessment of fluid responsiveness for patients in shock who are breathing passively on positive pressure ventilation. If preload is robust, the pulse pressure does not vary with respiration. In the example above, a breath is delivered with inspiration increasing intra-thoracic pressure and decreasing venous return. This results in decreased RV preload and output. Blood flows through the pulmonary circulation with a time delay (long arrow) and reaches the left heart with reduced LV preload and output. If preload is reduced (suggesting volume responsiveness), pulse pressure will increase with inspiration and decrease with exhalation. Top: Airway Pressure (purple) Bottom: Arterial Pressure Tracing (green). Abbreviations: LV = Left Ventricle, RV = Right Ventricle, PP = Pulse Pressure

Central Venous Pressure (CVP)
- Importance of CVP:
  - Assists in guiding hemodynamic interventions
    - In general, a normal CVP is 0–5 mmHg and it is often a good approximation of right atrial pressure; however, this can vary from patient to patient. Note also that goal CVP (e.g., when volume resuscitating a patient with shock) may differ according to the scenario (e.g., patient on positive pressure ventilation or not)
  - CVP is a dynamic and not a static measurement
- Relationship to IVC measurement:
  - When CVP < intraabdominal pressure, IVC will collapse
  - When CVP > intraabdominal pressure, IVC will remain distended
  - IVC compliance also dictates this relationship

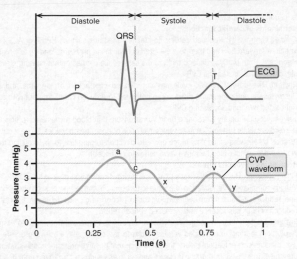

FIGURE 3.3: CVP waveform and correlation with electrical conduction in the heart. The CVP waveform has five distinct components: a wave (atrial contraction), c wave (right ventricular contraction), x descent (atrial relaxation with downward displacement of tricuspid valve with reduction in right atrial pressure), v wave (passive right atrial filling), and y descent (opening of tricuspid value with emptying of the right atrium into the right ventricle).

- Interpretation of CVP waveform: See Figure 3.3
  - a wave
    - Atrial contraction
    - Correlates with P wave on ECG
    - Disappears with atrial fibrillation
    - "Cannon a waves" are large a waves and a hallmark of AV dissociation in complete heart block or ventricular tachycardia
  - c wave
    - RV contraction against a closed tricuspid valve bulges into the right atrium
    - Correlates with the end of the QRS complex on ECG
  - x descent
    - Atrial relaxation and downward displacement of the closed tricuspid valve during RV contraction, which both reduce RA pressure
    - Occurs before the T wave on the ECG
  - v wave
    - Passive RA filling against a closed tricuspid valve during diastole increases RA pressure
    - Occurs after the T wave on the ECG
    - Tricuspid pathology such as tricuspid regurgitation leads to large v waves
  - y descent
    - The tricuspid valve opens and blood empties from the RA into the RV, leading to reduced RA pressure
    - Occurs before the P wave on the ECG
    - Loss of y descent suggests pathology such as tamponade with restricted RV filling

CRITICAL CARE MEDICINE

- CVP is influenced by cardiac function and venous return:
  - **Determinants of cardiac function:**
    - Cardiac contractility: Reduced cardiac contractility in states such as HFrEF or ACS can lead to impaired forward flow and therefore elevated cardiac filling pressures leading to a high CVP.
    - Heart rate: Both bradycardia and tachycardia can reduce cardiac output causing elevated right-sided pressures, increasing CVP.
    - Rhythm: The normal cardiac cycle has coordinated contraction of the atria and ventricles. Dysrhythmias and conduction disease can both lead to reduced cardiac output with consequent right-sided overload, increasing CVP.
    - Valve function: Properly functioning heart valves ensure that blood moves unidirectionally through the cardiovascular system. Diseased valves may open or close improperly, leading to reduced cardiac function by allowing blood flow in the opposite direction (regurgitant) or by requiring the heart to work harder to move blood across a valve narrowing (stenosis).
  - **Determinants of venous return:**
    - Filling pressure: Hypovolemia leads to reduced venous return and thus reduced CVP.
    - Venous compliance: Venodilation (e.g., due to furosemide) causes increased venous capacitance and reduced venous return, whereas venoconstriction (e.g., due to alpha agonists) causes reduced venous capacitance and increased venous return.
    - Respiration: Spontaneous negative pressure breathing reduces intrathoracic pressure during inspiration, leading to increased venous return to the right heart. Positive pressure breathing (i.e., mechanical ventilation) inverts the cycle such that positive pressure administration during a breath will increase intrathoracic pressure and reduces venous return to the right heart.

IVC Point-of-Care Ultrasound (POCUS)
- Description:
  - Common bedside assessment to aid in determining intravascular volume status
  - Like all ultrasound, it is user-dependent and requires proper measurement and interpretation
  - Along with CVP, PPV, passive leg raise, and other factors, can guide assessment of volume responsiveness
- How to measure the IVC using POCUS:
  - Location: Locate and measure the portion of the IVC just distal to the junction of the hepatic vein and the IVC, about 2 cm from the right atrium. See Figure 1.12 in Cardiology Chapter 1.
  - Measure the IVC diameter once at end expiration (largest diameter) and again at end inspiration (smallest diameter) to compare the two measurements
- IVC measurement interpretation:
  - IVC <2.1 cm and >50% collapsible estimates a CVP <3 mmHg
  - IVC <2.1 cm and <50% collapsible estimates a CVP ~8 mmHg (range 5–10)
  - IVC >2.1 cm and >50% collapsible estimates a CVP ~8 mmHg (range 5–10)
  - IVC >2.1 cm and <50% collapsible estimates a CVP >15 mmHg
- When IVC measurement may be inaccurate:
  - Increased intraabdominal pressure (e.g., ascites, pregnancy)
  - Positive pressure ventilation (e.g., ventilator or CPAP/bilevel)

Passive Leg Raise (PLR)
- Description:
  - Bedside maneuver and diagnostic test to predict fluid responsiveness
  - Used in conjunction with other hemodynamic and volume assessments such as IVC POCUS and PPV
  - Transiently increases venous return
  - Estimates roughly a 250cc bolus
- Technique:
  - Sit the patient up in 45-degree position
  - Then lay the patient flat and passively raise both legs at 45-degree angle
  - Maximal effect at 30–90 seconds
- Interpretation:
  - In the literature, a positive test is a 10% increase in cardiac output or stroke volume
  - At the bedside, because cardiac output and stroke volume are not directly measured, a positive test is often defined as a >10% increase in pulse pressure on an arterial line

APPROACHES AND CHIEF COMPLAINTS

Approach to Vascular Access

TABLE 3.1 · Flow Relationship Defined by the Poiseuille Equation	
$Flow\ (Q) = \dfrac{\pi Pr^4}{8\eta l}$	Q – flow rate P – pressure r – radius of tubing
$Flow \propto \dfrac{r^4}{l}$	η – fluid viscosity l – length of tubing

- Determinants of flow rate:
  - Catheter radius (larger radius $\rightarrow$ larger area $\rightarrow$ higher flows)
    - Small changes in radius have relatively large impacts on flow rates
    - Measured as French (Fr) vs. gauge
      - Two scales that reflect the diameter and therefore size of the lumen
        - Fr: Larger Fr catheters (i.e., higher number) have LARGER diameters
        - Gauge: Larger gauge catheters (i.e., higher numbers) have SMALLER diameters
  - Length of catheter (shorter catheter $\rightarrow$ higher flows)
  - Number of lumens (fewer lumens $\rightarrow$ higher flows)
  - Pressure difference (larger changes in pressure $\rightarrow$ higher flows rates)
    - Augment by using pressure bags, manually squeezing the bag, or increasing vertical distance between the fluid bag and the patient
  - Viscosity: More viscous products (i.e., blood) will flow more slowly
- Venous site selection:
  - Internal jugular (most common)
    - Pros: High placement success rate, low risk of pneumothorax with ultrasound guidance
    - Cons: Possible higher rate of bloodstream infections compared to subclavian
  - Subclavian
    - Pros: Likely lowest rates of bloodstream infections of the three sites
    - Cons: Highest rate of pneumothorax, decreased placement success rate with less experienced providers
  - Femoral
    - Pros: High placement success rate, no pneumothorax risk. Often used in trauma or codes given site is away from intubation or CPR
    - Cons: Possible higher rate of bloodstream infections given location, limits patient mobility
- Vascular access options for common patient scenarios:
  - Most patients in the ICU and medical wards:
    - Angiocath for peripheral venous access: Various sizes, including 14G, 16G, 18G, 20G, 22G
  - ICU patient with septic shock requiring vasopressors, multiple IV antibiotics, and other medications:
    - Triple-lumen central venous catheter: Contains three lumens which are 1 × 16G and 2 × 18G; catheter length from 15–30 cm selected based on patient size and insertion location
  - Gastrointestinal bleed requiring aggressive and rapid transfusion of multiple blood products:
    - MULTIPLE large-bore (often 16G or 18G) peripheral IVs
    - Alternative is an introducer or cordis, which are short catheters with large diameters, most commonly 8 Fr
  - Code blue $\rightarrow$ PEA arrest in a patient without IV access:
    - Intraosseous (IO) access into a long bone (often tibia) with a 15G tibial needle enabling rapid infusions; short-term use until other access can be obtained
  - Patient with endocarditis or osteomyelitis requiring long-term administration of antibiotics:
    - Peripherally inserted central catheter (PICC): Long catheters ranging from 30–60 cm in length; single-, double-, or triple-lumen options, with lumens being 4–5 Fr or 18G

CRITICAL CARE MEDICINE

Approach to Lactic Acidosis

- Description: Elevated serum lactate. Higher serum lactate levels are associated with higher mortality in both shock and nonshock patients
- Etiologies:
  - **Type A lactic acidosis** (most common): Systemic tissue hypoperfusion or hypoxemia (e.g., due to sepsis, ischemia)
  - **Type B lactic acidosis** (less common): Toxin-induced impairment of cellular metabolism and regional areas of ischemia. Ddx:
    - Seizures
    - Decreased gluconeogenesis:
      - Liver disease (decreased lactate clearance)
      - Metformin
    - Increased glycolysis:
      - Albuterol
      - Cocaine
      - Pheochromocytoma
      - Epinephrine
      - Warburg effect: Cancer cells tend to produce energy via glycoiysis and then lactic acid fermentation via anaerobic respiration given their high metabolic demands. Can present clinically as hypoglycemia and lactic acidosis in a patient with malignancy.
    - Impaired Krebs's cycle:
      - Thiamine deficiency
      - Mitochondrial toxicity
        - Alcohol
        - Medications (metformin, propofol, linezolid, NRTIs)
        - Toxins
        - Genetic mitochondrial disorders
- Treatment:
  - Type A lactic acidosis: Treat underlying cause
  - Type B lactic acidosis: Treat underlying cause if possible, remove offending medication, sometimes no treatment is indicated

Approach to Shock

- Important formulas:
  - MAP = CO x SVR
  - MAP = (HR x SV) x SVR

    MAP: Mean Arterial Pressure
    CO: Cardiac Output
    SVR: Systemic Vascular Resistance
    HR: Heart Rate
    SV: Stroke Volume
- Initial evaluation of shock (regardless of etiology):
  - EXAMINE THE PATIENT (most important)
    - Are extremities **warm** (vasodilated) or **cool** (vasoconstricted)?
    - Assess volume status (JVP, POCUS, passive leg raise)
    - Is the blood pressure real? As a rule of thumb, if radial pulse is present, then SBP >90 mmHg
  - Check labs
    - CBC, CMP (BMP + LFTs), troponin, lactate, CVO_2
  - Consider imaging and cardiac assessment
    - ECG, TTE, CXR; consider CT scans depending on the clinical concerns and hemodynamic trajectory
  - Consider infection
    - Blood cultures × 2, urinalysis with microscopy sputum culture or tracheal aspirate, sampling of other fluid (e.g., pleural, ascites fluid if indicated)

Approach to Analysis of an Arterial Blood Gas (ABG)

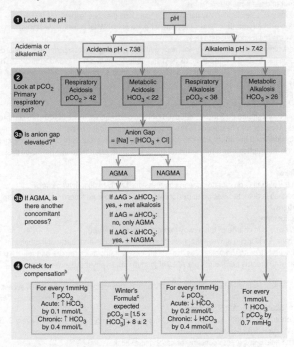

FIGURE 3.4: Approach to interpreting arterial blood gas. Evaluation of an arterial blood gas requires a different approach based on the primary derangement, with up to four steps: 1) Evaluate pH; 2) Evaluate pCO_2; 3) Evaluate anion gap and for a concomitant process (if appropriate); and 4) Check for compensation.

[a]Normal anion gap is patient-specific, approximated by the formula expected AG = 3x albumin (because a normal albumin is 4, normal AG is often said to be 12).

[b]When determining compensation there are several points to consider. First, the body never overcompensates, so the pH will never normalize in the absence of another primary disturbance. Second, respiratory compensation occurs more quickly based on changes in minute ventilation (RR × Vt), but metabolic compensation relies on the kidneys and therefore takes longer, resulting in the distinction between acute vs. chronic conditions.

[c]Metabolic acidosis compensation: Compare measured pCO_2 to expected pCO_2 based on Winter's formula. If measured pCO_2 is greater than expected, there is an additional respiratory acidosis. If measured pCO_2 is less than expected, there is an additional respiratory alkalosis.

Approach to Managing a Patient with Cardiac Arrest, aka "Code Blue"

- Three key principles:
  - Confirm code status
  - Provide high-quality chest compressions with minimal interruptions
  - Determine whether patient has a "shockable" rhythm (VT/VF) and shock EARLY if possible
- Approach to code leading:
  - The approach to code leading varies from provider to provider; however, one approach is to consider the code as having three phases: An initial phase focusing on setting up conditions for success (i.e., backboard, access, etc.) and establishing a rhythm for the code team, a second phase focused on establishing the etiology of the arrest, and a post-arrest phase.

CRITICAL CARE MEDICINE

Phase 1: Initial management and establishing a cardiac rhythm

Establish your and team members' roles
- Introduce your role clearly: "My name is _____ and I am the code leader."
- Gather crucial information: "Does the patient have a pulse? What is their code status?"
- Identify the team and delegate tasks:
  • Chest compressions, airway management, getting adequate IV access, performing critical diagnostics
  • Designate: 1) "Code whisperer" to help the code leader/assist in crowd control; 2) Timekeeper/ medication recorder; 3) Person to oversee medication administration (often a clinical pharmacist if available)

Chest compressions
- Place backboard and initiate chest compressions right away
- Compressions should be 2 inches deep (~5 cm) and performed at a rate of 100–120 compressions per minute. Allow for full chest recoil to promote venous return to the heart
- Identify additional providers who can switch in for subsequent rounds of chest compressions
- Minimize interruptions, as it takes several compressions to reach adequate perfusion pressure to vital organs

ECG leads/pads
- When the patient is on monitor, pause compressions briefly to do a rhythm check
- If Vfib/Vtach is detected, set up to perform an early shock per Advanced Cardiac Life Support (ACLS) algorithms

Airway management
- Identify who is in charge of the airway (often an anesthesiologist)
- Determine if advanced airway management is needed, such as endotracheal intubation
- Avoid overventilating the patient, as this will increase intrathoracic pressure and reduce preload
  • Goal of 10 breaths per minute per ACLS algorithm with an advanced airway in place

Access
- Obtain IV access. If unable to obtain robust IV access, then obtain intraosseous (IO) access.

Medications
- Give medications per ACLS algorithm
  • For either PEA or Vfib/Vtach arrest, give 1 mg epinephrine right away and then every 3–5 minutes
  • For Vfib/Vtach, also give amiodarone
- Consider fluid bolus unless concern for cardiogenic shock
- Consider 1 gram calcium chloride, 2–3 amps bicarb, 1 gram magnesium sulfate, 1 amp D50

Managing the room
- Summarize out loud frequently: Review patient one-liner, ACLS algorithm being used (e.g., "This is a 50yo man with CAD; we are in pulseless VT")

Phase 2: Diagnostics and determining etiology of arrest

Use the knowledge in the room
- Talk through "Hs/Ts" for PEA arrest (Table 3.2), invite thoughts from others in the room

End tidal CO_2 ($ETCO_2$)
- If $EtCO_2$ >10–20 mmHg, then chest compressions are adequate
- If $EtCO_2$ <10 mmHg, assess if chest compressions can be improved and/or consider reasons for poor ventilation and V/Q mismatch, such as PE
- If ROSC (Return of Spontaneous Circulation) is achieved, a sudden rise to >35–45 mmHg will typically occur, reflecting improved pulmonary perfusion and gas exchange

POCUS
- Can be used to help identify certain etiologies such as tamponade or pneumothorax
- Presence of right heart strain can suggest PE

Labs
- ABG with electrolytes/lactate, CBC, CMP, coags, type and cross, point-of-care glucose, troponin

Review existing data
- Ask a colleague to review the patient's chart to learn more about comorbidities, check recent labs, check ECG for QTc, review telemetry prior to the event, call primary team and update the patient's family

TABLE 3.2 • Etiologies and Management for PEA and Vfib/Vtach Arrests		
Pulseless Electrical Activity (PEA) Arrest		**Vfib/Vtach Arrest**
Differential diagnosis:		**Differential diagnosis:**
5 Hs	**5 Ts**	• Myocardial infarction (ACS)
1. Hypovolemia	1. Tension pneumothorax	• Arrhythmia
2. Hypoxia	2. Tamponade	• Scar/ischemia based
3. Hydrogen ions (acidosis)	3. Toxins	• Torsade de pointes
4. Hypo/hyperkalemia	4. Thrombosis (PE)	• Bradycardic arrest
5. Hypothermia	5. Thrombosis (ACS)	• Cardiomyopathy
Management:		**Management:**

• Start chest compressions right away
• When the monitors are on, pause compressions briefly and do a rhythm check
  • If not Vfib or Vtach, then it is a PEA arrest
• Follow ACLS algorithm for PEA arrest
		• Start chest compressions right away
		• When the monitors are on, pause compressions briefly and do a rhythm check
		  • If Vfib or Vtach on monitor, then follow this algorithm, including early defibrillation
		• Follow ACLS algorithm for Vfib/Vtach arrest

Phase 3: Post-arrest care and debriefing
Post arrest care
- Determine if ROSC obtained with return of pulse and/or sudden rise of $EtCO_2$ to >35–45 mmHg
- Assess mental status and responsiveness
  • If not responsive, intubate to protect airway (if not already done) and consider targeted temperature management (TTM)
    - If patient completely responsive, then do not need to cool
    - If any doubt, consult neurology for evaluation and consideration of TTM
- Assess hemodynamics: Give vasopressors and/or fluids to maintain MAP goal
  • MAP goal often >75 mmHg due to malfunctioning cerebral autoregulatory mechanisms
  • Etiology of low MAP can be multifactorial: Post-arrest vasodilation from cytokine storm, transient reduction in cardiac function, and possibly infectious etiology, depending on the clinical context
- Ensure adequate sedation and pain management, especially when intubated
- Pulmonary optimization:
  • Normocapnia with goal PCO_2 35–45 mmHg
  • Normoxia often SpO_2 92–96% or PaO_2 80–150 mmHg
- Obtain diagnostics:
  • Labs: POC glucose, CBC, CMP, coags, lactate, troponin, cultures, urine tox
  • Other studies: ECG, CXR, POCUS, consider CT scans (NCHCT, CTPE, CTAP)
- Determine disposition: ICU for most patients, cardiac catheterization lab if any concern for STEMI or other primary cardiac etiologies
- Notify family, next of kin, or other surrogate decision makers
- Notify attending(s)
- Write a code note
- Post-code debrief, ask for feedback
Targeted Temperature Management (TTM)
- Variable institutional practices about goal temperature, 33°C vs. 36°C given ongoing studies and debate about optimal goal
- Goal of avoiding hyperthermia is major driver to these protocols regardless of temperature goal
- Complications of cooling and rewarming: Hemodynamic changes, electrolyte shifts, coagulopathy
- TTM applied regardless of initial cardiac rhythm
- Protocol: Cool for 24 hours (from initiation), then at hour 24 gradually increase temperature to 37°C with passive rewarming, then maintain normothermia thereafter
  • Many institutions use internal cooling catheters, which are an effective means to reach targeted temperature
  • External cooling can also be achieved with ice packs, cooling blankets, NG lavage, IV saline methods
- Antipyretics are useful to prevent shivering and to prevent fevers/hyperthermia during rewarming
- Adequate sedation and sometimes paralysis are needed to prevent shivering

CRITICAL CARE MEDICINE

DISEASES AND PATHOPHYSIOLOGY

SIRS, Sepsis, Severe Sepsis, and Septic Shock

- Introduction:
  - Sepsis exists on a clinical spectrum of illness severity, with septic shock being the most severe
  - Two major clinical approaches to a patient with suspected sepsis:
    - qSOFA is an assessment score used to detect early sepsis. It is easily performed at the bedside and is best suited for triage and early assessments, as it is well validated in patients outside of the ICU.
    - Older definition using the Sepsis-2 guidelines remains the most widely used and preferred approach for grading the severity of sepsis in the ICU.
      - Note on Sepsis-3 guidelines (2016): SIRS and severe sepsis were dropped from these guidelines. Instead, Sepsis-3 defines sepsis as a rise in SOFA score of ≥ 2 points and septic shock as hypotension requiring vasopressors and an elevated lactate.
- Sepsis II definitions:
  - Systemic inflammatory response syndrome (SIRS): Must meet at least two of four criteria
    - Temp $<36°C$ or $>38°C$
    - HR >90 bpm
    - RR >20 breaths/min or P_aCO_2 <32 mmHg
    - WBC $>12K$ or $<4K$ or $>10\%$ bands
  - Sepsis: SIRS + suspected infection
  - Severe sepsis: Sepsis + acute organ dysfunction
    - Acute organ dysfunction
      - Hypotension (SBP <90 mmHg or MAP <70 mmHg)
      - Hypoxemia (P/F <300)
      - Oliguria (UOP <0.5 cc/kg/hr)
      - Renal injury (Cr increase >0.5)
      - Coagulopathy (INR >1.5)
      - Thrombocytopenia (Plt $<100K$)
      - Hyperbilirubinemia (Total bilirubin >4)
      - Lactate >2
      - New altered mental status
  - Septic shock: Hypotension due to sepsis despite adequate fluid resuscitation (classically 30 cc/kg), as well as signs of hypoperfusion
- Sequential Organ Failure Assessment (SOFA):
  - Alternative scoring system that can be used to predict the clinical outcome of critically ill patients and used in the Sepsis-3 guidelines. Takes into account Glasgow Coma Score (GCS), renal function, liver function, coagulopathy, and respiratory status (see Table 3.3)
  - qSOFA (Quick SOFA) is a bedside assessment for early detection of suspected sepsis
    - Criteria: 1 point for each
      - RR ≥ 22 breaths/min
      - Altered mentation
      - SBP ≤ 100 mmHg
    - Positive score is ≥ 2
    - Implications
      - Positive score should prompt evaluation for end-organ dysfunction and calculation of full SOFA score
      - Scores of 2–3 associated with higher in-hospital mortality
      - Easily identified at the bedside and can be repeated as clinical changes occur
      - Conflicting data on use in the ICU, may be more useful outside the ICU but research is ongoing
      - See Table 3.4 for types of shock and associated features
- Pathophysiology:
  - Infection causes proinflammatory cytokine storm (TNF-a, IL-1), "malignant intravascular inflammation"
  - In infection, microorganism factors such as bacterial cell wall components (LPS) and bacterial products (toxins) may cause inflammatory reaction
  - Inflammation leads to low systemic vascular resistance (SVR), fever, leukocytosis
  - Cellular injury occurs, which can lead to further organ dysfunction:
    - Tissue ischemia from metabolic autoregulatory failure and hypoperfusion
    - Mitochondrial dysfunction and cell death

- Management:
  - Antibiotics and infection control:
    - Start broad, empiric IV antibiotics **within 1 hour** of recognizing severe sepsis or septic shock
      - Consider healthcare exposure, immune status, prior culture data, risk of multi-drug resistant (MDR) organisms
      - See hospital-specific guidelines for empiric antibiotic choices based on local patterns of antimicrobial resistance
    - Special considerations:
      - If considering bacterial meningitis, should also co-administer steroids
      - Neutropenic fever empiric coverage includes anti-pseudomonal beta-lactam +/− MRSA coverage depending on the clinical situation
    - Collect blood cultures (×2) and urine cultures BEFORE starting antibiotics, if possible
    - Attempt to determine a source of infection based on history, physical exam, labs, cultures, and imaging. Consider additional imaging if needed to identify an occult source of infection
  - Intravenous fluid resuscitation:
    - Crystalloids are the initial preferred resuscitation agent
      - Usual resuscitation with 30 cc/kg of crystalloid
      - Normal saline is often first crystalloid used for hypovolemia and resuscitation; however, large volumes can cause hyperchloremic metabolic acidosis
      - Balanced solutions (lactated Ringer's [LR] or Plasma-Lyte) are isotonic solutions with less chloride than normal saline (NS) and are thus more physiologic and often used for larger volumes of infusion. Data also suggest a mortality benefit when used over NS for critically ill patients (SMART trial, *New Engl J Med* 2018).
    - Resuscitation goals:
      - MAP >65 mmHg for most patients
      - Maintain adequate RV filling pressure
        - Classically, guidelines had targeted CVP goals; however, CVP changes under a variety of patient conditions, such as if they are intubated (positive pressure ventilation) or not (negative pressure ventilation) as well as if RV dysfunction is present
      - Urine output >0.5 cc/kg/hr
    - Can use lactate clearance to help guide resuscitation and risk stratification
      - Higher lactate correlates with higher mortality
      - Trend and remeasure lactate during resuscitation
  - Vasopressors:
    - If still hypotensive despite adequate fluid resuscitation, add vasopressors
    - Norepinephrine is the first-line vasopressor for septic shock
    - Be aware of the patient's cardiac status and renal function when giving IVF, monitor for hypoxia with aggressive fluid resuscitation

TABLE 3.3 · Sequential Organ Failure Assessment (SOFA) Score					
Criteria	**0**	**1**	**2**	**3**	**4**
PaO$_2$/FiO$_2$	>400 mmHg	<400 mmHg	<300 mmHg	<200 mmHg	<100 mmHg
				with respiratory support	
Platelets (k/μL)	>150	<150	<100	<50	<20
Bilirubin (mg/dL)	<1.2	1.2–1.9	2.5–5.9	6–11.9	>12
Mean arterial pressure (MAP) or vasopressor requirement	≥70	<70	Dopamine <5 μg/kg/min *or* dobutamine (any dose)	Dopamine 5.1–15 μg/kg/min *or* epinephrine ≤0.1 μg/kg/min *or* norepinephrine ≤0.1 μg/kg/min	Dopamine >15 μg/kg/min *or* epinephrine >0.1 μg/kg/min *or* norepinephrine >0.1 μg/kg/min
Glasgow Coma Scale score	15	13–14	10–12	6–9	<6
Creatine (Cr) (mg/dL) or urine output (UOP)	Cr <1.2	Cr 1.2–1.9	Cr 2.0–3.4	Cr 3.5–4.9 *or* UOP <500 cc/day	Cr >5 *or* UOP <200 cc/day

CRITICAL CARE MEDICINE

CRITICAL CARE MEDICINE

TABLE 3.4 · Types of Shock

Types of Shock	Features*	Common Etiologies	Clinical Features	Additional Diagnostics	Approach to Treatment
Cardiogenic	↓↓CO ↑SVR ↑PCWP	Ischemia (ACS) Heart failure Dysrhythmias Cardiomyopathy Valvular disease Myocarditis	Peripheral vasoconstriction → **cool extremities** Increased JVP, S3/S4, pulmonary congestion and/or edema, LE edema, possible new murmur	Calculate and trend cardiac output/index using the Fick equation or $AVDO_2$ (see Cardiology Chapter 1)	**CO: Increase with inotropes, typically dobutamine** SVR: First, vasopressors (norepi) to maintain end-organ perfusion, then reduce SVR with inodilators (dobutamine) and later afterload reduction to offload LV PCWP: Use diuretics or dialysis to treat volume overload If ACS, revascularize (i.e., take the patient to the cath lab)
Distributive	↑CO ↓↓SVR ↓PCWP	Infection Anaphylaxis Adrenal insufficiency	Peripheral vasodilation → **warm extremities** Septic patients often febrile with leukocytosis Anaphylaxis with facial swelling, airway compromise, rash/urticaria, culprit ingestion, or exposure	Extensive history, physical exam, and consider additional imaging to identify potential source of infection (sepsis) or exposure (anaphylaxis)	**SVR and PCWP: Increase with fluids (30 cc/kg bolus) and vasopressors (first line: norepi, second line: vaso, third line: epi)** Septic: IV antibiotics, can consider adding steroids for refractory septic shock Adrenal insufficiency: Steroids Anaphylaxis: Epinephrine (first line), identify trigger, monitor and maintain patent airway
Hypovolemic	↓↓CO ↑SVR ↓PCWP	Hemorrhagic (trauma, GI bleed) Non-hemorrhagic (volume depletion from vomiting, diarrhea, poor PO intake, burns)	Peripheral vasoconstriction → **cool extremities** Identify source of bleeding or trauma Evaluate for signs of cirrhosis or high-risk GIB Volume depletion: Dry MM, poor skin turgor, delayed capillary refill	Serial CBCs, coags, type and screen Consider CT scan, endoscopy and colonoscopy if concern for GI bleed	**CO and PCWP: Increase with IVF resuscitation and blood products (goal Hgb >7 g/dL)** Maintain adequate vascular access Consider reversal of coagulopathy GIB: PPI, octreotide (if portal HTN), endoscopy/colonoscopy, IR embolization

(Continued)

TABLE 3.4 • Types of Shock (Continued)				
Types of Shock	Features*	Common Etiologies	Clinical Features	Additional Diagnostics	Approach to Treatment
Obstructive	$\downarrow\downarrow$**CO** $\uparrow$SVR $\downarrow/\uparrow$PCWP	Pulmonary embolism	PE: RV strain or failure on ECG or TTE, elevated JVP, hypoxemia, signs of DVT	CT with arterial phase contrast ("CT PE"), CXR, TTE, ECG, trop, BNP	Vasopressors (norepi, vaso) to maintain end organ perfusion
		Cardiac tamponade	Cardiac tamponade: Hypotension, elevated JVP, distant heart sounds, pulses paradoxus	Some scenarios require emergent management (e.g., empiric anticoagulation or needle decompression) without formal diagnostic studies	PE: Anticoagulation, possible advanced therapy (tPA, catheter-directed thrombolysis, ECMO)
		Tension pneumothorax	Tension PTX: Absent breath sounds, mediastinal shift away from PTX, respiratory failure		Tamponade: Pericardiocentesis, IVF for adequate preload
					PTX: Needle or tube decompression
Neurogenic	$\downarrow$CO $\downarrow$SVR $\downarrow$PCWP	Spinal cord injury Head trauma Anesthesia	Loss of vascular tone → peripheral vasodilation → **warm extremities**	NCHCT, CT Spine, MRI Brain/Spine	Vasopressors to restore tone
			*Sometimes listed as a subtype of distributive shock, since physiologic derangements are similar		IVF resuscitation
					Maintain normothermia

Bold $\downarrow\downarrow$ = Primary hemodynamic change.

Abbreviations; CO = cardiac output, SVR = systemic vascular resistance, PCWP = pulmonary capillary wedge pressure, norepi = norepinephrine, vaso = vasopressin, epi = epinephrine, ECMO = extracorporeal membrane oxygenation

CRITICAL CARE MEDICINE

Acute Respiratory Distress Syndrome (ARDS)

- Definition: Berlin Criteria (ARDS Definition Task Force, *JAMA* 2012)
  - Onset within 1 week (<7 days) of known insult or worsening respiratory symptoms
  - Bilateral infiltrates on CXR
  - Respiratory failure not fully explained by heart failure or volume overload (PCWP <18 mmHg)
    - This determination is often made clinically, as most patients do not have PA catheters
  - Hypoxemia
    - Severity of ARDS classified based on PaO_2/FiO_2 ratio, also called "P to F Ratio"
    - Calculated when PEEP $\geq$5 cm H_2O
- Etiology:
  - <u>Direct injury</u>: Pneumonia (bacterial, viral including COVID-19, fungal), aspiration, pulmonary contusion, DAH, inhalation injury, near drowning, post lung transplantation, acute drug toxicity (e.g., amiodarone)
  - <u>Indirect injury</u>: Sepsis, severe trauma, shock, DIC, pancreatitis, transfusion-related acute lung injury (TRALI)
- Pathophysiology:
  - Insult or injury directly to the lungs or as a result of systemic inflammation
  - Increased vascular permeability leads to pulmonary edema and protein leakage into the interstitium and alveoli. This causes stiff lungs, blood shunting, and increased dead space, ultimately resulting in hypoxemia.
- Treatment:
  - Treat the underlying cause of ARDS
  - Ventilation strategy: ARDSNet protocol (aka lung protective ventilation or low tidal volume ventilation) (*New Engl J Med* 2000)
    - Low tidal volume ventilation: 4–6 cc/kg of ideal body weight (IBW), which is based on gender and height
    - Permissive hypercapnia and respiratory acidosis: Tolerate pH as low as 7.25 if needed to reduce tidal volume
    - Relative hypoxemia: Goal >SpO_2 87% or PaO_2 >55 mmHg
    - Reduce injury and avoid barotrauma and atelectrauma: Keep peak and plateau pressures (P_{PL}) $\leq$30 cm H_2O on the ventilator
    - Use sedation as needed to promote ventilator synchrony (low TV and hypercapnia is uncomfortable for patients)
  - Refractory hypoxemia on ARDSNet protocol:
    - <u>Conservative fluid management</u>
      - Conservative fluid strategy with diuresis (goal CVP <4 mmHg, PCWP <8 mmHg) resulted in better oxygenation, fewer days on ventilator (FACTT study, *New Engl J Med* 2006)
      - "Dry lungs are happy lungs": Fluid restrict and use diuretics as needed while avoiding hypotension/hypoperfusion
    - <u>Proning</u>
      - Reduced mortality if proning done early (12–24 hr) and vigorously (at least 16 consecutive hours) (PROSEVA group, *New Engl J Med* 2013)
      - Note: PROSEVA definition is PaO_2/FiO_2 ratio <150 for severe ARDS
      - Suspected mechanism of benefit: Better matching of ventilation and perfusion, opening of dependent collapsed lung segments

TABLE 3.5 · ARDS Severity Classifications		
Severity	**PaO_2/FiO_2 Ratio**	**Mortality****
Mild	200–300	27%
Moderate	100–200	32%
Severe	<100*	45%

*PROSEVA (proning trial) definition is PaO_2/FiO_2 ratio <150 for severe ARDS.
**Mortality data from Berlin Definition paper, ARDS Definition Task Force, *JAMA* 2012

- Neuromuscular blockade/paralysis
  - Paralysis should be a patient-specific decision; requires higher sedation to RASS − 5 with the accompanying side effects and complications
  - Evidence:
    - ACURASYS Trial (*New Engl J Med* 2010): Paralysis with cisatracurium within 48 hours of onset of severe ARDS with continued infusion for 48 hours improved survival at 28 and 90 days, as well as increased ventilator-free days
    - ROSE Trial (*New Engl J Med* 2019): Early use of neuromuscular blockade with cisatracurium continuous infusion (48 hours) compared to usual care with light sedation for moderate to severe ARDS had no mortality benefit but was associated with more ICU-acquired weakness. Note: Possible that in the ROSE Trial the benefit of paralytic was offset by requirement for more sedation.
  - Mechanism of potential benefit: Unknown, thought to be due to decreased O_2 consumption from skeletal muscles and improving ventilator synchrony to enable low tidal volume/ARDSNet ventilation strategy that is known to improve mortality
- Inhaled nitric oxide (iNO)/epoprostenol (Flolan)
  - Inhaled nitrous oxide temporarily improves oxygenation, but no clear mortality benefit (Cochrane 2010)
  - Sometimes used as an FiO_2-sparing agent to avoid theoretical effects of high FiO_2 (>0.7) for prolonged periods if patient has refractory hypoxemia
- Recruitment maneuvers
  - Transiently increase PEEP to recruit atelectatic lung; typical maneuver: 40 cm H_2O for 40 seconds
  - Precautions and risks:
    - Must be used with caution; requires close bedside monitoring during maneuver
    - Patient can become transiently hypotensive, as increased intrathoracic pressures leads to decreased cardiac preload. May increase mortality by causing hemodynamic instability (ART Trial, *JAMA* 2017)
    - Increases risk of barotrauma with high intrapulmonary pressures
- ECMO (i.e., lung replacement therapy with extracorporeal membrane oxygenation)
  - Consider for severe refractory hypoxemia, often PaO_2/FiO_2 <50
  - Mortality benefit not yet proven
    - Improved survival shown in but confounded by treatment at a more experienced ARDS center in the CESAR Trial (*Lancet* 2009)
    - No mortality benefit in the EOLIA Trial (*New Engl J Med* 2018), but results questionable because despite trend towards benefit study was stopped early and was underpowered

Diabetic Ketoacidosis (DKA) and Hyperosmolar Hyperglycemic Syndrome (HHS)

DKA and HHS are medical emergencies that require prompt triaging, evaluation, and treatment, often in the ICU, due to the need for close monitoring, frequent lab draws, and IV insulin therapy.

Diabetic ketoacidosis (DKA)
- Definition:
  - Hyperglycemia (glucose >250 mg/dL), ketonemia, anion gap metabolic acidosis
- Clinical presentation:
  - Acute onset with symptoms of hyperglycemia (polyuria, polydipsia)
  - GI symptoms: Nausea, vomiting, abdominal pain
  - Fatigue, lethargy $\rightarrow$ coma if severe in later stages
  - Hypovolemia: Dry mucous membranes, reduced skin turgor, tachycardia, hypotension if severe
- Etiology:
  - Common: Infection, medication nonadherence, insufficient insulin, new-onset type 1 diabetes
  - Less common: Acute illness (MI, CVA, pancreatitis), substance use (especially cocaine), glucose pump malfunction, medications (SGLT2i, antipsychotics, steroids)
- Evaluation and diagnostics:
  - History: Focused history to determine underlying trigger
  - Physical exam: Vital signs, hemodynamic assessment, mental status, volume exam
  - Laboratory evaluation: Serum glucose, CBC with differential, BMP (calculate the anion gap), plasma osmolarity, serum ketones (often beta hydroxybutyrate), ABG (or VBG), urinalysis, ECG, CXR, +/− blood and urine cultures if signs of infection, HgA1c

- Management: Follow institutional guidelines if present. General principles are as follows:
  - <u>Fluids</u>
    - Resuscitation: Patients are volume depleted (deficit often 3–8 L) and require resuscitation; isotonic crystalloids (Plasma-Lyte or NS) given first for volume expansion
    - Avoiding hypoglycemia (later in course): When fingerstick glucose (FSG) <250 mg/dL, switch to dextrose-containing solution (often D5 1/2 NS)
  - <u>Electrolytes</u>
    - Potassium
      - Serum potassium can be low, normal, or elevated
        - Regardless, patients are total body potassium down if their pH is low
        - Both insulin deficiency and acidemia will raise serum potassium
      - Insulin administration and correction of acidemia will shift potassium intracellularly and risk hypokalemia and potentially fatal arrhythmias
      - Potassium repletion is based on current serum potassium
        - If K <3.3 mEq/L, replete K BEFORE giving insulin
        - If K 3.3–5.3 mEq/L, then given K (20–40 mEq/L of fluids) and insulin
        - If K >5.3 mEq/L, give insulin alone with close trending of serum K
    - Magnesium: Replete to >1.6 mg/dL to enable proper K repletion
    - Phosphorus: Goal >1.0 mg/dL
    - Bicarbonate: Use is not well studied, but can consider if pH <6.9
  - <u>Insulin</u>
    - Dosing: Intravenous bolus (0.1 units/kg or 5–10 units) and continuous drip (often started at 0.1 units/kg/hr); most institutions have titration protocols for DKA
    - Goal: Reduction of FSG by 10% or 50 mg/dL absolute points per hour
      - If not achieving goal, can either rebolus or increase gtt rate
    - Transitioning from gtt to SQ insulin:
      - When FSG <250 mg/dl, reduce gtt rate by 50% (and transition to dextrose containing solution, as noted earlier)
      - Determine basal SQ insulin dose
        - Note: Patients with DKA have HIGHER insulin needs acutely, often due to stressors such as infection, and thus some methods for estimating insulin needs will overestimate and may risk hypoglycemia
        - Total daily dose (TDD) is total insulin needs with roughly 50% given as basal and 50% as prandial
          - Method 1: Use home regimen to estimate needs
          - Method 2: Weight-based dosing with TDD = 0.5–0.6 units/kg
          - Method 3: If patient is on stable, low rate of insulin gtt (ideally <5 units/hr), take total insulin used over the last 6 hours × 4 to estimate TDD. Then take 80% of that calculation for safety purposes (this method will often overestimate insulin needs).
          - Combination method: Compare TDD from the methods earlier. If significant discrepancies exist, consider averaging or using the lower, more conservative estimate to avoid hypoglycemia.
          - Transition to basal insulin when 1) Anion gap closed; 2) Patient eating; and 3) FSG <250 mg/dL
            - Often requires delay until morning or evening to get the patient back on a normal medication schedule
          - Continue insulin drip until 1–2 hours AFTER basal SQ insulin dose is given to ensure overlap
          - Monitor FSG and labs to ensure anion gap does not reopen

Hyperosmolar hyperglycemic syndrome (HHS)
- Definition: Hyperglycemia (often FSG >600 mg/dL) without ketones or acidemia
- Clinical presentation:
  - Often more insidious onset than DKA with days of symptoms
  - Symptoms of hyperglycemia: Polyuria, polydipsia
  - Hypovolemia: Dry mucous membranes, poor skin turgor, tachycardia, hypotension if severe
  - Neurologic symptoms (including seizure and coma in severe cases) arise from high serum osmolarity due to extreme hyperglycemia

- Etiology:
  - Can be triggered by infection, medication nonadherence, MI, CVA, substance use, medications (steroids, antipsychotics)
- Evaluation and diagnostics:
  - Initial triage, evaluation, and diagnostics are the same as for DKA (see prior section)
  - Hemodynamic assessment, neurologic exam, and volume exam are essential
- Management: Principles of treatment and management of HHS are generally the same as in DKA with a focus on adequate and aggressive fluid resuscitation, close monitoring of electrolytes, and IV insulin therapy
  - Fluids
    - Patients with HHS are typically **more** profoundly dehydrated than those with DKA and require aggressive IVF resuscitation
    - Total body water deficits often approaching 5–10 liters
    - Based on corrected sodium, often have residual free water deficit needing hypotonic solutions even after patient is euvolemic
  - Electrolytes
    - Potassium: In the absence of acidemia, potassium depletion is less pronounced
    - Sodium: Hyponatremia from osmotically active glucose pulling in water requires calculating corrected sodium
      - $\text{Corrected Na} = \text{measured Na} + \left[2.4 \times \left(\dfrac{\text{serum glucose} - 100}{100} \right) \right]$
    - Osmolarity: Patients have hyperosmolarity, which is responsible for neurologic symptoms
      - $\text{Serum osmolarity} = \left(2 \times Na^+ \right) + \left(\dfrac{BUN}{2.8} \right) + \left(\dfrac{Glucose}{18} \right)$
    - Resolution of HHS, in addition to correction of electrolyte disturbances and hyperglycemia, includes resolution of any neurologic symptoms and serum osmolarity correction to usually <315 mg/dL
  - Insulin
    - General insulin management is the same as that for DKA
      - Intravenous bolus (0.1 units/kg or 5–10 units) + continuous drip (often started at 0.1 units/kg/hr)
      - Follow hospital-specific guidelines for insulin drip management
      - For transition from drip to SQ insulin, see the DKA section

CRITICAL CARE MEDICINE

COMMON COMPLICATIONS OF ICU ADMISSION

Post-Intensive Care Syndrome & Other Long-Term Physical and Cognitive Disability

- Definition: Generally defined as new or worsening cognitive, psychiatric, and/or physical function
  - Cognitive: Memory, executive function
  - Psychiatric: Depression, anxiety, PTSD
  - Physical: ICU-acquired weakness is most common
- Risk factors:
  - Pre-existing factors: Neuromuscular disorders, prior cognitive impairment, psychiatric disease, frailty, medical comorbidities
  - ICU-specific factors: Mechanical ventilation, delirium, sepsis, ARDS
- Management:
  - Daily sedation interruptions, delirium avoidance and management, early ambulation and physical therapy, nutritional optimization, avoidance of hypoglycemia and hypoxemia
  - Post-discharge treatment with physical therapy and rehab, occupational therapy, social support, mental health services
- Clinical importance:
  - Survivors of critical illness report lower quality of life (QOL) scores
  - Family members of survivors report lower QOL scores
  - Survivors of critical illness have higher likelihood of rehospitalization, higher unemployment rates, and higher overall mortality

Complications Associated with Mechanical Ventilation

- See "Intubation and Mechanical Ventilation" under *Key Medications and Interventions*

Delirium

- Definition: Sudden, acute onset, fluctuating changes in consciousness and cognition
  - Can be hypoactive (diminished responsiveness, apathy) or hyperactive (agitation)
- Importance:
  - Delirium increases hospital length of stay and mortality (3× in mechanically ventilated patients), long-term cerebral dysfunction, SNF placement, and dementia after ICU discharge
  - Common: Prevalence of 50% in ICU patients
- Risk factors:
  - Nonmodifiable: Older age, cognitive impairment/dementia, substance use disorder
  - Modifiable: Medications, pain, acute renal failure, critical illness, environment, weakness, extra drains, lines and tubes
- Assessment: CAM-ICU (Confusion Assessment Method): validated, RN-driven protocol
- Management:
  - Reverse underlying cause(s)
  - Maximize nutrition
  - Reorientation
  - Correct sensory deficits (e.g., replace hearing aids, glasses)
  - Limit extraneous stimuli in the environment
  - Promote normal sleep pattern
  - Avoid restraints if possible. Use bedside coaches/sitters
  - Pharmacologic management (if **all** earlier interventions fail): Use with caution, best indication is to protect patient/staff safety if pulling at devices or interfering with care; no evidence that antipsychotics reduce duration of delirium or mortality
    - Antipsychotics (haloperidol, quetiapine, risperidone)
    - Benzodiazepines **only** if withdrawal is suspected

Infections

Central line-associated bloodstream infections (CLABSI)

- Pathogens:
  - Typically skin flora with coagulase-negative staph, *S. aureus*, enterococci. Infections with Gram-negative organisms (*E. coli*, *Klebsiella*, *Pseudomonas*) less common
  - Often infection from skin colonization but can be from hematogenous spread from bloodstream infection occurring from another, distant focus
- Risk factors: Duration of use, catheter material, insertion conditions, site care, placement site (subclavian < internal jugular ≤ femoral), host immunodeficiency
- Clinical importance: Nosocomial infection associated with higher morbidity and mortality
- Management: Empiric systemic antibiotics, catheter removal. May need ID consultation depending on the organism/clinical situation.

Catheter-associated UTI (CAUTI)
- Definition: Culture growth of ≥1000 CFU/mL with symptoms compatible with UTI in a patient with an indwelling urethral or suprapubic catheter OR in a patient who had catheter (including condom catheters) removed within the past 48 hours
- Risk factors: Duration of catheterization, female sex, older age, DM, factors related to catheter insertion and care
- Pathogens: *E. coli, Enterococcus, Pseudomonas, Klebsiella, Candida*
- Treatment: Antibiotic selection based on risk factors for multi-drug resistant organisms and prior culture data. Obtain cultures prior to antibiotics if possible and narrow antibiotics based on sensitivities. Typical antibiotic duration 7–14 days. Replace or remove catheter.

Clostridium difficile
- Microbiology: Caused by spore-forming and toxin-producing Gram-positive anaerobic bacterium. Typically presents with diarrhea (≥3 stools in 24 hours). Can also cause more severe, fulminant disease with shock and toxic megacolon
- Diagnosis and Treatment: See Infectious Diseases Chapter 8

Ventilator-associated pneumonia (VAP)
- Definition: Pneumonia diagnosed >48 hours after intubation
- Diagnosis and treatment: See Infectious Diseases Chapter 8

DVT/PE
- Risk factors: ICU patients are considered high risk for VTE given immobility and severe inflammation
- Prophylaxis: Pharmacologic or mechanical prophylaxis indicated in most patients
- Contraindications for pharmacologic prophylaxis: Active bleeding, use of systemic anticoagulation, severe thrombocytopenia, recent or planned procedure, certain CNS lesions

Decubitus Ulcers
- Definition: Injury to skin and underlying tissue from prolonged pressure on the skin
- Risk factors: Bed rest, deconditioning, malnutrition, poor wound healing
- Treatment: Nursing-driven turning, nutritional optimization, padding pressure points

Malnutrition
- Risk factors: Critical illness often associated with increased catabolism and muscle breakdown
- Benefits of adequate nutrition: Maintains gut integrity and prevents bacterial translocation, reduces risk of stress ulcer formation, possibly reduces the risk of infection and may decrease mortality
- Treatment: Enteral nutrition within 48 hours is preferred; however, parenteral nutrition is necessary in some patients with contraindications to enteral nutrition

Critical Illness Polyneuropathy, Critical Illness Myopathy, and ICU-Acquired Weakness
- Risk factors: Mechanical ventilation, sepsis, prolonged use of paralytics, multiorgan failure, ARDS
- Clinical manifestations: Symmetric limb weakness (proximal > distal), respiratory muscle weakness leading to failure to wean ventilation, sparing of facial muscles
  - Critical illness polyneuropathy (CIP): Features as noted above
  - Critical illness myopathy (CIM): Features as noted above; sensory loss may be particularly suggestive, CK may be elevated
  - ICU-acquired weakness: Diagnosis of exclusion, first sign is often the failure to wean from mechanical ventilation, spares cranial nerves
- Management: Minimize sedation and neuromuscular blockade, treat underlying causes, rehabilitation with early mobilization and physical therapy

Anemia
- Importance:
  - Common: >95% of patients within 1 week of ICU admission
  - Associated with worse outcomes: Mortality, failure to wean from mechanical ventilation, MI
  - Risk and potential harm with blood transfusions
- Etiology: Often multifactorial including frequent lab draws, hematopoiesis inhibition from critical illness (bone marrow suppression), minor GI bleeding (stress ulceration)
- Management:
  - Conservative transfusion goals: Transfusion goal of >7 g/dL (restrictive) improved survival compared with a transfusion goal of >10 g/dL (liberal) (TRICC Trial, *New Engl J Med* 1999)
  - Avoid unnecessary lab draws or use pediatric tubes that require less volume
  - Avoid using venous access catheters for lab draws that increase the amount of discarded blood
  - Consider PPI, although recent evidence suggests increased risk of pneumonia and no change in mortality

CRITICAL CARE MEDICINE

KEY MEDICATIONS AND INTERVENTIONS

Respiratory Support

TABLE 3.6 · Supplemental oxygen delivery devices

Device	Flow	FiO₂	Advantages	Disadvantages
Nasal Cannula	1–6 LPM	25%–40% FiO_2 increases by 4% for every additional 1 LPM	Cheap Tolerable Common device	Variable FiO_2 delivery based on RR, V_t, mouth breathing
Simple Face Mask	6–10 LPM Flows >5 LPM will prevent rebreathing	35%–50%	Accessible Easy to use Common device Generates high FiO_2	Not as well tolerated, especially with delirious or anxious patients Not precise FiO_2 delivery: Depends on RR and mask fit
Non-rebreather (NRB)	10–15 LPM Flows >15 LPM ensure reservoir bag is always inflated	80%–95%	High FiO_2 delivery	Less tolerable for some patients Must have one valve open to ensure patient safety
High-Flow Nasal Cannula (HFNC)	10–60 LPM	21%–100%	High FiO_2 delivery with close titration Washes out dead space, decreasing work of breathing and RR Some PEEP at high flow rates	Variable FiO_2 delivery based on RR, V_t, mouth breathing Less mobile device

TABLE 3.7 · Noninvasive positive pressure ventilation (NIPPV)

Device	Settings	Indications	Clinical Uses	Contraindications
Continuous positive airway pressure (CPAP)	Airway pressure (constant throughout respiratory cycle)	Hypoxemia	Cardiogenic pulmonary edema* Hypoxemic respiratory failure Obstructive sleep apnea	- Unable to protect airway (encephalopathy, aspiration, vomiting, excessive secretions, UGIB) - At risk of losing airway (recent facial trauma or surgery, evolving obstruction with anaphylaxis or angioedema)
Bilevel positive airway pressure (BiPAP)	Inspiratory pressure (IPAP) Expiratory pressure (EPAP = PEEP)	Hypoxemia Hypercapnia	Cardiogenic pulmonary edema* Hypoxemic respiratory failure COPD exacerbations with hypercapnia Obesity hypoventilation syndrome (OHS) At risk of hypoventilation after extubation (COPD, OSA, OHS)	- NIPPV inappropriate to address the cause of respiratory failure (e.g., fixed upper airway obstruction) - Unable to tolerate mask or inconsistent with goals of care

*Mechanisms by which positive pressure improves cardiogenic pulmonary edema:
1. Increased intrathoracic pressures decreases preload
2. Increased alveolar pressure reduces filtration out of vessel via Starling forces: Positive pressure increases interstitial pressure that opposes intravascular hydrostatic pressure
3. PEEP reduces LV afterload by decreasing wall stress: Increased intrathoracic pressure reduces LV transmural pressure so that the LV does not have to overcome a negative pressure on the outside of the heart in order to contract inwards
4. Decreased LV transmural pressure also decreases myocardial oxygen consumption

Intubation and mechanical ventilation
- Purpose:
  - Relieve respiratory distress
  - Improve gas exchange for CO_2 (hypercarbia) and O_2 (hypoxemia)
  - Decrease work of breathing
  - Protect airway in cases of low GCS (<8), apnea, inability to clear secretions
- Indications: Typically try noninvasive forms of ventilation before progressing to invasive mechanical ventilation, except in the setting of altered mental status, cardiac arrest, or severe respiratory compromise with impending arrest. Following are other clinical situations where intubation and mechanical ventilation may be appropriate:
  - <u>Hypoxemic respiratory failure</u>: PaO_2 <55 mmHg
    - Common causes: Pneumonia, hemorrhage, ARDS, pulmonary edema
  - <u>Hypercarbic respiratory failure</u>: $PaCO_2$ >45 mmHg with acidemia pH <7.35
    - Common causes: COPD, asthma, hypoventilation
  - <u>Upper airway obstruction</u>:
    - Common causes: Tumor, angioedema, stenosis
  - <u>Severe acidemia with inability to compensate</u>:
    - Common causes: DKA, severe sepsis, other conditions with increased respiratory/ventilatory demands
  - <u>Neuromuscular weakness</u>:
    - Common causes: Amyotrophic lateral sclerosis (ALS), Guillan Barré Syndrome (GBS), toxins, myasthenia gravis
  - <u>To safely perform procedures or imaging</u> (relative indication)
  - <u>Hemodynamic instability</u> (relative indication)
- How to intubate:
  - There are various methods for intubation: Endotracheal vs. nasal, awake vs. paralyzed and sedated, direct visualization vs. video-assisted
  - Most common: Paralyzed and sedated orotracheal intubation by direct larnygoscopy (DL)
  - Often institution-specific protocols for who intubates: ED, anesthesia, and/or critical care–trained clinicians
  - Difficult intubations or those with airway obstructions often require backup support with ENT involvement or options for tracheostomy
- Ventilator modes and key parameters: See Table 3.8, Figure 3.5
- Complications of intubation:
  - Inability to intubate (often abnormal anatomy, severe obesity), inability to ventilate, hypotension (e.g., due to auto-PEEP physiology or sedation/induction medications → decreased vascular tone and SVR), aspiration (especially for patients who were not NPO prior), hypoxemia, arrhythmia
  - Risk factors: Conditions that reduce patients' ability to augment cardiac output such as aortic stenosis and pulmonary hypertension are risk factors for hemodynamic collapse during intubation, because induction medications reduce vascular tone
    - Placing an arterial line permits closer hemodynamic monitoring and earlier intervention in patients at risk for hemodynamic collapse
- Complications of mechanical ventilation:
  - Ventilator-associated pneumonia: Pneumonia diagnosed >48 hours after intubation; see hospital-acquired pneumonia and ventilator-associated pneumonia in Infectious Diseases Chapter 8
  - Laryngeal edema, ulceration: Consider tracheostomy after 14 days of intubation
  - Oxygen toxicity: Higher risk with higher FiO_2, often >0.7 (at present this is a theoretical concern based on lab studies without robust human evidence)
  - Oversedation and delirium: Particularly for patients with ARDS and those who require paralysis with deeper sedation goals
  - Barotrauma complications: Pneumothorax, subcutaneous emphysema
  - Ventilator-associated lung injury (VALI)
  - Diaphragmatic weakness: Atrophy from mechanical ventilation and muscle disuse

TABLE 3.8 · Ventilator Modes			
Variable	**Volume Control (VC)**	**Pressure Control (PC)**	**Pressure Support (PS)**
Independent Variables (what you set)	TV, RR, FiO_2, PEEP	Inspiratory pressure, time, PEEP, RR, FiO_2	Inspiratory pressure, PEEP, FiO_2
Dependent Variables (what changes)	Pressure	TV (and minute ventilation)	TV and RR (minute ventilation)
Tidal Volume	Same every breath	Depends on patient effort and lung compliance	Depends on patient effort and lung compliance
Airway Pressure	Depends on lung compliance	Same every breath: Peak Pressure = Inspiratory Pressure + PEEP	Same every breath
Respiratory Rate	Minimum set, but patient can trigger spontaneously	Minimum set, but patient can trigger spontaneously	Completely spontaneous
Flow Rate	Same every breath	Depends on patient effort and lung compliance	Depends on patient effort and lung compliance
Waveforms	Pressure – time Pressure – volume loop	Volume – time Flow – time	Volume – time
Notes	Mode for ARDS for lung protective ventilation	Minute ventilation can vary with changes in pulmonary compliance More comfortable so requires less sedation	Often a vent weaning and SBT mode Does not have mandatory minute ventilation

Abbreviations: TV = tidal volume, RR = respiratory rate, FiO_2 = fraction of inspired oxygen, PEEP = positive end-expiratory pressure, ARDS = acute respiratory distress syndrome, SBT = spontaneous breathing trial

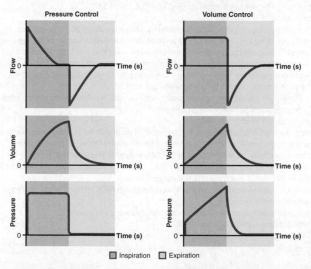

FIGURE 3.5: Volume control and pressure control modes in mechanical ventilation. Pressure, volume, and flow curves during inspiration (purple) and expiration (blue).

TABLE 3.9 · Key Parameters Affecting Oxygenation and Ventilation	
Parameters that Affect Oxygenation:	**Parameters that Affect Ventilation (CO_2):**

• FiO_2: Fraction of inspired air that is oxygen
• Mean airway pressure
  • Positive end expiratory pressure (PEEP): Positive pressure applied during exhalation
  • Peak inspiratory pressure (PIP)
  • Inspiratory/expiratory ratio (I:E ratio)
 	
*Increase PaO_2 by increasing FiO_2 and/or PEEP
 	
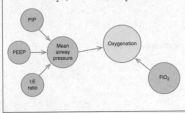
	• Respiratory rate (RR)
	• Tidal volume (TV)
	*Minute ventilation (MV) = RR × TV
	
	*Decrease $PaCO_2$ by increasing RR and/or TV (to increase minute ventilation)

Additional Parameters:

- Plateau pressure (P_{PL}): Surrogate for compliance (stiffness). Measured at end inspiration when there is no flow.
- Peak inspiratory pressure (PIP): Surrogate for compliance and airway resistance. Measured during inspiration when flow is present.
- Compliance ($\Delta V/\Delta P$): Stiffness of the lung, how it handles volume.
- Auto-PEEP: Measured with end-expiratory hold maneuver, PEEP *above* set value.
  - Occurs when breath is delivered before full expiration of the prior breath.
  - Can result in high intrathoracic pressure causing decreased cardiac preload and hypotension.
- Inspiratory/expiratory ratio (I:E ratio): Typically 1:2.
  - Inspiratory time is usually set, remainder is expiratory time.
  - Goal is to maximize E time in conditions like COPD with risk of auto-PEEP by reducing the RR.

- Managing refractory hypoxemia:
  - Mechanical: Increase FiO_2, increase PEEP, increase inspiratory time
  - Nonmechanical: Neuromuscular blockade (decrease ventilator dyssynchrony), prone positioning (improve V/Q mismatch), inhaled pulmonary vasodilator (e.g., nitrous oxide or prostacyclin), ECMO
- Criteria for extubation:
  - Perform daily assessment of readiness for spontaneous breathing trial (SBT)
  - Screening criteria for consideration of SBT:
    - Most important: Ensure that the reason why the patient was intubated in the first place has been resolved or is significantly improved
      - If not, then the patient requires ongoing mechanical ventilation
    - Minimal ventilator settings
      - FiO_2 <0.5 (which can be provided by other means)
      - PEEP <8 cm H_2O
    - Intact gag/cough. Ideal if the patient is also responding to commands but this is not always essential
    - Minimal secretions and ability to handle any secretions after extubation
    - Hemodynamically stable off vasopressors OR vasopressors titrating off and stable on low-dose pressors
    - If prolonged intubation (>5–7 days):
      - Consider checking "cuff leak" to assess for upper airway edema, which could lead to post-extubation stridor if present. This is more common in women, patients who are obese, and patients with prolonged courses or volume overload.

CRITICAL CARE MEDICINE

- Performing SBT:
  - All options are roughly equivalent to determine who will be successful and reduce risk of reintubation
  - SBT options:
    - <u>Favored approach</u>: 30–120 minutes of pressure support at PS 7 and PEEP 5
      - Note there is no evidence suggesting a benefit of checking ABG during an SBT
      - Note that longer SBTs are not necessarily better and may tire the patient out
    - <u>Alternate approach</u>: 30 minutes of T-piece with blow-by oxygen
      - Note: Patient must overcome resistance of T piece and circuit with this method
  - Rapid Shallow Breathing Index (RSBI)
    - RSBI = RR / Tidal Volume (in liters)
      - Slow, deeper breaths are more reassuring
      - RSBI >105 predicts extubation failure
- Deciding to discontinue mechanical ventilation:
  - Underlying reason for intubation is reversed or significantly improved
  - Patient must pass SBT
    - Hemodynamically stable throughout
    - Stable RR and TV (= stable MV) throughout
    - No desaturations
    - Stable $PaCO_2$ or $EtCO_2$
      - If increased, not ventilating sufficiently
    - Patient is awake, following commands, ideally wants to be extubated
    - Minimal secretions
    - Good cough and gag to clear secretions and protect airway
  - If patient tolerates SBT, consider extubation. If patient fails SBT, identify cause and correct it if possible.
- Rationale for extubation failure:
  - Physiology: Imbalance between respiratory load (what the lungs are being asked to do) and the combination of ventilatory muscle power and central drive to breathe
    - Increased respiratory load
      - Poor compliance
      - Increased dead space
      - Metabolic acidosis requiring higher minute ventilation
    - Muscle power diminished by deconditioning, often from prolonged intubation and mechanical ventilation
    - Reduced or impaired central drive to breathe, often from sedation
- Causes of extubation failure:
  - Post-extubation stridor
  - Respiratory muscle weakness
  - Aspiration
  - Mucus plugging
  - Pulmonary edema
    - Removal of positive pressure leads to increased preload and afterload
    - Consider diuresis especially in patients with HFrEF or impaired myocardial function
  - Failure to reverse the reason for intubation

Extracorporeal membrane oxygenation (ECMO)

- Definition: Temporary external bypass of the lungs and/or heart to treat life-threatening organ failure
- Types:
  - **Venovenous (VV)**: Treats hypoxemic/hypercarbic respiratory failure only. <u>No circulatory support</u>.
    - Blood is extracted from the venous system, externally oxygenated, CO_2 is removed, and it is returned to the venous system
    - Relies on patient's own cardiovascular system to support their hemodynamics
  - **Venoarterial (VA)**: Treats hypoxemic/hypercarbic respiratory failure and <u>provides circulatory support</u>.
    - Blood is extracted from the venous system, externally oxygenated, CO_2 is removed, and it is returned to the arterial system
    - Bypasses both the heart and the lungs

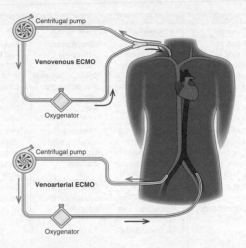

FIGURE 3.6: Venovenous (VV) and venoarterial (VA) extracorporeal membrane oxygenation. Top: Venovenous ECMO; Bottom: Venoarterial ECMO.

- Indications:
  - Severe pulmonary and/or cardiac failure causing refractory hypoxemic/hypercarbic respiratory failure or cardiogenic shock; should exhaust all less invasive treatments first
  - Etiology of organ failure is reversible (e.g., massive PE, ARDS) or with known definitive replacement planned (e.g., VADS, transplant)
- Contraindications:
  - Absolute: Etiology cannot be reversed and no definitive treatment options, other comorbidities that will prohibit survival
  - Relative: Thrombocytopenia, severe brain injury, severe comorbidities, life-limiting condition
- Complications:
  - Bleeding: Systemic heparization required and patients are also more coagulopathic with ECMO
  - Thrombosis: Cannula-associated thrombus, LV thrombus
  - Cannulation-related: Line infections, pneumothorax, leg ischemia with femoral artery insertion

Analgesia, Sedation, Paralytics, and Vasoactive Medications

This section includes key medications used in the ICU, including their indications, pharmacokinetics, and adverse effects. Typical dosing and dosing considerations will be provided. However, selecting the proper medication, dose, and route of administration requires clinical context and is patient-specific. Please use appropriate resources for dosing in clinical contexts and speak with your clinical pharmacists.

Pain management
- Goal: Control pain adequately to ideally achieve a maximally functional patient
  - Note: Does not mean zero pain, as this is often not possible to achieve, but the goal is to control pain as best as possible
- General principles:
  - See Table 3.10 for pain medications commonly used in the ICU
  - Try PRNs first to determine needs prior to starting drips
  - Treat pain first, as it can also be causing anxiety, delirium
  - Assess analgesic needs daily
  - Note: For patients on chronic opiates, best practice is to convert opiates to oral morphine equivalents (OME) and then convert this amount to the desired opiate using a conversion table. A dose reduction for incomplete cross-tolerance (often 25–50%) is then applied for patient safety, and the remainder total dose is divided into the number of doses per day with additional PRNs.
- Indications: Patient-reported pain, postoperative pain, trauma, chronic opioid use, decreased air hunger associated with certain modes of mechanical ventilation, neuromuscular blockade (paralysis)
- Adverse effects: Respiratory depression, constipation, withdrawal, nausea; adverse effects may be magnified when used with other sedatives such as benzodiazepines

TABLE 3.10 · Pain Medications Commonly Used in the ICU				
Agent	**Typical Dosing**	**Pharmacokinetics**	**Adverse Effects**	**Notes**
fentanyl	• Bolus/Load: 25–50 mcg • Initial Maintenance Drip Rate: 25–50 mcg/hr • Maintenance Drip Range: 25–300 mcg/hr	• MOA: Opioid receptor agonist • Onset: Seconds • Half-life: 1.5–6 hr • Metabolism: Liver • VD: Fat soluble • No active metabolites	• Constipation, drowsiness, tolerance • Opioid withdrawal with prolonged infusions • Skeletal muscle rigidity	• Fast onset • First line for pain and sedation in most intubated patients • Fat soluble = prolonged duration even after gtt off
morphine	• Bolus/Load: 2–4 mg • Initial Maintenance Drip Rate: 1–4 mg/hr • Maintenance Drip Range: 1–15 mg/hr	• Onset: 5–10 min • Half-life: 3–7 hr • Metabolism: Liver • VD: Water soluble • Excretion: Renal	• Histamine release leads to hypotension and itchiness	• Fast onset but slower than fentanyl • Accumulates in renal failure
hydro-morphone (Dilaudid)	• Bolus/Load: 0.25–1 mg • Initial Maintenance Drip Rate: 0.5–2 mg/hr • Maintenance Drip Range: 0.5–5 mg/hr	• Onset: 5 min • Half-life: 1–4 hr • Metabolism: Liver • VD: Water soluble • Excretion: Renal	• Safer in organ dysfunction than morphine	• Similar pharmacokinetics as morphine
ketamine	**Pain Dosing** • Bolus/Load: 0.25–0.5 mg/kg • Initial Maintenance Drip Rate: 0.05–0.25 mg/kg/hr • Maintenance Drip Range: 0.05–1 mg/kg/hr	• MOA: NMDA receptor antagonist • Metabolism: Liver • Excretion: Renal	• Dissociation • Agitation with emergence • Bronchorrhea • Hypertension more common than hypotension	• Often managed by pain and anesthesia services • Useful in opioid-tolerant patients

Abbreviations: MOA = mechanism of action, VD = volume of distribution

Sedation
- Goal: To ensure comfort while using the minimal amount of sedative/hypnotics possible
  - Ideally, patients should be calm, lucid, pain-free, and interactive
- General principles:
  - See Table 3.11 for medications commonly used for sedation in the ICU
  - Perform a daily sedation interruption (DSI) if possible
  - Assess pain and sedation needs daily
  - Target a sedation goal using a scale (often the Richmond Agitation and Sedation Scale [RASS])
    - Ideal is patient at RASS 0 (awake, cooperative)
    - Often initial goal is 0–2 in most patients and then reassess
    - For neuromuscular blockade/paralysis, requires RASS −5
      - Dexmedetomidine is not appropriate sedation in paralyzed patients; propofol or benzodiazepine is needed
- Indications: Ventilator dyssynchrony, anxiety not due to delirium, neuromuscular blockade, intracranial hypertension, refractory status epilepticus, severe respiratory failure, agitation when safety of the patient or providers is at risk, procedural sedation
- Adverse effects: Delirium, hypotension, dependence with subsequent risk for withdrawal, prolonged ICU stay

Neuromuscular blocking agents (NMBAs)
- General principles:
  - See Table 3.12 for commonly used neuromuscular blocking agents used in the ICU
  - Mechanism: Blocks acetylcholine-mediated transmission at the neuromuscular junction
- Indications: Severe ARDS/hypoxemia and severe ventilatory dyssynchrony not controlled by sedation. NMBAs paralyze the patient, so deep sedation (RASS −5) and adequate pain control are required

Vasopressors and inotropes
- Indications: To support blood pressure and contractility
- Medications: See Tables 3.13 and 3.14

TABLE 3.11 · Medications Commonly Used for Sedation in the ICU

Generic Name (Trade Name)	Typical Dosing	Pharmacokinetics	Adverse Effects	Notes

propofol	• Bolus/Load: 2 mg/kg
	• Maintenance Drip Range: 10–80 mcg/kg/min
		• MOA: Activates GABA receptors
		• Onset: 1 min
		• Half-life: 2–4 min
		• Metabolism: Liver
			• Hypotension, bradycardia, respiratory depression
			• Hypertriglyceridemia
			  • Reduce or consider switching if TG >500 mg/dL
			    • Factored into nutritional assessment
			• Pancreatitis
			• Propofol-related infusion syndrome (PRIS)
			  • Rare but fatal
			  • Higher risk in young (<18 yr), prolonged infusion (>3 days)
			  • Characterized by hypotension, renal failure, lactic acidosis
			  • Treatment: Stop propofol
				• Only used for intubated patients or sometimes procedural sedation with careful maintenance of airway

dexmedetomidine (Precedex)	• Bolus/Load: 0.1 mcg/kg over 10 min • Maintenance Drip Range: 0.2–1.5 mcg/kg/hr	• MOA: Central alpha-2 agonist • Onset: 5–10 min • Half-life: 1–2 hr • Metabolism: Liver • No active metabolites	• Hemodynamic instability (up or down), commonly hypotension and bradycardia • May obscure alcohol withdrawal adrenergic symptoms: If used for this indication patients still require GABA agonism (i.e., benzodiazepines) • Dependence if longer than 7 days, can cross-taper with clonidine to avoid withdrawal • Cannot achieve deep sedation, so is inappropriate for patients on NMBA	• Used as an adjunct agent for sedation and usually ineffective as primary agent • Also used in alcohol withdrawal or severe agitation • May reduce delirium if used overnight in ICU
midazolam (Versed)	• Bolus/Load: 0.5–2 mg • Initial Maintenance Drip Rate: 1–4 mg/hr • Maintenance Drip Range: 0.5–8 mg/hr	• MOA: GABA agonism • Onset: 2–3 min • Half-life: 2–4 hr • Metabolism: Liver • Excretion: Renal	• Respiratory depression • Hypotension if rapid infusion • Nausea/vomiting • Delirium • Patients develop dependence and can experience withdrawal after prolonged infusion	• Used for procedural sedation or for patients unable to tolerate propofol • Active metabolites: Lingering effects especially with organ dysfunction
ketamine	**Sedation Dosing** • Bolus/Load: 1–2 mg/ kg bolus • Maintenance Drip Range: 0.2–0.5 mg/kg/hr	• MOA: NMDA receptor antagonist • Metabolism: Liver • Excretion: Renal	• Dissociation • Agitation with emergence • Bronchorrhea • Hypertension more often than hypotension	• Often managed by pain and anesthesia services • Used for procedural sedation, adjunct sedation agent, and with propofol intolerance

CRITICAL CARE MEDICINE

CRITICAL CARE MEDICINE

TABLE 3.12 · Neuromuscular Blocking Agents

Generic Name (Trade Name)	Typical Dosing	Pharmacokinetics	Notes	Adverse Events
vecuronium	• Bolus/Load: 0.08–0.1 mg/kg • Maintenance Drip Range: 0.8–1.7 mcg/kg/min	• Duration: 45 min • Metabolism: Kidney, liver	Shorter acting than rocuronium	• Prolonged paralysis • Myopathy • Requires higher levels of sedation with associated side effects given required RASS -5
rocuronium	• Bolus/Load: 0.6–1.0 mg/kg • Maintenance Drip Range: 4–12 mcg/kg/min	• Onset: 60–90 sec • Duration: 25–60 min	Used for rapid sequence intubation (RSI) given quick onset of action	
cisatracurium (Nimbex)	• Bolus/Load: 0.1–0.2 mg/kg • Maintenance Drip Range: 0.5–10 mcg/kg/min	• Duration: 45–60 min • Metabolism: Hoffman degradation (immediate metabolization in the serum without reliance on organs)	Expensive and not always readily available	

TABLE 3.13 · Vasopressors

Generic Name (Trade Name)	Mechanism/ Receptor Binding	Clinical Effects	Usage	Typical Dose	Side Effects
epinephrine, "epi" (Adrenaline)	α1 (at high dose), α2, β1 (at low dose), β2	Increased HR Increased SVR Increased CO	Shock (cardiogenic, distributive), ACLS/cardiac arrest, bronchospasm, anaphylactic shock (first line)	ACLS: 1 mg IV q3–5min Anaphylactic shock: 0.1 mg IV or 0.3 mg IM ("EpiPen" is for IM only) Shock maintenance drip range: 0.1–0.5 mcg/kg/min	• Arrhythmias • Cardiac ischemia • Intracranial hemorrhage
norepinephrine (Levophed, "Levo")	α1 and β1 agonist	Increased SVR Increased CO	First-choice pressor for shock: Septic/distributive, cardiogenic, mixed	Maintenance Drip Range: 1–30 mcg/min or weight-based dosing	• Arrhythmia • Digital ischemia
vasopressin, "vaso" (Pitressin)	V1 and V2 receptors: ADH in kidney/spleen; generalized vasoconstriction via cAMP	Increased SVR Limited effect on PVR	Septic shock (second line), VT/VF/PEA arrest Shock in pulmonary HTN	Maintenance Drip Range: 0.01–0.04 units/min Max Maintenance Drip Rate: 0.07 units/min	• Coronary, peripheral vasoconstriction can lead to ischemia • Arrhythmias • Skin necrosis
phenylephrine (Neo Synephrine, "Neo")	α1 agonist	Increased SVR	Distributive shock, can be useful in tachyarrhythmias	Maintenance Drip Range: 20–200 mcg/min or 0.5–6 mcg/kg/min	• Renal or peripheral vasoconstriction can lead to hypoperfusion • Reflex bradycardia • Metabolic acidosis • Skin necrosis
Dopamine	Low dose (1–2 mcg/kg/min): D1 agonist Medium dose (5–20 mcg/kg/min): β1 > D1 agonist High dose: α1 > β1 > D1	Increased CO	Bradycardia and cardiogenic shock Can augment diuresis, although no clear protective benefit for the kidneys	Initial Maintenance Drip Rate: 2–5 mcg/kg/min Max Maintenance Drip: 20 mcg/kg/min	• Natriuretic effect • Tachycardia and arrhythmias at higher doses • Hyperglycemia

CRITICAL CARE MEDICINE

CRITICAL CARE MEDICINE

TABLE 3.14 · Inotropes					
Generic Name	Mechanism/ Receptor Binding	Clinical Effects	Usage	Typical Dose	Side Effects
dobutamine	Mainly β1 with some β2	Increased HR, SV and CO Decreases SVR	Increases cardiac output in cardiogenic shock	• Initial Maintenance Drip Rate: 0.5–1 mcg/kg/min • Maintenance Drip Range: 2–20 mcg/kg/min • Set rate based on desired SVR, hemodynamics and should NOT be titrated by nursing, only manual	• Tachycardia • Hypotension • Arrhythmias • Angina • Tachyphylaxis
isoproterenol	β1 and β2 agonist	Increased HR and CO	Intractable bradycardia, torsades not responding to magnesium (increased HR decreases QTc)	Bradyarrhythmia • Maintenance Drip Range: 2–10 mcg/min	• Vasodilation can decrease MAP and cause hypotension • Arrhythmias • Angina
milrinone	Inhibits phosphodiesterase III	Increased CO Decreases SVR and PVR	Similar to dobutamine	• Bolus/Load: 50 mcg/kg over 10 min • Maintenance Drip Range: 0.125–0.75 mcg/kg/min, decrease if renal dysfunction	• Hypotension • Arrhythmias • Accumulates in renal failure (relative contraindication)

KEY CLINICAL TRIALS AND PUBLICATIONS
Shock Management
- **SMART Trial**. *New Engl J Med* 2018;378(9):829–839.
  - Multicenter, cluster-randomized, multiple crossover trial that randomized over 15,000 critically ill adult patients to receive saline (0.9% sodium chloride) or balanced crystalloids (Lactated Ringer's solution or Plasma-Lyte A). Use of balanced crystalloids for fluid resuscitation in critically ill patients resulted in lower rate of the composite outcome of death from any cause, new renal replacement therapy, or persistent renal dysfunction than the use of saline.
- **Rivers Trial.** *New Engl J Med* 2001;345(19):1368–1377.
  - Single-center, parallel-group, randomized controlled clinical trial that randomized 263 patients with severe sepsis or septic shock to either early goal-directed therapy or standard care. Early goal-directed therapy included several goals in the ER prior to ICU admission: CVP 8–12 mmHg achieved with fluid boluses, MAP >65 mmHg achieved with vasopressors if necessary, $ScvO_2$ >70% achieved with PRBC transfusions and dobutamine if necessary, and urine output >0.5 mL/kg/hour. In this study, early goal-directed therapy for severe sepsis and septic shock showed mortality benefit vs. standard therapy. More recent studies have not shown this protocolized approach to be better than standard of care, likely because standard care involves many components of this process. However, targeting a CVP of 8–12 mmHg and transfusing pRBC for low $ScvO_2$ is no longer routine care.

Acute Respiratory Distress Syndrome (ARDS)
- **Berlin Definition**. *JAMA* 2012;307(23):2526–2533.
  - This paper defines the ARDS Berlin criteria based on a consensus process by a panel of experts convened in 2011.
- **ARMA.** *New Engl J Med* 2000;342(18):1301–1308.
  - Multicenter randomized controlled trial that randomized patients with ARDS to ventilation with a lung-protective strategy using lower tidal volumes of 6 mL/kg of predicted body weight (PBW) (goal plateau pressure 25–30 mmHg) vs. conventional mechanical ventilation using tidal volumes of 12 mL/kg of PBW (goal plateau pressure 45–50 mmHg). The use of low tidal volume ventilation (initial TV 6 mL/kg PBW) improved mortality and reduced ventilator-free days compared to traditional tidal volumes (12 mL/kg).
- **ALVEOLI Trial.** *New Engl J Med* 2004;351(4):327–336.
  - Multicenter, randomized controlled clinical trial that randomized 549 patients with ARDS to receive mechanical ventilation with either lower or higher PEEP levels, set according to different tables of predetermined combinations of PEEP and fraction of inspired oxygen. Among patients with ARDS who received low tidal volume ventilation of 6 mL/kg of predicted body weight and an end-inspiratory plateau pressure limit of 30 cm H_2O, there were no differences in clinical outcomes whether lower or higher PEEP levels were used.
- **ACURASYS.** *New Engl J Med* 2010;363(12):1107–1116.
  - Multicenter, double-blinded, placebo-controlled trial that randomized 340 patients with early severe ARDS (P/F <150) in French ICUs to cisatracurium-induced paralysis or placebo for 48 hours. Paralysis with cisatracurium within 48 hours of severe ARDS onset was associated with improved mortality.
- **FACTT Trial.** *New Engl J Med* 2006;354(24):2564–2575.
  - Multicenter, two-by-two factorial, randomized controlled trial that randomized 1000 patients with acute lung injury (ALI)/ARDS to a conservative fluid management strategy targeting a CVP <4 mmHg vs. a liberal fluid management strategy targeting a CVP 10–14 mmHg. The conservative fluid strategy improved lung function, decreased ventilator days, and decreased ICU days compared to a liberal fluid strategy, although there was no difference in mortality between groups.
- **PROSEVA Trial.** *New Engl J Med* 2013;368(23):2159–2168.
  - Multicenter, randomized, open-label trial that randomized 466 patients with severe ARDS to early (<36 hours after intubation) or lengthy (goal 16 hours/day) intermittent prone positioning versus a standard supine position. In patients with severe ARDS, early and prolonged proning was associated with improved 28-day mortality.

CRITICAL CARE MEDICINE

NOTES

Gastroenterology

4

Structure and Innervation of the GI Tract

- Components: The GI tract includes epithelial cells (specialized for absorption/secretion), muscularis mucosa (changes surface area for absorption/secretion), circular muscle (decreases the diameter of the lumen), and longitudinal muscle (shortens a segment of the GI tract)
- Extrinsic innervation: May be parasympathetic (excitatory, via the vagus/pelvic nerve) or sympathetic (usually inhibitory)
- Intrinsic innervation: Coordinates extrinsic signals and uses local GI reflexes to modify motility (via the myenteric plexus) and secretion/blood flow (via the submucosal plexus)

The Neuroendocrine System of the Gut

Classification of GI regulatory substances

- Hormones: Released from endocrine cells in the GI tract into the portal circulation. They enter the systemic circulation and then act on target cells
- Paracrines: Released from endocrine cells in the GI tract, diffuse locally, and then act on target cells
- Neurocrines: Synthesized by neurons in the GI tract, released by action potentials across the synaptic cleft, and then act on target cells

GI regulatory substances

- Gastrin: Hormone. Produced by G cells in the stomach, stimulated by high pH, stomach distention. Action: Increases H^+ secretion, gastric motility.
- Gastrin-releasing peptide (GRP): Neurocrine. Released from the vagus nerve and act on G cells. Action: Stimulates gastrin release.
- Histamine: Paracrine. Secreted by mast cells in the stomach. Action: Increases H^+ directly and by potentiating effects of gastrin/vagal nerve stimulation.
- Cholecystokinin (CCK): Hormone. Produced by I cells in the small intestine, stimulated by fatty acids/amino acids. Action: Stimulates pancreatic secretion, gallbladder contraction.

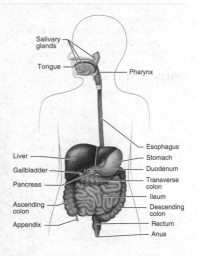

FIGURE 4.1: Anatomy of the gastrointestinal tract.

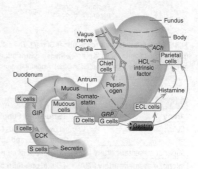

FIGURE 4.2: Locations and functions of the GI secretory cells. The secretory cells are indicated in blue and their secreted hormone products are shown with arrows and indicated in black. Abbreviations: Acetylcholine (Ach), hydrochloric acid (HCl), enterochromaffin-like (ECL), gastrin-releasing peptide (GRP), gastric inhibitory polypeptide (GIP), cholecystokinin (CCK), gastrin cells (G cells), delta cells (D cells).

- Secretin: Hormone. Produced by S cells in the small intestine, stimulated by fatty acids and low pH. Action: Increases pancreatic HCO_3^- and bile secretion.
- Glucose-dependent insulinotropic peptide (GIP): Hormone. Produced by K cells in the small intestine, stimulated by fatty acids, amino acids, and oral glucose. Action: Decreases gastric acid secretion, increases insulin release.
- Vasoactive intestinal polypeptide (VIP): Neurocrine. Released by the parasympathetic ganglia in the intestine, stimulated by stomach distention and the vagal nerve. Action: Stimulates pancreatic HCO_3^- secretion, inhibits H^+ secretion, promotes relaxation of sphincters.
- Somatostatin: Paracrine. Produced by D cells, stimulated by vagal stimulation and low pH. Action: Decreases gastric acid secretion, gallbladder contraction, and pancreatic secretion.

Gastric secretions
- HCl: Produced by parietal cells in the stomach. Stimulated by histamine, vagal stimulation (via ACh), and gastrin. Inhibited by somatostatin, prostaglandin, and chyme. Action: Decreases stomach pH to promote food digestion.
- Pepsin: Produced by chief cells in the stomach. Stimulated by vagal stimulation (via ACh), local acid. Action: Stimulates protein digestion.
- Bicarbonate (HCO_3^-): Neutralizes acid.

Vasculature of the GI Tract

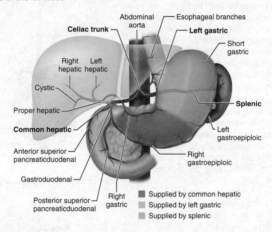

FIGURE 4.3: **Arterial supply to the upper GI tract.** The celiac trunk gives rise to the common hepatic artery (supplies the region shaded in purple), the left gastric artery (supplies the region shaded in green), and the splenic artery (supplies the region shaded in blue). Additional arterial branches supply the proximal duodenum, liver, gallbladder, pancreas, and spleen.

TABLE 4.1 · Vascular Supply to the Upper and Lower GI Tract	
Artery	**Structures Supplied**
Celiac	Low esophagus to the proximal duodenum; liver, gallbladder, pancreas, and spleen
Superior mesenteric artery (SMA)	Distal duodenum to the proximal two-thirds of the transverse colon
Inferior mesenteric artery (IMA)	Distal one-third of the transverse colon to the upper portion of the rectum

DIAGNOSTICS

TABLE 4.2 · Diagnostic Tests in Gastroenterology

Study	Indication	Procedure Details

Upper endoscopy (EGD)	• Diagnosis: Upper GI bleed (UGIB), iron-deficiency anemia, diarrhea with features of small bowel disease (e.g., celiac), refractory GERD, dysphagia, odynophagia, upper abdominal symptoms with alarm features (e.g., unintentional weight loss, early satiety)
	• Treatment:
	  - UGIB: Injections, thermals/cautery, mechanical clipping
	  - Varices: Variceal banding
	  - Achalasia, stenosis, strictures
	  - Pneumatic dilation, stent placement
	  - Malignancy: Stent placement, resection
	• Screening: Barrett's esophagus, upper GI malignancies in high-risk patients
		• Prep: NPO for >8 hr
		• Sedation: Options include moderate sedation, monitored anesthesia care, general anesthesia
		• Procedure: Endoscope inserted through the mouth and advanced through the esophagus, stomach, and as far as to the second portion of duodenum. Biopsies and therapeutics can be performed as indicated.
		• Push enteroscopy: Variation of an EGD that utilizes a longer endoscope, which makes it possible to advance beyond the ligament of Treitz and into the jejunum.

Colonoscopy	• Diagnosis: Lower GI bleed (LGIB), iron-deficiency anemia, lower GI symptoms (e.g., chronic diarrhea), evaluation for IBD
	• Treatment:
	  - LGIB: Injections, thermals/cautery, mechanical clipping
	  - Polyp removal
	  - Decompression of sigmoid volvulus/ colonic pseudo-obstruction
	  - Balloon dilation of strictures
	• Screening: Colorectal cancer (CRC)
		• Prep: Clear liquids × 1 day prior with bowel prep, NPO at least 2 hr
		• Sedation: Options include no sedation, moderate sedation, monitored anesthesia care, general anesthesia
		• Procedure: Colonoscope inserted through the anus and advanced through the rectum, large bowel, and small bowel up to the cecum/terminal ileum. Biopsies and therapeutics can be performed as indicated.

Flexible sigmoidoscopy	• Diagnosis: LGIB, iron-deficiency anemia, lower GI symptoms (e.g., chronic diarrhea), surveillance for IBD. • Treatment: Polyp removal • Screening: CRC (alternative to colonoscopy, q5yr)	• Prep: Less involved than colonoscopy: Enemas × 2 • Sedation: None (benefit over colonoscopy) • Procedure: Colonoscope inserted through the anus and advanced through the rectum and up to the distal 60 cm of the colon (up to the splenic flexure). Misses proximal/right-sided lesions. Thus, colonoscopy is preferred for CRC screening.
Capsule endoscopy	• Diagnosis only: Iron-deficiency anemia with normal EGD/colonoscopy, small bowel tumor, Crohn's disease.	• Prep: NPO for 12 hr • Procedure: The patient swallows a video capsule. An external wireless recorder captures images of the entire GI tract while the capsule is in transit, and then the footage is analyzed. Capsules are disposable and excreted with a bowel movement.

(continued)

TABLE 4.2 · Diagnostic Tests in Gastroenterology (*Continued*)

Study	Indication	Procedure Details

Endoscopic retrograde cholangiopancreatography (ERCP)	• Diagnosis/Treatment: Typically performed when both a diagnostic/ therapeutic indication are present, such as to evaluate and possibly treat the following conditions:
	  - Suspected biliary obstruction
	  - Suspected pancreatic/biliary malignancy
	  - Acute pancreatitis with cholangitis or biliary obstruction
	  - Choledocholithiasis
	  - Biliary dyskinesia
	  - Biliary strictures
	  - Pancreatic pseudocyst drainage
	• Limitation: Difficult to perform in Roux-en-Y anatomy
		• Prep: Pregnancy testing, coagulation studies, NPO for 8 hr
		• Sedation: Monitored anesthesia care or general anesthesia
		• Procedure: Combined endoscopic/ fluoroscopic procedure. Duodenoscope is advanced through the mouth and to the duodenum. A catheter is then inserted into the papilla of Vater and contrast is injected. X-rays are taken of the biliary tree and pancreatic duct. May perform sphincterotomy, stent placement, CBD stone extraction, and/or dilation of strictures.
		• Complications: >5% risk: Acute pancreatitis, bleeding, cholangitis/ sepsis, perforation

Endoscopic ultrasound (EUS)	• Diagnosis: Pancreatic cancer with FNA, choledocholithiasis, submucosal masses of stomach, duodenum, rectum. • Treatment: Pancreatic fluid collection drainage, celiac plexus neurolysis (improves pain control in pancreatic cancer)	• Prep: NPO for 8 hr • Sedation: Monitored anesthesia care, general anesthesia • Procedure: Endoscope with an ultrasound transducer is advanced through the mouth and down to the duodenum. Enables clearer view of the pancreas. Can be done in conjunction with FNA.
Magnetic resonance cholangiopancreatography (MRCP)	• Diagnosis only: Choledocholithiasis, biliary strictures, chronic pancreatitis, suspected congenital anomaly of pancreaticobiliary tract, preop/postop evaluation of biliary abnormalities	• Prep: NPO for 4 hr • Procedure: Same as MRI scan. Allows for better visualization of pancreaticobiliary tract
Barium swallow	• Diagnosis only: Dysphagia, esophageal perforation, hiatal hernia, malignancy, diverticula, esophageal motility disorders (e.g., achalasia, diffuse esophageal spasm)	• Procedure: The patient is put in a prone or supine position with tilt and then instructed to rapidly swallow barium contrast (100–200 cc). X-ray or fluoroscopy is used to evaluate the patient's swallow, enabling the localization of lesions and the initial identification of some esophageal pathologies. • Classic findings: "Bird beak" appearance of achalasia, "corkscrew sign" in diffuse esophageal spasm
Esophageal manometry	• Diagnosis only: Esophageal motility disorders (e.g., achalasia, hypercontractile esophagus, distal esophageal spasm)	• Procedure: Can be conventional or high resolution (more pressure sensors). A long tube is positioned in the esophagus terminating in the stomach. The patient is instructed to swallow, and then the system detects pressure changes generated by the esophagus or the upper/lower esophageal sphincter.
Ambulatory pH monitoring	• Diagnosis only: GERD	• Procedure: Options include a transnasally placed catheter or a wireless capsule that is fixed to the distal mucosa. pH sensor results are analyzed after 24 hr to 4 days.

APPROACHES AND CHIEF COMPLAINTS

Abdominal Pain

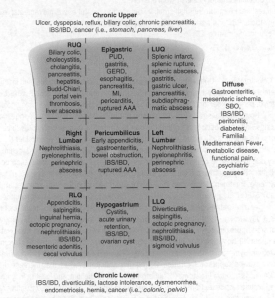

Chronic Upper
Ulcer, dyspepsia, reflux, biliary colic, chronic pancreatitis,
IBS/IBD, cancer (i.e., *stomach, pancreas, liver*)

RUQ
Biliary colic, cholecystitis, cholangitis, pancreatitis, hepatitis, Budd-Chiari, portal vein thrombosis, liver abscess

Epigastric
PUD, gastritis, GERD, esophagitis, pancreatitis, MI, pericarditis, ruptured AAA

LUQ
Splenic infarct, splenic rupture, splenic abscess, gastritis, gastric ulcer, pancreatitis, subdiaphragmatic abscess

Diffuse
Gastroenteritis, mesenteric ischemia, SBO, IBS/IBD, peritonitis, diabetes, Familial Mediterranean Fever, metabolic disease, functional pain, psychiatric causes

Right Lumbar
Nephrolithiasis, pyelonephritis, perinephric abscess

Pericumbilicus
Early appendicitis, gastroenteritis, bowel obstruction, IBS/IBD, ruptured AAA

Left Lumbar
Nephrolithiasis, pyelonephritis, perinephric abscess

RLQ
Appendicitis, salpingitis, inguinal hernia, ectopic pregnancy, nephrolithiasis, IBS/IBD, mesenteric adenitis, cecal volvulus

Hypogastrium
Cystitis, acute urinary retention, IBS/IBD, ovarian cyst

LLQ
Diverticulitis, salpingitis, ectopic pregnancy, nephrolithiasis, IBS/IBD, sigmoid volvulus

Chronic Lower
IBS/IBD, diverticulitis, lactose intolerance, dysmenorrhea,
endometriosis, hernia, cancer (i.e., *colonic, pelvic*)

FIGURE 4.4: **Differential diagnosis for abdominal pain based on area of pain.** Shown are the regions of the abdomen and the differential diagnosis for pain in each region. Of note, pain does not always localize precisely, so no matter the location of the pain, consider a broad differential diagnosis. Abbreviations: AAA, abdominal aortic aneurysm; IBD, inflammatory bowel disease; IBS, irritable bowel syndrome; SBO, small bowl obstruction; MI, myocardial infarction; PUD, peptic ulcer disease; RUQ, right upper quadrant; RLQ, right lower quadrant; LUQ, left upper quadrant; LLQ, left lower quadrant.

Nausea/Vomiting

Differential diagnosis:

- Neuropsychiatric:
  - Intracerebral: Increased intracranial pressure (ICP) due to malignancy, hemorrhage, abscess, hydrocephalus
  - Labyrinthine: Labyrinthitis, motion sickness, malignancy
  - Psychiatric: Anorexia, bulimia nervosa, depression (may be associated with delayed gastric emptying)
- Cardiopulmonary: Myocardial infarction, congestive heart failure (nausea/early satiety can be early symptoms), post-tussive emesis
- Gastrointestinal:
  - Obstructive: Pyloric obstruction, SBO, colonic obstruction, SMA syndrome
  - Inflammatory: Enteric infections (viral, bacterial), cholecystitis, cholangitis, pancreatitis, appendicitis, hepatitis
  - Altered function/functional: Gastroparesis, ileus, pseudo-obstruction, GERD, cyclic vomiting syndrome, cannabinoid hyperemesis syndrome
  - Other: Medications, pregnancy, uremia, DKA/HHS, thyroid disease

Diarrhea

- Definitions/mimics:
  - <u>Diarrhea</u>: Passage of abnormally liquid or unformed stools at an increased frequency from baseline
  - <u>Pseudo-diarrhea</u>: Frequent passage of <u>small</u> volumes of stool, often accompanied by tenesmus, sensation of incomplete evacuation, or rectal urgency; commonly associated with IBS or proctitis
  - <u>Fecal incontinence</u>: Involuntary fecal discharge, usually due to neuromuscular etiologies or anorectal structural etiologies; however, severe diarrhea may aggravate or result in fecal incontinence

- "Localizing" features: These features may be present, but are non-specific
  - Small intestine: Watery, large volume, associated with abdominal cramping, bloating, gas; fever, occult blood/inflammatory cells in stool are rare
  - Large intestine: Frequent, regular, small volume, often painful bowel movements; fever, bloody or mucoid stools, RBCs/inflammatory cells in stool are common
- Clinical features: See Table 4.3

Acute Diarrhea (<3 weeks)
Infection
Bloody:

- Shigella: Colonic infection. Outbreaks frequently occur in institutions (e.g., daycare) and in food supply (e.g., raw vegetables contaminated with feces). Transmission can also occur by sexual contact, contaminated food/water, or person to person. Incubation period averages 3 days. Treatment: Fluroquinolone.
- Salmonella: Nontyphoidal species cause gastroenteritis. Most commonly due to ingestion of infected poultry, eggs, milk products; less commonly due to contact with pets or reptiles. Incubation period <72 hours. Treatment: Self-limited, provide support/rehydration; if severe, consider fluroquinolone.
- Campylobacter: Infection that involves the jejunum, ileum, and often the colon and rectum. Transmission commonly due to ingestion of undercooked or raw meat, especially poultry. Incubation period averages 3 days. Higher risk for reactive arthritis if HLAB27+. Also a well-established and classic trigger for Guillain-Barré syndrome. Treatment: Self-limited, provide support/rehydration; if severe, consider azithromycin.
- *E. coli* O157/STEC ("Shiga toxin–producing *E. coli*"): Classically from exposure to undercooked food (especially beef) or petting zoos; person-to-person transmission can also occur. Incubation period averages 3 days (range 1–10 days). Classic presentation is diarrhea, abdominal pain, vomiting, and fever that start approximately 72 hours after ingestion, followed by conversion from watery to bloody diarrhea about 48 hours later. If TTP-HUS occurs (i.e., fever, hemolytic anemia, thrombocytopenia, AKI, neurologic symptoms), the onset is typically 1–2 weeks after the onset of diarrhea. Treatment: Self limited, provide support/rehydration. Do *not* give antibiotics, which may increase the risk of HUS.
- Yersinia: Can pass through the stomach, adhere to the gut epithelium, and localize in lymphoid tissue to evade the immune response. Transmission largely foodborne (especially pork consumption), but can also be due to consumption of untreated spring water, transmission from household pets, or in extremely rare cases from pRBC transfusions. Incubation averages 5 days. Clinically, can cause acute yersiniosis (febrile gastroenteritis) or a pseudo-appendicitis syndrome (fever, milder diarrhea, RLQ pain). Can also cause an autoimmune-type thyroiditis, pericarditis, or glomerulonephritis. Treatment: Self limited, provide support/rehydration; if severe use fluroquinolone or TMP-SMX.
- *Entamoeba histolytica* (amebiasis): Parasite transmitted via fecal-oral route. Clinically, causes bloody diarrhea, typically with subacute symptom onset (over 1–3 weeks). Can also cause liver abscesses. Diagnosis: O&P, stool antigen testing. Treatment: Metronidazole + paromomycin, diiodohydroxyquinoline, or diloxanide furoate.

Non-bloody:

- Any cause of bloody diarrhea can also present with non-bloody diarrhea
- Viruses:
  - Rotavirus: Transmitted via fecal-oral route with an incubation period of <48 hours. Most commonly infects young children or those with a sick household contact. The virus activates the enteric nervous system, releases direct enterotoxin, and destroys patches of the brush border (resulting in osmotic diarrhea). Classically presents with diarrhea, vomiting. Treatment: Self limited, provide support/rehydration.
  - Norovirus: Transmitted via fecal-oral route, by airborne droplets of vomit, or by contaminated food or water with an incubation period of <48 hours. The virus decreases intestinal brush border activity and reduces fat absorption. Classically presents with diarrhea, vomiting. Treatment: Self limited, provide support/rehydration.
- Bacteria:
  - *Clostridium perfringens*: Commonly due to consumption of improperly refrigerated meat. Incubation period averages 12 hours. Treatment: Self limited, provide support/rehydration.
  - *B. cereus*: Classically, infection is due to consumption of reheated rice. More commonly causes vomiting than diarrhea. Treatment: Self limited, provide support/rehydration.
  - *E. coli* ("traveler's diarrhea"/ETEC): Fecal-oral transmission. Causes malaise, anorexia, abdominal cramps, followed by sudden-onset diarrhea. Treatment: Self limited, provide support/rehydration; if severe, consider fluoroquinolone or azithromycin.
  - *Vibrio vulnificus*: Transmitted by consumption of infected shellfish; higher risk for infection if the patient has underlying disease or heavy alcohol use. Treatment: Self limited, provide support/rehydration; if severe, consider doxycycline or fluroquinolone.
  - *Clostridium difficile* (*C.diff*): See Infectious Diseases Chapter 8.

- Parasites:
  - Only test for parasites if diarrhea for 7+ days
  - <u>Giardia</u>: Transmission from contaminated water (e.g., outdoor streams), or can occur person-to-person (e.g., via sexual contact). Incubation period 7–14 days. Classic presentation is steatorrhea (foul-smelling, fatty stool) with long-standing malabsorption (symptoms may last up to 4 weeks). Treatment: Tinidazole or nitazoxanide; alternative is metronidazole.

Medications
- Medications that may cause diarrhea: Antibiotics (via side effects; also increase risk for *C. difficile* infection), laxatives, prokinetic agents, antacids, digitalis, colchicine, chemotherapy agents, alcohol

"Early chronic diarrhea"
- Malabsorption/inflammatory: Small intestine bacterial overgrowth (SIBO), celiac disease, exocrine pancreatic insufficiency
- Ischemia: Colonic ischemia
- Neuropathic: Diabetic autonomic neuropathy (DAN)
- Functional: Irritable bowel syndrome (IBS)

Chronic Diarrhea (>3 weeks)
- Work-up:
  - Use history/physical to determine the probable subtype of diarrhea (i.e., watery, fatty, or inflammatory)
  - Send further diagnostics from the stool based on the suspected subtype (watery = stool osms; fatty = fecal fat; inflammatory = stool RBC/WBC, consider fecal calprotectin)
  - Pursue additional testing based on narrowed differential diagnosis
- Etiologies: See Table 4.3

Diarrhea in a Patient with HIV and a Low CD4 Count
May be due to a common cause, but also consider the following broader differential diagnosis:
- Infectious etiologies:
  - Bacterial: *Campylobacter*, *Shigella*, *Salmonella*, *Escherichia coli*, *Clostridium difficile*
  - Mycobacteria: MAC (diarrhea, fever; treatment: macrolide + ethambutol or rifabutin)
  - Viral: CMV (CD4 <50 cells/μL; diarrhea, colitis, rarely perforation; treatment: PO valganciclovir)
  - Fungal: *Microsporidium*, disseminated histoplasmosis
  - Parasites: *Giardia, Entamoeba histolytica, Strongyloides, Cryptosporidium*
- Other:
  - HIV enteropathy
  - HIV-associated malignancy
  - Pancreatic insufficiency
  - Antiretroviral (ARV)-associated diarrhea
  - Other non-infectious causes of diarrhea (other medications, IBD, etc.)

GI Bleed

Upper GI bleed (UGIB, i.e., above the ligament of Treitz)
- Clinical features:
  - Hematemesis (bright red blood in vomit suggests a more rapid bleed; "coffee ground" emesis suggests a slower bleed)
  - Melena (black tarry stool, caused by degradation of hemoglobin by bacteria; typically patients have a high BUN dissociated from Cr with UGIB due to urea production from blood breakdown)
  - A brisk UGIB can cause bright red blood per rectum
- Causes of UGIB:
  - Peptic ulcer disease (50%)
  - Esophageal varices (10–30%)
  - Gastropathy, gastritis, duodenitis (15%)
  - Severe or erosive esophagitis (10%)
  - Mallory-Weiss tear (10%)
  - Other: Tumor, Dieulafoy's lesion (arterial malformation which can cause a massive UGIB), aortoenteric fistula (after aortic surgery; ask patients about prior aortic repairs), Cameron's lesion (linear erosion near a hiatal hernia), hemobilia, hemosuccus pancreaticus

TABLE 4.3 ·	Types of Chronic Diarrhea: Clinical Features, Diagnostics, and Etiologies			
	Secretory	**Osmotic**	**Malabsorptive**	**Inflammatory**
Diarrheal type	Watery*	Watery*	Fatty (excess flatulence, foul-smelling, floating)	Blood/pus in stool
Mechanism	Increased secretion or decreased absorption of water/electrolytes	Presence of poorly absorbed, osmotically active substance with resultant intraluminal water retention	Impaired nutrient absorption and impaired digestive function	Inflammation or invasive infections
Effect of fasting	No effect	No effect	Improves	Improves
Diagnostics	Low fecal osm gap (<50 mOsm/kg)**	High fecal osm gap (>125 mOsm/kg)**	Fecal fat	Fecal WBCs/RBCs, fecal calprotectin, colonoscopy with inflammation
Examples	• Alcohol use • Enterotoxins (e.g., cholera) • Bile acid malabsorption • SIBO • Medications • Nonosmotic laxatives • Early Crohn's • Endocrine disorders (e.g., thyroid) • Neuroendocrine tumors • Vasculitis	• Lactose/fructose malabsorption • Celiac disease • Osmotic laxatives • Sugar alcohols (e.g., mannitol, sorbitol)	• Lactose intolerance • Noninvasive parasite (e.g., giardia) • SIBO • Celiac sprue (gluten enteropathy) • Tropical sprue • Whipple disease • Pancreatic insufficiency • Medications (e.g., orlistat, acarbose) • Lymphatic damage • Mesenteric ischemia • Gastric bypass • Postresection diarrhea • Short bowel syndrome	• IBD • Diverticulitis • Invasive infections (e.g., *C. diff.*, yersiniosis, entamoeba) • Ulcerating viruses (e.g., CMV, HSV) • Neoplasia • Radiation colitis

*Chronic watery diarrhea may also be **functional**, most commonly due to IBS; organic causes of chronic diarrhea are suggested by weight loss >5 kg, nocturnal diarrhea, GIB, anemia, hypoalbuminemia, and elevated inflammatory markers.

**Fecal osmotic gap: 290 − 2(fecal sodium + fecal K). If <50 mOsm/kg suggests secretory, 50–125 mOsm/kg equivocal, >125 mOsm/kg suggests osmotic

Lower GI bleed (LGIB, i.e., below the ligament of Treitz)
  • Clinical features: Hematochezia (bright red blood per rectum)
  • Causes of LGIB:
    - Diverticulosis (30%)
    - Malignancy (20%), which often causes occult bleeding
    - Colitis (20%) – ischemic, IBD, radiation
    - Hemorrhoids (15%)
    - Other: Postpolypectomy, solitary rectal ulcer, angiodysplasia, arteriovenous malformation (AVM), pediatrics: Meckel's diverticulum

Obscure GI bleed (i.e., bleeding of unknown cause)
  • Definition: GIB with negative EGD/colonoscopy, which is often presumed to represent an unvisualized small bowel bleed
  • Causes of obscure GIB: Angiodysplasia is the most common cause
  • Diagnosis: Testing options include:
    - Repeat EGD/colonoscopy: Assesses for lesions that may have been missed on first attempt.
    - Capsule endoscopy: Now considered the first-line diagnostic test in the evaluation of obscure GI bleeds (except in the presence of a stricture, which increases the risk of capsule retention; consider deep enteroscopy instead in this setting).

- Technetium-labeled nuclear scan: Can detect general area of bleeding; requires follow-up study.
- Angiography: Can identify bleed if rate >0.5mL/min; allows for intervention such as selective mesenteric embolization, but contrast exposure is high.
- Push enteroscopy: Advancement of endoscope beyond the ligament of Treitz into the jejunum; angiodysplasia is the most common lesion that is found.
- Deep enteroscopy: Surveys the entire small bowel. Techniques include spiral enteroscopy, single- or double-balloon enteroscopy. Risk of small bowel perforation.

Approach to managing a patient with a GIB
- Assess hemodynamic stability and ability to resuscitate:
  - Verify IV access; patient should have at least two large-bore IVs
  - Ensure access to blood products (i.e., verify active type & screen; if rapid/hemodynamically significant bleed, consider activation of massive transfusion protocol)
- Obtain additional historical details and data:
  - History: Symptoms, timing, severity, risk factors, prior GIBs
  - ROS: Medications (anticoagulation, aspirin, NSAIDs; steroid use), *H. pylori* risk or history, alcohol use, history of liver disease
  - Exam: Vital signs, rectal exam; consider nasogastric lavage
  - Labs: CBC, PT/PTT, type & screen, BMP (look for isolated BUN elevation in UGIB), LFTs
- Treatment:
  - **Upper GIB:** Admit to the hospital. Place ≥2 large-bore IVs (18 gauge or larger), make patient NPO, fluid resuscitate, order type and screen, transfuse blood products as needed, and administer an IV PPI prior to EGD. If a variceal bleed suspected, also: 1) IV octreotide; 2) IV ceftriaxone; 3) Urgent EGD. If bleeding cannot be stopped by an EGD, consider embolization by interventional radiology or surgery.
  - **Lower GIB:** Usually self-limited, but manage as above with admission, fluid resuscitation, and transfusion of blood products if severe/ongoing. Can consider colonoscopy for ongoing bleeding or high-risk features within 24 hours.
  - **Transfusion threshold:**
    - Transfuse based on a Hgb threshold *only* if the patient is relatively stable and not demonstrating severe active bleeding at the bedside
    - Most commonly used transfusion threshold: Hgb <7 g/dL, which is associated with improved mortality compared to a higher transfusion threshold (TRICC Trial, *New Eng J Med* 1999)
    - Hgb <8 g/dL may be considered in patients with ongoing bleeding and/or acute coronary syndrome with ischemia

Jaundice
- Definition: Yellow discoloration of sclerae of the eyes, mucous membranes, and/or skin due to overproduction or inadequate clearance of bilirubin. Scleral icterus is usually evident if bilirubin >3 mg/dL, sublingual icterus if bilirubin >4 mg/dL, and skin is jaundiced if bilirubin >6 mg/dL.
- Diagnosis: Check whether bilirubin is unconjugated (indirect) or conjugated (direct) and then consider differential diagnosis for each type as below.
  - **Unconjugated (indirect) bilirubin:** Tightly bound to albumin and not water soluble so cannot be excreted; can cross blood–brain-barrier and cause neurologic deficits.
    - Differential diagnosis:
      - Excess production bilirubin: Hemolytic anemia
      - Reduced hepatic uptake of bilirubin or impaired conjugation: Gilbert's, Crigler-Najjar, diffuse liver disease (hepatitis, cirrhosis), medications (sulfonamides, penicillin, rifampin, radiocontrast)
        - Gilbert's: Autosomal dominant disorder that causes decreased activity of the uridine diphosphate glucuronyl transferase. Causes mild jaundice with fasting. Does not need to be treated.
        - Crigler-Najjar: Autosomal recessive disorder caused by mutations in the gene encoding for uridine diphosphate glucuronyl transferase (UGT1A1).
          - Type I: Infants with severe jaundice and kernicterus; requires liver transplantation
          - Type II: Adults. Treatment: Phenobarbital, clofibrate
  - **Conjugated (direct) bilirubin:** Loosely bound to albumin so water soluble, causing dark urine or pale stool when excreted
    - Differential diagnosis:
      - Decreased intrahepatic excretion of bilirubin: Hepatocellular disease (viral, alcoholic hepatitis, cirrhosis), inherited disorders (Dubin-Johnson, Rotor's syndrome), oral contraceptive pills, primary sclerosing cholangitis (PSC), primary biliary sclerosis (PBC), biliary atresia
      - Extrahepatic: Gallstones, pancreatic carcinoma, cholangiocarcinoma, periampullary tumors, extrahepatic biliary atresia

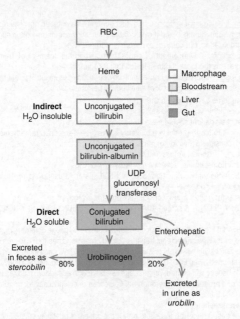

FIGURE 4.5: Breakdown and elimination of bilirubin. Bilirubin is derived from two main sources: approximately 80% is produced by the breakdown of hemoglobin in red blood cells (RBCs) and prematurely destroyed erythroid cells in the bone marrow, and the rest comes from the turnover of heme-containing proteins in other tissues (e.g., the liver, muscles). Macrophages break down RBCs and heme-containing products into heme, which is further degraded into unconjugated bilirubin. Unconjugated bilirubin, or indirect bilirubin, is not water soluble. Unconjugated bilirubin then enters the bloodstream bound to albumin. In the liver, bilirubin is conjugated with glucuronic acid by the enzyme glucuronyltransferase, making it water soluble. The conjugated form of bilirubin is the main form of bilirubin present in the "direct" bilirubin fraction. Finally, conjugated bilirubin is secreted into the bile canaliculus as part of bile and delivered to the small intestine, where it is metabolized by bacteria and ultimately eliminated in the feces as stercobilin or the urine as urobilin.

Approach to evaluating patients with suspected hepatic/biliary pathology
- Step 1: Take a thorough history.
  - Ask about alcohol use, medications (acetaminophen, ingestions, herbs, OCPs), family or personal history of autoimmune conditions, sexual history (for viral hepatitis risk factors), travel history, IVDU/needle sticks, tattoos, vaccination history
  - Review of systems: Perform a complete GI, GU, neurologic and infectious review of systems
- Step 2: Perform a physical exam
  - Vital signs
  - Neuro: Perform a full neurologic exam, including mental status assessment and evaluation for asterixis
  - HEENT: Evaluate for scleral icterus, assess for Kayser-Fleischer rings (Wilson's disease)
  - Skin: Evaluate for jaundice, spider angiomas, palmar erythema, gynecomastia, caput medusae
  - Abd: Evaluate for RUQ tenderness, hepatosplenomegaly, abdominal distension, fluid wave
- Step 3: Check LFTs and other labs as indicated
  - LFTs:
    - <u>Hepatocellular pattern</u>: Increased AST/ALT, normal or mildly increased AlkP
    - <u>Cholestatic pattern</u>: Increased AlkP (and GGT), normal or mildly increased AST/ALT
    - <u>Mixed hepatocellular and cholestatic pictures</u>: Both AST/ALT and AlkP are elevated
  - Additional labs to consider: See Table 4.4
- Step 4: For hepatocellular liver injury, consider the differential diagnosis and work-up in Table 4.5
- Step 5: For cholestatic liver injury, consider the differential diagnosis and work-up in Table 4.6

TABLE 4.4 · Laboratory Tests Commonly Ordered to Evaluate Patients with Liver Disease

Test	Relevance in Hepatic Disease
LFTs (AST, ALT, Tbili, AlkP)	• AST is released by damaged hepatocyte cells and damaged myocytes, whereas ALT is more specific to hepatocyte damage • The AST:ALT ratio can be useful for determining etiology, although it is not sensitive or specific. An AST:ALT ratio of 4:1 may suggest rhabdomyolysis, 2:1 may suggest alcoholic hepatitis, 1:1 is consistent with other hepatitis • ALT is typically greater in fatty liver disease • AST and ALT values may be normal or even low in patients with cirrhosis due to reduced hepatocyte function • AlkP elevations can be due to hepatobiliary disease or bone breakdown • Total bilirun can be elevated due to liver disease or other causes (e.g., hemolytic anemia). If elevated, check indirect vs. direct bilirubin to help frame the differential diagnosis (see earlier in this chapter)
AlkP, GGT	• Elevated GGT helps confirm hepatobiliary etiology (GGT is not elevated due to bone breakdown)
BMP, Mg^{2+}, Phos	• Sodium may be low in cirrhosis and is needed to calculate the MELDNa • Check creatinine to evaluate for AKI/HRS • Phosphate will be low if hepatic regeneration is occurring and may require repletion
CBC	• Assess for thrombocytopenia, which occurs with cirrhosis (but is not typical in acute liver injury)
Albumin, INR	• Markers of synthetic function • Albumin decreased in cirrhosis as the liver synthesizes albumin • INR elevated in cirrhosis as the liver produces factors I, II, V, VII, X, XI, XII, and XIII, which affect PT; PT is typically not prolonged until advanced liver damage
Ammonia	• Serum ammonia level is not well-correlated with mental status; however, ammonia is the pathophysiologic driver of cerebral edema
Other	• Hepatitis serologies to evaluate for viral hepatitis • ANA, SMA, and IgG to evaluate for autoimmune hepatitis • Antimitochondral antibody, IgM to evaluate for primary biliary cholangitis • Alpha-1 antitrypsin to evaluate for alpha-1 antitrypsin deficiency • Iron saturation and serum ferritin (increased), genetic testing for HFE mutations to evaluate for hemochromatosis • Alpha-fetoprotein (AFP), which can be useful for hepatocellular carcinoma (HCC) screening • Serum ceruloplasmin (decreased) and urinary copper (increased) to evaluate for Wilson's disease • MRCP to evaluate for primary sclerosing cholangitis • TTE, right heart catheterization to evaluate for portopulmonary hypertension

TABLE 4.5 · Differential Diagnosis and Evaluation of Hepatocellular Liver Injury

Differential diagnosis for hepatocellular liver injury	Diagnostic test(s) that can be used for evaluation

• Alcoholic hepatitis
• Nonalcoholic fatty liver disease (NAFLD)
• Viral hepatitis
• Medication-induced liver injury
• Autoimmune hepatitis
• Wilson's disease
• Hemochromatosis
• Alpha-1 antitrypsin deficiency
• Ischemia
• Conditions associated with pregnancy:
  - Hemolysis, elevated liver enzymes, low platelet count (HELLP) syndrome
  - Acute fatty liver of pregnancy (AFLP)
	• CAGE substance abuse screening tool
	• Hepatitis serologies
	• Medication review: acetaminophen, antibiotics, statins, antiepileptics
	• IgG, ANA, SMA, anti-LKM
	• Serum ceruloplasmin, urine copper
	• Ferritin, % iron saturation, HFE genetic testing
	• Alpha-1 antitrypsin level, genetic testing
	• RUQ ultrasound with doppler to rule out portal vein thrombus
	• Evaluation of pregnancy if indicated

Clues for etiology of hepatocellular liver injury based on time course & degree of AST/ALT elevation

Time course:
Acute:
  - Ischemic
  - Toxins, acetaminophen
  - Viral: Hepatitis A, E
Either acute or chronic:
  - Alcohol
  - Wilson's
  - Budd-Chiari
  - Hepatitis B, C
  - Autoimmune
Chronic:
  - NAFLD
  - Hemochromatosis
  - Alpha-1 antitrypsin

Degree of AST/ALT elevation:
• Mild (AST/ALT in low hundreds):
  - Alcohol use
  - NAFLD
  - Most autoimmune conditions
• Moderate (AST/ALT in high hundreds to low thousands):
  - Acute viral hepatitis
  - Biliary obstruction
• Severe (AST/ALT in thousands):
  - Ischemia (e.g., Budd Chiari, shock liver)
  - Toxicity (e.g., acetaminophen)

Workup of chronically elevated AST/ALT

• First-pass workup:
  - Discuss alcohol intake and recommend cessation
  - Review medication list and stop hepatotoxic medications
  - Hepatitis B surface antigen
  - Hepatitis C surface antibody
  - Iron, TIBC, ferritin
  - Advise weight loss if elevated BMI
• Second-pass workup:
  - RUQ ultrasound (to evaluate for NAFLD)
  - ANA, anti–smooth muscle
  - Ceruloplasmin (if patient <40 yr)
• If negative, rule out nonhepatic causes of elevated AST/ALT (e.g., muscle disorders, hypo/hyperthyroidism, celiac disease, adrenal insufficiency)
• Consider liver biopsy if >2-fold unexplained, persistent increase AST/ALT despite above workup

Stop EtOH & hepatotoxic medications; hepatitis serologies, weight loss
→ If asymptomatic, can observe 6 months
→ Repeat LFTs
— Abnormal → Ultrasound, ANA, smooth muscle antibody, ceruloplasmin → Rule out non-hepatic etiologies → Liver biopsy if AST + ALT >2 ULN
— Normal → Observation

TABLE 4.6 · Differential Diagnosis and Evaluation of Cholestatic Liver Injury

Differential diagnosis for cholestatic liver injury	Diagnostic test(s) that can be used for evaluation
Intrahepatic: • Medication-induced liver injury • Primary sclerosing cholangitis (PSC) • Primary biliary cirrhosis (PBC) • Infections: Fungal, tuberculosis, echinococcus • Conditions associated with pregnancy: - Intrahepatic cholestasis of pregnancy (ICP) **Extrahepatic:** • Gallstones • Malignancy • Primary sclerosing cholangitis (PSC) • Chronic pancreatitis • HIV cholangiopathy	• Medication review: Oral contraceptive pills, antibiotics, anabolic steroids, TPN • Antimitochondrial antibody (AMA) • Infectious workup/cultures • Evaluation of pregnancy if indicated • RUQ ultrasound • MRCP • ERCP

Workup of chronically elevated AlkP

- First-pass workup:
  - Check gamma-glutamyl transferase (GGT) (if biliary origin, both AlkP and GGT will be elevated)
  - Stop offending medications (if applicable) and recheck AlkP
- If AlkP still elevated, check RUQ ultrasound
- If dilated ducts seen, perform MRCP and/or ERCP to rule out obstruction
- If ducts appear normal, check anti-mitochondrial antibody (AMA), which is associated with primary biliary cholangitis (PBC)
  - If positive: Perform liver biopsy to confirm the diagnosis of PBC
  - If negative, consider liver biopsy and/or ERCP and assess for other etiologies

Check GGT to ensure biliary origin, Review medication list + stop offending medications

RUQ ultrasound

— Dilated ducts — Normal ducts —

MRCP/ERCP

Check anti-mitochondrial antibody (PBC)

— Pos — Neg —

Liver bx to confirm PBC

Liver bx/ERCP to eval for PSC, other etiologies

DISEASES AND PATHOPHYSIOLOGY

Esophagus

Gastroesophageal reflux disease (GERD)

- Pathophysiology: Decreased lower esophageal sphincter (LES) tone; may also have decreased esophageal motility, gastric outlet obstruction, and/or hiatal hernia
- Clinical features: Heartburn (i.e., burning sensation in the retrosternal area), regurgitation (i.e., perception of refluxed gastric content flowing up into the mouth or hypopharynx)
- Diagnosis: Treat empirically. Typically only perform EGD and/or ambulatory pH monitoring in patients who have refractory or alarm symptoms (e.g., new onset GERD at age >60 yr, dysphagia/odynophagia, weight loss, anorexia, GIB or iron-deficiency anemia, persistent vomiting, or GI malignancy in a first-degree relative)
- Treatment:
  - <u>Mild</u>: Lifestyle modifications (e.g., weight loss, eliminate dietary triggers, avoid lying down after eating, use of a wedge pillow)
  - <u>Moderate</u>: Add an H2 blocker
  - <u>Severe</u>: Switch to a PPI.
    - Potential side effects of PPI use: Increased risk of *C. diff* infection, osteoporosis, vitamin B_{12} deficiency
    - Consider the use of a long-term PPI in patients with refractory symptoms, recurrent GI bleeds, Zollinger-Ellison syndrome, Barrett's esophagus, severe esophagitis
  - <u>Refractory</u>: If no improvement with empiric treatment after 8 weeks, recommend EGD. Surgical options: Laparoscopic fundoplication or bariatric surgery if obesity is contributing.
- Complications: Erosive esophagitis, stricture, Barrett's esophagus, increased risk of esophageal cancer

Barrett's esophagus

- Pathophysiology: Normal squamous epithelium that lines the esophagus changes to columnar epithelium with goblet cells like intestinal cells, typically due to repeated exposure to stomach acid from GERD. Can progress to esophageal adenocarcinoma.
- Diagnosis: Guidelines from various societies differ; overall, should consider screening patients with multiple risk factors for adenocarcinoma (male sex, older age, white, chronic GERD, obesity, hiatal hernia, smoking, first-degree relative with GI malignancy).
- Treatment:
  - PPI indefinitely
  - If no dysplasia present: Surveillance EGD every 3–5 yr
  - If low- or high-grade dysplasia present: Remove with radiofrequency ablation, photodynamic therapy, cryotherapy or endoscopic resection. Perform repeat endoscopy for surveillance within 3–12 months (timing based on severity and whether the dysplasia was deemed to be eradicated)

Esophageal motility disorders

- Classification: First differentiate oropharyngeal dysphagia (difficulty *initiating* a swallow) vs. esophageal dysphagia (sensation of obstruction several seconds *after* swallowing)
- Clinical features:
  - Dysphagia with <u>solids only</u> is often due to a <u>mechanical obstruction</u>
    - Intermittent: Esophageal rings or webs (Plummer-Vinson syndrome, Schatzki's ring), eosinophilic esophagitis
    - Progressive with chronic heartburn/GERD, no weight loss: Peptic stricture
    - Progressive, age >50 yr, weight loss: Esophageal carcinoma, Zenker's diverticula
  - Dysphagia with <u>solids and liquids</u> is often due to a <u>motility problem</u>
    - Intermittent: Esophageal rings
    - Intermittent, with chest pain (similar to angina pain): Diffuse esophageal spasm (DES)
    - Progressive, with heartburn/GERD and skin tightening: Scleroderma
    - Progressive, with regurgitation of food and saliva, weight loss: Achalasia
- Diagnosis:
  - Barium swallow. Perform an EGD prior if the patient has a history of radiation, caustic injury, esophageal cancer, or stricture to avoid the risk of perforation
  - EGD: Used to detect structural abnormalities
  - Esophageal manometry: If the barium swallow and EGD are normal, esophageal manometry may be used to diagnose a motility disorder
- Treatment:
  - EGD with dilation of strictures and rings
  - Diffuse esophageal spasm: First line, PPI; second line, calcium channel blocker; third line, botulinum injection
  - Achalasia: First line, dilation, surgical or endoscopic myotomy of LES; second line, botulinum injection; third line, nitrates

Esophagitis

- Infectious esophagitis: *Candida albicans* is the most common fungal etiology (treatment: fluconazole or itraconazole). Other etiologies include HSV (treatment: acyclovir) or CMV (treatment: ganciclovir).
- Medication-induced esophagitis: Several hours after taking oral medications (e.g., commonly occurs with alendronate, doxycycline, aspirin). Treatment: Stop offending medication if possible.
- Eosinophilic esophagitis: Typical presentation is an atopic man in mid-30s who presents with dysphagia. Diagnosis: Eosinophils on biopsy plus exclusion of other causes of eosinophils in the esophagus (including infections, medications, connective tissue diseases, esophageal Crohn's). Treatment: PPI +/− topical steroids (delivered as orodispersible tablet or as an inhaled formulation).

Esophageal hiatal hernia

- Sliding hiatal hernias (type I): Most common type of hiatal hernia (>95%). Causes displacement of the gastroesophageal junction above the diaphragm. Typically due to benign anatomic causes. Associated with an increased risk of GERD. Treatment: No treatment unless symptomatic.
- Paraesophageal hiatal hernia (type II–IV): Less common cause of hiatal hernia (<5%). Type II involves the gastric fundus herniating through a defect in the diaphragm while the GE junction remains below the diaphragm; type III has features of both I and II; type IV involves a diaphragmatic defect large enough to allow other organs to also protrude in the hernia sac (e.g., colon, spleen, pancreas, small intestine). Complications: Volvulus, strangulation, obstruction. Treatment: Elective surgical repair if symptomatic; emergent surgical repair if volvulus, uncontrolled bleeding, obstruction, strangulation, or respiratory compromise.

Other

- Mallory-Weiss tear: Forceful vomiting causes upper GI mucosal tear; classic history is initial non-bloody emesis for several episodes followed by development of hematemesis. Treatment: EGD with thermal coagulation, Hemoclips, or band ligation.
- Boerhaave syndrome: Forceful vomiting causes esophageal transmural tear with chest pain, odynophagia, fever, subcutaneous emphysema, and possibly shock. Diagnosis: Contrast esophagram (with water-soluble gastrografin) or CT chest/abdomen/pelvis. Pleural fluid may reveal low pH, high amylase. Treatment: Admit to the ICU, NPO, IV PPI/antibiotics, drainage of fluid collection; requires thoracic surgery if evidence of clinical deterioration, extension of perforation, or certain complications.

Stomach

Peptic ulcer disease (PUD)

- Pathophysiology: Ulcers that develop in the stomach or duodenum. Common risk factors include *H. pylori* infection, NSAID use
- Clinical features: Asymptomatic (70%), abdominal pain, bleeding. Features differ based on the ulcer location:
  - Gastric ulcer: NSAIDs, *H. pylori*, high malignant potential (*always biopsy!*), eating does NOT help
  - Duodenal ulcer: *H. pylori* 90%, low malignant potential (don't need biopsy), eating relieves pain
- Diagnosis:
  - Endoscopy: Low-risk gastric ulcers (e.g., young person on NSAIDs) and duodenal ulcers do not typically require follow-up; high-risk patients (including gastric ulcers with inadequate-quality biopsy) require repeat endoscopy in 8–12 weeks
  - *H. pylori* testing:
    - <u>*H. pylori* IgG antibody test</u>: Positive if any prior exposure (i.e., cannot differentiate active vs. prior infection); however, a negative result is very helpful. Highest-yield clinical use is if never tested or treated before and high pre-test probability for infection; no role if known prior *H. pylori* infection.
    - <u>Urea breath test</u>: Identifies active infection. Costly. Used to confirm infection if pre-test probability low, to confirm eradication (eradication should be confirmed for *all* patients, approximately 4 weeks after treatment), or to assess for reinfection. Less accurate in patients taking a PPI, bismuth, or antibiotics, or during active PUD bleeding.
    - <u>Fecal antigen test</u>: Identifies active infection. Less expensive. Used to confirm infection if pre-test probability low, to confirm eradication (eradication should be confirmed for *all* patients, approximately 4 weeks after treatment), or to assess for reinfection. Less accurate in patients taking a PPI, bismuth, or antibiotics; the impact on accuracy of active bleeding may depend on the assay used.
    - <u>EGD with biopsy</u>: Gold standard, identifies active infection. Less accurate in patients taking a PPI, bismuth, or antibiotics, or during active UGIB.

- Treatment:
  - Supportive care: Stop ASA, NSAIDs, restrict alcohol use, smoking cessation
  - Acid suppression: PPIs (first line; more rapid at promoting ulcer healing); H2 blockers, antacids
  - Eradicate *H. pylori*, if present. Guidelines now recommend triple therapy only in regions where *H. pylori* clarithromycin resistance is known to be <15% and in patients with no previous history of macrolide exposure. Quadruple therapy is an appropriate first-line treatment, and the paradigm is shifting toward quadruple therapy as first line for most patients due to resistance.
    - <u>Triple therapy</u>: PPI BID + clarithromycin 500 mg BID + amoxicillin 1000 mg BID *or* metronidazole 500 mg BID for 14 days
    - <u>Quadruple therapy</u>: PPI BID + bismuth 420 mg QID + metronidazole 500 mg QID + tetracycline 500 mg QID for 10–14 days
- Key association: *H. pylori* infection is also associated with gastric MALT lymphoma. First-line treatment is *H. pylori* treatment, followed by serial endoscopies.

Gastritis

- Atrophic gastritis: Two forms 1) *H. pylori* associated (treat *H. pylori*); 2) Autoimmune (not curable; can lead to pernicious anemia requiring lifelong vitamin B_{12} replacement).
- Metaplasia (chronic) atrophic gastritis: Precancerous lesion of the gastric mucosa associated with *H. pylori*. Treat *H. pylori*. Risk factor for adenocarcinoma; unclear if *H. pylori* eradication can affect the natural history of gastric intestinal metaplasia/progression to gastric cancer.
- Eosinophilic gastritis/gastroenteritis: Rare inflammatory disorder characterized by eosinophilic infiltration of the stomach and/or duodenum (most commonly). Treatment: Elimination diet, steroids.
- Lymphocytic gastritis: Rare, benign, chronic inflammatory condition, associated with *H. pylori* and Celiac disease. Treat *H. pylori*.

Gastroparesis

- Clinical features: Delayed stomach emptying; early satiety, postprandial fullness, nausea/vomiting, pain, bloating, weight loss
- Diagnosis: Perform EGD and upper GI barium radiography first to rule out an obstruction. Then perform a gastric emptying study while off all medications that can affect motility (e.g., opiates). Evaluate for the cause of gastroparesis with work-up such as: HgA1c, TSH, +/− ANA or additional testing for neuroautonomic etiologies based on the clinical context.
- Treatment: Dietary changes, diabetes control, metoclopramide (side effects: parkinsonism, tardive dyskinesia), erythromycin, prucalopride (off-label). For refractory symptoms, consider PEG placement for decompression and feeding or gastric pacemaker for diabetic gastroparesis.

Gastric outlet obstruction

- Pathophysiology: Obstruction of the gastric outlet by malignancy, PUD, strictures, caustic injury
- Clinical features: Nausea/vomiting, epigastric pain, early satiety; "succussion splash" on physical exam
- Diagnosis: EGD to diagnose and identify cause
- Treatment: Depends on the cause of obstruction; sometimes need nasogastric tube placement, PPI, endoscopic dilation, stenting or surgery

Bariatric surgery

- Indication: Can be offered to patients with an elevated BMI (typically >35) despite diet/exercise and lifestyle interventions
- Procedure: Surgical procedure. There are several different types/approaches.
- Potential complications:
  - Restrictive complications: Band slippage, staple-line leakage
  - Malabsorptive complications: Cholelithiasis, nephrolithiasis (due to increased urine oxalate excretion), dumping syndrome, short bowel syndrome, SBO, fistulas, stricture
  - Nutritional complications: Micronutrient deficiencies
  - Bleeding-related complications: Marginal ulcers

Small Bowel
Inflammatory Bowel Disease (IBD)

TABLE 4.7 · Features of Ulcerative Colitis vs. Crohn's Disease		
	Ulcerative Colitis (UC)	**Crohn's Disease**
Age of onset	Bimodal: 15–30 yr or 60–80 yr (*elderly patients can have new-onset IBD!*)	
Tobacco	• Tobacco decreases risk of disease (may flare when stop smoking)	• Tobacco increases risk of disease
Location/Pathology	• Rectal involvement in all cases and then ascends up the colon contiguously • Mucosal/submucosal • Crypt abscesses	• Entire GI tract mouth to anus with "skip" lesions. Ileal involvement >50% of time. • Transmural • Granulomas (noncaseating)
Common GI manifestations	• Bloody diarrhea • Tenesmus	• Diarrhea ($+/-$ bloody) • Crampy abdominal pain
Extraintestinal manifestations	• Uveitis, episcleritis • Ankylosing spondylitis (30-fold increased risk, independent of bowel disease severity) • Pyoderma gangrenosum (neutrophilic ulcerative skin lesion(s); parallels bowel disease activity in only ~50% of cases) • Erythema nodosum (tender tibial nodules; often parallels bowel disease activity) • Primary sclerosing cholangitis ([PSC]; 90% of patients with PSC have underlying UC; however, only 5% of patients with UC have PSC, which is similar to the prevalence of PSC in patients with Crohn's disease)	
Complications	• Marked increased risk of colon cancer • Hemorrhage • Toxic megacolon	• Slight increased risk of colon cancer, can also increase the risk for other GI malignancies • Fistulas • Abscesses • Obstruction • Cholelithiasis (due to decreased bile acid absorption) • Nephrolithiasis (due to increased colonic oxalate absorption)
Surgery	• Curative	• For complications such as stricture

- History:
  - Even if you suspect IBD, always rule out infection first! Take a good travel and dietary history, ask about recent antibiotic use, assess risk factors for being immunocompromised.
  - Ask about extraintestinal manifestations of IBD (see Table 4.7)
  - Quantify diarrhea and ask about tenesmus (fecal urge; suggests rectal involvement)
  - Ask about family history of autoimmune disease or IBD
- Diagnosis:
  - General: CBC with differential, BMP, INR
  - Rule out infection: Bacterial stool culture, Shiga toxin, *E. coli* 0157, *C. diff*, *Giardia*, O+P. Viral colitis (e.g., CMV) will not be evident on culture, so take biopsies during colonoscopy to rule out.
  - ESR, CRP, and fecal calprotectin are inflammatory markers that can be elevated in IBD flares. It is helpful to check at baseline when the patient is asymptomatic and then again if there is concern for an IBD flare.
  - Imaging:
    - Before initial colonoscopy in the inpatient setting, consider an abdominal plain film to ensure that there are no anatomic variations that would make colonoscopy more dangerous. There is no need for imaging if the patient is stable as an outpatient.
    - CT abdomen/pelvis is indicated in patients with severe pain to rule out complications of IBD, such as toxic megacolon, perforation, intraabdominal abscess, or bowel obstruction. Imaging can also be used to help rule out other causes of hematochezia, such as mesenteric ischemia.
  - Colonoscopy with biopsies is always indicated when evaluating for a new diagnosis of IBD

- Treatment:
  - <u>Induction therapy</u>: Steroids (prednisone, budesonide). These should only be used for induction, not maintenance; patients with IBD should <u>not</u> be placed on oral steroids indefinitely.
  - <u>Maintenance therapy</u>: Depends on the severity and extent of disease
    - Mild/moderate disease: 5-ASA, sulfasalazine
    - Severe disease: TNF-alpha inhibitor (e.g., infliximab, adalimumab), thiopurines (azathioprine, 6-MP), methotrexate, anti-integrin (vedolizumab), IL-12/23 inhibitor (ustekinumab), JAK inhibitor (tofacitinib)
  - <u>IBD flare</u>: Depends on the severity. For severe flares:
    - Consider hospital admission
    - Diagnostics/labs:
      - Rule out infection: Stool culture, *C. diff* testing, stool O&P, fecal calprotectin
      - Prepare for the possibility of a rescue therapy with a biologic: Place PPD, send hepatitis serologies, perform cocci testing if risk factors, consider checking levels of antibiotics to biologic if prior exposure to biologics (e.g., infliximab ab)
    - Initiate IV corticosteroids; use symptoms, stool count/quality, and inflammatory markers (usually on hospital day 3 and 5) to predict corticosteroid failure and, if high probability of corticosteroid failure, consider surgical consultation and rescue therapy (e.g., infliximab)
    - Other aspects of care: Nutrition workup/consult, administer VTE prophylaxis (highly inflammatory state is prothrombotic; administer even if stools are bloody), control pain with APAP or tramadol (do not use opiates unless perioperative, as they may increase all-cause mortality in patients with IBD)
- Surveillance: Patients with UC and Crohn's colitis have an increased risk of colorectal cancer. Therefore, begin screening colonoscopies 8–10 yr after the initial diagnosis, and continue screening every 1–2 yr.

Malabsorption

Celiac disease

- Pathophysiology: Immune-mediated inflammatory disease of the small intestine resulting from sensitivity to gluten (wheat) and gluten-related proteins.
- Clinical features: Steatorrhea (bulky, floating, foul-smelling stool), malabsorption (weight loss, nutritional deficiency), associated with dermatitis herpetiformis (papules and vesicles on the forearms, knees, scalp, or buttocks).
- Diagnosis: IgA tissue transglutaminase (tTG) antibody AND duodenal biopsies with blunted villi while the patient is consuming gluten.
- Treatment: Gluten-free diet

Small intestinal bacterial overgrowth (SIBO)

- Pathophysiology: Over-colonization of the small bowel with microbes.
- Clinical features: Watery diarrhea, bloating, flatulence, micronutrient deficiency. Most common in setting of motility disorders and chronic pancreatitis, although any disorder altering mucosal defenses can precipitate SIBO. Nutritional deficiencies can be severe and symptomatic (e.g., B_{12} deficiency, hypocalcemia) in the setting of jejunoileal bypass or short bowel syndrome.
- Diagnosis: Positive carbohydrate breath test or endoscopy with jejunal aspirate $>10^3$ organisms. Sometimes may initiate treatment empirically instead.
- Treatment: Rifaximin × 14 days (to reduce small intestinal bacteria), correct micronutrient deficiencies

Short bowel syndrome

- Pathophysiology: Dysregulation of electrolytes, fluids, and proteins/nutrients as a result of a large portion of the small intestine being resected or diseased, typically with <2 meters remaining.
- Clinical features: Diarrhea, bloating, weight loss
- Treatment: Diet high in complex carbs, modest in fat and oxalate (to reduce calcium oxalate nephrolithiasis); oral rehydration; antidiarrheals.

Carbohydrate malabsorption

- Pathophysiology: Lactose malabsorption is most common; fructose malabsorption can also occur.
- Clinical features: Bloating, diarrhea
- Treatment: Dietary restriction, lactase supplementation for lactose intolerance

Whipple's disease

- Pathophysiology: Malabsorptive diarrheal disease caused by *Tropheryma whipplei*.
- Clinical features: Chronic diarrhea, malabsorption, abdominal discomfort, weight loss, and arthralgias; rarely CNS involvement, skin hyperpigmentation, and endocarditis can occur.
- Diagnosis: Small bowel biopsy with PAS stain and PCR for *T. whipplei*. May also obtain tissue/fluid from a site of extraintestinal manifestation (e.g., CSF, vitreous fluid, cardiac valve, peripheral blood).
- Treatment: Ceftriaxone or penicillin for 2–4 weeks, followed by TMP-SMX for 1 yr.

Vitamin Deficiencies

TABLE 4.8 • Vitamin Deficiencies: Causes and Clinical Features

Deficiency	Cause	Clinical Features
Vitamin A*	Diet/malabsorption	Night blindness, dry skin, immunosuppression
Vitamin B₁ (thiamine)	Heavy alcohol use (glucose can't break down, no ATP)	Wernicke-Korsakoff (nystagmus, ophthalmoplegia, ataxia), wet beriberi (heart failure), dry beriberi (neuropathy)
Vitamin B₃ (niacin)	Carcinoid syndrome (low tryptophan due to use in serotonin), Hartnup disease, isoniazid	Pellagra: 3Ds = Diarrhea, Dermatitis (sun-exposed areas, looks like sunburn), Dementia + glossitis
Vitamin B₆ (pyridoxine)	Isoniazid, oral contraceptives	Seizures, neuropathy, sideroblastic anemia
Vitamin B₉ (folic acid)	Inadequate dietary intake (rare in countries with folate-fortified foods), pregnancy, medications (e.g., methotrexate, phenytoin, sulfonamides), alcohol	Macrocytic anemia (folate is required for synthesis of nitrogenous bases in DNA and RNA)
Vitamin B₁₂ (cobalamin)	Malabsorption (meat/dairy, years), lack intrinsic factor (pernicious anemia, gastric bypass)	Macrocytic anemia, nerve damage due to abnormal myelination
Vitamin C	Diet (lack of fruits/vegetables)	Scurvy (results from collagen synthesis defect in absence of vitamin C) – swollen gums, bruises, corkscrew hairs, poor wound healing
Vitamin D*	Diet/malabsorption, CKD, lack of sun	Rickets (children), osteomalacia (adults); hypocalcemic tetany
Vitamin E*	Diet/malabsorption	Sensory/motor neuropathy (can mimic vitamin B₁₂ deficiency), hemolytic anemia (vitamin E is an antioxidant that protects RBCs from free radical damage)
Vitamin K*	Diet/malabsorption, prolonged antibiotic exposure (disrupts vitamin K synthesis by intestinal bacteria)	Evidence of hemorrhage/bleeding (e.g., easy bruising, melena, hematuria)
Zinc deficiency	Diet/malabsorption, IBD, cystic fibrosis, sickle cell disease, liver disease, renal disease	Alopecia, loss of smell, dermatitis, impaired wound healing

*Fat-soluble vitamins

Other Conditions that Affect the Small Bowel

Microscopic colitis

- Epidemiology: Age of diagnosis typically 45–65 yr; more common in females than males
- Etiology: Chronic inflammatory disease of the colon with two histologic subtypes: 1) Lymphocytic and 2) Collagenous colitis. Associated with autoimmune diseases, NSAIDs, tobacco use.
- Clinical features: Chronic, watery, non-bloody diarrhea.
- Diagnosis: Colonoscopy with biopsy showing lymphocytic or collagenous colitis. Workup should include ruling out infectious causes (check stool studies) and celiac sprue (check serologies).
- Treatment: 1) Stop NSAIDs (or other offending medications); 2) Loperamide for symptoms; 3) Budesonide for active disease. Second-line agents include cholestyramine, bismuth, and biologics if needed.

Irritable bowel syndrome (IBS)

- Pathophysiology: Idiopathic and multifactorial, sometimes considered a functional disorder. Associated with female sex, depression, anxiety, fibromyalgia.
- Clinical features: Subtypes are IBS-C (constipation), IBS-D (diarrhea), IBD with mixed bowel movements.
- Diagnosis:
  - Exclude other organic etiologies through history and labs: Fecal calprotectin, stool studies, celiac disease studies.
  - Colonoscopy is typically not needed, but should be considered for alarm features: Age >50 yr, GI bleeding, weight loss, progressive abdominal pain, lab abnormalities, family history of IBD, colon cancer.
  - Rome IV criteria: Abdominal pain at least once per week for ≥3 months with ≥2 symptoms related to defecation, change in stool frequency, change in stool form.

- Treatment:
  - For all subtypes: Education/reassurance, low FODMAP diet, dicyclomine for abdominal cramping, encapsulated peppermint oil
  - IBS-D: Loperamide, cholestyramine, 5HT-3 antagonists, rifaximin, TCAs, SNRI
  - IBS-C: Polyethylene glycol (MiraLAX), psyllium, prucalopride, plecanatide, lubiprostone, linaclotide, SSRI (not paroxetine), SNRI
  - IBS-M: Fiber supplementation

Mesenteric ischemia

- Definition: Ischemia affecting the small intestine is generally referred to as mesenteric ischemia, while ischemia affecting the large intestine is referred to as colonic ischemia; mesenteric ischemia can be subdivided into acute and chronic subtypes.

Acute mesenteric ischemia

- Pathophysiology: Can be caused by arterial embolism (50%; e.g., Afib), arterial thrombosis (15–25%; e.g., atherosclerosis), venous thrombosis (5%; e.g., in setting of infection, hypercoagulability, malignancy), nonocclusive (20–30%; e.g., hypoperfusion, such as in hypotensive patient)
- Clinical features: Severe abdominal pain out of proportion to physical findings; anorexia, vomiting, mild GI bleed
- Diagnosis: CT angiogram
- Treatment: IV fluids, anticoagulation, broad-spectrum antibiotics. Arterial: Early surgical laparotomy with embolectomy. Venous: Anticoagulation. Nonocclusive: Treat underlying cause.

Chronic mesenteric ischemia

- Pathophysiology: Atherosclerosis can cause abdominal angina
- Clinical features: Dull pain that typically starts about one hour after eating; can cause food anxiety with subsequent weight loss
- Diagnosis: CT angiogram
- Treatment: Antiplatelet therapy, surgical revascularization

Carcinoid syndrome

- Pathophysiology: Neuroendocrine tumor that secretes serotonin
- Clinical features: 1) Flushing, 2) Diarrhea, 3) Wheezing, 4) Right-sided valvular heart disease (pathognomonic plaque-like deposits of fibrous tissue)
- Diagnosis: Increased urine 5-HIAA; imaging for tumor localization (e.g., CT, somatostatin receptor imaging) with EGD/colonoscopy if primary site remains undetermined
- Treatment: Surgical removal of the tumor. If not resectable, octreotide injection (long-acting release), telotristat, loperamide

Colon
Diverticular Disease
Diverticulosis

- Pathophysiology: Multiple outpouchings of colonic mucosa/submucosa through areas of focal weakness in the setting of increased intraluminal pressure, particularly in the sigmoid colon.
- Clinical features: Asymptomatic or LLQ pain, bloating. More common in elderly patients and those who consume a low-fiber diet
- Diagnosis: CT, colonoscopy
- Treatment: High-fiber diet

Diverticular bleed

- Pathophysiology: Painless hematochezia due to the exposure of the vasa recta over time as the diverticulum herniates
- Treatment: Usually self-limited. If bleeding does not stop, perform colonoscopy to evaluate for the site of active bleeding or visible vessel. Consider angiography with embolization if the bleeding site cannot be identified on colonoscopy. Surgery is a last resort.

Diverticulitis

- Pathophysiology: Inflammation/focal necrosis due to erosion of the diverticular wall by increased intraluminal pressure or inspissated food particles.
- Clinical features: LLQ pain, fever, leukocytosis
- Diagnosis: No imaging needed, can consider CT abd/pelvis if there is concern for complications such as abscess, obstruction, fistula, or perforation
- Treatment: Ciprofloxacin and metronidazole for 7–10 days. Recommend colonoscopy 6–8 weeks later to rule out colon cancer if the patient has not had a colonoscopy in the past year. Do NOT need to avoid nuts, seeds, and popcorn (this myth has been debunked). Elective surgery controversial.

Other Diseases Affecting the Colon

Angiodysplasia of the colon (AV malformations, vascular ectasia)

- Clinical features: Tortuous dilated veins in the colon can rupture and cause a lower GI bleed. Classic association is Heyde's syndrome (triad of aortic stenosis, acquired vWF deficiency due to shear stress from the aortic valve, and GI bleeding from angiodysplasia)
- Diagnosis: Colonoscopy
- Treatment: Bleeding is typically self-limited

Ischemic colitis

- Definitions: Ischemia in the mesenteric distribution specifically affecting the large intestine
- Pathophysiology: Colonic hypoperfusion in the setting of hypotension (e.g., MI, aortoiliac surgery)
- Clinical features: Sudden abdominal pain, diarrhea, hematochezia
- Diagnosis: CT abd/pelvis with contrast. Early colonoscopy shows patchy segmental ulcerations
- Treatment: Usually just supportive care; if severe and necrotic bowel, may need surgical resection

Colonic polyps

- Adenoma: Premalignant. Three subtypes: 1) Tubular adenoma, 2) Tubulovillous adenoma, 3) Villous adenoma (most worrisome)
- Serrated: 1) Hyperplastic polyp (benign), 2) Sessile serrated polyp (premalignant), 3) Traditional serrated adenoma (premalignant)
- Other: 1) Hamartomatous polyp (variable potential for transformation); 2) Inflammatory polyp (benign).
  - After premalignant polyps are removed, typically recommend closer interval surveillance colonoscopy (interval depends on size and number).

Sigmoid volvulus

- Pathophysiology: Occurs when a loop of the sigmoid bowel twists around its own mesentery, resulting in obstruction and underperfusion.
- Clinical features: Insidious onset of abdominal pain, nausea, and distension, eventually with severe continuous abdominal pain and colicky episodes. More common age >70 yr, M>F, patients with comorbid neuropsychiatric diseases.
- Diagnosis: CT abd/pelvis with "whirl pattern" (dilated sigmoid around mesocolon/vessels) and "bird-beak" appearance of adjacent colonic segments; if not present, absence of rectal gas, separation of sigmoid walls, and two transition points are suggestive.
- Treatment: Emergent surgery if peritonitis/perforation. If stable, sigmoidoscopy to diagnose and detorse the twisted segment, followed by surgery.

Cecal volvulus

- Pathophysiology: Occurs when a segment of the cecum rotates/torses, resulting in obstruction and underperfusion. More common in younger women.
- Clinical features: Presentation varies widely from insidious abdominal pain/vomiting to abdominal catastrophe
- Diagnosis: CT abd/pelvis with "whirl pattern," as with sigmoid volvulus, but with the anatomic location at the cecum.
- Treatment: Primarily surgical management

Radiation proctitis

- Pathophysiology: Inflammation of the rectum as a result of damage due to pelvic radiation (e.g., for prostate cancer, cervical cancer)
- Clinical features:
  - Acute: Diarrhea, mucus discharge, urgency, and tenesmus within 6 weeks of radiation
  - Chronic: Same symptoms >9 months after radiation exposure. Chronic radiation proctitis can cause bleeding. Treat with endoscopic argon plasma coagulation (APC).
- Diagnosis: Diagnosis of exclusion. Endoscopic findings are nonspecific (pallor with friability, telangiectasia); biopsy demonstrates submucosal fibrosis.
- Treatment: Supportive care, sucralfate enemas, hyperbaric oxygen

Hemorrhoids

- Pathophysiology: Varicose veins of the anus/rectum. Risk factors include constipation, pregnancy, portal hypertension, and obesity.
- Clinical features: Bright red blood on the toilet paper when wiping.
  - External: Dilated veins from inferior hemorrhoidal plexus distal to dentate line (sensate area) – *painful*!
  - Internal: Dilated submucosal veins of superior rectal plexus above dentate line (insensate area) – *painless*!
- Treatment: Sitz bath, ice packs, stool softeners, topical steroids. If internal hemorrhoids are severe, can pursue rubber band ligation or surgery.

GASTROENTEROLOGY

Gallbladder and Biliary Tract
Gallbladder Stone Diseases
Cholelithiasis
- Etiology: Stone in the **gallbladder**
- Clinical features: Patients may be asymptomatic or develop biliary colic
- Diagnosis: RUQ ultrasound
- Treatment: Elective cholecystectomy, if symptomatic
- Types of stones: *Cholesterol*: Obesity, multiparity, OCPs, rapid weight loss. *Pigmented*: Hemolysis, cirrhosis, biliary infections, TPN

Cholecystitis
- Etiology: Stone in the **cystic duct**
- Clinical features: Acute inflammation of the gallbladder wall which causes RUQ pain, N/V, fever, leukocytosis, +Murphy's sign (inspiratory arrest during deep palpation of RUQ)
- Diagnosis: RUQ ultrasound, if inconclusive consider HIDA scan
- Treatment: IVF, NPO, IV antibiotics. Then early cholecystectomy (within 24–48 hr). If poor surgical candidate, achieve drainage with a percutaneous cholecystostomy.

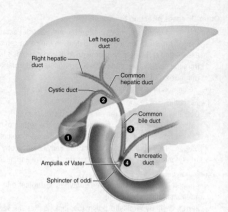

FIGURE 4.6: Anatomy of the biliary tree and the types of gallbladder stone disease. Shown is the biliary tree and the passage of gallstones through this system: 1) Cholelithiasis; 2) Cholecystitis; 3) Choledocholithiasis; 4) Cholangitis. Of note, cholangitis can be due to obstruction from a gallstone or another cause (see chapter text).

- Subtypes:
  - <u>Acalculous cholecystitis</u>: Cholecystitis in the absence of a stone. More common in patients that are very ill (e.g., ICU patients, burn patients). Treatment: If necrosis, perforation, or emphysematous cholecystitis, needs emergent cholecystectomy or percutaneous drainage.
  - <u>Emphysematous cholecystitis</u>: Infection of the gallbladder with gas-forming bacteria. Ultrasound shows air-fluid levels and gas shadows. Treatment: IVF, antibiotics, early cholecystectomy
- Post-cholecystectomy syndrome: Persistent abdominal pain post-operatively or months/years later due to a retained stone or extrabiliary problem. Patients also may have bile salt wasting and diarrhea. Diagnosis: RUQ ultrasound, MRCP, or ECRP. Treatment: Bile acid sequestrants.

Choledocholithiasis
- Etiology: Stone in the **common bile duct**
- Clinical features: Abdominal pain, fever. Labs notable for initial transaminitis followed by a cholestatic elevation. RUQ ultrasound may show biliary dilatation.
- Treatment: High risk: ERCP with removal of stone, followed by elective cholecystectomy. Intermediate risk: MRCP, if positive proceed to ERCP. Low risk: If gallstones/sludge seen on RUQ ultrasound, consider elective cholecystectomy.

Cholangitis
- Etiology: Infection of the biliary ducts due to obstruction (stone, tumor, stricture), biliary stasis, or bacterial overgrowth.
- Classic symptoms: Charcot's triad: 1) RUQ pain, 2) Jaundice, 3) Fever. Reynold's pentad: The prior triad and in addition: 4) Septic shock, 5) Altered mental status
- Diagnosis: RUQ ultrasound, hyperbilirubinemia, leukocytosis, mild elevation serum transaminases
- Treatment: IV antibiotics, IVF. Perform ERCP with sphincterotomy, stone extraction, and/or stenting within 24–48 hours

Other Diseases of the Biliary Tree
- Biliary cysts: Cysts in the biliary tree. Clinically, can cause abdominal pain, recurrent cholangitis, pancreatitis, and increased risk for cholangiocarcinoma. Diagnosis: Ultrasound, ERCP with biopsy. Treatment: Surgical resection
- Bile duct stricture: May be benign or malignant, and can cause obstructive jaundice. Treatment: Endoscopic dilation, percutaneous transhepatic biliary drain, stenting, or surgical bypass.
- Biliary dyskinesia: Motor dysfunction of the sphincter of Oddi. Causes recurrent biliary colic without evidence of gallstones. Diagnosis: HIDA scan with administration of cholecystokinin (CCK) to determine the gallbladder ejection fraction. Treatment: Laparoscopic cholecystectomy, sphincterotomy.

Pancreas
Acute pancreatitis
- Etiology: Premature activation of pancreatic digestive enzymes causes autodigestion of pancreatic tissue
- Causes: **GET SMASHED** – **G**allstones (40%), **Et**OH (30%), **T**rauma, **S**corpion, **M**umps, **A**utoimmune, **S**teroids, **H**ypertriglyceridemia (>1000 mg/dL)/**H**ypercalcemia, **E**RCP (post-procedure), **D**rugs (sulfonamides, thiazides, lisinopril, furosemide, antiretrovirals)
- Clinical features:
  - Symptoms: Epigastric pain that radiates to the back, often worse after eating. Also fever, nausea/vomiting
  - Classic signs: Hemorrhagic: 1) Grey Turner (flank ecchymosis), 2) Cullen (periumbilical ecchymosis), 3) Fox (nontraumatic ecchymosis over the inguinal ligament)
- Diagnosis: Need two of three criteria: 1) Typical pancreatic abdominal pain, 2) Elevation in lipase or amylase >3× ULN, 3) Imaging findings of acute pancreatitis.
- Prognosis: Multiple scoring systems exist, including the following:
  - BISAP: 5-point score to predict mortality (BUN >25 mg/dL, GCS <15, SIRS, age >60 yr, pleural effusion)
  - Ranson's criteria: Uses age, admission labs, and labs at 48 hours to predict mortality
- Treatment:
  - Make patient NPO, administer early aggressive IVF (5–10 cc/kg, Lactated Ringer's preferred), replete electrolytes, provide pain control
  - Gallstone pancreatitis: Early ERCP, followed by cholecystectomy after recovery
- Complications:
  - Pancreatic necrosis: If suspect sterile fluid collection, monitor closely, antibiotics controversial. If infection suspected, give IV antibiotics and pursue surgical debridement.
  - Pancreatic pseudocyst: Fluid collection 2–3 weeks after acute pancreatitis. Risk rupture, infection, obstruction. Treatment: Observation if minimal symptoms/no pseudoaneurysm. If symptomatic or rapidly enlarging, drain percutaneously, endoscopically, or surgically.
  - Other complications of acute pancreatitis: ARDS, pancreatic ascites, pleural effusions, ascending cholangitis, ileus, renal failure, hemorrhagic pancreatitis, abdominal compartment syndrome.

Chronic pancreatitis
- Etiology: Persistent inflammation of the pancreas with fibrotic tissue replacing pancreatic parenchyma, leading to endocrine/exocrine dysfunction. Heavy alcohol consumption is the most common cause (>80%); gallstones usually don't cause chronic pancreatitis. Consider the diagnosis of cystic fibrosis in young patients without a history of heavy alcohol use.
- Clinical features: Chronic intermittent abdominal pain, diabetes, steatorrhea (fat in the stool due to lack of pancreatic enzymes)
- Diagnosis: CT abd/pelvis or MRCP – calcifications, dilated main pancreatic duct. ERCP is the gold standard but it is not routinely performed. Labs are *not* helpful and lipase/amylase are often normal!
- Treatment:
  - Nonoperative: Alcohol and smoking cessation, pain control, pancreatic enzyme supplementation, frequent small low-fat meals
  - Operative: Pancreatojejunostomy (pancreatic duct drainage to decompress the dilated duct), total pancreatectomy with auto-islet cell transplant, or denervation (celiac plexus block)

Autoimmune pancreatitis (AIP)
- Subtypes:
  - Type 1 ("lymphoplasmacytic sclerosing pancreatitis"): IgG4-related autoimmune pancreatitis. Most patients have another concurrent IgG4-related condition, such as sclerosing cholangitis or lymphadenopathy. Often presents as a pancreatic mass or as painless jaundice; can be mistaken for pancreatic cancer.
  - Type 2 ("idiopathic duct–centric chronic pancreatitis"): Much more rare than type 1. IgG4 may be elevated or normal. Sometimes associated with IBD.
- Clinical features: Abdominal pain, pancreatic mass or enlargement with obstructive jaundice, extrapancreatic manifestations (e.g., IBD, IgG-4 associated cholangitis, lung nodules, Sjogren's)
- Diagnosis: **HISORt** criteria (**H**istology, **I**maging, **S**erology [IgG4 >2× ULN], **O**ther organ involvement, **R**esponse to steroids therapy). "Sausage-like pancreas" is buzzword for CT findings for AIP.
- Treatment: Steroids

Liver
Acute Liver Failure (ALF)

- Definitions:
  - <u>Acute liver injury (ALI)</u>: AST/ALT >100 IU/L
  - <u>Acute liver failure (ALF)</u>: All three criteria must be present – 1) Coagulopathy (INR >1.5), 2) Hepatic encephalopathy, 3) No preexisting liver disease
- Etiology:
  - Major causes: Ischemic hepatitis (e.g., shock liver, Budd-Chiari, hepatic artery thrombus or vaso-spasm), drug- or toxin-induced liver injury (e.g., acetaminophen, *Amanita* mushrooms), viral hepati-tis, autoimmune hepatitis (See Table 4.9)
  - Other causes: Fulminant Wilson's disease, malignancy with infiltration, pregnancy-related, hemo-phagocytic lymphohistiocytosis (HLH)
  - Conditions that do <u>not</u> typically cause ALF: Alcohol-related liver disease, hemochromatosis, NAFLD, alpha-1 antitrypsin deficiency, PSC, PBC
- Workup:
  - Viral: Hepatitis A IgM, hepatitis B surface ag/ab/core, hepatitis C virus antibodies, hepatitis C RNA, HSV, EBV, CMV, varicella zoster antibodies, hepatitis E IgM
  - Other labs: Acetaminophen level, toxicology screen, ceruloplasmin, urine copper (patients <35 yr), pregnancy test, ANA, anti-SMA, IgG, HIV, amylase/lipase
  - Complete abdominal ultrasound with Doppler
  - If hepatic encephalopathy is present, consider NCHCT to rule out brain herniation
- Complications: Neurologic (hepatic encephalopathy, herniation), pulmonary (ARDS), cardiac (high-output heart failure), hepatic (hypoglycemia, lactic acidosis, coagulopathy), bone marrow suppression, adrenal insufficiency, renal failure (thought to be due to cytokine-induced damage)
- Prognosis: Multiple prognostic scoring systems are available (e.g., King's College Criteria)
- Treatment:
  - Supportive care:
    - N-acetylcysteine (NAC): Historically only used to treat acetaminophen-related ALF, but there is emerging evidence to consider use of NAC for all patients with ALF
    - Continuous renal replacement therapy (CRRT) if needed
    - Intracranial hypertension prevention/treatment if needed: Hypertonic saline and then mannitol, goal Na 145 mEq/L, elevate head of bed, intubate if needed
    - Prophylactic antibiotics
    - Phosphate repletion
    - Glucose monitoring/dextrose administration
    - Enteral feeding
    - Frequent neurologic checks. Of note, lactulose is *not* used to treat hepatic encephalopathy in ALF
  - Treat the underlying cause of ALF: See Table 4.9
  - Consider liver transplantation if low probability of recovery

TABLE 4.9 · Etiologies of Acute Liver Failure (ALF) and Recommended Treatments	
Etiology of Acute Liver Failure (ALF)	**Treatment**
Acetaminophen (and potentially all patients)	N-Acetylcysteine (NAC)
Hepatitis B infection	PO antiviral
Amanita mushroom poisoning	Early administration of activated charcoal; silibinin and penicillin G
Budd-Chiari	Transjugular intrahepatic portosystemic shunt place-ment, surgical decompression, or thrombolysis
Herpes simplex virus infection	IV acyclovir
Wilson disease	Plasma exchange may temporize; requires liver transplantation
Autoimmune hepatitis	Steroids controversial in the presence of ALF

Cirrhosis and its Complications

Decompensated cirrhosis

- Decompensated cirrhosis: Defined by any one of: ascites, hepatic encephalopathy, and/or variceal bleed
- Etiologies of new decompensated cirrhosis: Infection, insults to the liver (drugs, toxins, herbs, shellfish), GI bleeding, ischemia/clotting (e.g., Budd-Chiari)
- Clinical features: Cirrhosis can cause clinical manifestations that affect almost any organ system (see Figure 4.7)

Portal hypertension

- Definition: Pressure gradient of >6 mmHg between the portal and hepatic veins
- Pathophysiology: 1) Increased resistance to portal flow at the level of the sinusoids due to disruption of blood flow by scarring/formation of parenchymal nodules; 2) Increased portal venous blood flow resulting from splanchnic circulation in response to nitric oxide release
- Etiologies: Intrahepatic (i.e., cirrhosis; much less commonly schistosomiasis, massive fatty change, diffuse fibrosing granulomatous disease such as sarcoidosis, amyloidosis, or infiltrative malignancy, and diseases of the microcirculation such as nodular regenerative hyperplasia); can also occur due to prehepatic (e.g., portal vein thrombosis) and posthepatic (e.g., Budd-Chiari, severe right-sided heart failure, constrictive pericarditis) causes

Ascites

- Description: Accumulation of excessive fluid in the peritoneal cavity. See differential diagnosis for ascites in Table 4.10. Cirrhosis is the most common cause of ascites (85%).
- Pathophysiology: 1) Portal hypertension (high hydrostatic pressure); 2) Hypoalbuminemia (low oncotic pressure); in addition, splanchnic dilatation results in lower systemic blood pressure, activating the RAAS system and resulting in additional fluid and sodium retention
- Diagnosis: Perform a paracentesis; the ascites fluid characteristics can inform the differential diagnosis for the cause of ascites fluid accumulation (See Table 4.10)
- Treatment: 1) Salt restrict <2 g/day, 2) Furosemide + spironolactone, 3) Paracentesis

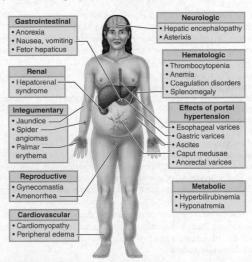

Gastrointestinal
- Anorexia
- Nausea, vomiting
- Fetor hepaticus

Renal
- Hepatorenal syndrome

Integumentary
- Jaundice
- Spider angiomas
- Palmar erythema

Reproductive
- Gynecomastia
- Amenorrhea

Cardiovascular
- Cardiomyopathy
- Peripheral edema

Neurologic
- Hepatic encephalopathy
- Asterixis

Hematologic
- Thrombocytopenia
- Anemia
- Coagulation disorders
- Splenomegaly

Effects of portal hypertension
- Esophageal varices
- Gastric varices
- Ascites
- Caput medusae
- Anorectal varices

Metabolic
- Hyperbilirubinemia
- Hyponatremia

FIGURE 4.7: Systemic clinical manifestations of liver cirrhosis. Cirrhosis can cause clinical manifestations that affect almost every organ system.

TABLE 4.10 · Differential Diagnosis for the Cause of Ascites Based on Ascites Fluid Characteristics		
	SAAG* <1.1	SAAG* >1.1
Ascitic fluid protein <2.5 g/dL	Nephrotic syndrome	Cirrhosis
Ascitic fluid protein >2.5 g/dL	Malignancy, tuberculosis	R-sided heart failure, Budd-Chiari

* Serum ascites albumin gradient (SAAG) = Serum albumin concentration (g/dL) – Ascites albumin concentration (g/dL)

Spontaneous bacterial peritonitis (SBP)
- Spontaneous vs. secondary bacterial peritonitis:
  - <u>Spontaneous bacterial peritonitis (SBP)</u>: Infection of ascites, without an evident surgically treatable intraabdominal source, which almost always occurs in patients with cirrhosis and ascites
  - <u>Secondary bacterial peritonitis</u>: Infection of ascites in the presence of a surgically treatable intraabdominal source, due to peritonitis with or without perforation. It is <u>crucial</u> to distinguish these conditions, because secondary bacterial peritonitis requires intraabdominal surgery, whereas surgery can be harmful for patients with SBP.
- Pathogenesis: Translocation of bacteria from the gut lumen across the intestinal wall
- Microbiology: *E. coli, Klebsiella, S. pneumoniae*
- Clinical features: Ascites due to cirrhosis with fever, abdominal pain/tenderness, and/or altered mental status; however, >10% of patients have no symptoms, and thus clinical suspicion should be high and ascitic fluid should be sampled for essentially all admitted patients with cirrhotic ascites
- Diagnosis: 1) Ascitic fluid with PMNs >250 cells/mm³, 2) Positive ascitic fluid bacterial culture, 3) Absence of a cause of secondary bacterial peritonitis (Gram stain with a large number of bacteria can be suggestive of secondary bacterial peritonitis; if suspicion is high for secondary bacterial peritonitis but imaging does not reveal a source, then perform repeat paracentesis at 48 hours)
- Treatment: Ceftriaxone or cefotaxime
- Prophylaxis: Antibiotic prophylaxis with ciprofloxacin or trimethoprim-sulfamethoxazole is indicated for patients with a prior episode of SBP, prior variceal hemorrhage, or ascitic fluid protein concentration <1 g/dL

Hepatohydrothorax
- Description: Presence of pleural effusion on CXR in the presence of ascites and in the absence of another reason to have a pleural effusion (e.g., cardiac, pulmonary, or pleural disease)
- Pathophysiology: Due to leakage of ascitic fluid through diaphragmatic defects; R-sided defects are more common since the L-sided diaphragm is thicker and more muscular
- Clinical features: Dyspnea, cough, pleurisy, hypoxemia. Hepatohydrothorax are 80% R-sided, 15% L-sided, 5% bilateral
- Diagnosis: CXR; thoracentesis with pleural fluid sampling demonstrates transudative fluid similar to ascitic fluid with a low protein concentration (<2.5 g/dL), SAAG >1.1 g/dL
- Treatment: 1) Medical management identical to ascites (i.e., sodium restriction, diuresis), 2) If refractory to medical management, consider other therapies such as recurrent thoracenteses or TIPS

Portosystemic shunts (collaterals and varices)
- Pathophysiology: Portal hypertension results in reversal of blood flow from the portal to systemic circulation, causing dilation of collateral vessels and development of new vessels
- Locations: Esophagus/stomach (esophageal varices, gastric varices, portal hypertensive gastropathy), rectum (hemorrhoids), periumbilical/abdominal wall collaterals (caput medusae: dilated subcutaneous veins extending from the umbilicus laterally)
- Management of esophageal varices:
  - Prescribe beta blockers for the prevention of variceal bleeding
  - Perform surveillance EGD for varices at an appropriate interval (See Table 4.11)
  - Modify routine management of GIB if concerned for variceal bleeding: Two large-bore IVs, PPI, type and screen *plus* ceftriaxone 1 g IV daily and octreotide 50 mcg IV bolus plus 50 mcg/hr infusion
  - Consider TIPS for uncontrolled bleeding if low MELDNa score and no pulmonary hypertension

Splenomegaly
- Description: Enlargement of the spleen to as large as 1000 gm
- Pathophysiology: Long-standing congestion of the spleen due to portal hypertension
- Complications: Thrombocytopenia (due to sequestration; low TPO production also contributes); less commonly can cause pancytopenia

TABLE 4.11 · EGD Surveillance for Patients with Cirrhosis	
Disease Status	**Interval for Surveillance EGD**
Compensated, no varices	Every 2–3 yr
Compensated, small varices	Every 1–2 yr
Decompensated	Annually

Hepatic encephalopathy (HE)

- Description: Not a single clinical entity; spectrum of disturbances in consciousness/mental status, ranging from subtle sleep-wake and behavioral changes to deep coma/death, likely due to combination of reversible metabolic encephalopathy, brain atrophy, and brain edema.
- Pathophysiology: Ammonia is the most well-documented contributing neurotoxin. It is thought to alter neuronal electrical activity and increase intracellular osmolarity, which contributes to increased cerebral edema
- Clinical features: Confusion, asterixis (flap), hyperreflexia, fetor hepaticus (musty breath)
- Grading (West-Haven): 1) Sleep-wake disturbance, 2) Dissociation, asterixis, 3) Marked confusion, 4) Coma
- Triggers for worsening HE: Infection, GIB, portal vein thrombosis, medications (e.g., benzodiazepines, opioids), inappropriate lactulose dosing
- Treatment: 1) Lactulose prevents ammonia absorption; 2) Rifaximin kills ammonia-producing gut flora; 3) Zinc deficiency is common so zinc supplementation is sometimes administered, but benefit for HE is understudied.

Hepatopulmonary syndrome

- Etiology: Hypoxemia and intrapulmonary vascular dilatation in the presence of liver disease; occurs in up to 30% of patients with decompensated cirrhosis
- Pathophysiology: Intrapulmonary vascular dilatations allow rapid blood flow through the capillary bed and do not provide enough time for oxygen diffusion, resulting in shunt physiology (Q>>V). Since blood flow is dependent (i.e., shifts with gravity) in the lungs, flow in the lung bases increases when sitting upright (Q). Therefore, for patients with hepatopulmonary syndrome, shunting and symptoms worsen when sitting in the upright position
- Clinical features: Dyspnea; easier to breathe while lying flat (platypnea) and worsening arterial oxygen saturation if upright (orthodeoxia)
- Diagnosis: PaO_2 <80 mmHg on room air, echo with intrapulmonary shunting
- Treatment: Supplemental oxygen, liver transplantation

Portopulmonary hypertension

- Description: Pulmonary hypertension in the presence of portal hypertension; present in 5–9% of liver transplant candidates
- Pathophysiology: Poorly understood; seems to relate to pulmonary vasoconstriction/remodeling in presence of portal hypertension
- Clinical features: Symptoms are variable, most commonly dyspnea, clubbing, fatigue, chest pain, syncope
- Diagnosis: TTE may be suggestive; confirm with right heart catheterization
- Treatment: Patients may be candidates for pulmonary artery hypertension therapy based on functional class (e.g., prostacyclin analogues, endothelin antagonists, phosphodiesterase inhibitors); avoid TIPS due to the risk of worsening right heart failure

Hepatorenal syndrome (HRS)

- Description: Renal failure occurring in patients with liver failure who have no other morphologic or functional reasons for renal impairment
- Pathophysiology: Decreased renal perfusion pressure due to systemic (including splanchnic) vasodilatation and resultant hypoperfusion/RAAS activation
- Subtypes:
  - Type 1: More severe; doubling of baseline Cr to >2.5 mg/dL in a period of <2 weeks
  - Type 2: Less severe; usually associated with diuretic-refractory ascites
- Diagnosis:
  - Hepatic disease with portal hypertension
  - AKI (prior definitions required Cr >1.5 mg/dL; however, this is evolving)
  - Absence of any other apparent cause of AKI (e.g., shock, nephrotoxic drugs, obstruction; obtain renal ultrasound to evaluate for obstruction, urinalysis to evaluate for proteinuria or RBC)
  - No improvement in function after albumin challenge (i.e., cessation of diuretics plus IV albumin 1 g/kg/day for 2 days)
- Treatment: **MOA** (**M**idodrine, **O**ctreotide, **A**lbumin); if critically ill, use norepinephrine and albumin; consider TIPS or dialysis for bridge to transplant in patients who fail medical therapy

Other clinical features of cirrhosis

- Hypoestrogenism: 1) Spider angiomas, 2) Palmar erythema, 3) Gynecomastia, 4) Testicular atrophy, 5) Amenorrhea, 6) Low libido
- Decreased hepatic synthetic/biochemical function: Hypoalbuminemia, decreased clotting factors (leading to INR prolongation)
- Thrombocytopenia: Results from splenic sequestration, decreased TPO production; suggestive lab abnormality for the presence of portal hypertension

Healthcare maintenance in cirrhosis
- Hepatocellular carcinoma (HCC) screening: Patients with cirrhosis have an increased risk of HCC; screen with q6mo abdominal imaging (e.g., abdominal ultrasound or quad phase CT) and serum AFP
- Hepatic osteodystrophy: Osteoporosis, osteopenia. Check DEXA, calcium, and vitamin D.
- Immunizations: Hepatitis A, hepatitis B, influenza, 23-valent pneumococcal polysaccharide vaccine (PSSV23)
- Avoidances: Alcohol, oysters/raw shellfish (due to risk of *Vibrio* infection in setting of relative immunocompromise), opioids; minimize use of acetaminophen (up to 2 grams/day is classic limit, although evidence for this limit is lacking), NSAIDs, sedating medications (e.g., benzodiazepines)
- Nutrition: Muscle wasting is common; high-protein diet is critical

Scoring systems used for the assessment of prognosis in liver cirrhosis
- Model for End-Stage Liver Disease (MELD)-Sodium (Na) Score:
  - Definition: A scoring system for assessing the severity of chronic liver disease that uses lab values including: serum bilirubin, creatinine, INR, and sodium to predict 3-month survival
  - Clinical uses:
    - Scores range from 6–40, with higher scores correlating with increased severity of liver dysfunction and higher 3-month mortality.
    - In 2002, MELD-Na was accepted by the United Network of Organ Sharing (UNOS) for prioritization of patients awaiting liver transplantation in the United States.
- Child-Pugh:
  - Definition: A scoring system to assess the prognosis of chronic liver disease, mainly cirrhosis. The score employs five clinical measures of liver disease: Total bilirubin, serum albumin, prothrombin time, ascites, and hepatic encephalopathy.
  - Clinical uses:
    - MELD-Na is more widely used, given its better prognostic value, but Child-Pugh is still referenced and utilized in some settings (e.g., HCC treatment guidelines in oncology).

Etiologies of Liver Disease
Alcohol-Induced Liver Disease
Alcoholic hepatitis
- Clinical features: Jaundice, anorexia, fever, tender hepatomegaly
- Diagnosis: Moderate elevation in transaminases (AST:ALT ratio ≥ 2) in a patient with a history of prolonged and heavy alcohol use (often >100 g/day for >20 yr); requires exclusion of other causes of liver disease
- Management:
  - Evaluate for other causes of acute hepatitis (e.g., HBsAg, anti-HBs, anti-HBc, Hep A IgM, acetaminophen level, RUQ ultrasound with Doppler)
  - Rule out mimics, such as sepsis due to intraabdominal source or SBP (should obtain blood culture; UA, urine culture; paracentesis for culture, cell count/differential, total protein, albumin)
  - Calculate MELD-Na and Maddrey's discriminant function (MDF)
    - MDF = 4.6 * (patient's PT in seconds − control PT in seconds) + patient serum total bilirubin
    - If steroids are indicated (MDF >32; indicates severe alcoholic hepatitis and 1-month mortality 35–45%), plan for steroid administration in consultation with hepatology; typical dose is prednisolone 40 mg/day for 28 days
    - Calculate the Lille score at day 7. If >0.45, suggests nonresponsiveness to steroids and steroids can be stopped
    - Pentoxifylline is an alternative to steroids if there are contraindications to steroid use, although this is controversial (STOPAH Trial, *New Eng J Med* 2015)
  - If AKI is present, consider gentle fluid resuscitation
  - Consider peptic ulcer prophylaxis, particularly if steroids will be used
  - Nutritional supplementation with thiamine, folate, and a multivitamin. Adequate nutrition is the most important intervention for alcoholic hepatitis survival and has the best data. It is not just about micronutrient deficiencies but also about ensuring adequate macronutrients. Protein intake in particular should be encouraged. Often these patients don't feel well enough to eat and may not eat enough, so enteral feeding can be considered.

Alcoholic cirrhosis
- Epidemiology: Cirrhosis develops in 10–25% of patients with chronic heavy alcohol use
- Treatment: Alcohol cessation, liver transplantation if eligible (typically requires >6 months of abstinence from alcohol to be considered)

Drug/Toxin-Induced Liver Injury

Acetaminophen

- Epidemiology: Most common cause of intrinsic drug-induced liver injury. Can occur due to accidental overdose, intentional overdose, co-ingestion with alcohol or other substances
- Diagnosis: Measure APAP level at 4 and 16 hours after ingestion. If timing unclear, draw immediately upon presentation and 4 hours later (levels may be negative up to 4 hours after ingestion)
- Treatment: N-acetylcysteine (NAC), consult poison control/toxicology

Other medications that cause liver injury

- Medications: Antibiotics (amoxicillin-clavulanate), antiepileptic drugs (phenytoin, valproate), antituberculosis drugs (isoniazid, rifampin), NSAIDs, azathioprine, *Amanita* mushroom poisoning

Infectious Etiologies of Liver Disease

Hepatitis A virus (HAV), Hepatitis E virus (HAE)

- HAV: Fecal–oral transmission. Patients may be asymptomatic or present with malaise, fatigue, nausea/vomiting. Diagnosis: HAV IgM. Treatment: Supportive, does not cause chronic hepatitis.
- HEV: Fecal–oral transmission, especially waterborne. Diagnosis: HEV IgM. Treatment: 1) Acute: Supportive care; infection can be much more severe in pregnant women. 2) Chronic: Chronic infection is almost exclusively seen in immunocompromised hosts; treat with ribavirin for 12 weeks in nonpregnant patients.

Hepatitis D virus (HDV)

- Pathophysiology: Parenteral (IVDU, blood), sexual, and vertical transmission. Vertical transmission is the most common. Requires the outer envelope of HbsAg for replication; if coinfection with hepatitis B occurs, can present as acute hepatitis; if superinfection occurs, can exacerbate chronic hepatitis B
- Diagnosis: HDV RNA, HDV IgM, IgG
- Treatment: Supportive care

Hepatitis B virus (HBV)

- Transmission: Parenteral (IVDU, blood), sexual, and vertical. Adults typically do *not* progress to chronic hepatitis B; children very frequently progress to chronic hepatitis B.
- Detection and interpretation of serologic results: See Figures 4.8, 4.9; Tables 4.12, 4.13
- Treatment:
  - Acute HBV: No treatment for acute HBV
  - Chronic HBV: Therapy is often lifelong and non-curative. Indications for treatment of chronic HBV:
    - Compensated cirrhosis and DNA >2000 IU/mL
    - Decompensated cirrhosis or acute liver failure with any detectable DNA
    - Immune active: 1) HBeAg positive: ALT ≥2× ULN and HBV>20,000 IU/mL; 2) HBeAg negative: ALT ≥2× ULN and HBV >2000 IU/mL
    - Other populations: Patients on chronic immunosuppressive therapy, pregnant women with high viral loads, patients with HCC, patients with HCV coinfection who are being treated for HCV
  - Agents:
    - Tenofovir (TDF, TAF): Lower rates of resistance; can be used in patients with decompensated cirrhosis.
    - Entecavir: Lower rates of resistance; do not use with lamivudine-resistant HBV; can be used in patients with decompensated cirrhosis.
    - Lamivudine: High rates of resistance so generally less preferred; can be used in patients with decompensated cirrhosis.
    - Interferon (INF-alpha): Can only be used in young patients with compensated liver disease

TABLE 4.12 · Interpretation of Hepatitis B Serologic Test Results			
HBsAg	Anti-HBc	Anti-HBs	Interpretation
Neg	Neg	Neg	Uninfected, not immune.
Neg	Neg	Pos	Immune due to vaccine.
Neg	Pos	Pos	Immune due to natural infection. · Obtain HBV DNA if immunocompromised.
Pos	Pos	Neg	Interpretation requires IgM anti-HBc. · If positive, acute HBV. · If negative, chronic HBV.
Neg	Pos	Neg	Four possibilities: Resolved infection (most common), false positive, low-level chronic infection, resolving acute infection. · Obtain HBV DNA, especially if immunocompromised.

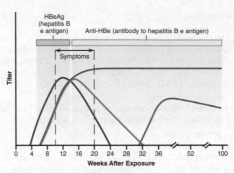

- HBsAg (hepatitis B surface antigen)
- IgM anti-HBc (immunoglobulin M to hepatitis B core antigen)
- Total anti-HBc (total antibody to hepatitis B core antigen)
- Anti-HBs (antibody to hepatitis B surface antigen)

FIGURE 4.8: Acute hepatitis B virus infection with typical recovery serologic course. Acute hepatitis B is diagnosed by detecting hepatitis B surface antigen (HBsAg) and IgM core antibody (IgM anti-HBc), or in the window period (i.e., when neither HBsAg nor its antibody [anti-HBs] can be detected in the serum) by IgM anti-HBc alone. IgM core antibodies are lost within 24–32 weeks of the onset of illness, whereas total antibody to hepatitis B core antigen (total anti-HBc) and anti-HBs persist. The hepatitis B e antigen (HBeAg) is initially positive, and then antibody to the hepatitis E antigen can later be detected.

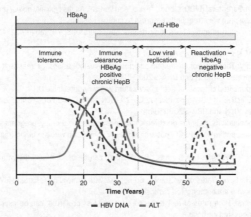

FIGURE 4.9: Natural course of chronic hepatitis B infection. There are several phases of chronic hepatitis B infection. During the immune tolerance phase, hepatitis B e antigen (HBeAg) is present, there are high hepatitis B virus DNA (HBV DNA) titers, and ALT is normal without evidence of active liver disease. During the immune clearance phase, HBeAg is still present. HBV DNA and ALT levels are typically both high and/or fluctuating. Due to the immune clearance phase, HBeAg is seroconverted, and then only antibody to the hepatitis B e antigen (anti-HBe) is detected during the subsequent phases. Most patients then enter a period of low viral replication, which is characterized by the absence of HBeAg, the presence of anti-HBe, low hepatitis B viral titers, low ALT, and little or no inflammation on liver biopsy. Some patients later have reactivation of their hepatitis B virus, characterized by absence of HBeAg and presence of anti-HBe (high and/or fluctuating; demonstrated as a dotted line on the right side of the figure).

TABLE 4.13 · Hepatitis B Testing Parameters		
Test	Description	Indicates
HBSAg	Surface antigen; detectable 1–2 wk after infection; will not be detected if virus is cleared	Whether patient is infected with Hep B, regardless of whether acute or chronic
Anti-HBs	Antibody to surface antigen; will be present after vaccination or clearance of Hep B	Whether patient is immune to Hep B, regardless of how immunity was conferred
HBeAg	Envelope antigen; suggests active viral replication and usually is associated with high Hep B DNA levels	Risk of infectivity/transmission (i.e., higher risk)
Anti-HBe	Antibody to envelope antigen; suggests decreased viral replication, but some strains develop a pre-core mutation and will have persistent viral replication despite antibody	Risk of infectivity/transmission (i.e., lower risk)
Anti-HBc	Antibody to Hep B core; positive during a "window" period when HB_sAg may be decreasing and undetectable but anti-HB_sAg levels are also still too low to detect	Whether the patient has been exposed to hepatitis B
IgM anti-HBc	IgM antibody to Hep B core	Whether the patient has been exposed to hepatitis B within 6 mo; particularly useful during the "window period"
Anti-HBc (IgG)	IgG antibody to Hep B core	Whether the patient has been exposed to hepatitis B; if patient is immune, this test can determine whether prior infection (positive result) or vaccine (negative result) conferred immunity
Viral load	HBV DNA measured by PCR; if persistent for >6 wk, more likely progression to chronic Hep B	Presence of hepatitis B

Hepatits C virus (HCV)
- Transmission: Mainly parenteral (IVDU)
- Screening: CDC and USPSTF recommend universal HCV screening at least once age 18–79 yr
- Symptoms: Most patients are asymptomatic or report non-specific symptoms (e.g., fatigue)
- Conditions associated with HCV infection:
  - Cryoglobulinemia: IgM against HepC IgG that causes vasculitis of the skin (palpable purpura, Raynaud's), kidneys (MPGN), nerves (motor-sensory axonopathy), and joints (arthralgias)
  - Porphyria cutanea tarda: Fragile, photosensitive, painless vesicles on the dorsum of hand
- Diagnosis: Check HCV antibody. If positive:
  - Check HCV viral load; if viremic, check genotype (1–6, 1a most common in United States [70%])
  - Screen for HAV/HBV and vaccinate; provide counseling about reducing alcohol consumption and mechanisms to reduce forward transmission (e.g., avoidance of needle sharing, condom use)
  - Fibrosis assessment: Affects decision for HCC screening and treatment choice
- Treatment: Treatment for HCV is curative and recommended for all patients with HCV! Treatment regimen depends on HCV genotype and whether the patient has cirrhosis
  - Direct-acting antivirals (DAAs)
    - Protease inhibitors ("P" = previr)
    - NS5B inhibitors ("B" = buvir)
    - NS5A inhibitors ("A" = asvir)
  - Regimen: NS5A + NS5B inhibitor
    - Velpatasvir/sofosbuvir (Epclusa): One pill daily for 12 weeks, can be used for all genotypes. First-line for treatment-naïve patients with no or compensated cirrhosis.
  - Regimen: NS5A + protease inhibitor
    - Pibrentasvir/glecaprevir (Mavyret): Three pills daily for 8 weeks. First line for treatment-naïve patients with no or compensated cirrhosis.
    - Elbasvir/Grazoprevir (Zepatier): One pill daily for 12 weeks. First line for patients with CKD
  - Monitor LFTs during treatment, as rarely patients can develop hepatic decompensation
  - Sustained viral response (SVR) = Undetectable viral load 12 weeks after completion of therapy

Other viruses that cause liver injury
- Viruses: EBV, CMV, HSV, VZV. See additional details in Infectious Diseases Chapter 8

Autoimmune Etiologies of Liver Disease

Autoimmune hepatitis

- Epidemiology: F:M = 4:1, associated with other autoimmune conditions
- Clinical features: Variable presentation from asymptomatic to acute liver failure
- Diagnosis:
  - Type 1: +ANA, +anti-smooth muscle (65%), +anti-actin, +anti-mitochondrial (with PBC overlap), anti-SLA/LP (10–30%), anti-dsDNA (25–35%), +pANCA
  - Type 2: +ALKM-1, +/−ALC-1
  - Liver biopsy
- Treatment: Steroids +/−azathioprine. Indications: AST>10× ULN, AST>2× ULN and IgG level >2× ULN, bridging fibrosis, cirrhosis. Advanced disease may require liver transplantation.

Metabolic Etiologies of Liver Disease

Nonalcoholic fatty liver disease (NAFLD)/nonalcoholic steatohepatitis (NASH)

- Risk factors: Associated with obesity, HLD, DM2
- Clinical features: Patients are usually asymptomatic but 10–20% of patients progress and develop cirrhosis (especially patients with NASH, which is an advanced form of NAFLD)
- Diagnosis: Can make presumptive diagnosis but need liver biopsy for definitive diagnosis. Histology appears similar to cirrhosis due to alcohol use, but patient reports no/minimal alcohol use.
- Treatment: Control risk factors for insulin resistance, weight loss, consider bariatric surgery. OK to use statins. Vitamin E is sometimes used for nondiabetic NASH.

Wilson's disease

- Pathophysiology: Autosomal recessive mutation of the *ATP7B* gene that encodes for ceruloplasmin (copper-binding protein needed for excretion); therefore, copper accumulates in the liver and blood. Typical age of onset is 5–35 yr.
- Clinical features:
  - Liver: Acute hepatitis, cirrhosis, liver failure
  - Eyes: Kayser-Fleischer rings, yellow rings in cornea
  - CNS: Copper deposits in the basal ganglia which can cause extrapyramidal signs (parkinsonism), depression, paranoia
  - Renal: Aminoaciduria, nephrocalcinosis
  - Hemolytic anemia: Caused by sudden release of copper from liver cells
- Diagnosis: Low serum ceruloplasmin, high urine copper, molecular test for mutation in *ATP7B* gene
- Treatment: Penicillamine or trientine (chelator), zinc (prevents dietary copper uptake), liver transplantation

Hemochromatosis

- Pathophysiology: Autosomal recessive disease of iron absorption; excess iron is absorbed in the gut and accumulates as ferritin and hemosiderin in organs, causing fibrosis
- Clinical features: Bronze diabetes (deposits in the pancreas), arthralgias, hepatomegaly, impotence, restrictive cardiomyopathy, arrhythmias
- Diagnosis: Ratio of iron to TIBC ≥45%, ferritin >150 ng/mL (women) and >200 ng/mL (men). Definitive diagnosis = HFE gene testing with C282Y polymorphism
- Treatment: Repeat phlebotomy for patients with ferritin >500 ng/mL, evidence of tissue injury, or increased tissue iron by imaging/biopsy. Target ferritin to normal range. Counsel patients to avoid raw seafood (increased risk of *Vibrio* infection). Liver transplantation may be necessary.

Alpha-1 antitrypsin deficiency

- Pathophysiology: Autosomal recessive disease that causes deficiency in alpha-1 antitrypsin production
- Clinical features: Lung (emphysema) and liver disease (cirrhosis, HCC, hepatitis)
- Diagnosis: Low serum alpha-1 antitrypsin
- Treatment: Liver transplantation

Cholestatic Liver Diseases

Primary biliary cholangitis (PBC)

- Etiology: Immune-mediated destruction of intrahepatic bile ducts, most common in females 40–50 yr
- Clinical features: Fatigue, pruritus, jaundice
- Diagnosis: At least two of following: AlkP >1.5× ULN, +anti-mitochondrial antibody, liver biopsy with destruction of interlobular bile ducts and destructive cholangitis
- Treatment: First line: ursodiol slows progression. Second line: obeticholic acid in compensated cirrhosis. For advanced disease, liver transplantation.

Primary sclerosing cholangitis (PSC)
- Etiology: Fibroinflammatory disorder of bile ducts, most common in men 20–30 yr. 80% patients have IBD (UC)
- Clinical features: Patients are usually asymptomatic or may develop pruritus, abdominal pain, cholangitis
- Diagnosis: MRCP or ERCP: "Beads on a string" of intrahepatic and extrahepatic ducts. Liver biopsy: Fibrous obliteration of the small bile ducts with an "onion skin" appearance on pathology
- Treatment: No effective treatment. Progressive disease that requires liver transplantation. High association with cholangiocarcinoma: Screen with q6–12mo LFTs, Ca19-9, MRCP

Pregnancy-Related Liver Diseases
Hyperemesis gravidarum: First trimester, severe vomiting, elevated ALT. Treatment: Hydration.
Intrahepatic cholestasis of pregnancy: Second or third trimester. Pruritis. ALT 10× ULN. Treatment: Ursodiol.
Preeclampsia: Third trimester. Hypertension, edema, proteinuria. Mild increase ALT. Treatment: Delivery.
HELLP syndrome: Third trimester. Features of preeclampsia with microangiopathic hemolytic anemia. Treatment: Delivery.
Acute fatty liver of pregnancy (AFLP): Features of preeclampsia with coagulation abnormalities (also more hepatic encephalopathy and hypoglycemia than HELLP). Treatment: Delivery.

Vascular Etiologies of Liver Disease
Portal vein thrombosis
- Etiology: Blood clot in the hepatic portal vein, which can lead to increased pressure in the portal venous system and reduced blood supply to the liver
- Diagnosis: RUQ ultrasound with Doppler
- Treatment: Chronic PVT does not require treatment. Can consider anticoagulation for acute PVT after evaluation for varices.

Budd-Chiari syndrome
- Etiology: Occlusion of the hepatic venous outflow by a thrombus. Associated with hypercoagulable states, such as polycythemia vera, pregnancy/OCPs, paroxysmal noctural hemoglobinuria
- Clinical presentation: Severe RUQ pain, hepatomegaly, ascites, jaundice, acute liver failure
- Diagnosis: RUQ ultrasound with Doppler or hepatic venography
- Treatment: Thrombolysis (i.e., anticoagulation) is first line; other options include percutaneous angiography with stenting, TIPS, surgical shunting, liver transplantation

Other Pathologies Affecting the Liver
Hypoperfusion
- Shock liver: Hypotension causes hypoperfusion of the liver; labs are notable for an elevated AST/ALT with relatively normal bilirubin/AlkP. Transaminases should normalize in 1–2 weeks. Treat underlying condition (e.g., treat sepsis to prevent further hypotension)

Hepatic cysts and abscesses
- Hepatic cysts: Usually benign and no follow-up/treatment is required; surgical removal can be considered if the cysts are causing symptoms; if many cysts, consider the diagnosis of autosomal dominant polycystic kidney disease.
- Hydatid liver cysts: The tapeworm *Echinococcus granulosus* can be transmitted from dogs to humans, and cause cysts in the liver that have "eggshell" calcifications. Treatment: Surgical resection (pre-inject with ethanol prior to surgery to kill the tapeworm first!), then metronidazole or albendazole after surgery.
- Pyogenic liver abscess: Pus-filled area in the liver, often due to a polymicrobial infection (*E. coli, Klebsiella, Proteus, Enterococcus*, anaerobes). Symptoms: Fever, malaise, anorexia, nausea/vomiting. Diagnosis: RUQ ultrasound or CT abd/pelvis. Treatment: IV antibiotics, drain (percutaneous vs. surgical depending on the number and size).

Benign liver tumors
- Hepatic hemangioma: Most common benign liver tumor. May increase in size with pregnancy or estrogen, but mechanism unknown. No treatment is required.
- Focal nodular hyperplasia (FNH): Second most common benign liver tumor. Predominantly in women of reproductive age. Not associated with OCP use. No treatment required.
- Hepatocellular adenoma: Benign liver tumor that typically affects women and is associated with OCP use; low malignant potential. Treatment: Stop OCPs. Resect tumors >5 cm or if symptomatic.

KEY MEDICATIONS AND INTERVENTIONS

Overlap of Diagnostic and Therapeutic Interventions in Gastroenterology

Several diagnostic tests commonly used by gastroenterologists also have therapeutic potential; for information about EGD, colonoscopy, ERCP, and other modalities, refer to the Diagnostics section of this chapter.

Paracentesis

- Indications: 1) All patients with new-onset ascites of uncertain cause, 2) All patients with preexisting ascites in whom SBP is suspected, 3) All patients with cirrhosis and ascites who are being admitted to the hospital
- Variations: Diagnostic (obtain small sample for testing), therapeutic (large-volume paracentesis)
- Tests to consider: See Table 4.14
- Relative contraindications: Fluid <2 cm deep from abdominal wall, severe thrombocytopenia (platelet count <50K/μL), DIC; no specific INR cutoff for patients with cirrhosis
- Complications: Complications of fluid shifts (e.g., hypotension, AKI), abdominal wall hematoma, intraabdominal bleeding, wound infection, persistent leak from the puncture site

TABLE 4.14 · Laboratory Tests Commonly Ordered to Evaluate Ascites Fluid	
Test	**Notes**
Albumin	• Required for SAAG calculation
Total protein	• <1 g/dL: Indication for SBP prophylaxis • >1 g/dL: Suggestive of secondary bacterial peritonitis
LDH	• LDH >ULN for serum suggests secondary bacterial peritonitis
Glucose	• Glucose <50 mg/dL suggests secondary bacterial peritonitis
Carcinoembryonic antigen (CEA)	• CEA >5 mg/mL suggests hollow viscus perforation
Alkaline phosphatase	• AlkP >240 U/L suggests hollow viscus perforation
Amylase	• Amylase >5× ULN for serum suggests pancreatic ascites or hollow viscus perforation
Triglyceride	• Triglyceride >200 mg/dL suggests chylous ascites
Cytology	• Used to assess for malignant ascites • Yield improves with multiple samples (typically >3)
Bacterial culture	• Used for the diagnosis of SBP • High load of bacteria suggests secondary bacterial peritonitis
Gram stain	• High load of bacteria suggests secondary bacterial peritonitis
Mycobacterial culture	• Used to assess for mycobacterial infection

Transjugular Intrahepatic Portosystemic Shunt (TIPS)

- Concept: Placement of a TIPS (via angiographic techniques) creates a low-resistance channel between the hepatic vein and an intrahepatic branch of the portal vein and thus helps to reduce elevated portal pressure (Figure 4.10)
- Indications: Bleeding related to portal hypertension, management of refractory ascites
- Contraindications:
  - <u>Absolute contraindications</u>: Congestive heart failure, severe pulmonary hypertension, severe tricuspid regurgitation, multiple hepatic cysts, active systemic infection, biliary obstruction
  - <u>Relative contraindications</u>: Obstruction of all hepatic veins, hepatocellular carcinoma (especially if centrally located), portal vein thrombosis, thrombocytopenia (platelets <20K/μL)
- Complications:
  - Intraprocedural complications: Cardiac arrhythmias, liver capsule puncture
  - Postprocedural complications: Hepatic encephalopathy, heart failure, liver failure, infection, TIPS dysfunction

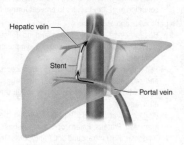

Hepatic vein

Stent

Portal vein

FIGURE 4.10: **Transjugular intrahepatic portosystemic shunt (TIPS).** TIPS is a shunt or bypass used to connect two veins within the liver – the portal vein and the hepatic vein – in order to treat portal hypertension.

Medications

TABLE 4.15 · Key Medications in Gastroenterology				
Class	**Examples**	**Mechanism**	**Uses**	**Side Effects**
Histamine-2 blockers	cimetidine ranitidine famotidine nizatidine	Reversibly inhibits the histamine H2 receptors → H^+ secretion by parietal cells	PUD, gastritis, mild GERD	• *Cimetidine* inhibits cytochrome P-450, has antiandrogenic effects, and crosses blood–brain barrier and placenta • Cimetidine and ranitidine → renal excretion of creatinine • All other H2 blockers largely free of these effects
Proton pump inhibitors (PPIs)	omeprazole, lansoprazole, esomeprazole, pantoprazole, dexlansoprazole	Irreversibly inhibits H^+/K^+ ATPase in stomach parietal cells	PUD, gastritis, GERD, Zollinger-Ellison syndrome, *H. pylori*, stress ulcer prophylaxis	• Increased risk of *C. difficile* infection, pneumonia, acute interstitial nephritis • Decreased Mg^{2+} and Ca^{2+} absorption (might mediate increased fracture risk in elderly)
Antacids	aluminum hydroxide, calcium carbonate, magnesium hydroxide	Neutralizes hydrochloric in the stomach	Dyspepsia, mild GERD	• May affect absorption, bioavailability, or urinary excretion of other drugs (by altering gastric pH, urinary pH, or gastric emptying) • All agents carry a risk of hypokalemia
Antidiarrheal	bismuth subsalicylate	Exhibits both antisecretory and antimicrobial action	Dyspepsia, traveler's diarrhea (including prophylaxis), *H. pylori* eradication	• Avoid concurrent use of other salicylates
	loperamide	μ-opioid receptor agonist, slows gut motility	Diarrhea	• Constipation, nausea
Antiulcer	sucralfate	Forms a viscous pastelike substance with GI exudates that locally coats the gastric lining to protect against peptic acid, pepsin, and bile salts	PUD (especially duodenal ulcers)	• Hyperglycemia has been reported in diabetics • Use with caution in renal failure as sucralfate is an aluminum complex

(continued)

TABLE 4.15 • Key Medications in Gastroenterology (*Continued*)				
Class	**Examples**	**Mechanism**	**Uses**	**Side Effects**
Antiemetic	ondansetron (Zofran)	5-HT3 antagonist (central acting); decreased vagal stimulation	Nausea/vomiting, especially postop or related to chemotherapy	• QT prolongation • Serotonin syndrome • Headache, constipation
	metoclopramide (Reglan)	D2 receptor antagonist (central acting); increases GI tract response to Ach with resultant increased LES tone, motility, and gastric emptying	Gastroparesis, persistent GERD	• Drowsiness (dose-related) • Nausea • Dystonic reaction (dose-related) • Drug-induced parkinsonism • Tardive dyskinesia
Somatostatin analog	octreotide	Mimics effects of somatostatin in multiple axes; inhibits secretion of splanchnic vasodilatory hormones resulting in decreased splanchnic blood flow	Acute variceal bleeds, carcinoid tumors and crisis, acromegaly, neuroendocrine tumors (e.g., VIPoma)	• Depends on indication; more side effects when used for acromegaly • Diarrhea, nausea, abdominal discomfort • Hyperglycemia • Bradycardia
Laxative	lactulose	Provides osmotic load to draw water into GI lumen; bacterial degradation of lactulose results in an acidic pH that inhibits diffusion of NH_3 into the blood (by causing the conversion of NH_3 to NH_4^+), in turn reducing hepatic encephalopathy	Hepatic encephalopathy, constipation	• Diarrhea • Gas • Nausea

KEY CLINICAL TRIALS AND PUBLICATIONS

GI Bleed

- **Transfusion Strategies for Acute Upper Gastrointestinal Bleeding.** *N Engl J Med* 2013;368:11–21.
  - Randomized controlled trial that randomized 921 patients with severe acute UGIB to a restrictive transfusion strategy (transfuse for Hgb <7 g/dL) or a liberal transfusion strategy (transfuse for Hgb <9 g/dL). The restrictive strategy reduced further bleeding, and a subgroup analysis revealed improved survival with the restrictive strategy for patients with cirrhosis and Child-Pugh A or B disease (but not Class C). Of note, exclusion criteria included massive exsanguinating bleeding, ACS, CVA/TIA, recent trauma/surgery, or LGIB.
- **COGENT.** *N Engl J Med* 2010;363:1909–1917.
  - Double-blind, randomized controlled trial that randomized patients on clopidogrel and aspirin to receive omeprazole vs. placebo. Prophylactic PPI reduced the rate of upper GI bleed.

Barrett's Esophagus

- **Radiofrequency Ablation in Barrett's Esophagus with Dysplasia.** *N Engl J Med* 2009;360:2277–2288.
  - Sham-controlled randomized controlled trial assessing whether endoscopic radiofrequency ablation could eradicate dysplastic Barrett's esophagus and decrease the rate of neoplastic progression. RFA had a high rate of complete eradication of both dysplasia and intestinal metaplasia and a reduced risk of disease progression.

Pancreatitis

- **Compared with Parenteral Nutrition, Enteral Feeding Attenuates the Acute Phase Response and Improves Disease Severity in Acute Pancreatitis.** *Gut* 1998;42:431–435.
  - Randomized controlled trial comparing TPN vs. enteral nutrition in patients with acute pancreatitis. Enteral nutrition improved disease severity and clinical outcomes.

Diverticulitis

- **AVOD.** *Br J Surg* 2012;99:532–539.
  - Nonblinded, placebo-controlled, randomized controlled trial comparing antibiotic vs. placebo for treatment of acute uncomplicated diverticulitis. Antibiotic treatment did not accelerate recovery or prevent complications or recurrence.

Cholecystectomy

- **ACDC.** *Ann Surg* 2013;258:385–393.
  - Parallel-group, open-label, randomized controlled trial comparing early laparoscopic cholecystectomy (<24 hours) versus initial antibiotics and delayed surgery (7–45 days). Early surgery had lower morbidity and healthcare costs.

IBD

- **SONIC.** *N Engl J Med* 2010;362:1383–1395.
  - Double-blind randomized controlled trial assessing the safety and efficacy of infliximab and azathioprine alone or in combination for patients with Crohn's disease. Combination therapy or infliximab monotherapy were more likely to have steroid-free remission than azathioprine monotherapy.

Functional Bowel Disorders

- **Cognitive-Behavioral Therapy Versus Education and Desipramine Versus Placebo for Moderate to Severe Functional Bowel Disorders.** *Gastroenterology* 2003;125:19–31.
  - Randomized controlled trial comparing CBT versus education and desipramine (TCA) versus placebo in treatment of female patients with functional bowel disorders (IBS, functional abdominal pain, constipation). CBT is effective and desipramine is effective when taken adequately and in certain clinical subgroups.

Alcoholic Hepatitis

- **STOPAH.** *N Engl J Med* 2015;372(17):1619–1628.
  - Prospective multicenter randomized, double-blind trial in 65 hospitals in the UK comparing the use of prednisone, pentoxifylline, combination prednisone-pentoxifylline, or placebo in patients with severe alcoholic hepatitis. Neither prednisolone nor pentoxifylline reduced all-cause mortality at 28 days. Prednisolone was associated with a nonsignificant mortality benefit at 28 days but no benefit at 90 days or 1 yr.

Cirrhosis Management

- **Norfloxacin vs. Ceftriaxone in the Prophylaxis of Infections in Patients with Advanced Cirrhosis and Hemorrhage.** *Gastroenterology* 2006;131:1049–1056.
  - Randomized controlled trial assessing oral norfloxacin vs. IV ceftriaxone for the prevention of bacterial infection in cirrhotic patients with UGIB. IV ceftriaxone was more effective than oral norfloxacin.

GASTROENTEROLOGY

NOTES

Endocrinology

5

ANATOMY AND PHYSIOLOGY

Endocrine Axes

- Organization: There are five parallel endocrine axes in the hypothalamic-anterior pituitary regulatory system (Figure 5.1)
- Chapter organization: For the remainder of this chapter we will organize anatomy, physiology, pathophysiology, and treatments by endocrine axis

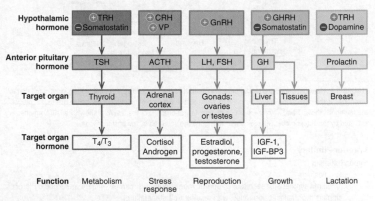

FIGURE 5.1: Endocrine axes in the hypothalamic–anterior pituitary regulatory system. There are five parallel endocrine axes in the hypothalamic–anterior pituitary regulatory system that control the biosynthesis and release of **1)** thyroid hormone, **2)** glucocorticoids, **3)** the sex steroids estradiol and testosterone, **4)** growth hormone, and **5)** prolactin. (⊕) indicates stimulatory action and (⊖) indicates inhibitory action. Abbreviations: TRH, thyrotropin-releasing hormone; TSH, thyroid-stimulating hormone; T_4, thyroxine; T_3, triiodothyronine; CRH, corticotropin-releasing hormone; VP, vasopressin; ACTH, adrenocorticotropic hormone; GnRH, gonadotropin-releasing hormone; FSH, follicle-stimulating hormone; LH, luteinizing hormone; GHRH, growth hormone-releasing hormone; GH, growth hormone; IGF-1, insulin-like growth factor-1; IGF-BP3, insulin-like growth factor binding protein-3.

PITUITARY

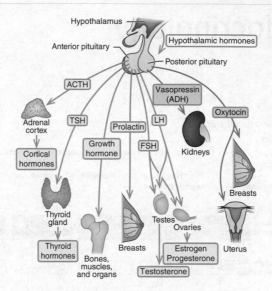

FIGURE 5.2: Hormones secreted by the pituitary gland and their functions. The pituitary is a small gland that is positioned in the base of the brain. The pituitary controls the function of most other endocrine glands, secreting the hormones shown here, which each act on distinct target organ(s) or tissues. As is shown, certain hormones are secreted by the anterior lobe, whereas other hormones are secreted by the posterior lobe.

Anterior Pituitary

Hypopituitarism

- Etiologies:
  - Impaired synthesis or secretion of one or more hormones; can be primary or secondary (process impairs hypothalamic hormones, with resultant pituitary failure)
  - Primary: Traumatic (e.g., head injury), neoplastic (e.g., adenoma), infiltrative/inflammatory (e.g., sarcoidosis), vascular (e.g., sickle cell disease, pregnancy-related), infections (e.g., histoplasmosis, TB), development/structural (e.g., dysplasia)
  - Secondary: Hypothalamic dysfunction or stalk interruption due to aforementioned processes
- Clinical features: Depends on which hormones are lost and the extent and duration of deficiency
- Hormone deficiencies:
  - ↓ Growth hormone (GH): Fatigue, increased fat mass, decreased muscle mass, growth retardation (children). Clinically this is measured using GH suppression testing with oral glucose tolerance and finding an elevated IGF-1.
  - ↓ Luteinizing hormone (LH)/follicle-stimulating hormone (FSH): Hypogonadotropic hypogonadism (infertility, amenorrhea, impotence)
  - ↓ Thyroid-stimulating hormone (TSH): Hypothyroidism, growth retardation (children)
  - ↓ Adrenocorticotropic hormone (ACTH): Secondary adrenal insufficiency (hypocortisolism; relative preservation of mineralocorticoid production)
  - ↓ Prolactin: Inability to lactate
- Diagnosis: Get pituitary MRI. Typically there are low levels of anterior pituitary hormones and thus low levels of target-organ hormones (e.g., low TSH, low free T_4). Pearl: Hormone levels that are within normal lab ranges may be "inappropriately normal" based on the clinical context. For example, if free T_4 is very low, then a normal TSH level would be inappropriately normal, since in this setting TSH should be elevated.
- Treatment: Replace deficient hormones. Adrenal insufficiency and hypothyroidism are the most important to treat. Patients in need of glucocorticoid replacement require careful dose adjustment in times of stress (e.g., acute illness).

Pituitary Tumors
- Approach:
  - Is there mass effect?
  - Is the tumor causing hormone excesses or deficiencies? Assess clinically for syndromes of cortisol, prolactin, growth hormone, and thyroid excess or deficiency and test accordingly
  - Is the tumor likely to grow and cause problematic mass effect? Obtain MRI brain and repeat over time as needed (interval time to repeat study determined by tumor size)
- Differential diagnosis:
  - Pituitary adenomas (can occur as part of MEN1 syndrome – See Table 5.1)
    - Microadenomas: <1 cm, incidentally found in approximately 10% of patients with brain MRIs
    - Macroadenomas: ≥1 cm
  - Rathke cleft cysts
  - Craniopharyngiomas
  - Meningiomas
  - Metastatic disease
- Symptoms:
  - Can cause mass effect: Headache, visual changes (optic chiasm compression can lead to bitemporal hemianopia)
  - Can cause hypopituitarism and DECREASED hormone levels (see hypopituitarism section above)
  - Tumors can also be functional and cause INCREASED hormone levels:
    - ↑Prolactin (most common): Hyperprolactinemia
      - Symptoms: Hypogonadism (due to inhibition of GnRH) leading to amenorrhea, decreased libido, infertility, galactorrhea
      - Diagnosis: Elevated prolactin (>200–250 ng/mL strongly suggests prolactinoma)
      - Differential diagnosis: Physiologic hypersecretion (e.g., pregnancy), drug-induced (e.g., antipsychotics), primary hypothyroidism, systemic disorders (e.g., renal failure, cirrhosis), compression of the pituitary stalk (with resultant disruption of dopamine inhibition), secretory pituitary tumor (obtain pituitary MRI to evaluate for tumor)
      - Treatment:
        - If asymptomatic and microadenoma: Treatment isn't always necessary and can follow with brain MRIs
        - If symptoms or macroadenoma: Dopamine agonists (bromocriptine/cabergoline; caution in patients on antipsychotic medications), typically surgery is NOT needed unless medical management is inadequate to control symptoms
    - ↑Growth hormone: Acromegaly
      - Symptoms: Large jaw/hands/feet/tongue, frontal bossing, cardiomegaly
      - Diagnosis: Elevated IGF-1 (oral glucose tolerance test to confirm) followed by pituitary MRI
      - Treatment:
        - Surgery (transsphenoidal tumor resection) or radiation
        - Dopamine agonists (e.g., somatostatin analogues)
        - Pegvisomant (GH receptor antagonist) can be used if surgery or radiation are not possible
    - ↑ TSH: Very rare – see "hyperthyroidism" in later section
    - ↑ACTH: Cushing's disease
      - Definition: Excess ACTH secretion from pituitary tumor = Cushing disease, which is the most common cause of Cushing syndrome (refers to hypercortisolism regardless of cause)
      - Symptoms: Proximal muscle weakness, facial plethora, wasting of the extremities with increased fat in the abdomen and face, wide purplish striae, bruising with no obvious trauma, dorsocervical and supraclavicular fat pads, DM2 due to insulin resistance, neuropsychiatric symptoms
      - Diagnosis:
        - Step 1: Establish whether the patient has hypercortisolism: Late-night salivary cortisol, 24-hour urinary free cortisol excretion, or overnight 1 mg dexamethasone suppression test
        - Step 2: Differentiate ACTH-dependent from ACTH-independent Cushing syndrome by measuring ACTH
          - If ACTH is low (ACTH-independent), it is typically due to a cortisol-secreting adrenal adenoma, adrenal carcinoma, or bilateral multi-nodular adrenal hyperplasia. Get a CT adrenal protocol to evaluate the adrenal glands
          - If ACTH is high (ACTH-dependent), it is typically due to a pituitary adenoma. Get a pituitary MRI followed by petrosal sinus sampling as appropriate
      - Treatment: For Cushing's disease from a pituitary adenoma, consider surgery (transsphenoidal resection of the involved pituitary)

Posterior Pituitary

↓Antidiuretic hormone (ADH): Diabetes insipidus (DI)
- Etiology: ADH channels do not function to reabsorb water, either due to inadequate ADH (central) or lack of response to ADH at the kidneys (nephrogenic)
  - Central DI:
    - Low posterior pituitary production of ADH
    - Etiologies: Idiopathic (~50% of cases in adults), acquired (trauma/surgery, neoplasms, infiltrative/infectious [Langerhans, sarcoidosis, tuberculosis], vascular), congenital malformations, genetic
  - Nephrogenic DI:
    - Normal ADH production but the renal tubules do not respond to ADH appropriately
    - Etiologies: Medications (lithium, cisplatin), metabolic (hypercalcemia, hypokalemia), ureteral obstruction
- Clinical features: Polyuria (>3 liters urine output in 24 hours), polydipsia. High serum osms, low urine osms
- Diagnosis:
  - Confirm polyuria with 24-hr urine volume (typically >3 L/day); urine is typically hypotonic (<300 mosm/kg); exclude glucosuria as cause
  - Differentiate between primary polydipsia (excessive fluid intake) and DI: history, serum sodium, and plasma osms can be helpful. Further testing that can be considered:
    - Water deprivation test: Withhold fluids and measure urine osmolality (should follow strict protocol with weights, urine osm, and endocrine input): Increase in UOsm = primary polydipsia. Stable = DI.
    - Hypertonic saline infusion test
    - Plasma copeptin proAVP (CPAVP) measurement
  - Differentiate between central and nephrogenic DI:
    - ADH (desmopressin) challenge: Increase UOsm >50% = Central DI. Stable = Nephrogenic DI.
- Treatment:
  - Central DI: Desmopressin (DDAVP), chlorpropamide increase ADH secretion and enhances effect
  - Nephrogenic DI: No good treatments. Sodium restriction and thiazide diuretics can be useful.
  - Pearl: Patients with central DI who don't have access to water and are hospitalized can develop severe hypernatremia. While hospitalized, monitor strict intake/output.

↑ADH: Syndrome of inappropriate ADH (SIADH)/syndrome of inappropriate antidiuresis (SIAD)
- Etiology: Ectopic production of ADH by a tumor (e.g., small cell lung cancer), CNS trauma, pulmonary infection, medications (e.g., SSRIs, chlorpropamide, oxytocin, morphine, vincristine, desmopressin), postoperative
- Clinical features:
  - Low serum Na^+ and osms because retain free water; normal or high urine sodium and osms
  - Acute symptoms: Lethargy, somnolence, seizures, coma, death
- Diagnosis: Check serum/urine sodium and osms. Rule out other causes of hyponatremia – SIADH is a diagnosis of exclusion.
- Treatment:
  - Fluid restriction is the mainstay of treatment in most cases
  - Central: Consider desmopressin
  - Peripheral: Consider thiazide diuretic
  - Lithium-induced: Stop lithium if possible

TABLE 5.1 · Multiple Endocrine Neoplasia (MEN) Syndromes

Type	Mutation	Clinical Manifestations
1	MENIN inactivation	• Parathyroid hyperplasia • Pancreatic islet cell neoplasia • Pituitary adenoma
2A	RET protooncogene	• Medullary thyroid carcinoma • Pheochromocytoma • Parathyroid hyperplasia
2B	RET protooncogene	• Medullary thyroid carcinoma • Pheochromocytoma • Mucosal and gastrointestinal neuromas

THYROID

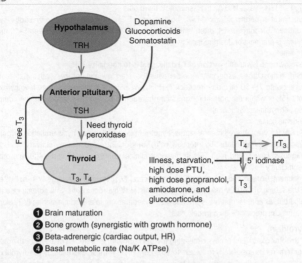

FIGURE 5.3: **Hypothalamic–pituitary–thyroid axis.** Shown is the hypothalamic–pituitary–thyroid axis, which regulates the production of thyroid hormones. The enzyme 5′ iodinase converts the biologically inactive thyroxine (T_4) to the active form of thyroid hormone, triiodothyronine (T_3). Conversion of $T_4 \rightarrow T_3$ can be inhibited by environmental conditions (illness, starvation) or medications (propylthiouracil [PTU], propranolol). T_4 can also be converted to reverse T_3 (rT_3), which is a biologically inactive metabolite of thyroxine. Green arrows indicate stimulatory actions, and red lines indicate inhibitory actions. Abbreviations: TRH, thyrotropin-releasing hormone; TSH, thyroid-stimulating hormone; T_4, thyroxine; T_3, triiodothyronine; rT_3, reverse triiodothyronine.

Hypothyroidism

- Etiologies:
  - <u>Primary</u>:
    - Hashimoto's thyroiditis
      - Most common cause of hypothyroidism in developed countries
      - Autoimmune thyroid destruction: >90% patients have positive thyroid peroxidase antibodies (TPO)
      - Patients can be hyperthyroid initially then hypothyroid
      - Thyroid exam: Firm, painless
      - No imaging required unless concern for a thyroid nodule
    - Subacute viral thyroiditis (de Quervain's)
      - Viral infection presents with very tender thyroid. ↑ESR, jaw pain
      - Patients are initially hyperthyroid, then hypothyroid; typically return to euthyroid, but not always
      - Treatment: NSAIDs, ASA for pain. Self-limited over a 2–4 month period
    - Reidel's thyroiditis
      - Rare, chronic inflammatory disease of the thyroid gland characterized by a dense fibrosis that replaces the normal thyroid parenchyma
      - Can cause neck tightness, dyspnea, hoarseness, cough. May invade local anatomic structures
      - Thyroid exam: Firm, "hard as wood," fixed, nontender, often misdiagnosed as malignancy
    - Iatrogenic: Surgical destruction of the thyroid gland, post-radiation or after radioactive iodine, medications (lithium, amiodarone)
    - Iodine deficiency: Most common cause of hypothyroidism (and goiter) worldwide
  - <u>Central</u>:
    - Hypothalamic or pituitary failure: TSH can be inappropriately normal, but T_3/T_4 are low
- Clinical features:
  - Fatigue, weakness, lethargy, cold intolerance, heavy menstruation, weight gain, constipation, slow mentation, depression, carpal tunnel syndrome, dry skin, coarse hair, hoarseness, myxedema (non-pitting edema due to increased glycosaminoglycans), bradycardia

- Diagnosis:
  - $\downarrow T_4/T_3$, $\uparrow$TSH. +anti-TPO Ab in Hashimoto's thyroiditis
  - Subclinical hyperthyroidism: $\uparrow$TSH, normal free T_4 and T_3 with no or only subtle symptoms. Treatment is controversial; often initiate treatment if TSH >10 mU/L or between 5–10 mU/L if the patient is pregnant or desiring fertility
- Treatment:
  - Levothyroxine (synthetic version of T_4) daily; goal is to normalize TSH
  - Pearl: In most cases, especially for older patients, "start low and go slow" with initial levothyroxine dose, giving 25–50 mcg/day; recheck TSH in 6 weeks and continue to titrate levothyroxine dose until TSH is within the normal range. Supratherapeutic dosing risks cardiovascular complications (e.g., arrhythmias, ischemia)
- Myxedema coma:
  - Clinical features: Altered mental status, hypothermia, hypotension, hypoventilation, hyponatremia, hypoglycemia. Precipitated by infection, cold, stressor, untreated hypothyroidism
  - Diagnosis: Low T_4 and high TSH in the right clinical context. Check cortisol to rule out adrenal insufficiency
  - Treatment: Consult endocrinology. Supportive care, IV T_4 (careful with large IV T_4 bolus, especially in the setting of CAD/CV risk factors), co-administer IV hydrocortisone until adrenal insufficiency is ruled out, as adrenal reserve is often low in myxedema coma and administering IV T_4 alone in that context can precipitate an adrenal crisis.

Hyperthyroidism

The term "thyrotoxicosis" (i.e., excess circulating thyroid hormone) is preferred over "hyperthyroidism," as the latter term refers specifically to excess thyroid hormone synthesis/secretion by the thyroid gland. In practice, "hyperthyroidism" is often used to describe thyrotoxicosis, however, and hyperthyroidism is in fact the most common cause of thyrotoxicosis.

- Etiologies:
  - Graves' disease
    - Epidemiology: Most common cause of thyrotoxicosis (60–75%). Common in women age 20–40 yr.
    - Pathophysiology: Autoimmune antibody stimulates TSH receptor $\rightarrow \uparrow T_3$, T_4.
    - Symptoms (in addition to symptoms of hyperthyroidism):
      - Thyroid: Diffusely enlarged, nontender thyroid, may have bruit
      - Exophthalmos (eyes pop out), pretibial myxedema (fibroblasts in eye/shin express TSH receptor stimulated by Graves' antibodies $\rightarrow$ deposition of connective tissue containing water-binding protein-mucopolysaccharide complexes $\rightarrow$ non-pitting edema)
    - Diagnosis: Thyroid ultrasound (enlarged, increased vascularity); thyroid-stimulating antibodies (if inconclusive, can get radioiodine uptake scan which will show diffuse increased uptake)
  - Multinodular goiter/toxic adenoma
    - Pathophysiology: Pituitary tumor secretes TSH and/or there is resistance to thyroid hormones
    - Thyroid exam: Bumpy, irregular, asymmetric
    - Diagnosis: Radioiodine uptake scan: Patchy uptake because some thyroid cells are hyperfunctioning, whereas other thyroid cells atrophy
  - Thyroiditis
    - Clinical features: Thyrotoxic phase of thyroid inflammation. Often transient hyperthyroidism for 2–6 weeks, then clinically hypothyroid after 6–12 weeks. May require therapy for both hyper- and then hypothyroidism during course. The majority of patients ultimately return to euthyroid state.
      - <u>Painful</u>: Inflammatory (de Quervain or subacute granulomatous thyroiditis) infection (post-URI), radiation
      - <u>Painless</u>: Postpartum (+TPO, subsequent hypothyroidism), silent or drug-induced thyroiditis
  - Molar pregnancy: Rare, due to HCG binding to the TSH receptor. Pregnancy test will be positive.
  - Iatrogenic: Use of levothyroxine (T_4) or liothyronine (T_3) for weight loss
- Clinical features: Nervousness, insomnia, tremor, heat intolerance, diarrhea, palpitations, muscle weakness, brisk reflexes, weight loss, lid lag, arrhythmias, hypertension

- Diagnosis:
  - $\downarrow$TSH, $\uparrow T_3$ and/or T_4 (for most causes, sufficient to order only TSH and free T_4)
    - Subclinical hyperthyroidism: $\downarrow$TSH, normal free T_4 and T_3 with no or only subtle symptoms. Consider repeat labs in 3 months. If TSH persistently <0.1 mU/L consider treatment if patient is >65 yr, has cardiac risk factors, and/or has osteoporosis.
  - Determine the cause of hyperthyroidism (initially try to rule out Graves')
    - TRAb for Graves' disease (if not clinically apparent)
    - Radioiodine uptake scan if etiology unclear (contraindicated in pregnancy and breastfeeding)
      - High uptake: If diffuse pattern: Graves'; if nodular/patchy pattern: Multinodular, toxic adenoma
      - Low uptake: Thyroiditis, recent iodine load (e.g., contrast, amiodarone)
- Treatment:
  - Beta blockers (propranolol, atenolol): For acute symptom management regardless of etiology. Propranolol also decreases $T_4 \rightarrow T_3$ conversion.
  - Methimazole, PTU: Inhibit T_4 synthesis at very high doses.
    - Methimazole typically preferred because once-daily regimen and PTU causes more hepatotoxicity, but methimazole is contraindicated during the first trimester of pregnancy.
    - For both, check baseline CBC with differential, LFTs, TSH. Risk of agranulocytosis that is dose-dependent (check CBC again if fever/sore throat)
  - Radioactive iodine (RAI): Careful in Graves' disease (may cause worsening of ophthalmopathy unless pretreated with steroids, so typically treat with methimazole first), contraindicated in pregnancy
  - Surgery: Typically done for patients with obstructive goiter, less common for Graves'. Side effect: Permanent hypothyroidism, recurrent laryngeal nerve injury, hypocalcemia if parathyroid glands removed/damaged.
- Thyroid storm:
  - Definition: Easy to meet numerical criteria for thyroid storm, which are nonspecific. True thyroid storm typically occurs in the setting of untreated/poorly treated hyperthyroidism with a precipitating event (e.g., surgery, trauma, infection, DKA, MI, childbirth, iodine load, amiodarone)
  - Symptoms: Tachycardia, fever, and GI symptoms (nausea, vomiting, abdominal pain). Many consider CNS dysfunction (e.g., agitation, psychosis, coma) a requirement for thyroid storm.
  - Treatment: Consult endocrinology. Supportive care (IVF, cooling blankets, acetaminophen), propranolol, steroids, and/or PTU (reduces T_4 to T_3 conversion), bile acid sequestrants (block enterohepatic recycling of thyroid hormones). Only consider treatment with iodine in consultation with endocrinology (blocks release of T_4/T_3 from the thyroid gland but can have rebound effect and can limit long term treatment options).

Sick Euthyroid Syndrome
- Pathophysiology: Illness causes caloric deprivation and an increased inflammatory state, which may lead to abnormal thyroid function tests
- Diagnosis: Check all TFTs (TSH, total T_4, free T_4, T_3). Interpret thyroid studies in hospitalized patients carefully.
- Treatment: Often no treatment needed and instead repeat TFTs in the outpatient setting once the acute illness resolves. Administering levothyroxine is not helpful unless there are other signs/symptoms consistent with hypothyroidism.
- Pearl: If TSH undetectable or >20 mU/L, suggests true thyroid disease

Thyroid Nodule
- Etiologies:
  - Benign follicular epithelial cell adenomas (common, present in 5–10% of adults)
  - Malignant tumors: Papillary carcinomas (80–90%), follicular carcinomas (5–10%), medullary thyroid cancer (<10%), other (1–2%)
- Clinical features: Palpable nodule, symptoms from mass effect; alternatively, may note as an incidental finding on imaging
- Diagnosis: First check thyroid-stimulating hormone (TSH)
  - If TSH is high or normal: Get thyroid ultrasound (to assess features of nodule, evaluate for other nodules/lymph nodes). If a concerning features, biopsy with a fine needle aspiration (FNA)
  - If TSH is low: Check FT_4, T_3, and thyroid uptake and on a ^{131}iodine scan
    - If functioning "hot" thyroid nodule: Treat hyperthyroidism (with medication vs. ablation/resection)
    - If nonfunctioning "cold" thyroid nodule: Biopsy and surgically resect if needed
- Multinodular goiter: Diagnose using the same principles described above for single thyroid nodules. Higher risk of malignancy. Consider surgery if compressive symptoms.

ENDOCRINOLOGY

ADRENAL GLAND

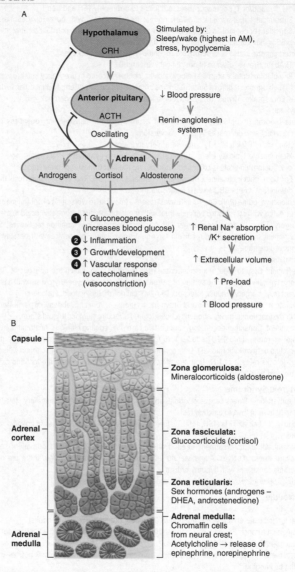

A

Hypothalamus
CRH

Stimulated by:
Sleep/wake (highest in AM),
stress, hypoglycemia

Anterior pituitary
ACTH
Oscillating

↓ Blood pressure

Renin-angiotensin
system

Adrenal
Androgens   Cortisol   Aldosterone

❶ ↑ Gluconeogenesis
(increases blood glucose)
❷ ↓ Inflammation
❸ ↑ Growth/development
❹ ↑ Vascular response
to catecholamines
(vasoconstriction)

↑ Renal Na⁺ absorption
/K⁺ secretion

↑ Extracellular volume

↑ Pre-load

↑ Blood pressure

B

Capsule

Adrenal
cortex

Adrenal
medulla

Zona glomerulosa:
Mineralocorticoids (aldosterone)

Zona fasciculata:
Glucocorticoids (cortisol)

Zona reticularis:
Sex hormones (androgens –
DHEA, androstenedione)

Adrenal medulla:
Chromaffin cells
from neural crest;
Acetylcholine → release of
epinephrine, norepinephrine

FIGURE 5.4: Hypothalamic–pituitary–adrenal axis and adrenal hormone production. A) Shown is the
hypothalamic–pituitary–adrenal axis, which regulates the production of adrenal hormones. ACTH activates the
production of androgens, cortisol, and aldosterone in the adrenal gland. Aldosterone production is also regulated
by the renin angiotensin aldosterone system (RAAS). Green arrows indicate stimulatory actions, and red lines
indicate inhibitory actions. B) The adrenal gland consists of the outer cortex and the inner medulla. The cortex
is further divided into three layers: the glomerulosa, the fasciculata, and the reticularis. Each of these layers
produces different hormones, as shown. Abbreviations: CRH, corticotropin-releasing hormone; VP, vasopressin;
ACTH, adrenocorticotropic hormone; DHEA, dehydroepiandrosterone.

Primary Hyperaldosteronism

- Etiologies:
  - <u>Primary</u>: Adrenal disorders. Labs notable for high aldosterone, which is independent of renin.
    - Adrenal hyperplasia
    - Adrenal adenoma (Conn's syndrome)
    - Adrenal carcinoma (very rare)
    - Glucocorticoid-remediable aldosteronism (GRA): ACTH-dependent rearranged promoter driving high aldosterone
  - <u>Secondary</u>: Extra-adrenal disorders. Labs notable for high aldosterone which is dependent upon renin.
    - Renovascular disease: Renal artery stenosis (common in young women), malignant hypertension
    - States with low effective arterial volume: CKD, CHF, cirrhosis
    - Bartter's syndrome (defective $Na^+/K^+/2Cl^-$ [NKCC] transporter) or Gitelman's syndrome (defective renal Na^+/Cl^- transporter)
    - Renin-secreting tumor (rare)
- Clinical features:
  - Hypertension (~20% cases; primary hyperaldosteronism is a common cause of resistant hypertension)
  - Hypokalemia (10–40% cases; potassium is normal for many patients)
  - Metabolic alkalosis
  - Mild hypernatremia
- Diagnosis: Check AM plasma renin and aldosterone
  - <u>Low renin, low aldosterone</u>: Non-aldosterone mineralocorticoid excess (e.g., Cushing's syndrome, exogenous mineralocorticoids, chronic licorice ingestion, Liddle's syndrome)
  - <u>Low renin, high aldosterone, high aldo/renin ratio (>20)</u>: Suspect primary hyperaldosteronism
    - Perform salt suppression test to confirm
    - Perform adrenal CT or MRI
      - If unilateral lesion, likely an adenoma. Treat adenoma with surgical resection.
      - If no lesion seen or bilateral adrenal lesion, consider adrenal venous sampling to help localize an adenoma. If no localization, then likely hyperplasia or glucocorticoid-remediable aldosteronism (GRA)
  - <u>High renin, high aldosterone, low aldosterone/renin ratio (<10)</u>: Suspect secondary hyperaldosteronism (see differential diagnosis earlier)
  - Pearl: Hold aldosterone receptor antagonists (e.g., spironolactone) and ACEi/ARBs 24–48 hours prior to blood draw during this evaluation if possible (can cause false-negative or normal results)

Cushing's Syndrome

- Definitions:
  - Cushing's syndrome: Excess cortisol regardless of cause
  - Cushing's disease: Cushing's syndrome due to pituitary ACTH hypersecretion
- Etiology:
  - Exogenous glucocorticoids is the most common cause of Cushing's syndrome
  - Pituitary adenoma that secretes ACTH (aka Cushing's disease): Most common endogenous cause of Cushing's syndrome. High ACTH, which can be suppressed with high-dose dexamethasone. Confirm diagnosis with inferior petrosal sinus sampling.
  - Adrenal adenoma/tumor that secretes cortisol: Low ACTH
  - Ectopic ACTH production (e.g., paraneoplastic secretion of ACTH can occur in small cell lung cancer, carcinoid tumors, medullary thyroid cancer): High ACTH and high-dose dexamethasone cannot suppress it
- Clinical features: Moon facies, buffalo hump, truncal obesity, muscle weakness with thin extremities (protein catabolism), abdominal striae (cortisol impairs collagen secretion), hypertension (subsequent mineralocorticoid access), DM2 (upregulation of gluconeogenesis), immune suppression (inhibits IL2, histamine), bruising, facial plethora, depression/anxiety, amenorrhea (inhibition of gonadotropin release)

- Diagnosis:
  - **Step 1**: Screen for Cushing's syndrome: Start initially with 1 mg (low-dose) overnight dexamethasone suppression test (synthetic corticosteroid that usually inhibits ACTH and decreases cortisol). Can also consider checking a 24-hour urine free cortisol (use for shift workers or patients on estrogen therapy) or late-night salivary cortisol.
    - For 1 mg dexamethasone suppression, if dexamethasone suppresses ACTH and cortisol is <1.8 mcg/dL, can exclude Cushing's syndrome and stop workup
    - Otherwise proceed with workup (but note false positives with alcohol use, obesity, and psychological disorders). An elevated AM cortisol (>2 mcg/dL) suggests Cushing's syndrome.
  - **Step 2**: Determine the etiology of the Cushing's syndrome: Measure ACTH
    - <u>Low ACTH</u> = ACTH-independent Cushing's syndrome. Ddx: Exogenous steroids vs. adrenal adenoma/tumor. Perform CT abd/pelvis to evaluate the adrenal glands and surgically remove the adrenal adenoma/tumor if present.
    - <u>High ACTH</u> = ACTH-dependent Cushing's syndrome: Evaluate for pituitary ACTH production (aka Cushing's disease) vs. ectopic ACTH production (e.g., from a lung tumor). Can do high-dose (8 mg) dexamethasone suppression test to differentiate etiologies or proceed directly to brain MRI. For high-dose dexamethasone suppression text, interpret as follows:
      - High-dose dexamethasone causes ACTH suppression (>50% suppression): Pituitary adenoma. Obtain pituitary MRI and conduct inferior petrosal sinus sampling.
      - High-dose dexamethasone does not cause ACTH suppression (<50% suppression): Ectopic ACTH-producing tumor (tumor most often in the lungs; sometimes can be difficult to locate). Consider CT C/A/P or an octreotide, MIBG SPECT, or DOTATATE PET/CT scan.
- Treatment:
  - Surgical resection of the pituitary adenoma, adrenal tumor, ectopic ACTH-secreting tumor
  - Possible initiation of hydrocortisone replacement after surgery to achieve physiologic levels
  - Etaconazole and metyrapone can be given if medical therapy is preferred or needed prior to surgery (inhibit cortisol biosynthesis)

Adrenal Insufficiency (AI)

- Etiologies:
  - <u>Primary</u>:
    - Autoimmune: Antibody against adrenal enzymes (most common)
    - Vascular: Adrenal hemorrhage, thrombosis, trauma
    - Infectious: Tuberculosis (adrenal calcification), CMV, histoplasmosis
    - Medications: Ketoconazole, rifampin, etomidate
    - Deposition diseases: Amyloid, sarcoidosis, hemochromatosis
    - Metastatic disease: Lung/breast cancer can go to the adrenals
  - <u>Secondary</u>:
    - Hypopituitarism (any primary or secondary cause)
    - Glucocorticoid therapy (typically consider if >3 weeks of ≥20 mg prednisone or equivalent, or long-term use of ≥10 mg prednisone or equivalent); suppression of the HPA axis is the most common cause of AI
- Clinical features:
  - Fatigue (most common), nausea/vomiting, lethargy, hypoglycemia, hypercalcemia, eosinophilia (rare), abdominal pain, anorexia
  - Primary only: Skin hyperpigmentation in areas of friction and/or sun exposure (MSH is a by-product of ACTH synthesis), hyperkalemia, hyponatremia (due to mineralocorticoid deficiency and diminished suppression of ADH by low cortisol)
- Diagnosis:
  - **Step 1:** Check early AM cortisol
    - If AM cortisol <3 μg/dL very concerning, if >18 μg/dL rules out adrenal insufficiency
    - Random cortisol level within the reference range does not rule out adrenal insufficiency
  - **Step 2:** Perform a standard cosyntropin stimulation test with 250 mcg cosyntropin
    - Can be performed at ANY time of day
    - Normal response is cortisol >18 μg/dL 60 minutes after administration of cosyntropin
  - **Step 3:** Determine etiology: Check plasma ACTH, plasma renin, serum aldosterone
    - High ACTH, high plasma renin, low aldosterone suggests primary adrenal insufficiency. Consider adrenal imaging, adrenal autoantibodies (e.g., steroid autoantibodies, marker for adrenalitis).
    - Low-normal ACTH, normal plasma renin, normal aldosterone suggests secondary adrenal insufficiency. Consider pituitary MRI, check other pituitary hormones.

- Treatment:
  - Primary: Oral corticosteroid (hydrocortisone or prednisone) and mineralocorticoid (fludrocortisone)
  - Secondary: Oral corticosteroid only; no mineralocorticoid needed
  - Stress-dose steroids:
    - Counsel patients to increase steroid dose 2–3× for minor stressors (e.g., minor illness)
    - For major stressors, often need 10× steroid dosing (aka "stress dose steroids")

Congenital Adrenal Hyperplasia

21-hydroxylase deficiency

- Pathophysiology: Autosomal recessive genetic disorder. Most common congenital adrenal hyperplasia (90% cases). Depending on the severity of enzyme deficiency, there is **classic CAH** (which is further subdivided into virilizing or salt-wasting forms) and **nonclassic CAH**. Enzyme deficiency causes an inability to produce cortisol (and aldosterone in the salt-wasting forms), which leads to low cortisol, low or normal aldosterone, and high ACTH, and thus to increased adrenal stimulation which results in high DHEA.
  - Classic CAH
    - More severe form
    - Virilizing features: XX karyotype: Ambiguous genitalia, normal ovaries/uterus, XY karyotype: Precocious puberty
    - Salt-wasting: Hypotension, hyperkalemia because of lack of aldosterone; emesis/dehydration in first 2–4 weeks of life
  - Nonclassic CAH
    - More mild form
    - Presents later in life with signs of androgen excess and without neonatal genital ambiguity; some patients are asymptomatic
- Diagnosis: High levels of 17-OH progesterone, which is the normal substrate for 21-hydroxylase (test for stimulated levels)
- Treatment: Administer steroids and mineralocorticoids, which turn off excess ACTH via a negative feedback loop. Can consider surgical correction of female genitalia, if abnormal.

17-hydroxylase deficiency

- Clinical features: Hypertension, hypokalemia. XX karyotype: Phenotypic female, lack of secondary sexual development. XY karyotype: Complete male pseudohermaphorditism; characterized by external female genitalia with a blind-ending vagina but without a uterus or fallopian tubes.
- Diagnosis: High aldosterone, low cortisol, low DHEA

11-hydroxylase deficiency

- Clinical features: Hypertension, hypokalemia. XX karyotype: Labial fusion. XY karyotype: Precocious puberty.
- Diagnosis: Low aldosterone, low cortisol, high DHEA

Pheochromocytoma

- Definition: Catecholamine-producing tumor derived from sympathetic or parasympathetic nervous system, rare (0.1% of patients with hypertension). Can occur in childhood or later in life.
- Etiology: 50% hereditary (e.g., associated with MEN2, von Hippel-Lindau disease, neurofibromatosis type 2, somatic RET mutations).
- Clinical features: **"5Ps"**, which occur in spells: **P**ressure (hypertension), **P**ain (chest pain, headache), **P**erspiration, **P**alpitations (tachycardia), **P**allor (vasoconstriction). Paroxysms generally last less than an hour, may be precipitated by positional changes, medications, surgery.
- Diagnosis:
  - Low suspicion: 24-hour urine metanephrines and creatinine (more specific)
  - High suspicion: Fasting plasma free metanephrines (more sensitive)
  - If urine/serum metanephrines are elevated, then obtain adrenal imaging with CT or MRI with contrast
- Treatment:
  - Start with alpha blockade (phenoxybenzamine): give alpha blocker <u>before</u> beta blocker, titrate BP <130/90 mmHg
  - Then add beta blocker to treat reflex tachycardia if needed (never start before adequate alpha-blockade due to risk of hypertensive crisis); target HR 60–80 bpm
  - Surgical resection of the tumor, after adequate alpha blockade and volume expansion have been achieved (typically requires weeks)

Adrenal Masses

Incidentally discovered adrenal mass

- Epidemiology: Common (at least 2% in the general population, more common with increasing age)
- Differential diagnosis:
  - <u>Nonfunctioning mass</u>: Benign adenoma (most common), hemorrhage, lipoma, cyst, malignancy (metastasis from another site more common than primary adrenal malignancy)
  - <u>Functioning mass</u>: Pheochromocytoma, adenoma or carcinoma that produces catecholamine, aldosterone, or cortisol
- Diagnosis:
  - Consider need to screen for excess hormones (consider pheochromocytoma, hyperaldosteronism, and cortisol secretion)
  - Identify patients who are at risk for malignancy (risk factors: >4 cm adrenal mass, patient with known malignancy)
  - Imaging characteristics (density <10 Hounsfield units [HU] on CT suggests adrenal adenoma, and makes malignancy much less likely)
  - Almost never biopsy an adrenal mass

Adrenocortical carcinoma

- Epidemiology: Rare, associated with excessive production of adrenal hormones and local mass effect (abdominal fullness). Typically poor prognosis.

REPRODUCTIVE ENDOCRINOLOGY

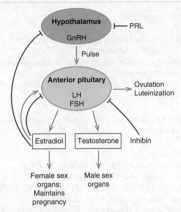

FIGURE 5.5: **Hypothalamic–pituitary–gonadal axis.** Shown is the hypothalamic–pituitary–gonadal axis, which regulates the production of the sex hormones estradiol and testosterone. Green arrows indicate stimulatory actions, and red lines indicate inhibitory actions. Abbreviations: GnRH, gonadotropin-releasing hormone; LH, luteinizing hormone; FSH, follicle-stimulating hormone; PRL, prolactin.

Females

Menstrual Cycle

- Follicular phase (day 0–13): From the onset of menses to the LH surge. The follicle develops during this phase. Estradiol inhibits FSH and LH during this phase and promotes endometrial healing. Rising estradiol causes menstruation to end.
- Ovulation (day 14): The dominant follicle secretes estradiol. Estradiol increases above a level such that it now positively feeds back to increase LH/FSH, and the resultant LH surge causes ovulation.
- Luteal phase (day 15–28): The corpus luteum produces estrogen. If the corpus luteum is not fertilized, it involutes and progesterone production declines. If it is fertilized, the zygote secretes bHCG, which sustains the corpus luteum.

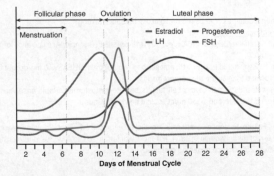

FIGURE 5.6: **Concentrations of hormones throughout the menstrual cycle.** The menstrual cycle is regulated by the complex interactions of four hormones: estrogen, progesterone, luteinizing hormone (LH), and follicle-stimulating hormone (FSH). There are three phases, as described in the text.

Amenorrhea

Primary amenorrhea

- Definition: Absent menses at age 15 yr
- Etiologies:
  - Genetic (50%): Turner's syndrome (XO karyotype) – patients may have a webbed neck, coarctation of the aorta. Diagnosis: High FSH, check karyotype.
  - Hormonal (35%): Low sex hormones due to excessive exercise, anorexia, craniopharyngioma. Diagnosis: Low FSH, consider brain MRI.
  - Anatomic/structural (15%): Müllerian agenesis, transverse vaginal septum, imperforate hymen. Diagnosis: Transvaginal ultrasound.

Secondary amenorrhea

- Definition: Absent menses for >3 months in women with previously regular menstrual cycles or >6 months if irregular menstrual cycles
- Etiologies:
  - Pregnancy (always rule out first!)
  - Ovarian: Polycystic ovarian syndrome (PCOS), ovarian failure (↑FSH)
  - Hypothalamic: Stress, exercise, systemic illness, and weight loss can result in functional hypothalamic amenorrhea (disruptions in pulsatile release of hypothalamic GnRH)
  - Pituitary: Prolactinoma (↑prolactin), empty sella syndrome
  - Endocrine: Hypo/hyperthyroidism, diabetes, obesity (normal FSH/LH but anovulation because progesterone dysregulation)
  - Uterine: Asherman's syndrome post dilation and curettage (D&C)
- Diagnosis: Urine pregnancy test, FSH, LH, prolactin, estradiol, TSH. Abnormal findings will guide management. If normal: Progesterone challenge can further assess estrogen status and functional anatomy. If progesterone challenge provokes menses, then the patient has a normal estrogen state; consider hyperandrogenism.

Hyperandrogenism syndromes

Polycystic Ovarian Syndrome (PCOS)

- Symptoms: Weight gain, male pattern baldness, acne, oligomenorrhea. Risk endometrial cancer due to unopposed estrogen.
- Criteria: Need two of the following: 1) Oligomenorrhea/anovulation; 2) Clinical/biochemical evidence of hyperandrogenism (hirsutism, acne); 3) Polycystic ovaries on pelvic ultrasound
- Diagnosis:
  - Diagnosis of exclusion (rule out thyroid dysfunction, congenital adrenal hyperplasia, hyperprolactinoma)
  - Labs/imaging not required for diagnosis unless needed to satisfy diagnostic criteria and/or to rule out other diagnoses (e.g., rapid-onset hirsutism with concern for malignancy)
  - If PCOS is diagnosed, also screen patient for diabetes, HLD, HTN, and OSA
- Treatment:
  - Oral contraceptive pills
  - Weight loss
  - Metformin if diabetes or impaired oral glucose tolerance testing

Other causes of hirsutism/virilization

- Congenital adrenal hyperplasia (CAH, e.g., 21-hydroxylase deficiency): Accumulation of 17-OH-progesterone → DHEA
- Adrenal neoplasm: Rapid hair growth, amenorrhea, virilization. If DHEA >7.0 mg/dL, get CT abdomen/pelvis protocoled to evaluate the adrenal glands.
- Ovarian neoplasms: Sertoli-Leydig cell tumors secrete testosterone. Rapid-onset acne, hirsutism, amenorrhea. If testosterone >150 ng/dL, obtain pelvic ultrasound.

Infertility

- Definition: Failure to conceive after 12 months of unprotected sex (~2×/wk) in women <35 yr and after 6 months in women ≥35 yr. For most women in 20s to low 30s one menstrual cycle = approximately 25% chance of getting pregnant.

- Etiologies:
  - Issues with ovulation: PCOS, anovulation. Diagnosis: 1) Day 21 progesterone, 2) FSH: Check ovulatory reserve (high FSH suggests less reserve), 3) Anti-Müllerian hormone, 4) Pelvic ultrasound (check if follicles present).
  - Blocked transport of the egg getting from the ovaries to the uterus: Pelvic inflammatory disease (PID), tuberculosis (particularly in endemic areas), fibroids, adhesions. Diagnosis: Hysterosalpingogram.
  - Idiopathic: Endometriosis
  - Semen analysis: Volume, motility, morphology. Diagnosis: Semen analysis. Ddx azospermia (no sperm): Cystic fibrosis, XXY Klinefelter's.
- Diagnosis: Both partners should be evaluated concurrently for causes of infertility. For females, evaluate ovulatory function (midluteal progesterone) and for anatomic abnormalities (hysterosalpingogram). For males, perform semen analysis.
- Treatment:
  - Clomiphene (selective estrogen receptor modulator [SERM]—inhibits estrogen binding at hypothalamus/pituitary so release FSH/LH): Increases ovulation 2–3 fold
  - If the patient has PCOS, metformin can improve fertility
  - Assisted reproductive technologies, such as intrauterine insemination, in vitro fertilization (IVF):
    - Use GnRH agonist leuprolide to shut down LH
    - Give FSH to target the release of 10 eggs; evaluate with pelvic ultrasound and estradiol levels
    - Give LH to cause ovulation
    - Harvest eggs approximately 36 hours later. Can freeze as eggs (without insemination) or embryos (inseminate prior to freezing).

Males
Physiology: GnRH pulse elicits pulses of LH/FSH. LH acts on Leydig cells → Testosterone. FSH acts on Sertoli cells → Spermatogenesis. Testosterone decreases with age.

Hypogonadism
- Primary hypogonadism: Testicular failure, causing decreased testosterone and sperm production. Ddx: Klinefelter's syndrome XXY, mumps orchitis, sequelae of radiation therapy, testicular trauma or torsion.
- Secondary hypogonadism: Insufficient GnRH production by hypothalamus or deficient LH/FSH production by anterior pituitary. Ddx: Pituitary tumor/infiltrative disease, prolactin excess, Kallmann's syndrome (associated with anosmia), OSA, obesity, idiopathic. Iatrogenic: Exogenous testosterone (often used for body building/energy/libido without frank hypogonadism), chronic opiates, steroids.
- Clinical features: Decreased morning and spontaneous erections, decreased libido, gynecomastia, decreased axillary or genital hair, decreased mood/energy, problems with sleep and memory.
- Diagnosis:
  - General screening is not recommended. In men with specific signs and symptoms, two early AM testosterone levels (fasting if possible) below reference range is indicative. In men with obesity, free testosterone can be measured since obesity lowers sex hormone–binding globulin (SHBG) leading to falsely low total testosterone. If low, check LH/FSH.
    - Elevated LH/FSH with low testosterone reflects primary hypogonadism.
    - Low/normal LH/FSH with low testosterone reflects secondary hypogonadism. Additional workup with prolactin, screening for hemochromatosis, consider pituitary imaging if evaluation suggestive of pituitary pathology.
  - Low testosterone common in chronic disease (e.g., ESRD, advanced COPD, HIV, malignancy), typically due to central hypothalamic–pituitary defects (low/normal LH/FSH).
- Treatment: Can give testosterone replacement. If the patient is overweight, weight loss also increases testosterone levels.

Gynecomastia
- Etiology: Excess estrogen or increased estrogen/androgen ratio.
- Clinical features: Increase in breast size. Usually bilateral, can be benign in adolescents, patients with certain chronic medical conditions (e.g., cirrhosis, malnutrition, CKD), obesity (pseudogynecomastia), or associated with certain medications (e.g., anabolic steroids, spironolactone). Concerning features include unilateral, nontender, fixed breast masses.
- Diagnosis: Review history and medications. If features concerning for malignancy (e.g., unilateral, palpable mass), order a mammogram. If no clear cause, also consider testicular exam, bHCG, estradiol, testosterone, LH, and prolactin.

ENDOCRINE PANCREAS

Diabetes Mellitus

- Definition:
  - HgA1c $\geq$6.5%
  - Fasting glucose $\geq$126 mg/dL $\times$ 2 readings
  - Random glucose >200 mg/dL $\times$ 2 (or $\times$ 1 if acute metabolic decompensation)
- Classifications:
  - Type 1 diabetes (DM1): Destruction of islet cells causing absolute insulin deficiency (Table 5.2)
  - Type 2 diabetes (DM2): Insulin resistance, abnormal insulin secretion, excessive hepatic glucose production, and abnormal fat metabolism (Table 5.2)
  - Prediabetes (pre-DM2): HgA1c 5.7–6.4% or impaired fasting glucose (100–125 mg/dL). Recommend diet/exercise, add metformin in certain cases
  - Maturity-onset diabetes of the young (MODY): Autosomal dominant forms of DM due to defects in genes that regulate insulin secretion
  - Gestational diabetes (GDM): Hyperglycemia during second or third trimester of pregnancy without previous diagnosis of diabetes
- Clinical features: See Table 5.2
- Acute complications of diabetes: Diabetes ketoacidosis (DKA) and hyperosmolar hyperglycemic state (HHS) – see Critical Care Chapter 3 for additional details
- Chronic complications of diabetes: See Table 5.3
- Patterns of glucose response
  - Dawn phenomenon: Increased nocturnal secretion of growth hormone causes AM hyperglycemia. Treatment adjustment: Increase PM insulin.
  - Somogyi effect: Low overnight blood sugar causes rebound and AM blood sugar is high. Treatment adjustment: Decrease PM insulin.
- Approach to managing a patient with DM1:
  - Insulin is the mainstay of therapy; oral agents used for DM2 are ineffective for DM1. Can consider the use of a continuous glucose monitor and insulin pump.
- Approach to managing a patient with DM2:
  - Generally, goal = HgA1c <7.0%, especially early in disease. Guidelines recommend individualized HgA1c goals with decreasing life expectancy, increasing microvascular complications, difficulties with hypoglycemia, etc. (e.g., may increase HgA1c to <8.0% in older patients).
  - Recommended management steps:
    - **Step 1:** Discuss and optimize non-pharmacologic management
      - Lifestyle changes: Diabetes self-management education and support is particularly effective when offered in a person-centered, team-based care setting
      - 5–15% weight loss if elevated body mass index (BMI)
      - Moderate to vigorous intensity aerobic activity for 150 minutes/week
      - Smoking cessation
      - Consider weight loss medications or bariatric surgery if BMI is very elevated
    - **Step 2:** Start a medication and add additional agents if needed (See Table 5.3)
      - Typically metformin is first line unless contraindicated (e.g., GFR<30). Titrate up slowly to allow for adjustment to side effects, up to max dose metformin 1000mg BID or 850 mg TID.
      - Add additional agents if needed based on medical comorbidities (e.g., CV risk factors, CKD, obesity), risk of hypoglycemia, cost. Common considerations:
        - Established or high-risk cardiovascular disease: GLP-1 receptor agonists, SGLT2 inhibitors
        - Best HgA1c-lowering medications: Metformin, GLP-1RA, sulfonylureas, TZDs
        - CKD (GFR 30–60 or UACr >3–30 mg/g): SGLT2 inhibitors
        - If concern for hypoglycemia: DPP4-inhibitors, GLP-1 agonists, SGLT2 inhibitors, TZD (avoid sulfonylureas)
        - If weight is a concern: GLP-1 agonist and SGLT2 inhibitor (evidence for weight loss)
      - If needed, start insulin
        - Consider starting insulin at 0.1–0.2 units/kg/day or 10 units/day if initial HgA1c >9–10%, but caution with renal dysfunction since insulin is cleared by the kidneys ($\rightarrow$ longer half-life with lower GFR).
        - Types of insulin (Figure 5.7)
          - Rapid-onset: Aspart, lispro, glulisine
          - Short: Regular
          - Intermediate: NPH (dosed BID)
          - Long: Detemir, glargine, degludec
          - Concentrated: U-500 (500 units/mL): Consider if total daily insulin dose 200–300 units/day

- Approach to managing a patient with gestational diabetes:
  - Pregnant women should be screened for gestational diabetes between 24–28 weeks of pregnancy with an oral glucose tolerance test (OGTT)
  - If gestational diabetes is diagnosed, repeat OGTT 4–12 weeks postpartum to confirm resolution of hyperglycemia
  - Patients with a personal history of GDM should have lifelong screening for diabetes q1–3 yr as they are at increased risk of DM

TABLE 5.2 • Clinical Features and Management of Type 1 vs. Type 2 Diabetes Mellitus		
	Type 1 Diabetes (DM1)	**Type 2 Diabetes (DM2)**
Epidemiology	5–10% cases Typical onset <20 yr	90–95% cases Typically adult onset
Pathophysiology	Autoimmune destruction of pancreatic beta cells, which causes insulin **deficiency**	Insulin **resistance**, impaired secretion, abnormal fat metabolism, excessive hepatic glucose production
Genetic associations	Some genetic predisposition Associated with HLA-DQ/DR	Stronger genetic concordance than DM1 No HLA association
Screening/ diagnosis	No screening; send diagnostics if symptoms of hyperglycemia • Check islet cell autoantibodies (ICAs). GAD-65 most common. If high suspicion, also consider others: IA-2, insulin, zinc transporter (ZnT-8). • If absence of autoantibodies, consider mature-onset diabetes of the young (MODY) vs. acquired (pancreatitis, neoplasia, cystic fibrosis, hemochromatosis). Minority of patients with DM2 (5–10%) can also have positive ICAs.	Screen for DM2 starting at age 45 yr every 3 yr. Consider starting to screen earlier if risk factors for DM2 (obesity, first-degree relatives DM2, history of gestational diabetes, PCOS, HTN, HLD)
Clinical features	Polyuria, polydipsia, fatigue, weight loss, blurred vision, fungal infections, neuropathy. Patients with DM2 can also be asymptomatic.	
Treatment	Lifelong insulin • Start 0.5 units/kg → ½ long-acting, ½ pre-meal; consider continuous subcutaneous insulin infusions if not at HgA1c goal, significant glycemic variability, severe or asymptomatic hypoglycemia	**Pre-DM2 (HgA1c 5.7–6.4):** 5-yr risk of DM 25%. Diet, exercise, consider metformin if age <60 yr, BMI >35, or gestational DM **DM2 (HgA1c >6.5):** First line: Metformin + weight loss/diet Second line: SGLT2i or GLP-1 RA for most patients. If HgA1c remains above target add additional agent: • DPP-4i (preferred in patients with heart failure) • SU or TZD (generally cheaper; avoid TZD if patient has heart failure) • Basal insulin

TABLE 5.3 • Microvascular and Macrovascular Complications of Diabetes	
Microvascular Complications of DM *Glycemic control reduces and slows the progression of microvascular complications of DM	**Macrovascular Complications of DM** *Glycemic control does not always reduce macrovascular complications of DM
• **Nephropathy**: Glomerular hyperfiltration → thick glomerular basement membrane → albuminuria • **Retinopathy**: Cataracts, retinopathy, glaucoma • **Neuropathy**: Peripheral and autonomic (impotence, overflow incontinence secondary to neurogenic bladder, gastroparesis)	• **Coronary artery disease** • **Peripheral vascular disease** • **Stroke/TIA**

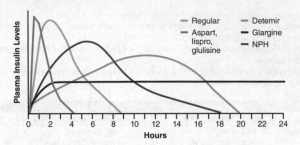

FIGURE 5.7: Plasma insulin levels over time for each type of insulin.

Hypoglycemia

- Etiology:
  - In patients with DM: Excess insulin, oral hypoglycemics, renal failure (which causes reduced insulin clearance)
  - In nondiabetes:
    - Increased insulin (factitious insulin intake [high insulin, low C-peptide], insulinoma)
    - Decreased glucose production: Adrenal insufficiency, hypopituitarism, cirrhosis, renal failure, sepsis, severe malnutrition
- Symptoms: Typically, patients symptomatic if glucose <55 mg/dL
  - Hyperadrenergic symptoms: Sweating, tremors, anxiety, tachycardia
  - CNS symptoms: Headache, confusion, can progress to obtundation, seizures and death
- Diagnosis:
  - History and medication review are critical
  - In nondiabetics: Repeat glucose, also check insulin, C-peptide, pro-insulin, beta-hydroxybutyrate, insulin secretagogue screen
- Treatment:
  - Glucose-containing foods or administer dextrose. Also treat underlying cause.
  - If patient has history of alcohol use disorder, give thiamine before glucose to reduce the risk of Wernicke-Korsakoff Syndrome
- Hypoglycemia unawareness:
  - Insufficient counterregulatory autonomic response. History of hypoglycemia increases risk
  - Management: Relax glycemic targets (e.g., target HgA1c 8.0% in some patients), avoidance of hypo-glycemia may reverse unawareness. Consider continuous glucose monitor (CGM).

TABLE 5.4 · Medications Used for the Treatment of Diabetes

Medication Class	Examples	Expected Decrease in HgA1c with Monotherapy (%)	Mechanism of Action	Advantages	Disadvantages
Alpha-glucosidase inhibitor	acarbose miglitol	0.5–0.8	Lowers glucose by blocking breakdown of carbohydrates in the intestine	• Weight neutral	• GI side effects • TID dosing
Biguanides	metformin	1.0–2.0	Decreases hepatic glucose production; decreases insulin resistance in the periphery	• Weight neutral to weight loss • No hypoglycemia • Low cost • Potential ASCVD benefit	• GI side effects common • Contraindicated with renal insufficiency (eGFR <30) • Associated with B12 deficiency, duration dependent • Risk of lactic acidosis (rare)
DPP-4i	linagliptin saxagliptin sitagliptin	0.5–0.8	Increasing insulin synthesis/release from pancreatic beta cells	• Weight neutral	• Possible increased risk of heart failure with saxagliptin • Joint pain
Glucagon-like peptide 1 receptor agonist (GLP-1 RA)	dulaglutide exenatide liraglutide lixisenatide semaglutide	0.5–1.5	Enhances glucose-dependent insulin secretion by the pancreatic beta cell; slows gastric emptying	• Reduction in major adverse cardiovascular events • Weight loss • No hypoglycemia • Benefit in NASH	• Most require injection • GI side effects common
SGLT2i	canagliflozin dapagliflozin empagliflozin ertugliflozin	0.5–0.7	Reduces renal tubular absorption of glucose so more glucose expelled in urine	• Reduced cardiovascular mortality in patients with established CVD • Improved renal outcomes in patients with nephropathy • No hypoglycemia • Weight loss	• UTIs, vulvovaginal candidiasis, balinitis • Bone fractures • Euglycemic DKA (rare)
Sulfonylureas (SU)	chlorpropamide glyburide glipizide glimepiride	1.0–2.0	Stimulates pancreatic beta cells to release insulin	• Rapidly effective	• Hypoglycemia • Weight gain • Concern in patients with CAD (glimepiride may be safer)

(Continued)

TABLE 5.4 • Medications Used for the Treatment of Diabetes *(Continued)*

Medication Class	Examples	Expected Decrease in HgA1c with Monotherapy (%)	Mechanism of Action	Advantages	Disadvantages
Thiazolidine-diones (TZD)	pioglitazone	0.5–1.4	Decreases insulin resistance in the muscle, fat, and liver	• Improved lipid profile • Potential ASCVD benefit in patients without heart failure • Benefit in NASH	• Fluid retention, heart failure, weight gain • Bone fractures • Potential increase in bladder cancer
Insulin	Rapid: Aspart, lispro, glulisine Short: Regular Intermed: NPH Long: Detemir, glargine, degludec Concentrated: U-500 (500 units/mL)	1.5–3.5	Helps cells break down glucose	• Rapidly effective • No dose limit	• Requires injections • Risk of hypoglycemia (higher risk with human insulin NPH or premixed formulations vs. analogs) • Weight gain

KEY CLINICAL TRIALS AND PUBLICATIONS

Thyroid Disease

- **Guidelines for the treatment of hypothyroidism: Prepared by the American Thyroid Association task force on thyroid hormone replacement.** *Thyroid* 2014;24(12):1670–1751.
  - Guidelines about hypothyroidism management.
- **2016 American Thyroid Association guidelines for diagnosis and management of hyperthyroidism and other causes of thyrotoxicosis.** *Thyroid* 2016;26(10):1343–1421.
  - Guidelines about hyperthyroidism and other thyrotoxicosis management.

Diabetes

- **Diabetes Control and Complication Trial (DCCT).** *N Engl J Med* 1993;329(14):977–986. Follow-up: *N Engl J Med* 2000;342(6):381–389.
  - Multicenter randomized controlled trial that randomized 1441 patients with type 1 diabetes to intensive vs. conventional glycemic control therapy. Patients who kept their blood glucose levels as close to normal as safely possible with intensive diabetes treatment as early as possible in their disease had fewer diabetes-related health problems after 6.5 yr (including diabetic retinopathy, development of kidney and cardiovascular disease), compared to patients who used conventional treatment. Long-term follow-up of these patients demonstrated that these benefits persisted. After 30 yr of follow-up, the group that had tightly controlled blood glucoses in the study had a 32% reduction in major cardio-vascular events, suggesting that better control early in DM1 can prevent cardiovascular disease.
- **UK Prospective Diabetes Study (UKPDS).** *Lancet* 1998;352:837–853. Follow up: **Holman et al.** *N Engl J Med* 2008;359(15):1577–1589.
  - Multicenter randomized controlled trial that randomized 3867 patients with newly diagnosed DM2 to intensive vs. lenient glycemic control therapy. A follow-up study 10 yr later found that the inten-sive glucose control group had a lower risk of MIs and death from any cause. Patients who under-went intensive glycemic control (fasting glucose <108 mg/dL) had a 25% reduction in microvascular complications, but there was no effect on macrovascular disease or mortality between treatment groups.
- **Nice-Sugar Study**. *N Engl J Med* 2009;360(13):1283–1297.
  - Multicenter, nonblinded, randomized controlled trial that randomized 6104 patients with diabetes who had been admitted to an intensive care unit and were expected to stay at least 3 days to intensive glucose control (goal glucose 80–108 mg/dL) vs. liberal glucose control (<180 mg/dL). Intensive glucose control led to <u>more</u> deaths than the conventional approach, suggesting more permissive glucose control with glucose <180 mg/dL is preferred in the ICU setting.

Diabetes Prevention

- **Diabetes Prevention Program (DPP).** *N Engl J Med* 2002;346(6):393–403.
  - Multicenter, double-blind, randomized controlled trial that randomized 3234 middle-aged adults to intensive lifestyle counseling (dietary changes and 150 minutes of exercise per week for a weight loss goal of ≥7%) versus usual care. The intensive lifestyle counseling reduced the onset of diabe-tes by 58% compared to usual care. Metformin treatment reduced the onset of diabetes by 31%. These benefits persisted though the study's 15-yr follow-up.

NOTES

Nephrology

ANATOMY AND PHYSIOLOGY

Renal Anatomy

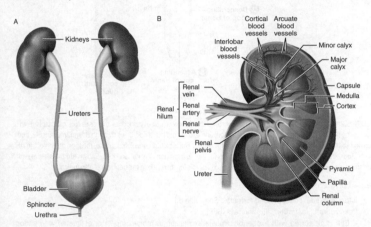

FIGURE 6.1: **Anatomy of the urinary tract and kidney**. A) The organs of the urinary system include the kidneys, ureters, bladder, and urethra. The function of the urinary system is to filter the blood and create urine as a waste by-product. B) The kidney has an outer region called the renal cortex and an inner region called the medulla. The renal columns are connective tissue extensions that radiate from the cortex to the medulla and separate the renal pyramids and papillae. The papillae are bundles of collecting ducts that carry urine made by the nephron to the calyces for excretion. The renal hilum is the entry and exit site for the blood vessels, nerves, lymphatics, and ureters.

Renal Physiology

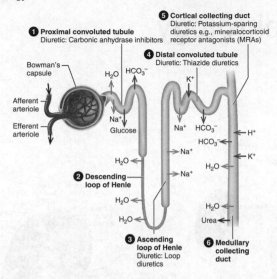

FIGURE 6.2: **Diagram of the nephron.** The nephron is the functional unit of the kidney that uses four mechanisms to process the filtrate: filtration, reabsorption, secretion, and excretion. First, blood flows through Bowman's capsule, and fluid and solutes are filtered out to form a glomerular filtrate. The proximal convoluted tubule, the loop of Henle, the distal convoluted tubule, and the collecting ducts are sites for the reabsorption of water and ions. Shown are the sites at which ions are moved in each segment. The site where each diuretic functions along the nephron is also indicated.

Renal Formulas

- Important renal concepts and formulas: See Table 6.1
- Pearls about glomerular filtration rate (GFR):
  - GFR is measured with exogenous substances (inulin or radioisotopes) or estimated with endogenous substances (creatinine or cystatin C)
  - In clinical practice, estimated GFR (eGFR) is calculated using the Chronic Kidney Disease Epidemiology Collaboration (CKD-EPI) formula, which has the best accuracy in persons with normal eGFR, or using the Modification of Diet in Renal Disease (MDRD) equation. These equations have largely replaced the Cockcroft-Gault equation.
  - eGFR is most accurate when a patient is in a steady state (i.e., has a stable sCr). When interpreting eGFR, consider common scenarios that affect the result, such as muscle mass, medication effect (e.g., TMP/SMX), or dynamic states (e.g., early AKI).
  - If eGFR accuracy is critical, consider calculating eGFR with cystatin C, a freely filtered molecule that is not affected by muscle mass.

TABLE 6.1 · Important Renal Concepts and Formulas		
Concept	**Formula**	**Description**
Clearance	$C_{plasmaofx} = U_x * V/P_x$	mL of plasma cleared of substance X over a specific amount of time
Renal blood flow (RBF)	(1) $RPF = C_{PAH} = [U]_{PAH} * V/[P]_{PAH}$ (2) $RBF = RPF / 1 - Hct$	The clearance of PAH is used to estimate RPF, then RPF is used to estimate RBF
Glomerular filtration rate (GFR)	$GFR = [U]_{inulin} * V/[P]_{inulin}$ $GFR = K_f[(P_{GC} - P_{BS}) - (\pi_{GC} - \pi_{BS})]$	The clearance of inulin is used to estimate GFR

Abbreviations: C_x: Clearance of X, U_x: Urine concentration of X, V: Urine volume, P_x: Plasma concentration of X, RPF: Renal plasma flow, PAH: Para-aminohippurate, Kf: Filtration coefficient, P_{GC}: Hydrostatic pressure in glomerular capillary, P_{BS}: Hydrostatic pressure in Bowmen's space, π_{GC}: Oncotic pressure in the glomerular capillary, π_{BS}: Oncotic pressure in the glomerular capillary

DIAGNOSTICS

TABLE 6.2 · Urinalysis Tests and Interpretation				
Test	Purpose	Clinical Significance	False negative results*	False positive results*
Leukocytes	Detects presence of pyuria	• Infection • Bladder tumor • SLE • Medication effect	• Elevated urine glucose, protein, ketones, specific gravity • Certain oxidizing antibiotics (e.g., cephalexin, nitrofurantoin)	• Contamination
Nitrite	Detects evidence of bacteriuria	• Bacterial infection	• Elevated specific gravity, pH <6.0, vitamin C	• Contamination
Urobilinogen	Detects hepatic damage or obstruction; aids in differentiation between obstructive and hemolytic jaundice	• Low: May suggest biliary obstruction (due to less than typical amounts of conjugated bilirubin reaching the intestine for conversion to urobilinogen) • High: Hemolysis, hepatobiliary disease		• Elevated nitrite levels • Phenazopyridine
Protein	Detects glomerular disease or damage. Urine dipstick is sensitive for albumin, but has very low sensitivity for non-albumin proteinuria (e.g., tubular protein, immunoglobulins)	• Primary or secondary renal damage	• Urine that is acidic or dilute • Dipstick best detects albumin so may miss non-albumin protein (e.g., abnormal antibodies produced by plasma cells in multiple myeloma)	• Urine that is alkaline or concentrated • Phenazopyridine
pH	Assesses renal function for excretion of acids and ability to maintain acid–base balance	• Acid-base disturbances • Renal tubular acidosis (RTA)		
Blood	Detects presence of free hemoglobin, myoglobin, or RBCs	• Hgb: Extensive/rapid intravascular hemolysis • Myoglobin: Skeletal muscle trauma (e.g., rhabdomyolysis, seizure) • RBC: See "hematuria below" or "Trauma, infection, stone, malignancy or GN"	• Elevated specific gravity • Captopril • Vitamin C	• Menstrual bleeding • If assessing for blood, myoglobin can cause a false positive

NEPHROLOGY

(*Continued*)

TABLE 6.2 • Urinalysis Tests and Interpretation (*Continued*)				
Test	Purpose	Clinical Significance	False negative results*	False positive results*
Specific gravity	Assesses renal ability to concentrate/dilute urine	• <u>Low</u>: Diabetes insipidus, renal disease, increased fluid intake, diuresis • <u>High</u>: Hypovolemia, low effective circulating volume (heart failure, cirrhosis, nephrotic syndrome), SIADH, contrast dye	• Alkaline urine	• IV contrast
Ketone	Assesses for evidence of stressors (which cause incomplete fat metabolism)	• Fever • Starvation • Diabetic ketoacidosis	• Delay in urine examination	• Elevated specific gravity • Some medications (e.g., mesna, levodopa, phenolphthalein)
Bilirubin	Detects hepatic damage or obstruction; aids in differentiation between obstructive and hemolytic jaundice	• Hepatobiliary disease • Hyperthyroidism • Septicemia	• Chlorpromazine • Selenium	• Phenazopyridine
Glucose	Detects evidence of hyperglycemia (and therefore, often, diabetes)	• Hyperglycemia (usually due to diabetes) • Proximal tubule dysfunction (Fanconi syndrome) • SGLT2 inhibitors Of note, glucosuria in the setting of normal serum glucose may indicate Fanconi syndrome.	• Elevated specific gravity • Uric acid • Vitamin C	• Ketones • Levodopa

* False positive results are caused by false elevations in the given parameter. False negative results are caused by a false depression in the parameter.

APPROACHES AND CHIEF COMPLAINTS
Proteinuria
- Definition:
  - Urine protein to creatinine ratio (UPCR) >150 mg/g or 24-hr protein >150 mg
    - Greater than 3 g/24 hr is *nephrotic-range* proteinuria
  - Urine albumin to creatinine ratio (UACR) >30 mg/g or 24-hr albumin excretion >30 mg
    - 30–300 mg/g is termed microalbuminuria
    - >300 mg/g is termed macroalbuminuria
- Etiology:
  - Glomerular proteinuria: Increased glomerular permeability; due to primary glomerulonephritis (GN) or GN secondary to systemic illness (e.g., diabetes)
  - Tubular proteinuria: Impaired tubular reabsorption due to tubular dysfunction; seen in tubular interstitial injury from systemic illness, congenital disease, endogenous toxins or exogenous toxins (e.g., beta-lactam antibiotics)
  - Overflow proteinuria: Impaired resorptive ability of the proximal tubule; due to excess filtration and/or production of proteins (e.g., hemolysis, rhabdomyolysis, Bence-Jones protein in multiple myeloma, amyloidosis)
  - Other: Fever, exercise, orthostatic proteinuria (i.e., proteinuria only when standing; benign/self-limited, typically occurs in young people)
- Diagnosis:
  - Spot tests: UPCR, UACR, or dipstick; dipstick detects albumin ranges from 1+ (30–100 mg/dL) to 4+ (>1000 mg/dL)
  - 24-hour urine is rarely needed, but may be useful in establishing the accuracy of spot tests and quantifying a baseline level of proteinuria in a patient with persistent proteinuria; however, it is cumbersome and susceptible to collection error
- Pearls:
  - Multiple myeloma and other light-chain diseases will produce proteinuria without significant albuminuria; therefore, UACR or dipstick will be "falsely" negative (or unexpectedly mild)
  - Dilution and high pH may also yield false-negative dipstick results. Specific gravity should be greater than >1.005 and pH <8 for accurate results.
  - Persistent proteinuria is associated with progression of kidney disease, and thus is often a treatment target and a surrogate outcome in the treatment of kidney disease. One needs to identify the underlying cause and treat. ACEi/ARBs are often used to improve proteinuria.

Hematuria
- Types:
  - Microscopic hematuria: Normal appearing urine with ≥ 2 RBCs/HPF detected in the UA → Consider glomerular disease
  - Gross hematuria: Visibly abnormal appearing urine with RBCs on microscopy → More likely urologic disease (e.g., trauma, infection, stones, malignancy, PKD)
  - Mimics of gross hematuria: Menstruation or other uterine sources of bleeding, medications (e.g., pyridium, phenytoin, rifampin), foods (e.g., beets), metabolites (e.g., bile, porphyrin, methemoglobin)
  - Causes of UA positive for blood without hematuria on microscopy: Hemolysis, rhabdomyolysis
- History: The following clues may inform the differential diagnosis:
  - Gross hematuria (e.g., visible blood in the urine) → More likely urologic but may also be caused by IgA nephropathy or renal vasculitis
  - Concurrent dysuria → UTI, malignancy, stone
  - Recent URI → IgA nephropathy if SYNpharyngitic (i.e., at the same time as the infection) vs. post-infectious GN (usually occurs 2-3 weeks after)
  - Family history (polycystic kidney disease, Alport's syndrome, benign familial hematuria)
  - Flank pain → Stones
  - Recent vigorous exercise → Exercise-induced hematuria
  - Travel → Urinary schistosomiasis, renal tuberculosis
  - Timing:
    - Beginning of urination → Urethra
    - End of urination → Bladder/Prostate
    - Throughout urination → Kidney/Ureter
  - Transient or persistent → Transient asymptomatic hematuria occurs in young patients and can be benign

NEPHROLOGY

- Workup: Repeat UA and urine microscopy, then evaluate urine sediment
  - <u>Glomerular</u>: Dysmorphic RBCs, acanthocytes ("Mickey Mouse ears"), brown urine, proteinuria, AKI, systemic symptoms → Get renal ultrasound and refer to nephrology for evaluation and possible biopsy
  - <u>Non-glomerular</u>: Bright red blood, blood clots, isomorphic erythrocytes
    - If evidence of UTI, treat and repeat UA in 6 weeks
    - If complaining of acute flank pain, rule out nephrolithiasis or PKD with non-contrast CT abd/pelvis (alternative: renal ultrasound)
    - If gross hematuria, age >40 yr for men, age >50 yr for women, or risk factors for urological malignancy (e.g., smoking, occupational dye exposure, chronic cystitis, pelvic irradiation, cyclophosphamide use) → Get CT urogram and refer to urology for evaluation and possible cystoscopy
    - Can start with renal ultrasound and cystoscopy if age <60 yr, <30 pack-yr smoking history, and <25 RBCs/hpf on urine microscopy (intermediate risk)
    - Can recheck UA within 6 months prior to imaging and cystoscopy if age <40 yr for men, age <50 yr for women, <10 pack-yr smoking history, and <10 RBCs/hpf on urine microscopy (low risk)

Uremia

- Definition: Syndrome of symptoms and metabolic derangements thought to be due to retained toxins in renal failure (i.e., not attributable to abnormal fluid volume, electrolyte levels, or decreased renal synthetic function)
- Clinical features:
  - Symptoms: Fatigue, sleep disturbances, decreased mental acuity, nausea, decreased appetite, changes in smell and taste, pruritis, cramping, restless legs, serositis (e.g., pericarditis), seizures, coma
  - Metabolic changes: Sexual dysfunction, reduced body temperature, insulin resistance, increased protein-muscle catabolism, platelet dysfunction, leukocyte dysfunction, reduced muscle membrane potential
- Diagnosis: Primarily based on a combination of symptoms related to uremia, history of severe AKI or advanced CKD, and elimination of other potential causes of symptoms. Typically, elevated BUN and serum creatinine are present; however, the degree of elevation is highly variable between different individuals and clinical scenarios.
- Treatment:
  - Long-term management of uremia requires dialysis or kidney transplantation
  - Dialysis is indicated for morbid and life-threatening uremic symptoms, including malnutrition, pericarditis, bleeding, mental status changes, seizures and refractory pruritis
  - Symptomatic management may be more appropriate depending on the patient's goals of care
    - <u>Pain</u>: Synthetic opioids (e.g., fentanyl, methadone, hydromorphone) are preferred to avoid neurotoxic metabolites produced by less synthetic opioids and prodrugs (e.g., meperidine, codeine, tramadol and morphine), which accumulate harmful metabolites in renal dysfunction
    - <u>Nausea</u>: Haloperidol has more data for efficacy but must be dose-reduced. Ondansetron also has some data for efficacy. There is concern for limited efficacy and increased risk of EPS with metoclopramide.
    - <u>Pruritis</u>: Emollients are first-line treatment. Topical analgesics (e.g., capsaicin) may be trialed. Other treatments include antihistamines and gabapentin.
    - <u>Cramping</u>: May be treated with benzodiazepines or haloperidol, but caution must be exercised with dosage

DISEASES AND PATHOPHYSIOLOGY

Renal Dysfunction

Acute Kidney Injury (AKI)

- Definition:
  - Serum Cr increase $\geq$ 0.3 mg/dL within 48 hours
  - Serum Cr increased to $\geq$ 1.5$\times$ baseline within the prior 7 days
  - Urine volume <0.5 mL/kg/h for 6 hours

Pre-renal (decreased renal perfusion)

- Etiologies: Hypovolemia (poor PO intake, diuresis, hemorrhage), vasodilation (sepsis, anaphylaxis), poor effective circulating volume (heart failure, cirrhosis, nephrotic syndrome), contrast, medications (ACE inhibitors, ARBs, NSAIDs), abdominal compartment syndrome
- Clinical features: BUN/Cr >20:1, fractional excretion of sodium (FENa) <1%, urine osmolality >500 mOsm/kg H_2O, urine Na^+ <20 mEq/L, benign sediment, few hyaline casts, no cellular casts

Intra-renal (direct injury to renal tissue)

Acute tubular necrosis (ATN)

- Etiologies:
  - Ischemia: Prolonged or severe hypoperfusion (e.g., from hemorrhage or sepsis)
  - Toxic: Pigment (rhabdomyolysis, hemolysis), paraproteins (multiple myeloma), medications (aminoglycosides, cisplatin, foscarnet, pentamidine, tenofovir), IV contrast
- Clinical features: "Muddy brown" granular casts; usually FENa >2%
- Pearl: Ischemic ATN lies on a spectrum of decreased renal perfusion along with "pre-renal" AKI; a single patient (or even a single kidney) may exhibit both pre-renal and ATN pathophysiology in tandem

Acute interstitial nephritis (AIN)

- Etiologies:
  - Medications: Antibiotics, especially beta-lactams, NSAIDs, and PPIs
  - Infection: Streptococcal infection, diphtheria, CMV, EBV, tuberculosis, hantavirus, leptospirosis
  - Systemic autoimmune disease: Sjögren's, sarcoidosis, SLE, IgG4 disease
- Clinical features:
  - Rash, eosinophilia, WBC casts
  - Eosinophils in the urine are not specific or sensitive (low diagnostic value); instead of ordering urine eos, if high suspicion for AIN, stop the culprit medication and consider a kidney biopsy

Acute Glomerulonephritis

- Etiologies: Several causes listed under "Nephrotic Syndrome" and "Nephritic Syndrome"
- Clinical features: Proteinuria, hypertension, hematuria, RBC casts

Post-renal (obstruction of urinary tract)

- Etiology: Benign prostatic hyperplasia (BPH), malignancy, strictures, stones, functional urinary retention, congenital abnormalities. Typically, AKI is caused by obstruction of *bilateral* kidneys.
- Clinical features: Increased PVR by ultrasound or Foley, hydronephrosis on ultrasound or CT

General Approach to the Diagnosis and Management of AKI

- Step 1: Address any urgent management needs (e.g., treat severe hyperkalemia, hypoxemia due to pulmonary edema)
- Step 2: Confirm baseline Cr and diagnose the etiology. See differential diagnosis above and in Figure 6.3. Volume exam suggesting hypovolemia may suggest a pre-renal cause. Obtain a bladder scan to rule out postrenal causes. Get a UA with microscopy. Consider checking the fractional excretion of sodium (FENa), which can help differentiate pre-renal AKI from ATN.
  - Pearl: Most AKI in the hospital will be pre-renal due to hypovolemia, intra-renal due to ATN, or postrenal due to obstruction. Thus, a majority of inpatient AKI can be resolved with fluids and/or a Foley catheter.
- Step 3: Treat the underlying cause (e.g., give fluids if pre-renal, place Foley if post-renal)
- Step 4: Monitor for complications. Check electrolytes, evaluate volume status, reassess for uremia regularly. AKI can cause CKD progression in patients with baseline kidney dysfunction.
- Step 5: Avoid factors that may worsen AKI or complications. Avoid nephrotoxic medications and adjust dosing of renally excreted medications.
- References:
  - KDIGO Work Group. KDIGO clinical practice guideline for acute kidney injury (Kidney Int Suppl 2012;2(1):1–138)
  - Mercado et al. Acute kidney injury: Diagnosis and management (Am Fam Physician 2019;100(11): 687–694)

NEPHROLOGY

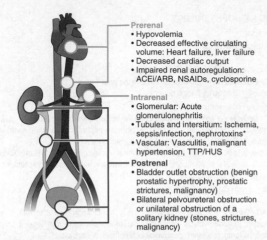

FIGURE 6.3: **Etiologies of acute kidney injury (AKI)**. This diagram depicts the etiologies of AKI, divided into pre-renal (green), intrarenal (blue), and postrenal (pink) etiologies. *Nephrotoxins include both exogenous substances (e.g., aminoglycosides, iodinated contrast, cisplatin, PPIs, NSAIDs) and endogenous substances (e.g., damage due to rhabdomyolysis, hemolysis, multiple myeloma). Abbreviations: ACEi, angiotensin-converting enzyme inhibitor; ARB, angiotensin receptor blocker; NSAID, nonsteroidal antiinflammatory drug; TTP/HUS, thrombotic thrombocytopenic purpura/hemolytic uremic syndrome.

Chronic Kidney Disease (CKD) and End-Stage Renal Disease (ESRD)

- Definitions:
    - CKD: Any of the following signs of kidney disease lasting >3 months
        - GFR <60 mL/min/1.73 m^2
        - Albuminuria >30 mg/g or 30 mg/24 hr
        - Urine sediment suggesting kidney damage (e.g., tubular casts, hematuria with dysmorphic RBCs)
        - Electrolyte abnormalities attributed to tubular disease
    - Or the following:
        - Abnormalities on histology from a kidney biopsy
        - Structural kidney disease on imaging
        - History of kidney transplantation
- Stages:
    - GFR category:
        - G1: eGFR >90 mL/min/1.73 m^2
        - G2: eGFR 60–90 mL/min/1.73 m^2
        - G3a: eGFR 45–59 mL/min/1.73 m^2
        - G3b: eGFR 30–44 mL/min/1.73 m^2
        - G4: eGFR 15–29 mL/min/1.73 m^2
        - G5: eGFR <15 mL/min/1.73 m^2
    - Albuminuria category:
        - A1: UACR <30 mg/g
        - A2: UACR 30–300 mg/g
        - A3: UACR >300 mg/g
    - ESRD: Term that typically refers to patients with CKD who have either:
        - GFR <15 mL/min/m^2
        - Requirement of long-term dialysis or history of kidney transplant
- Etiologies:
    - <u>Systemic disease</u>: Diabetes, hypertension, glomerulonephritis due to autoimmune, infectious or inflammatory disease, polycystic kidney disease, malignancy, nephrotoxin exposure
    - <u>Primary kidney disease</u>: Primary glomerulonephritis, renal artery stenosis, chronic urinary obstruction, congenital kidney disease

- Treatment:
  - Treat the underlying cause of kidney disease
  - Prevent progression of kidney damage
  - Avoid nephrotoxic medications and adjust dosing of renally excreted medications
    - NSAIDs are a particularly common nephrotoxic medication
    - Most antibiotics need dose adjustment for decreased renal function
  - Manage complications
    - Renal diet: Na^+ 2–3 g/day, low K^+, low phos, fluid restriction (if anuric generally 1.5 L/day max)
  - Prepare for renal replacement when GFR is severely decreased
    - See dialysis section below
    - Includes referring for transplant evaluation and preparing access for dialysis
    - Consider a tool to predict the probability of dialysis or transplant for a patient with CKD stage G3 to G5
- References:
  - Chen TK et al. Chronic kidney disease diagnosis and management: A review (JAMA 2019;322(13): 1294–1304).
  - KDIGO Work Group. KDIGO 2012 clinical practice guideline for the evaluation and management of chronic kidney disease (Kidney Int Suppl 2013;3(1):1–150).

Dialysis/Access

Types of dialysis

- Hemodialysis (HD):
  - Blood is pumped along a semipermeable membrane across which electrolytes, water, and toxins are removed by diffusion into another fluid being pumped along the other side of the membrane (dialysate). The composition of the dialysate solution and a number of dialysis specifications are adjusted to meet individual clearance needs.
  - Water is filtered across the membrane by pressure
  - Usually performed over 2–4 hours, three times per week in a dialysis center
  - <u>Pros</u>: Frequent contact with providers, can be initiated emergently
  - <u>Cons</u>: Hypotension, circuit needs anticoagulation, need vascular access
- Continuous renal replacement therapy (CRRT):
  - Continuous venovenous hemodialysis (CVVHD) is dialysis performed continuously
  - Indicated for hemodynamically unstable patients requiring dialysis, e.g., patients requiring pressors
  - Only performed in the ICU
- Peritoneal dialysis (PD):
  - Peritoneum used as semipermeable membrane for removal of water and toxins from the blood via diffusion into intraperitoneal dialysate
  - <u>Pros</u>: Performed at home, "gentler" fluid and electrolyte shifts
  - <u>Cons</u>: Increased risk of hyperglycemia, peritonitis and catheter-associated infections; several con- traindications related to abdominal anatomy

Indications for dialysis

- Acute indications for dialysis: **"AEIOU"**
  - **A**cidosis
  - **E**lectrolytes (e.g., hyperkalemia)
  - **I**ntoxication (e.g., methanol, lithium, ASA, ethylene glycol)
  - Volume **O**verload
  - **U**remia
- Indications for dialysis in CKD:
  - Development of signs and symptoms of uremia, especially malnutrition
  - Complications of CKD that become refractory to medical management

Dialysis access

- Arteriovenous fistula (preferred): Needs 3–4 months to mature after placement; lowest infectious risk
- Arteriovenous graft: Typically needs 1 month to mature, although newer grafts can be accessed in 2 to 3 days; moderate infectious risk
- Central venous catheter: Can access immediately after placement, may be a temporary catheter or a permanent tunneled dialysis catheter placed by IR; highest infectious risk

NEPHROLOGY

- Peritoneal dialysis catheters:
  - Placed by general surgery, IR, or interventional nephrology laparoscopically
  - Ideally allow 2 weeks for surgical wound healing at catheter placement site to avoid dialysate leaks from peritoneal cavity; however, "urgent start peritoneal dialysis" can be initiated with low volume, supine exchanges for patients requiring dialysis sooner to avoid a temporary venous dialysis catheter placement
  - Need to start off with low volumes then increase slowly over 1–2 months to full prescription

Renal transplant

- Transplant referral: Usually consider when eGFR is between 20 and 30 mL/min/1.73 m^2
  - Evaluation includes months-long extensive biopsychosocial assessment
  - Transplant is generally contraindicated if there is concern for limited medical prognosis or ability to adhere to medical treatment
  - Waiting time for living and deceased donor transplants ranges from 1–5 yr depending on the region (USRDS Annual Report 2019)

Management of Complications Associated with Advanced CKD/ESRD

Blood pressure/volume

- Pathophysiology of hypertension in CKD: Complex and multifactorial, attributed to reduced nephron mass, increased Na^+ retention, extracellular volume expansion, activation of hormones (RAAS) and the sympathetic nervous system, and endothelial dysfunction
- Goal blood pressure: Generally <130/80 mmHg. This may be more liberal when accounting for certain factors, such as the degree of kidney disease, dialysis tolerance, polypharmacy, adverse effects of medication, and history of transplant.
- Treatment:
  - Sodium restriction is a key element of BP control. Fluid restriction becomes more important when GFR is severely reduced.
  - Patients should monitor PO intake and weight. Dry weight is estimated by exam and maintained through diuresis or ultrafiltration during dialysis.
  - Pharmacotherapy:
    - Diuretics
      - If a patient is still urinating, diuretics can assist with volume management
      - Diuretics depend on reaching active concentrations in the tubule lumen; higher doses are required with worsening renal function as urea competitively binds to the Organic Anion Transporter 1 (OAT1) which transports the diuretics into the tubular lumen
      - Most diuretics cause net fluid loss by preventing tubular sodium reabsorption
      - Loop diuretics will often be necessary if eGFR <30 mL/min/1.73 m^2 (Efficacy in reduced eGFR: bumetanide > furosemide > metolazone > chlorthalidone > hydrochlorothiazide).
    - ACE inhibitors/ARBs
      - First-line antihypertensive in CKD, especially with proteinuria and relatively preserved native kidney function
      - Can cause hyperkalemia
      - Increase in creatinine after starting agents is not necessarily indicative of kidney injury; generally should not be discontinued unless eGFR decreases by >30%
      - Combination ACE/ARB associated with increased renal decline and generally contraindicated (ONTARGET study *Lancet* 2008)
    - Calcium channel blocker (CCB)
      - Do not need dose modification for renal clearance
      - Relatively few adverse effects, can cause lower extremity edema
      - Preferred class in CKD after ACE/ARB and diuretics; can reduce proteinuria
    - Beta-blockers
      - Typically used if secondary prevention of cardiac events is warranted
      - Agents with combination alpha/beta antagonism are preferred to avoid metabolic effects of beta blockers, e.g., carvedilol and labetalol
      - Nonrenal clearance is preferred, e.g., carvedilol
    - Clonidine
      - No renal dose adjustment
      - Often used for hypertension on days between dialysis sessions
      - Associated with rebound hypertension when discontinued or doses missed

Anemia
- Pathophysiology: Results from decreased erythropoietin (EPO) production, EPO resistance, and decreased RBC lifespan
- Treatment:
  - Goal Hgb 10–11.5 g/dL
  - Check iron studies in CKD patients with anemia
  - Guidelines recommend for transferrin saturation >30%, ferritin >500 ng/mL, though practice patterns vary widely and less stringent targets may be used (e.g., transferrin saturation >20% and ferritin >100 ng/mL)
    - Ferritin can be increased with inflammatory states too
    - Rule out GI bleeding if you detect iron deficiency
  - Iron supplementation
    - IV iron is preferred in patients on hemodialysis. PO supplementation causes constipation, adds to pill burden, and is minimally absorbed compared to IV formulations.
    - Iron sucrose (Venofer) and ferric gluconate (Ferrlecit) are the most commonly used formulations
    - IV iron can cause anaphylaxis when first given; provide a test dose and administer slowly for patients who are IV iron naive
  - Erythropoietin-stimulating agents (ESAs)
    - Give if patient is iron replete but remains below Hgb goal
    - Three formulations:
      - Epoetin alfa (Epogen). 3× per week during HD or weekly in non-HD CKD.
      - Darbepoetin alfa (Aranesp). Weekly during HD or monthly in non-HD CKD.
      - Methoxy polyethylene glycol-epoetin beta (Mircera). Every 2 weeks.
  - RBC Transfusion
    - Uses:
      - Consider pRBC transfusion if ESAs are contraindicated or unsuccessful
      - Administer pRBCs if anemia is symptomatic or severe (Hgb <7 g/dL)

Bone mineral metabolism
- Pathophysiology: Mineral bone disorder is due to secondary hyperparathyroidism, which has two main contributing factors:
  - Decreased 1-alpha-hydroxylase (made by the kidney) → decreased activation of 25-hydroxy vitamin D to 1,25-dihydroxy vitamin D → decreased Ca^{2+} absorption → decreased serum Ca^{2+} level → increased PTH
  - Poor phosphate excretion → elevated phosphate → increased PTH and decreased 1,25-dihydroxy vitamin D
- Manifestations of CKD mineral bone disorder:
  - Mineral and hormone abnormalities
    - Increased phosphate
    - Increased PTH
    - Decreased 1,25-dihydroxy vitamin D
  - Structural bone abnormalities
    - Renal osteodystrophy: Range of abnormal bone pathology, bone turnover, and mineralization; includes osteomalacia, adynamic bone disease, and osteitis fibrosa cystica
    - Increased alkaline phosphatase: Reflects osteoblast activity and bone turnover
    - Increased FGF23: Secreted by osteocytes and involved in phosphate regulation
  - Calcification of blood vessels and soft tissue
- Management of CKD mineral bone disorder:
  - Phosphate
    - Phosphate level should ideally be within the normal range, though levels <5.5 mg/dL are often tolerated by providers
    - Phosphate binders are used to lower phosphate by preventing absorption of dietary phosphate
    - Calcium-based phosphate binders (data below from ST. PETER et al. *AJKD* 2018)
      - Calcium acetate (Phoslo) 667 mg/tablet; 34% of ESRD patients on this medication, cheap ($678/user-yr), strongest binder
      - Calcium carbonate (Tums), cheap
    - Non-calcium-based phosphate binders
      - Sevelamer (Renvela) 800 mg/tablet; preferred by some due to absence of calcium, 54% of ESRD patients on this medication, expensive ($2000–$4000/user-yr).
      - Lanthanum carbonate (Carbrenol); 5% ESRD patients on this medication, expensive ($5000/user-yr).
      - Iron-based phosphate binders: Ferric citrate and sucroferric oxyhydroxide. May be preferred if iron supplementation is needed.

NEPHROLOGY

- Calcium
  - Keep corrected Ca^{2+} within normal range
  - Dialysate can be adjusted to address low or high Ca^{2+} levels
  - Consider measuring ionized calcium (iCa) in patients with significant hypoalbuminemia, acidemia, or hyperphosphatemia
- Vitamin D
  - All CKD patients should be screened and treated for vitamin D deficiency or insufficiency (check 25-hydroxy vitamin D level). 1,25-dihydroxy vitamin D is not routinely measured in practice.
  - Treat with cholecalciferol or ergocalciferol unless hypercalcemia or significant hyperphosphatemia is present
- PTH
  - Guidelines recommend that PTH remain within 2–9× the upper limit of normal (~150–600 pg/mL) in HD patients
  - Practice varies and treatment in non-HD patients is controversial
  - Treatment: Active vitamin D analogs or calcimimetics are prescribed for severely elevated or rising PTH with replete 25-hydroxy vitamin D
    - Active vitamin D: Analogs of 1,25-dihydroxy vitamin D
      - Calcitriol (Rocaltrol). PO. Usually used for non-HD patients.
      - Paricalcitol (Zemplar). Administered IV. Usually given with HD.
      - Doxicalciferol (Hectorol). Administered IV. Usually given with HD.
    - Calcimimetics: Competitive binder of Ca^{2+} sensing receptor, which regulates PTH release. Usually used when active vitamin D analogues are inadequate or contraindicated due to hypercalcemia. More expensive than active vitamin D analogues. Side effects: Can cause hypocalcemia, nausea and vomiting.
      - Cinacalcet (Sensipar) – PO; in use since 2004
      - Etelcalcetide (Parsabiv) – IV; given with HD
    - Parathyroidectomy: Reserved for severe and refractory hyperparathyroidism in CKD

Glomerular Diseases

Glomerular diseases are divided into two patterns (nephrotic and nephritic) based on clinical features, including urine sediment and degree of proteinuria. Nephrotic and nephritic syndrome can be caused by diseases that only affect the kidney (primary) or systemic diseases (secondary).

Nephrotic Syndrome

- Pathophysiology: Syndrome of abnormal glomerular permeability and consequent proteinuria with associated symptoms and metabolic abnormalities
- Clinical features:
  - **Nephrotic range proteinuria**
    - >3 g/day or urine protein-to-creatinine ratio (UPCR) > 3 g/g
    - Leads to negative nitrogen balance and muscle wasting which may be obscured by edema
    - ACE inhibitors and ARBs are usually prescribed to reduce proteinuria
  - **Edema**
    - Due to decreased oncotic pressure (hypoalbuminemia) and increased Na^+ absorption in the distal nephron
    - Often includes morning periorbital edema
    - Treated with dietary sodium restriction and loop diuretics
  - **Hypercoagulability**
    - Due to many causes, including protein C and S deficiency and a compensatory increase in the production of procoagulant factors by the liver
    - Most commonly manifests as lower extremity DVT
    - PE and renal vein thrombosis are other important manifestations
    - Prophylactic anticoagulation is considered when serum albumin is <2 g/L
      (Gordon-Cappitelli et al. *CJSN* 2020)
  - **Hyperlipidemia**
    - Clinical significance is controversial; however, patients with nephrotic syndrome have significantly increased rates of cardiovascular events; statin medications may be given.
  - **Increased infection risk**
    - People with nephrotic syndrome should receive the pneumococcal vaccine.

Glomerular Pathologies Commonly Associated with Nephrotic-Range Proteinuria

Minimal change glomerulopathy (MCG, "minimal change disease")
- Epidemiology: Most common cause of nephrotic syndrome in children, less common in adults
- Pathophysiology:
  - Defined by nephrotic-range proteinuria and kidney biopsy with little or no change to the glomerular structure on light microscopy
  - Primary MCD is idiopathic
  - Secondary MCD may be associated with atopic disease, mononucleosis, Hodgkin's lymphoma, medications (e.g., NSAIDS, interferon, lithium)
- Treatment: Steroids 4–8 weeks, good prognosis

Focal segmental glomerulosclerosis (FSGS)
- Epidemiology: Most common cause of nephrotic syndrome in black adults
- Pathophysiology:
  - Defined by proteinuria and scarring in scattered glomeruli on biopsy
  - Primary FSGS may result from genetic mutations in podocyte proteins
  - Secondary FSGS is associated with HIV ("collapsing" type), obesity, heroin use
- Treatment:
  - Steroids or calcineurin inhibitors: 40–60% achieve remission, others have refractory disease and often advance to ESRD.
  - Can recur in the transplanted kidney and is thought to be due to a soluble factor that has yet to be identified.
  - Plasmapheresis can be utilized to remove this soluble factor to help prevent recurrence.

Membranous glomerulopathy (MGN, "membranous nephropathy")
- Epidemiology: Second most common cause of nephrotic syndrome in U.S. adults after diabetic nephropathy
- Pathophysiology:
  - Primary MGN is associated with the anti-phospholipase A2 receptor (anti-PLA2R) antibody; majority of cases are primary
  - Causes of secondary MGN: SLE, hepatitis B, solid tumor malignancy (lung, breast, and GI carcinomas), medications (penicillamine, NSAIDs, mercury, captopril)
- Diagnosis: Diagnosis requires a kidney biopsy, which shows deposits of IgG and C3
- Clinical features: Higher propensity for thromboembolic events (particularly renal vein thrombosis)
- Treatment: Up to one-third of patients will experience spontaneous remission; treatment with immunosuppression is considered for patients with a poor prognosis.
  - <4 g protein/day: Good prognosis for remission
  - 4–8 g protein/day: Possible chance of remission
  - >8 g protein/day: Poor chance of remission, start treatment immediately

Other Systemic Disorders Associated with Nephrotic-Range Proteinuria
- Diabetes:
  - Leading cause of glomerular disease and kidney failure in the United States
  - Hyperglycemia causes hyperfiltration through the glomeruli, leading to strain, scarring, proteinuria, and, eventually, a decrease in eGFR
  - Glycemic control and treatment of proteinuria may slow CKD progression
- Amyloidosis:
  - Abnormally-folded proteins deposit in the glomeruli resulting in impaired function and proteinuria
  - Dialysis-related amyloidosis is not typically a cause of nephrotic syndrome
- HIV-associated nephropathy (HIVAN):
  - Manifests as hematuria, proteinuria, edema with enlarged kidneys
  - Collapsing FSGS on pathology
  - Glucocorticoids for treatment are controversial
- Lupus nephritis:
  - Divided into six subclasses (class I–VI) based histological appearance. Nephrotic syndrome typically seen in class III to VI. Also see Rheumatology Chapter 9.
    - Class I: Minimal mesangial LN (no changes on light microscopy)
    - Class II: Mesangial proliferative LN (mesangial changes on light microscopy)
    - Class III: Focal LN (<50% of glomeruli involved)
    - Class IV: Diffuse LN (>50% of glomeruli involved)
    - Class V: Lupus membranous nephropathy (diffuse capillary wall thickening)
    - Class VI: Advanced sclerosing LN (90% sclerosing glomeruli, often bland urine sediment)

Nephritic Syndrome

- Pathophysiology: Syndrome of symptoms and findings caused by inflammation of glomeruli
- Clinical features:
  - Oliguria/AKI
  - Hematuria with RBC casts
  - Subnephrotic range proteinuria (<3 g/24 hr)
  - Edema
  - Hypertension

Glomerular Pathology Associated with Nephritic Syndrome

Post-streptococcal glomerulonephritis

- Epidemiology: More common in children
- Pathophysiology: Glomerular damage is due to deposition of anti-streptococcal Ab in the glomeruli, so hematuria, hypertension, edema begin 1–3 weeks after infection with *Streptococcus* bacteria
- Diagnosis: Anti-streptolysin O may be elevated; low complement
- Treatment: Supportive: Antihypertensives, loop diuretics, steroids if severe; majority of cases self-resolve in weeks to months

IgA nephropathy (Berger disease)

- Pathophysiology: Caused by deposition of dysregulated IgA immune complexes
- Clinical features:
  - Usually immediately preceded by or co-presenting with respiratory or GI infection ("syn-pharyngitic" hematuria as opposed to post-streptococcal GN, which occurs weeks after pharyngitis); can also be "silent" and go undetected for years
  - Manifests as episodic gross hematuria (more common in patients <25 yr) or persistent microscopic hematuria (more common in patients >25 yr)
  - Can be primary or secondary to systemic IgA vasculitis
- Diagnosis: Mesangial deposits of predominantly IgA immune complexes on biopsy. Complement levels are often normal.
- Treatment: No effective treatment, some advocate for steroids or fish oil; most patients have good prognosis

Membranoproliferative GN

- Pathophysiology: Hypercellularity and thickening of GBM on light microscopy
  - Type I (subendothelial GN): Immune complex mediated, typically caused by infections (e.g., HBV, HCV, endocarditis, schistosomiasis)
  - Type II (dense deposit disease): Complement mediated, rare, typically in children, but also occurs in adults with monoclonal gammopathy
- Treatment: Treat underlying cause, immunosuppression with steroids if idiopathic

Rapidly progressive (crescentic) glomerulonephritis (RPGN)

- Clinical features: Acute decline in renal function over days to weeks due to severe glomerular injury
- Diagnosis: Light microscopy with crescents in >50% of glomeruli due to fibrin formation and macrophages. Pathology and immunopathology distinguish between the three major etiologies:
  - Anti-GBM disease: Autoantibody to type IV collagen; called Goodpasture's syndrome when kidney and lung are involved. Linear immunofluorescence. Treatment: Cyclophosphamide, steroids, plasmapheresis.
  - Immune complex disease: Can be caused by systemic infections (e.g., post-streptococcal glomerulonephritis, infective endocarditis), systemic immune complex disease (e.g., IgA vasculitis, SLE) or primary GN (e.g., IgA nephropathy). Granular immunofluorescence.
  - Pauci-immune disease: Due to small-vessel vasculitis (GPA, EGPA, MPA) or can be drug-induced (penicillamine, hydralazine). Absence or paucity of glomerular staining for immunoglobulins. Most are ANCA-positive (80%)

Other Diseases Affecting the Kidney
Renal Tubular Acidosis (RTA)

RTA Type I (Distal)
- Pathophysiology: Defect in collecting tubule's ability to excrete H^+ due to congenital causes, multiple myeloma, autoimmunity, amphotericin B toxicity
- Labs: Urine pH >5.5; hypokalemia (secrete K^+ instead of H^+); non-anion gap metabolic acidosis
- Clinical features: ↑Risk kidney stones (increased calcium and phosphate excretion into alkaline urine)
- Treatment: Sodium bicarb to correct acidosis; phosphate salts promote excretion of titratable acid

RTA Type II (Proximal)
- Pathophysiology: Carbonic anhydrase mutation → HCO_3^- is not reabsorbed. Associated with multiple myeloma (rule out!), lead poisoning, amyloid, Fanconi syndrome
- Labs: Urine pH <5.5; hypokalemia; non-anion gap metabolic acidosis. Fanconi: +glycosuria.
- Clinical features: No risk of kidney stones like type I; risk of hypophosphatemic rickets
- Treatment: Sodium restriction increases Na^+ resorption in proximal tubule with bicarb asbsorbed as well. Do not give bicarb because it will be excreted.

RTA Type IV (Hyperkalemic)
- Pathophysiology: Hypoaldosteronism or lack of collecting tubule response to aldosterone; common with interstitial renal diagnosis or diabetic nephropathy
- Labs: Acidic urine; hyperkalemia, non-anion gap metabolic acidosis. No stones.

Other Diseases Affecting Renal Tubular Absorption

Renal papillary necrosis
- Etiology: Poor medullary perfusion resulting in ischemia and necrosis. Most often bilateral. Caused by vascular disease (diabetes), vasoconstriction (NSAIDs), vascular occlusion (sickle cell).
- Treatment: Stop offending agent, treat the underlying disease

Hartnup Syndrome
- Etiology: Rare autosomal recessive inborn error of amino acid metabolism. Impaired amino acid absorption in the gut and proximal renal tubule causing variable losses of proteins (e.g., tryptophan).
- Clinical features: Variable. Can be similar to pellagra: Dermatitis, diarrhea, ataxia, psychiatric findings
- Diagnosis: Elevated amino acids in the urine
- Treatment: Supplemental nicotinamide if symptomatic

Fanconi Syndrome
- Etiology: Primary (idiopathic) or secondary proximal tubule dysfunction causing defective transport of glucose, amino acids, Na^+, K^+, phosphorus, uric acid, bicarb. Causes include genetic (Wilson's disease, galactosemia), acquired damage from heavy metals, connective tissue disorders, hematologic malignancies (monoclonal gammopathy), and medications (tenofovir, carbonic anhydrase inhibitors).
- Clinical features: Glucosuria, phosphaturia (rickets, osteomalacia), proteinuria, polyuria, dehydration, hypercalciuria, hypokalemia
- Treatment: Treat the underlying cause if possible. Electrolyte and vitamin D supplementation may be required.

Renal Cystic Diseases

Renal cysts
- Classification: Categorized as simple or complex based on imaging appearance
  - Simple cysts (thin walled, fluid filled, no enhancement) are very common with advancing age. Typically benign, but may need intervention if size or location causes pain or impaired renal function.
  - Complex cysts (enhancement, solid components) have a high risk of malignancy; may require partial or total nephrectomy for tissue examination

Autosomal Dominant Polycystic Kidney Disease (ADPKD)
- Etiology: Mutation in PKD1 or PKD2 (chromosome 16), most common hereditary kidney disease in the United States
- Clinical features:
  - Onset of hypertension, hematuria, nephrolithiasis in young adulthood (PKD1) or in middle age (PKD2)
  - Increased risk for extrarenal diagnoses: Circle of Willis berry aneurysm (risk factor for subarachnoid hemorrhage), hepatic cysts, diverticula, abdominal hernias, and consequences of HTN (e.g., CVD)
- Diagnosis: Combination of family history, genetic testing, and ultrasound showing bilateral kidneys with cysts
- Treatment: No curative treatment. Control hypertension, manage pain (from cyst rupture or pressure). The majority of patients will require dialysis or a kidney transplant.

NEPHROLOGY

Renal Vascular Diseases

Renal artery stenosis

- Etiology: Majority of cases are due to atherosclerosis, most others are due to fibromuscular dysplasia (often in young women, 50% bilateral, can be hereditary). Renal artery narrowing and subsequent RAAS activation causes renovascular hypertension.
- Clinical features: Early or medication-refractory hypertension (i.e., uncontrolled HTN on three antihypertensives including a diuretic); abdominal bruits on exam
- Diagnosis: Duplex ultrasound, CTA, or MRA
- Treatment:
  - Treat hypertension with ACE inhibitor/ARB, plus diuretic
  - Consider revascularization with stent or endarterectomy if there is high chance of benefit or high risk of complications (e.g., rapid progression of disease, recurrent flash pulmonary edema, medical therapy not tolerated or ineffective, bilateral disease with declining kidney function)

Hypertensive nephrosclerosis

- Etiology: Sclerosis of the tubulointerstitial, glomerular, and vascular spaces due to genetic predisposition and chronic hypertension
- Clinical features: Presents with two distinct clinical courses defined as benign or malignant:
  - <u>Benign nephrosclerosis</u>: Most often seen in African Americans with high-risk APOL1 genotypes, preceding hypertension, thickening of glomerular afferent arterioles; presents as mild ↑Cr elevation, microscopic hematuria, mild proteinuria
  - <u>Malignant nephrosclerosis</u>: Rapid decrease in renal function with severe hypertension → Markedly elevated BP (papilledema, cardiac decompensation, CNS findings), renal abnormalities (rapid ↑Cr, proteinuria, hematuria, RBC/WBC casts, microangiopathic hemolytic anemia)
- Treatment: Control blood pressure

Renal vein thrombosis

- Etiology: Can result from systemic inflammation or prothrombotic state (e.g., nephrotic syndrome, carcinoma, trauma, pregnancy/OCPs), extrinsic compression, trauma
- Clinical features: Evidence of decreased renal perfusion (rising Cr, decreased urine output, hypertension) and renal injury (hematuria, proteinuria)
- Diagnosis: Duplex ultrasound, CTA, MRA
- Treatment: Consider thrombolysis/thrombectomy or anticoagulation based on clinical severity

Thrombotic microangiopathy (TMA)

- Etiology: Syndrome of microangiopathic hemolytic anemia, low platelets, and organ injury; most often due to TTP and atypical HUS; can also result from HUS, APLS, scleroderma renal crisis, malignant hypertension, pregnancy (HELLP/preeclampsia). Also see Hematology/Oncology Chapter 7.
- Diagnosis: Thrombi and fibrin accumulation in capillaries on glomerular biopsy
- Treatment: Treat underlying cause. Plasma exchange if TTP.

Stones and Obstructions

Nephrolithiasis (kidney stones)

- Types:
  - Calcium stones (80%): Radiodense. Calcium oxalate (90%, envelope shape, malabsorption) or calcium phosphate (10%, hyperparathyroidism, RTA).
  - Uric acid stones (10%): Radiolucent, flat square plates. Hyperuricemia due to gout, tumor lysis syndrome
  - Struvite stones (5–10%): Radiodense; rectangular prisms, staghorn morphology. Recurrent UTIs by protease-producing organism (*Proteus, Klebsiella, Serratia, Enterobacter* convert urea to ammonia, which combines with magnesium or phosphorus to form struvite calculi).
  - Cystine stones (1%): Poorly visualized by x-ray, hexagon-shaped crystals. Screen with urinary cyanide nitroprusside.
- Clinical features: Acute renal colic (sudden onset, can't sit still, cramping abdominal/flank pain in waves), nausea/vomiting, dysuria, +/− fever/chills
- Diagnosis:
  - UA with microscopy (evaluate for microscopic/gross hematuria, crystals)
  - Imaging (confirm diagnosis, stone size/location, assess for hydronephrosis): Noncontrast CT abd/pelvis if nephrolithiasis has not been previously established (superior sensitivity, specificity), ultrasound is useful to avoid radiation in patients who may be pregnant

- Treatment:
  - Acute treatment:
    - IVF, pain control (NSAIDs > morphine), medical expulsive therapy with an alpha blocker
    - Urgent stone removal required if:
      - Stone unlikely to pass: Stone >10 mm, GU anatomical abnormality
      - Infection: UTI, sepsis
      - Severe symptoms: Intractable pain or nausea/vomiting
    - If stone not removed urgently, consider follow-up imaging in 14 days to monitor stone position
- Prevention:
  - Adequate fluid intake (goal >2 L urine output/24 hr)
  - If high risk for stone recurrence (large stone burden, non-calcium stone, abnormal urological anatomy, history of GI disease or bariatric surgery, family history), then refer for metabolic assessment to tailor preventive measures
  - Almost all patients with nephrolithiasis should adhere to a low-sodium diet, which reduces calcium excretion. Other dietary changes may be beneficial based on urine lab abnormalities.
  - Pharmacologic treatments include thiazides for hypercalciuria, allopurinol for hyperuricemia, alkali supplementation for hypocitraturia

Urinary tract obstruction
- Etiology:
  - Lower tract: Neurogenic bladder (e.g., due to diabetes), bladder cancer, BPH, prostate cancer, urethral stricture, blood, stone, trauma
  - Upper tract:
    - Intrinsic: Kidney stones, blood clots, sloughed papillary, tumor, ureteral stricture
    - Extrinsic: Pregnancy, tumor, abdominal aortic aneurysm, retroperitoneal fibrosis, endometriosis, hematomas, IBD, diverticulitis
- Clinical features: Renal colic and pain (especially if acute), oliguria, recurrent UTIs, hematuria/proteinuria, renal failure
- Diagnosis:
  - Renal ultrasound
  - Advanced diagnostics: Intravenous pyelography (IVP) for ureteral obstruction, voiding cystourethrography for lower tract obstruction, cystoscopy for bladder
- Treatment:
  - Lower tract: Foley Catheter, BPH medications (e.g., alpha-blockers; 5-alpha-reductase inhibitor)
  - Upper tract: Ureteral stent via cystoscopy if possible, otherwise percutaneous nephrostomy tube

Fluids, Electrolytes, and Acid/Base Disorders
For each electrolyte, we will discuss the normal regulation and then discuss what happens when levels of the electrolyte are too low or too high.

Sodium
Sodium homeostasis (Na$^+$ 135 to 145 mmol/L)
- Extracellular Na$^+$ concentration reflects water homeostasis: Hyponatremia and hypernatremia are caused by too much/too little water. Total Na$^+$ content reflects Na$^+$ homeostasis
- Sodium is actively pumped out of cells: Na$^+$ is the main cation in the extracellular fluid (ECF); most sodium reabsorption occurs at the proximal tubule
- Sodium homeostasis (RAAS):
  - Decreased ECF volume $\rightarrow$ Decreased renal perfusion $\rightarrow$ $\uparrow$Renin by juxtaglomerular (JGA) cells $\rightarrow$ ACE activates angiotensin II
  - Angiotensin II then increases ADH and aldosterone secretion, which increases net Na$^+$ reabsorption and water is absorbed with the Na$^+$
  - Aldosterone is secreted by the adrenal gland: Na$^+$/H$_2$O reabsorbed, H$^+$/K$^+$ secreted
- Water homeostasis (ADH):
  - Increased plasma osmolarity $\rightarrow$ Osmoregulators in the hypothalamus stimulate thirst and secretion of ADH
  - ADH increases H$_2$O permeability at the principal cells $\rightarrow$ Promotes water absorption (and also stimulates thirst!)

NEPHROLOGY

Hyponatremia (Na$^+$ <135 mEq/L)
- Etiologies: See Figure 6.4. History is key!
  - <u>Acuity</u>: Has the hyponatremia occurred within the last 48 hours (e.g., postoperatively with a normal preoperative baseline)?
  - <u>Volume</u>: Fluid intake, diet, urinary changes, extrarenal losses (e.g., diarrhea or hemorrhage)
  - <u>PMH</u>: Active renal, endocrine, pulmonary or neurologic disease
  - <u>Medications</u>: Especially diuretics and recent medication changes
  - <u>Social history</u>: Use of alcohol, MDMA, other illicit substances
- Clinical features: Signs/symptoms predominantly neurologic: Headache, delirium, hyperactive deep tendon reflexes, seizures, coma
- Diagnosis: See Figure 6.4 and the steps below

Step 1: Is sodium the problem (e.g., is the blood hypotonic)? Check serum osms.
Sodium is the major solute in the blood, so if sodium is low then the serum osms should also be low unless another process is contributing to the serum mOsms. Test = serum osms.
- High serum osms (>295 mOsm/kg):
  - Hypertonic hyponatremia: Low sodium is an appropriate response to the presence of excess osmotic substrate, e.g., glucose, mannitol, maltose/sucrose (IVIG)
  - Correct for hyperglycemia: If glucose >100 mg/dL, for every additional 100 mg/dL, add 1.6 to Na$^+$ (e.g., if glucose 300 mg/dL and Na$^+$ 132 mEq/L then add 1.6(2) = approximately 135 mEq/L corrected)
- Normal serum osms (280–295 mOsm/kg):
  - Pseudohyponatremia (normal amount of Na$^+$ in water; however, there is a higher-than-normal amount of another non-aqueous substance, e.g., paraprotein, lipids, or bilirubin, causing underestimation of the Na$^+$ concentration). May also be due to a mixed hypotonic and hypertonic process
- Low serum osms (<280 mOsm/kg): True hyponatremia. Proceed to step 2.
  - If the measured serum osms are normal but the calculated osms are low, it is because a solute not included in the calculated estimate is present and being measured, e.g., ethanol or toxic alcohol

Step 2: Is the kidney responding appropriately (e.g., is ADH off)? Check urine osms.
ADH causes increased reabsorption of free water at the collecting ducts. In hyponatremia, ADH should be repressed if the kidneys are responding appropriately to get rid of excess free water. Test = urine osms.
- If urine osms <100 mOsm/kg: This indicates that the problem is not in the kidney, and instead it relates to how much water or salt the patient is consuming.
  - Too much water = Primary polydipsia (12 to 20 L/day): Psychosis, ecstasy, marathon running. Will produce copious urine in the absence of extrarenal fluid loss.
  - Too little solute = "Beer potomania"/"tea and toast diet" deficient in solute. In this case, the kidney cannot produce as much dilute urine to remove excess free water as someone with normal solute intake. This will often be a contributor in patients with concomitant hypovolemia.
- If urine osms ≥100 mOsm/kg: Proceed to Step 3
  - Pearl: If intermediate urine osms, or even if low, think about tubular dysfunction due to diuretics, AKI or CKD. In severe renal disease, the kidney can't concentrate urine appropriately, and this may cause hyponatremia. Isosthenuria, or a urine specific gravity similar to serum concentration (1.006 to 1.012), may be an early clue.

Step 3: Is ADH "on" for a hemodynamic reason (e.g., low effective arterial blood volume)? Check volume status and UNa.
- Hypovolemia: Hypovolemia → RAAS activation → ADH "on" and increases renal free H$_2$O absorption. Signs: Orthostatic hypotension, dry mucous membranes, decreased skin turgor.
  - Typically urine Na$^+$ <20 mEq/L if extrarenal losses (e.g., vomiting, diarrhea, third-spacing)
  - Urine Na$^+$ may be higher if patient on diuretics or if tubular dysfunction is present (e.g., ATN advanced CKD)
- Hypervolemic: ADH "on" due to perceived low volume at the JGA (e.g., heart failure, cirrhosis, nephrotic syndrome)
  - Typically urine Na$^+$ <20 mEq/L with heart failure, cirrhosis, nephrotic syndrome, hypoalbuminemia
  - Urine Na$^+$ may be higher in advanced CKD or while taking diuretics

Step 4: Is ADH "on" for a non-hemodynamic reason? Consider euvolemic etiologies of hyponatremia.
- "Inappropriate" causes of ADH activity:
  - Syndrome of inappropriate ADH (SIADH)
    - Diseases: CNS, pulmonary, malignancy (especially SCLC)
    - Medications: SSRIs, antiepileptic drugs, chemotherapy
    - Cortical stimulation: Pain, nausea, psychosis
  - Endocrine: Hypothyroidism, mineralocorticoid deficiency, glucocorticoid deficiency

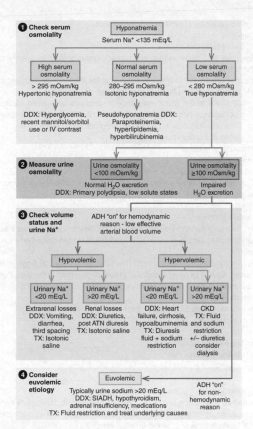

FIGURE 6.4: **Workup of hyponatremia**. This diagram depicts one strategy to work up hyponatremia. See the text for additional details.

- Treatment of hyponatremia:
  - General principles:
    - Don't correct too quickly! Unless acute (confirmed duration <48 hr, usually postoperatively) or presenting with severe symptoms (seizure, coma). Overcorrection can cause central pontine demyelination (see below).
    - Goal for correction is 6–8 mEq/24 hr. Do not correct sodium more than 8 mEq/24 hr if hyponatremia has been present for >48 hours or an unknown duration of time.
    - If Na^+ <120 mEq/L: Consider nephrology consult, check Na^+ q2–4 hours when beginning correction
    - If severe symptoms or Na^+ <115 mEq/L: Nephrology consult, check q1-2 hours when beginning correction
    - Electrolyte-free water clearance (EFWC) can be used to estimate urinary free water excretion (and effective concentrating activity of ADH)
      - EFWC = Urine output × [1 − (Urine Na^+ + Urine K^+ / P)/Plasma Na^+]
      - Gives volume of water free of osmotically active electrolytes "cleared" from plasma. If negative, kidneys are concentrating urine and hypertonic saline will likely be needed. If positive, kidney is correcting and hyponatremia may improve with isotonic fluids or salt tabs
      - Assumes consistent urine concentration (usually true in SIADH, usually <u>not</u> true in hypovolemia or heart failure)
    - Pearl: Giving potassium will increase serum sodium because the potassium is an exchangeable ion and will be transported intracellularly in exchange for sodium, so account for this when calculating fluids for sodium correction to avoid overcorrection

- Treatment of non-acute hyponatremia by volume status:
  - Hypovolemia
    - If mild, trial IV fluids and recheck
    - Monitor urine free water output and recheck serum sodium frequently to avoid sodium overcorrection
    - May need to give DDAVP to slow correction after volume repletion if patient is overcorrecting; hypertonic saline will likely be needed for subsequent correction
    - If hyponatremia is severe (due to magnitude or symptoms) and hemodynamics are stable, volume resuscitation can be done gently with hypertonic saline and DDAVP, especially if SIADH is still on differential diagnosis, but do this in consultation with nephrology
  - Euvolemia (often due to diuretics or SIADH)
    - Address underlying cause
    - Free water restriction
    - Sodium tabs with loop diuretics or oral urea
    - Consider demeclocycline or vasopressin antagonists (tolvaptan and conivaptan) if refractory to conservative measures
  - Hypervolemic
    - Free water restriction
    - Diuresis with loop diuretics may be helpful and is often necessary to treat hypervolemia
    - Vasopressin antagonists may be useful in heart failure but can cause liver injury in patients with cirrhosis
- Complication of hyponatremia correction that is too rapid: Central pontine demyelination
  - Pathophysiology: Caused by osmotic shift due to sodium correction in the brain that has adapted to hypotonic environment over 1–2 days. Usually clinical effects occur days after sodium overcorrection.
  - High-risk populations:
    - Very low sodium <110 mEq/L (in most cases)
    - Concurrent hypokalemia
    - Liver disease
    - Malnourished patients
    - Patients with heavy alcohol use

Hypernatremia (Na$^+$ >145 mEq/L)
- Etiologies:
  - Extra-renal water imbalance μOsm >600 mOsm/kg
    - Inadequate free water intake (e.g., due to altered mental status, inadequate fluid replacement)
    - Increased sodium intake (e.g., IV sodium bicarb, tube feeds, or TPN administration)
    - Extrarenal free water loss (e.g., vomiting, diarrhea)
  - Renal free water loss
    - Diuresis due to medications (usually loop diuretics) or osmotic diuresis (hyperglycemia, azotemia, mannitol)
    - Diabetes insipidus (DI): Inadequate ADH activity, μOsm <600 mOsm/kg.
      - Two causes:
        - Nephrogenic DI: Kidney is ADH-resistant. μOsm <300 mOsm/kg. Does not respond to water deprivation and decreased response to desmopressin. Differential diagnosis: Lithium, hypercalcemia, hypokalemia, tubulointerstitial disease
        - Central DI: Pituitary is not secreting endogenous ADH. Urine remains dilute with water deprivation, responds to desmopressin. Differential diagnosis: Brain trauma, neurosurgery, tumor, CNS infection
      - Diagnosis: Water deprivation test: Patient is deprived of water for 12–16 hours with serum sodium and serum Osm ideally achieving upper limit of normal. Normally ADH should be maximally released and urine osmolality should rise above 600 mOsm/kg. If not increased, DI is present. Desmopressin can be administered to further differentiate between nephrogenic and central DI; >50% increase in urine osms after desmopressin administration is consistent with central DI.
- Symptoms: Neurologic: altered mental status, restlessness, weakness, confusion, seizures, coma

- Diagnosis: Assess volume status, careful review of fluid intake and output, urine osms
- Treatment:
  - Address the underlying cause
  - Replace free water deficit
    - Most easily done with IV D5W. Goal correction rate is no more than 10 mEq/24 hr. Less data about overcorrection than in hyponatremia
    - Free water deficit can be estimated by multiplying total body water (TBW) $\times$ [(serum Na$^+$/ goal Na$^+$) − 1]. TBW: 0.6 $\times$ body weight in kg; varies depending on age, sex, and muscle mass.
    - Accounting for urinary free water loss using electrolyte free water clearance will help prevent under-replacement [EFWC = Urine output $\times$ (1 − (Urine Na$^+$ Urine K$^+$) / Plasma Na$^+$)]
  - Address volume depletion if present
    - Can do this with separate isotonic fluid administration or "mixing" isotonic fluid with free water (e.g., D5 ¼ normal saline is roughly 25% isotonic fluid and 75% electrolyte-free water)

Calcium

Calcium regulation (Ca^{2+} 8.5–10.5 mg/dL)

- Physiology: Most calcium is bound to albumin; free ionized calcium is the physiologic active form under control of PTH
  - Calcium levels are affected by albumin and pH
  - Hypoalbuminemia: Total calcium + [(4 − albumin) $\times$ 0.8]
  - High serum pH: Normal total Ca^{2+} but ionized Ca^{2+} low
- Hormones/molecules regulating calcium:
  - **PTH:** ↓Ca^{2+} or ↓Mg^2→ ↑PTH (from chief cells) → Net ↑Ca^{2+}, ↓PO4^{3-}
    - Bone: PTH → Ca^{2+} and PO4^{3-} release from bones
    - Kidney: PTH → ↑ Ca^{2+} reabsorption (distal tubule) + ↓PO4^3 reabsorption (proximal tubule)
    - Gut: PTH → ↑1,25-dihydroxy vitamin D by stimulating 1-α-hydroxylase in kidney → ↑Gut absorption of Ca^{2+} + PO4^3
  - **Vitamin D:** D$_3$ from sun, D$_2$ ingested → 25-OH vitamin D in the liver → 1,25(OH)$_2$ vitamin D in kidney. ↑PTH, ↓PO4^{3-}, ↓Ca^{2+}→ ↑ Activated vitamin D → Net ↑Ca^{2+}, ↑PO4^{3-}
    - Bone: Activated vitamin D → Bone resorption of both Ca^{2+} and PO4^{3-}
    - Gut: Activated vitamin D → Absorption of both Ca^{2+} and PO4^3
  - **Calcitonin:** Parafollicular cells (C cells) of thyroid (relatively minor effect) ↑Ca^{2+}→ ↑Calcitonin → ↓Bone resorption of Ca^{2+}. Opposes action of PTH ("tones down Ca^{2+}").

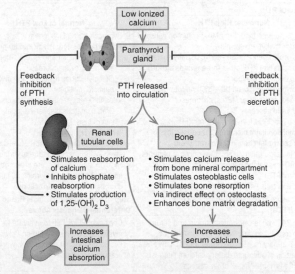

FIGURE 6.5: Calcium homeostasis. The parathyroid gland, renal tubular cells, bones, and intestine all play a role in calcium regulation. Green arrows indicate positive inputs and red bars indicate negative feedback.

Hypercalcemia (Ca^{2+} >10.5 mg/dL after correcting for serum albumin)
- Etiologies: See Table 6.3
- Clinical features: "Stones, bones, groans, psychiatric overtones"
  - Stones: Nephrolithiasis, nephrogenic DI → polyuria
  - Bones: Osteopenia, osteitis fibrosa cystica (occurs in severe hyperparathyroidism only)
  - Groans: Abdominal pain, nausea/vomiting, constipation, pancreatitis
  - Psychiatric overtones: Fatigue, depression, confusion, coma
- Diagnosis: See Table 6.3
- Treatment:
  - Address underlying etiology, withhold offending medications
  - Calcium <12 mg/dL corrected:
    - If patient asymptomatic, often don't need immediate treatment but monitor closely. If symptoms of rising calcium, try fluids first.
    - If etiology due to hyperparathyroidism, parathyroidectomy is curative in most patients. Refer for surgery; if declined/deferred, can offer cinacalcet or bisphosphonates.
  - Calcium >12 mg/dL corrected:
    - Aggressive normal saline repletion (4–6 L/day): Increased urine output = increased renal calcium secretion. Use furosemide cautiously, typically only if evidence of volume overload.
    - Calcitonin: Acts rapidly (hours) but tachyphylaxis in 1–2 days so less effective long term
    - Bisphosphonates: Slower onset of action (~2 days): Inhibits osteoclasts. Caution in renal failure.
    - Consider hemodialysis for rapid calcium correction if Ca^{2+} >18 mg/dL
    - Special use therapies: Phosphate (may increase risk of calciphylaxis), glucocorticoids (certain malignancies, vitamin D excess, sarcoidosis)

TABLE 6.3 · Evaluation of Hypercalcemia

Step 1: Corrections/Considerations	
· Correct for albumin if albumin is low. · High pH can also affect calcium binding (higher pH = higher affinity of albumin for calcium → less free calcium). · In patients with conditions of increased protein binding (e.g., hyperalbuminemia, paraproteinemia), first check ionized calcium (iCa), as serum calcium level may be artificially elevated.	
Step 2: Check PTH	
Normal or High PTH	**Normal or Low PTH**

· Primary hyperparathyroidism: Most common cause of *asymptomatic* hypercalcemia
   - Parathyroid adenoma (80–90%): Usually solitary gland secreting PTH (other three glands atrophy due to negative feedback)
   - Parathyroid hyperplasia (10–15%): All four glands enlarged; sporadic or MEN syndromes
   - Parathyroid cancer (<1%)
 · Familial hypocalciuric hypercalcemia (FHH): Autosomal dominant disorder that causes loss of calcium sensor function in the parathyroid
 · Tertiary hyperparathyroidism: Can occur in patients with ESRD (multigland hyperplasia from chronic stimulus of PTH)
 · Lithium: Can cause altered PTH secretion
	· Hypercalcemia of malignancy:
	   - PTHrp-mediated: PTHrP can be produced by certain malignancies (e.g., lung, head and neck, ovarian, breast)
	   - Osteolytic bone lesions: Bone metastases, multiple myeloma
	 · Vitamin D – dependent hypercalcemia:
	   - Granulomatous diseases (fungal, TB, sarcoidosis, lymphoma)
	   - Vitamin D intoxication
	 · Ingestions of large amount of calcium/milk-alkali syndrome: Often due to antacid use
	 · High bone turnover: Acute prolonged immobilization, hyperthyroidism, thiazide diuretics, vitamin A intoxication

Step 3: Measure Fractional Urinary Calcium Excretion (FECa)	**Step 3: Send Additional Tests Based on the Differential Diagnosis Above**
· Check a 24-hr urine calcium/creatinine and serum calcium/creatinine concurrently to calculate the fractional urinary calcium excretion (FECa). Low FECa in the setting of adequate dietary calcium suggests FHH. FECa is normal for all other causes.	· Consider SPEP/UPEP to evaluate for multiple myeloma, CT Chest/Abdomen/Pelvis to evaluate for occult malignancy, workup for granulomatous diseases, etc.

Hypocalcemia (Ca^{2+} <7.0 mg/dL after correcting for serum albumin)

- Etiologies: See Table 6.4
- Clinical features:
  - Seizures, muscle spasms (tetany)
  - Trousseau's sign (inflate BP cuff → carpal spasm)
  - Chvostek's sign (tap facial nerve → contraction facial muscles)
  - Hypotension
  - Long QT
  - Renal osteodystrophy (from secondary hyperparathyroidism)
- Diagnosis: See Table 6.4
- Treatment:
  - Correct the underlying etiology
  - Replete calcium:
    - If severe/symptomatic or acute: IV calcium gluconate +/− calcitriol; replete Mg^{2+} if needed
    - If mild/asymptomatic: Oral calcium, ensure magnesium and vitamin D repleted if needed
    - Chronic renal failure: Oral calcium, phosphate binder, calcitriol

TABLE 6.4 · Hypocalcemia Workup

Step 1: Corrections/Considerations
· Correct for albumin if albumin is low
· High pH (higher pH = higher affinity of albumin for calcium and less free calcium)
· In patients with conditions of increased protein binding (e.g., hyperalbuminemia, paraproteinemia), first check ionized calcium (iCa), as serum calcium level may be artificially elevated

Step 2: Check PTH	
Normal-High PTH	**Normal or Low PTH**
· Secondary hyperparathyroidism - Chronic renal failure (most common cause). Normal kidneys activate vitamin D to enable calcium absorption and excrete PO_4, so patients with renal disease often have low calcium and high phosphorus. · Vitamin D deficiency: Low dietary intake, malabsorption (e.g., celiac disease), liver disease, lack of sun exposure · Hyperphosphatemia and other extravascular deposition (e.g., bone metastases, pancreatitis)	· Destruction of parathyroid glands (e.g., iatrogenic complication of neck surgery, autoimmune, infiltrative diseases) · Abnormal parathyroid development (e.g., DiGeorge syndrome) · Altered calcium regulation (e.g., Ca^{2+}-signaling receptor mutation) · Hungry bone syndrome (rapid profound hypocalcemia after parathyroidectomy for severe primary hyperPTH) · Hypomagnesemia causes functional, reversible parathyroid hypofunction and must be corrected first

Magnesium

Magnesium homeostasis (Mg^{2+} 1.8–2.5 mg/dL)

- Distribution:
  - 99% intracellular, two-third of that in bones
  - 1% extracellular, 30% bound of that to albumin
- Regulation:
  - Intake: Passive intestinal absorption
  - Storage: Intracellular shift by insulin and glucocorticoids
  - Excretion: Inhibited by ADH, PTH, and hypomagnesemia

Hypomagnesemia (Mg^{2+} <1.8 mg/dL)

- Clinical features:
  - Neurologic: Tremors, hyperreflexia, seizures, altered mental status
  - ECG: Prolonged QT, T-wave flattening, torsade de pointes
  - Often also hypocalcemia (low PTH), hypokalemia (in muscle/myocardium Mg^{2+} and K^+ move together)
- Etiology:
  - Poor intake: Alcohol use, diarrhea, short bowel, fasting, malabsorption
  - Intracellular shift: Insulin, hungry-bone (post-parathyroidectomy), pancreatitis, catecholamine excess
  - Renal wasting: Alcohol, diuretics, calcineurin inhibitors, aminoglycosides, cisplatin, amphotericin B, Gitelman syndrome
- Treatment: Mild: PO magnesium oxide. Severe: IV magnesium sulfate

Hypermagnesemia (Mg^{2+} >2.5 mg/dL)
- Clinical features: Loss of deep tendon reflexes (earliest sign), nausea, weakness, ECG similar to hyperkalemia (increased PR interval, widened QRS, peaked T)
- Etiology:
  - Endogenous: Renal failure, burns/trauma, adrenal insufficiency, rhabdomyolysis
  - Exogenous: Magnesium enemas, excessive PO supplementation, IV magnesium for treatment of other pathology (e.g., preeclampsia)
- Treatment:
  - Stop exogenous magnesium
  - Give IV calcium gluconate for cardioprotection
  - Consider IVF/furosemide, dialysis if anuric

Potassium
Potassium regulation (K^+ 3.5–5.0 mEq/L)
- Distribution:
  - 98% intracellular, maintained by Na^+/K^+ ATPase
- Extracellular K^+ shift:
  - Acidosis (especially without anion gap)
  - Alpha adrenergic stimulation
  - Hypertonicity
  - Intracellular release (rhabdomyolysis, hemolysis, TLS)
- Intracellular K^+ shift:
  - Insulin
  - Alkalosis
  - Beta-2 adrenergic agonists (via Na^+/K^+ ATPase)
- Secretion of K^+: Via ROMK transporter, driven by voltage created from sodium reabsorption in the distal nephron
  - Aldosterone: Increases sodium reabsorption via ENac transporter in the distal nephron, increasing potassium excretion
  - Volume expansion: Increases distal nephron sodium delivery, but is usually compensated by decrease in aldosterone, which negates the effect on serum potassium level
  - Magnesium: Inhibits loss of potassium in the distal nephron in the absence of aldosterone

Hypokalemia (K^+ <3.5 mEq/L)
- Etiology:
  - Intracellular shift:
    - Insulin and beta-2 adrenergic stimulation are most common
    - Other causes include hypothermia, alkalemia, increased blood cell production, barium, chloroquine, cesium, hypokalemic periodic paralysis
  - Extrarenal losses (transtubular potassium gradient [TTKG] <3 or urine K <20 mEq/day):
    - Diarrhea or other fecal loss. Less commonly profuse sweating.
  - Renal losses (TTKG >7 or urine K >20 mEq/day):
    - Excess mineralocorticoid activity: Primary hyperaldosteronism, renin-secreting tumor, renovascular disease, Liddle's syndrome, licorice
    - Increased distal-tubule sodium delivery:
      - Alkalemic: Emesis, nasogastric suction, diuretics, Barter's, Gittleman's
      - Acidemic: Renal tubular acidosis, diabetic ketoacidosis (after treatment with insulin)
    - Hypomagnesemia
    - Amphotericin
- Clinical features:
  - Arrhythmias (prolonged conduction, U waves, flattened T waves; can have normal ECG)
  - Muscular: Weakness, ileus, rhabdomyolysis

- Diagnosis:
  - **Step 1:** Repeat serum K^+ and check Mg^{2+}
  - **Step 2:** Assess volume and acid–base status
  - **Step 3:** Rule out common causes of cellular potassium shift (see potassium regulation section above) by history
  - **Step 4:** Obtain transtubular potassium gradient (TTKG) = [Urine K / Plasma K] × [Plasma Osm / Urine Osm] to help differentiate extrarenal vs. renal losses
    - Pearl: Normal urinary K excretion has significant circadian variation, limiting utility of spot urine K measurement
- Treatment:
  - Potassium repletion
    - Mild: Oral potassium repletion
    - Severe: IV potassium repletion
      - Do not give more than 20 mEq/hr via central line or 10 mEq/hr via peripheral line, as it is very irritating to blood vessels
      - Avoid dextrose-containing solutions which will cause intracellular K^+ shift precipitated by insulin release
    - Rule of thumb: 10 mEq KCl → increase of 0.1 mEq/L serum K^+, replete with half as much potassium in the setting of renal dysfunction
  - Treat underlying cause; stop medications that exacerbate hypokalemia if possible (e.g., diuretics, amphotericin B)
  - Must treat hypomagnesemia as well

Hyperkalemia (K^+ >5.0 mEq/L)
- Etiology:
  - AKI or CKD (usually eGFR <20 mL/min/1.73 m²)
  - Spurious: Hemolysis due to tourniquet, small-bore needles, mechanical trauma
  - Extracellular shift: Tissue injury (hemolysis, tumor lysis, rhabdomyolysis), acidosis (especially non-anion gap metabolic acidosis), alpha adrenergic stimulation, hypertonicity
  - Medications: ACE inhibitors, ARBs, potassium-sparing diuretics, NSAIDs, calcineurin inhibitors, trimethoprim, beta blockers
  - Hyporeninemic hypoaldosteronism: Diabetic nephropathy, interstitial renal disease
  - Tubular disease: SLE, sickle cell, chronic urinary obstruction, amyloidosis, post-transplant
  - Primary adrenal insufficiency
- Clinical features:
  - Paresthesias, fasciculations, weakness, paralysis
  - EKG changes
    - Evolution of EKG changes with increasing hyperkalemia (rate of K^+ change more important than K^+ concentration): Peaked T wave → ST depression → PR prolongation and P wave flattening → QRS widening → "Sine wave" → Vfib or asystole
    - An EKG can be normal minutes before a fatal arrhythmia! A normal EKG should not slow treatment.
- Treatment: **"C BIG K D**rop"
  - **C**alcium gluconate – Stabilizes myocardial membrane (careful if patient on digoxin). Effect lasts for up to 1 hour.
  - **B**eta-agonist (usually 10 mg of nebulized albuterol)
  - **B**icarbonate (increases pH) – Shifts K^+ into cells, quick fix
  - **I**nsulin / **G**lucose – Requires frequent subsequent glucose measurement, especially in patients with impaired renal function (and decreased insulin excretion).
  - **K**ayexalate (sodium polystyrene sulfonate) – Salt which binds potassium in the intestinal lumen, preventing absorption. Usually works over hours to days. Has risk of GI complications in patients with ileus, colitis, or with prolonged administration. If available, patiromer or zirconium cyclosilicate are safer alternatives.
  - **D**iuretic (Loop diuretic, e.g., furosemide) – Causes urinary loss of potassium
  - **D**ialysis – Used in ESRD, severe AKI or emergent cardiotoxicity

Phosphate
Phosphate regulation (PO_4^{3-} 3.0–4.5 mg/dL)
- Distribution: Most phosphorus is in the bones (85%), remainder is in the soft tissues (15%)
- Phosphate absorption: Vitamin D controls phosphate absorption in the GI tract
- Phosphate excretion: PTH inhibits phosphate absorption in the kidney, thus promoting excretion in the urine

Hypophosphatemia (PO^{4-} <3.0 mg/dL)
- Etiology:
  - Decreased intestinal absorption: Alcohol use, vitamin D deficiency, malabsorption, excessive antacid use, TPN
  - Increased renal excretion: Excess PTH, hyperglycemia, ATN, hypokalemia, hypomagnesemia, Fanconi's syndrome
  - Other: Refeeding syndrome, respiratory alkalosis, steroids, DKA, hungry bone syndrome
- Clinical features:
  - Mild: Patients are usually asymptomatic
  - Severe: Can affect many organ systems: Neurologic (confusion, numbness), MSK (weakness, osteomalacia), heme (hemolysis), cardiac (cardiomyopathy, myocardial depression), rhabdomyolysis, anorexia
- Diagnosis: Low serum phosphate. Also check Cr. Consider checking PTH, vitamin D.
- Treatment:
  - Mild: Oral supplementation (milk, Neutra-Phos, K-Phos)
  - Severe: IV sodium phosphate or potassium phosphate

Hyperphosphatemia (PO^{4-} >4.5 mg/dL)
- Etiology:
  - Decreased renal excretion because of renal insufficiency (most common), bisphosphonates, hypoparathyroidism, vitamin D toxicity, tumor calcinosis
  - Increased phosphate supplementation
  - Rhabdomyolysis, cell lysis, acidosis
- Clinical features: Metastatic soft tissue calcification, hypocalcemia
- Diagnosis: High serum phosphate. Also check Cr. Consider checking PTH, vitamin D.
- Treatment:
  - Phosphate binders (bind phosphate in the bowel and prevent absorption)
  - Hemodialysis if the patient is in renal failure or becoming severely hypocalcemic

Acid–Base Disorders

First, a reminder of the normal values:
pH = 7.4 ± 0.05
$PaCO_2$ = 40 ± 5 mmHg
HCO_3^- = 24 mEq/L (typically normal range 22–30 mEq/L)
Normal Anion Gap = Albumin x 2.5 (so typically 8–12 is normal)

Example Case:
pH 7.19, $PaCO_2$ 26, HCO_3^- 9, anion gap 17

Follow these steps:
- Check pH: Acidemia pH <7.4, Alkalemia pH >7.4
  - Example: 7.19 = Acidemia
- Check $PaCO_2$: If the same direction as pH (either both high or both low) then primary metabolic process is present; if they are going in the opposite directions, then primary respiratory process is present
  - Example: $PaCO_2$ = 26, so both pH and $PaCO_2$ are low, indicating a primary metabolic acidosis
- Check compensation: Respiratory compensation occurs in hours, whereas metabolic compensation takes days
  - Example: Since we have a primary metabolic acidosis, use Winter's formula to check compensation. Expected $PaCO_2$ = $1.5(HCO_3^-) + 8 ± 2$ ... so expected $PaCO_2$ = 1.5(9) + 8 = 21... but in this case the actual $PaCO_2$ was 26. If the actual $PaCO_2$ is higher than calculated $PaCO_2$ then the patient has a combined metabolic acidosis + respiratory acidosis.
- What is the anion gap? Anion gap = $Na^+ - (Cl^- + HCO_3^-)$. The expected anion gap = 2.5 × albumin.
  - Example: Our patient has an anion gap of 17, which is elevated, so there is a metabolic anion gap acidosis here

- Check the "gap-gap" (delta anion gap/delta HCO_3^-)? Compare change in anion gap (calculated anion gap − expected anion gap) to the change in HCO_3^- (24 − measured HCO_3^-). Anion gap change/bicarb change should be between 1 and 2 if only an anion-gap metabolic acidosis is present.
  - If anion gap change/bicarb change <1 (bicarb decreased more than expected) → There is also a normal anion gap acidosis lowering the bicarb
  - If anion gap change/bicarb change >2 (bicarb decreased less than expected) → There is also metabolic alkalosis raising the bicarb
  - Example: Here, the delta-delta was: (calculated AG 17 − expected AG of 10) / (24 − HCO_3^- of 9) = 7/15 = 0.45. Therefore, the ratio is <1, indicating a concurrent normal anion gap acidosis.
  - **Thus:** We have a mixed gap/nongap metabolic acidosis and respiratory acidosis (triple acid–base problem)

Respiratory Acidosis

↓pH, ↑$PaCO_2$, (Delayed compensation:↑HCO_3^-)

- Clinical features: Somnolence, confusion, myoclonus, headache, papilledema
- Etiology: Hypoventilation due to acute/chronic lung disease, airway obstruction, opioids or other ingestion causing hypoventilation, respiratory muscle weakness
  - Acute: Minimal to no renal compensation; each 10 mmHg ↑$PaCO_2$ → ↓0.08 pH, ↑1mEq/L HCO_3^-
  - Chronic: Renal compensation (↑HCO_3^- reabsorption); each 10 mmHg ↑$PaCO_2$ → ↓0.03 pH, ↑4 mEq/L HCO_3^-
- Treatment: Treat underlying problem (e.g., COPD/asthma → bronchodilators, opioid-induced → naloxone); support with BiPAP or intubation if severe acidosis and/or respiratory fatigue

Metabolic Acidosis

↓pH, ↓HCO_3^-, (Immediate respiratory compensation = Hyperventilation ↓$PaCO_2$)

- Clinical features: Hyperventilation (Kussmaul's respirations if pH <7.2); decreased cardiac output and tissue perfusion due to decreased response to catecholamines
- Calculate anion gap (AG): **Anion Gap = Na^+ − (Cl^- + HCO_3^-)**
  - Increased anion gap: There are mnemonics like "MUDPILES" or "GOLD MARK," but simpler to consider four buckets:
    • Ketoacidosis (DKA, starvation, alcohol use)
      - Pearl: SGLT2 inhibitors are associated with *euglycemic* ketoacidosis (glucose <200 mg/dL). A normal serum glucose does not rule out ketoacidosis if these medications are being taken!
    • Lactic acidosis (hypoperfusion, bowel ischemia, seizures)
      - L-lactic acidosis = Hypoperfusion and type B causes
      - D-lactic acidosis = Bacterial overgrowth, DKA or propylene glycol infusion. Of note, D lactic acidosis is NOT measured by laboratory lactate measurement.
    • Renal failure (decreased excretion of NH_4^+ and other acids)
    • Intoxication (aspirin, methanol, ethylene glycol)
      - Check osmolar gap (Measured serum osms − calculated serum osms)
      - Calculated serum osms = 2(Na^+) + Gluc/18 + BUN / 2.8 + EtOH / 4.6
      - Pearl: Measure serum ethanol and incorporate into the serum Osm calculation to avoid a false-positive osmolar gap if it is present.
  - Normal anion gap: Check urine anion gap = Urine (Na^+ + K^+ − Cl^-)
    • Renal losses (positive urine anion gap): Proximal/distal tubular acidosis, acetazolamide, spironolactone
    • GI or other extra-renal losses (negative urine anion gap): Saline administration, diarrhea, pancreatic or small bowel fistulas or drains
    • Hypoaldosteronism
- Appropriate respiratory compensation? **Winter's formula: $PaCO_2 = 1.5(HCO_3^-) + 8 \pm 2$**
  - If $PaCO_2$ falls within the excepted range, then the patient just has a metabolic acidosis
  - If the actual (i.e., measured) $PaCO_2$ is higher than the calculated $PaCO_2$ using Winter's formula, then the patient has a metabolic acidosis + respiratory acidosis
  - If the actual (i.e., measured) $PaCO_2$ is lower than the calculated $PaCO_2$ using Winter's formula, then the patient has a metabolic acidosis + respiratory alkalosis
- Treatment: Treat the underlying cause; PO alkali supplementation (sodium bicarb, sodium citrate, potassium citrate) for chronic causes; IV sodium bicarb if pH <7.1

Mixed Acidosis

↓pH, ↑$PaCO_2$, ↓HCO_3^-

NEPHROLOGY

Respiratory Alkalosis

↑pH, ↓$PaCO_2$, (Delayed compensation: ↓HCO_3^-)

- Clinical features: Decreased cerebral blood flow: dizziness, anxiety; tetany (indistinguishable from hypocalcemia), arrhythmias if severe
- Etiology: Hyperventilation due to anxiety, pulmonary embolism, pneumonia, asthma, salicylates (early toxicity), pregnancy (due to progesterone), cirrhosis, sepsis, high altitude
  - Acute: No renal compensation. Each 10 mmHg ↓$PaCO_2$ → ↑0.08 pH, ↓2 mEq/L HCO_3^-
  - Chronic: Renal compensation (less HCO_3^- absorb). Each 10 mmHg ↓$PaCO_2$ → ↑0.03 pH, ↓5 mEq/L HCO_3^-
- Treatment: Correct underlying cause; inhaled mixture containing CO_2 or breathe into a brown paper bag; do not need to correct in pregnancy

Metabolic Alkalosis

↑pH, ↑HCO_3^- (Immediate respiratory compensation = Hypoventilation: ↑$PaCO_2$)

- Clinical features: No characteristic signs/symptoms; history most helpful
- Etiology:
  - Saline-sensitive (urine chloride <15 mEq/L): ECF contraction and hypokalemia; Ddx includes vomiting, loop/thiazide diuretics, NGT suction, and villous adenoma of colon (via diarrhea with high Cl^- content)
  - Saline-resistant (urine chloride >15 mEq/L): ECF expansion and HTN; Ddx includes primary hyperaldosteronism, Cushing's, active diuretic use, stimulant or laxative abuse
- Treatment: Treat underlying cause; normal saline restores ECF volume if volume contracted; spironolactone helps if volume expanded

Mixed Alkalosis

↑pH, ↓$PaCO_2$, ↑HCO_3^-

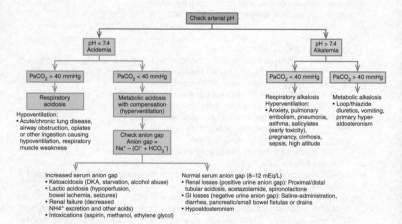

FIGURE 6.6: Approach to acid–base problems. Evaluation of acid-base disturbances begins with an evaluation of pH, followed by an evaluation of $PaCO_2$. Calculation for appropriate compensation can help determine if multiple concurrent acid-base disturbances are present.

KEY MEDICATIONS AND INTERVENTIONS

TABLE 6.5 · Key Medications in Nephrology				
Medication Class	**Examples**	**Mechanism**	**Use**	**Side Effects**
Diuretics				
Thiazide diuretics	• hydrochlorothiazide • chlorthalidone • chlorothiazide • metolazone • indapamide	Inhibits sodium reabsorption via Na^+Cl^- transporter in the distal convoluted tubule	• Treatment of uncomplicated hypertension • Treatment of edema in combination with loop diuretics • Prevention of recurrent nephrolithiasis due to hypercalciuria	• Hyponatremia • Hyperglycemia • Hyperlipidemia • Hyperuricemia • Hypercalcemia • Hypovolemia
Loop diuretics	• furosemide (Lasix) • bumetanide (Bumex) • torsemide • ethacrynic acid	Inhibits sodium reabsorption via Na^+-K^+-$2Cl^-$ transporter in thick ascending loop of Henle	• Treatment of hypertension in persons with decreased renal function • Edema • Heart failure • Hyperkalemia • Hypercalcemia with edema	• Ototoxicity • Hyponatremia • Hypokalemia • Hypomagnesemia
Potassium-sparing diuretics	• amiloride • triamterene	Blocks ENaC sodium channels in the principal cells of the collecting tubule	• Hypokalemia in patients on loop or thiazide diuretics • Polyuria in lithium-induced DI (amiloride)	• Hyperkalemia • Metabolic acidosis • Nephrolithiasis (triamterene)
Mineralo-corticoid receptor antagonists (also called "potassium-sparing")	• spironolactone • eplerenone	Competitively inhibits mineralocorticoid receptor of ENaC sodium channels in the collecting tubule	• Resistant hypertension • Hypertension in primary hyperaldosteronism • Heart failure refractory to optimal treatment • Ascites • Anti-androgen hormonal therapy (spironolactone)	• Hyperkalemia • Metabolic acidosis
Carbonic anhydrase inhibitors	• acetazolamide	Inhibits carbonic anhydrase, leading to excretion of sodium bicarbonate	• Hypervolemia with metabolic alkalosis and alkalemia • Metabolic alkalosis while weaning mechanical ventilation	• Metabolic acidosis
Osmotic diuretic	• mannitol	Promotes osmotic diuresis due to inability to be reabsorbed	• Hyponatremia • Increased ICP	• Hyperosmolality • Hypervolemia and hyponatremia if not filtered due to renal impairment

(Continued)

NEPHROLOGY

TABLE 6.5 · Key Medications in Nephrology (*Continued*)

Medication Class	Examples	Mechanism	Use	Side Effects
Medications used to treat metabolic complication of CKD				
Erythropoiesis-stimulating agents (ESAs)	• epoetin alfa • darbepoetin alfa • methoxy polyethyline glycol-epoetin beta	Directly stimulates red blood cell production and maintenance	• Treatment of anemia due to kidney disease • Rule out iron deficiency anemia before starting ESAs	• Hypertension • Venous access thrombosis • Potentially increased risk of malignancy and thrombosis if supratherapeutic levels are targeted
Phosphate binders	**Calcium based:** • calcium acetate (Phoslo) • calcium carbonate (Tums) **Non-calcium based:** • sevelamer (Renvela) • lanthanum carbonate (Carbrenol) **Iron-based phosphate binders:** • ferric citrate (Auryxia) • sucroferric oxyhydroxide (Velphoro)	Ionically binds phosphate in the gut to prevent dietary absorption	• Treatment of hyperphosphatemia	• Metabolic acidosis (sevelamer) • Hypercalcemia (calcium acetate and calcium citrate)
Vitamin D analogs	• calcitriol (Rocaltrol) • paricalcitol (Zemplar) • doxercalciferol (Hectorol)	Replaces deficient activated 1,25-OH vitamin D	• Treatment of secondary hyperparathyroidism (usually due to CKD)	• Hypercalcemia • Hyperphosphatemia
Alkali supplements	• sodium bicarbonate • sodium citrate (Bicitra- rapidly metabolized to bicarb)	Exogenous supplementation of alkaline compounds or compounds with alkaline metabolites	• Treatment of metabolic acidosis due to CKD	• Bloating (sodium bicarb) • Increased absorption of aluminum
Potassium lowering agents	• patiromer (Veltassa) • sodium zirconium cyclosilicate (Lokelma)	Binds potassium in the GI tract and thus causes more fecal potassium secretion	• Chronic hyperkalemia	• Patiromer: Constipation, low K^+/Mg^{2+}, abdominal pain • Sodium zirconium cyclosilicate: Edema, low potassium

(Continued)

TABLE 6.5 · Key Medications in Nephrology (*Continued*)				
Medication Class	Examples	Mechanism	Use	Side Effects
Calcium-lowering medications				
Hormone	• calcitonin	Inhibits osteoclast activity	• Treatment of acute hypercalcemia (Note: significant tachyphlaxis after 24-48 hours of administration)	• Hypersensitivity • Rhinitis • Hypocalcemia
Bisphosphonates	• zoledronic acid • alendronate • pamidronate	Interferes with osteoclast recruitment and function	• Osteoporosis • Hypercalcemia	• GI irritation • Infusion reaction • AKI (zoledronic acid) • Osteonecrosis of the jaw, especially in patients with multiple myeloma or metastatic bone disease
RANK-L inhibitor	• denosumab	Prevents osteoclast development through RANK-L inhibition	• Hypercalcemia when zoledronic acid is ineffective or contraindicated due to renal impairment • Osteoporosis	• Hypocalcemia
Calcimimetics	• cinacalcet (Sensipar) • etelcalcetide (Parsabiv)	Competitively binds the Ca^{2+} sensing receptor, which inhibits PTH secretion	• Primary hyperparathyroidism • Secondary hyperparathyroidism when vitamin D analogs are contraindicated due to hypercalcemia or hyperphosphatemia	• Hypocalcemia • Increased urinary calcium (risk for nephrolithiasis) • Unlike with parathyroidectomy, bone mineral density is not improved with cinacalcet

NEPHROLOGY

KEY CLINICAL TRIALS AND PUBLICATIONS

Acute Kidney Injury

- **STARRT-AKI.** *N Eng J Med* 2020;383:240–251.
  - Open-labeled, randomized, controlled trial among critically ill patients with AKI who were randomized 1:1 to accelerated versus standard initiation of renal replacement therapy. Accelerated renal replacement strategy did not improve 90-day mortality when compared to a standard strategy.

Renal Artery Stenosis

- **CORAL.** *N Eng J Med* 2014;370(1):13–22.
  - Multicenter, randomized, controlled trial that randomized patients with severe atherosclerotic renal artery stenosis and hypertension or CKD to undergo renal artery stenting with optimal medical therapy vs. optimal medical therapy alone. Among patients with atherosclerotic renal artery stenosis and hypertension or CKD, renal artery stenting did not reduce risk of a composite cardiovascular and renal clinical outcome.

Timing of Dialysis Initiation in CKD

- **IDEAL.** *N Eng J Med* 2010;363(7):609–619.
  - Multicenter randomized controlled trial that randomized adults with progressive CKD and eGFR <15 mL/min/1.73 m^2 to receive early initiation of dialysis vs. late initiation of diagnosis (usual care). Early initiation of dialysis did not improve survival, risk of CV events, or several dialysis-related outcomes when compared to initiation based on symptoms or eGFR <7.

Hemoglobin Targets in Patients with CKD

- **TREAT.** *N Eng J Med* 2009;361(21):2019–2032.
  - Multicenter, double-blinded, randomized, placebo-controlled trial that randomized patients with CKD, DM2, and anemia to receive darbepoetin or placebo. The darbepoetin group received therapy to maintain a Hg >13 g/dL, while the placebo group received rescue darbepoetin if hemoglobin fell below 9 g/dL. Targeting a hemoglobin of >13 g/dL with the use of erythrocyte-stimulating agents did not confer a survival benefit, but was associated with increased risk of stroke.

Hyperkalemia

- **AMETHYST-DN.** *JAMA* 2015;314(2):151–161.
  - Phase 2 multicenter, open-label, dose-ranging, randomized controlled trial among patients with DM2, CKD, and hyperkalemia on RAAS inhibitors. Patients were stratified by baseline serum potassium and randomized to one of three starting doses of patiromer. Among these patients, patiromer starting doses of 4.2–16.8 g BID resulted in statistically significant decreases in serum potassium level after 4 weeks of treatment, lasting through 52 weeks.

SGLT2 Inhibitors in Diabetic Kidney Disease

- **CREDENCE.** *N Eng J Med* 2019;380(24):2295–2306.
  - Prospective, double-blind, randomized controlled trial that randomized patients with DM2, albuminuria, and reduced GFR to the SGLT2 inhibitor canagliflozin or placebo. Canagliflozin 100 mg/day reduced risk of kidney failure and cardiovascular events among these patients.

ACE Inhibitor-ARB Combination

- **VA-NEPHRON D.** *N Eng J Med* 2013;369(20):1892–1903.
  - Multicenter, randomized, double-blind, placebo-controlled trial that randomized patients with diabetes with proteinuria to receive losartan 100 mg PO daily plus either lisinopril 10–40 mg PO daily or placebo. The addition of lisinopril to losartan did not prevent kidney function decline but did increase risk of hyperkalemia and AKI compared to losartan plus placebo. The trial was stopped early due to safety concerns.

Statins in ESRD

- **4D.** *N Eng J Med* 2005;353:238–248.
  - Multicenter, double-blind randomized controlled trial that randomized patients with DM2 and ESRD on maintenance hemodialysis to receive atorvastatin 20 mg PO daily vs. placebo. Atorvastatin did not improve risk of a composite cardiovascular outcome.

NOTES

NOTES

Hematology and Oncology

7

HEMATOLOGY

Hematopoiesis
Hematopoietic stem cells can differentiate into either a myeloid or lymphoid lineage (Figure 7.1)

Myeloid
- Megakaryocytes make thrombocytes (aka platelets): **Critical for clotting. Lack nuclei. Platelet lifespan: 7–10 days.**
- Erythrocytes (aka RBCs): **Carry oxygen. Lack nuclei. RBC lifespan: 120 days.**
- Mast cells: **Involved in allergic response. Numerous purple cytoplasmic granules.**
- Granulocytes:
  - Neutrophils (PMNs): **Critical part of innate immune system. Release cytokines. 3–5 lobes, if fewer lobes then may be immature band form. PMN lifespan: 7 days.**
  - Basophils: **Express IgE receptors. Abundant dark blue cytoplasmic granules.**
  - Eosinophils: **Two lobes with red granules.**
  - Monocytes: **Phagocytic – enter tissue and become macrophages. Large with "horseshoe" nucleus and sky-blue cytoplasm.**

Lymphoid
- Lymphocytes: **Small, round cells with dark blue cytoplasm**
- Natural killer (NK) cells: **Part of the innate immune system. Granulated cells that induce apoptosis when triggered by Toll-like receptors.**
- T cells: **Involved in cell-mediated immunity. Made in the bone marrow, mature in the thymus.**
- B cells: **Involved in humoral (antibody-driven) adaptive immunity. Produce and secrete antibodies that activate the immune system to destroy pathogens. Made in the bone marrow, mature in lymph nodes or the spleen.**

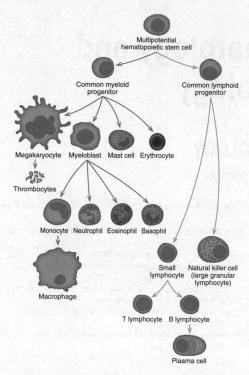

FIGURE 7.1: Normal human hematopoesis. The multipotential hematopoietic stem cell can differentiate into a common myeloid or lymphoid progenitor. Each of these cells can further differentiate into cells in the myeloid or lymphoid lineage, respectively.

The Coagulation Cascade

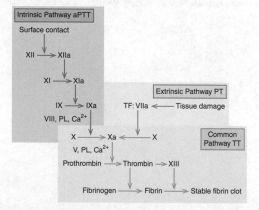

FIGURE 7.2: The coagulation cascade. The intrinsic pathway and extrinsic pathways converge in the common pathway. Abbreviations: Activated partial thromboplastin time (aPTT), prothrombin time (PT), thrombin time (TT), clotting factor in the activated form (a), tissue factor (TF), platelet membrane phospholipid (PL), calcium ions (Ca^{2+}).

DIAGNOSTICS

Evaluation of a Peripheral Blood Smear

Evaluate a peripheral blood smear using a systematic and thorough approach:

- Examine the entire feathered edge first: Large things (e.g., platelet clumps, blasts) can sometimes end up on the feathered edge so look for these first so you don't miss them. See Figure 7.3A.
- Find the monolayer. Start at the very edge of the feathered edge with the microscope on 10x. Move back towards the body of the slide until the cells form a smooth monolayer.
- Evaluate WBCs:
  - Normal and pathologic WBC morphologies are shown in Figure 7.3B
  - Note any morphology changes (toxic changes, reactive lymphocytes) and any abnormal cell populations (e.g., blast cells, which have a large nucleus, immature chromatin, a prominent nucleolus, scant cytoplasm, and few or no cytoplasmic granules)
- Evaluate RBCs:
  - Normal and pathologic RBC morphologies are shown in Figure 7.3C
  - Evaluate the RBC size: Microcyte = small; macrocyte = large
  - Evaluate the hemoglobin distribution:
    - Hypochromasia = light RBCs with more central pallor. Often present with iron deficiency anemia.
    - Polychromasia = darker RBCs. Often present with reticulocytosis/regeneration.
  - Evaluate the RBC shape: Acanthocytes, schistocytes, spherocytes, etc.
  - Evaluate for red cell inclusions:
    - Nuclei: Not typically present in RBCs; presence suggests vigorous bone marrow response or myelophthisic process
    - Basophilic stippling: Blue dots in the RBC; common in lead poisoning
    - Howell-Jolly bodies: Blue inclusions from nuclear remnants common with splenic dysfunction
    - Parasites: E.g., malaria, babesiosis
  - Note red cell distribution: Agglutination, rouleaux formation
- Evaluate platelets:
  - First check the feathered edge for platelet clumps as these will invalidate a low platelet count (i.e., pseudothrombocytopenia)
  - Note the platelet size

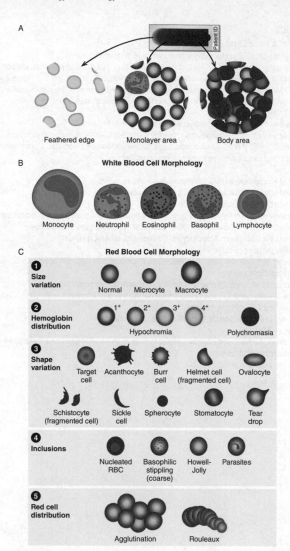

FIGURE 7.3: **Blood smear preparation and features.** A) A blood smear has a thumbprint appearance. The body of the smear is the thickest part where cells are densely packed. The cells become more thinly spread until you reach the monolayer, the area where the red cells form a single layer with little space between them. It is easiest to count and view cells by looking at the monolayer. At the far edge of the smear is the feathered edge, where there are large white spaces between cells and there is a reticulated appearance. B) Normal mature white blood cell morphology. C) Normal and pathologic red blood cell morphology.

APPROACHES & CHIEF COMPLAINTS

See approach to anemia, thrombocytopenia, and bleeding disorders in the Diseases and Pathophysiology Section below.

DISEASES & PATHOPHYSIOLOGY: NON-MALIGNANT HEMATOLOGY

First, some terminology and then we'll dive into each of these conditions separately below:

TABLE 7.1 · Terminology for Abnormal Cell Counts		
Cell type	Too Few Cells	Too Many Cells
WBC	Leukopenia	Leukocytosis
RBC	Anemia	Polycythemia
Platelets	Thrombocytopenia	Thrombocytosis

WBC Disorders

Leukopenia

- Definition: Low WBC ($<$4K/µl). If absolute neutrophil count (ANC) $<$1000/µl, that is called neutropenia and carries an increased risk of infection. Severe neutropenia is when the ANC $<$500/µl.
- Differential diagnosis:
  - Infection: Often causes leukocytosis, but can cause leukopenia
  - Malignancy: Bone marrow infiltration
  - Inflammatory/autoimmune conditions: SLE, others
  - Medications: Chemotherapy, antibiotics, anti-epileptics, and substances (e.g., alcohol) can all be myelosuppressive
- Treatment: Treat underlying condition. Patients with ANC $<$500/µl typically require urgent workup even if asymptomatic.

Leukocytosis

- Definition: High WBC ($>$10K/µl)
- Differential diagnosis:
  - Infection
  - Malignancy: If very high WBC, consider acute leukemia
  - Inflammatory/autoimmune conditions
  - De-margination: Stress response, steroids
- Treatment: Treat underlying condition. Leukocytosis itself does not require treatment except in hyperleukocytosis related to leukemia, for which hydroxyurea and leukapheresis may be indicated.

RBC Disorders

Anemia

- Definition: Low hemoglobin (Hg $<$13 g/dL in men, Hg $<$12 g/dL in women)
- Symptoms: Fatigue, shortness of breath, dizziness, bleeding, pallor
- Work-up:
  - Check reticulocyte count
    - Low retic count (reticulocyte index $<$2) $\rightarrow$ Decreased RBC production
    - Normal/high retic count (reticulocyte index $>$2) $\rightarrow$ RBC loss or increased RBC destruction
  - If underproduction, check MCV and help refine differential diagnosis. Review differential diagnosis for each category below and ask the patient relevant questions.
  - Check peripheral blood smear, which can also help inform the differential diagnosis:
    - RBC morphologies:
      - Spherocytes = autoimmune hemolytic anemia (AIHA), splenomegaly, post-splenectomy, hereditary spherocytosis, hemoglobin C, hemoglobinopathies
      - Schistocytes = disseminated intravascular coagulation (DIC), hemolytic uremic syndrome (HUS), thrombocytopenic purpura (TTP), scleroderma renal crisis, vasculopathies, valvular heart disease, obstetric or hypertensive emergencies
      - Burr cells (echinocytes) = renal disease, artifact
      - Spur cells (acanthocytes) = liver disease
    - Pancytopenia +/– blasts = aplastic anemia, myelodysplastic syndrome (MDS), leukemia
  - Check additional studies based on differential diagnosis (e.g., macrocytic anemia – check folate, B12, TSH, ask about alcohol use, review the patient's medication list, etc.)

Anemia due to decreased RBC production
Normal reticulocyte index (<2%). Think of three buckets: Microcytic, normocytic, macrocytic
1. **Microcytic (MCV <80 fL)**
   - Iron deficiency anemia:
     - Etiologies: Blood loss (e.g., menorrhagia, GI bleed), malabsorption
     - Diagnosis: ↓Fe, ↓Ferritin, ↑TIBC. Smear with hypochromia, anisocytosis (varied size), poikilocytosis (varied shaped)
     - Treatment: PO or IV iron. Every other day PO iron dosing is preferred, take on an empty stomach
   - Sideroblastic anemia:
     - Etiologies: Hereditary (X-linked) or acquired (e.g., lead, alcohol use, vitamin B6 deficiency, isoniazid, chloramphenicol, INH, myelodysplastic syndromes)
     - Diagnosis: ↑Fe, ↓TIBC. Ringed sideroblasts in marrow. Patient may have fatigue, insomnia, hypertension
     - Treatment: Pyridoxine (B6). Stop culprit agent (e.g., lead chelation, stop medication)
   - Anemia of chronic inflammation:
     - Pathophysiology: Inflammatory states (e.g., infection, autoimmune disease, heart failure, liver disease) upregulate hepcidin, which is an acute phase reactant, and leads to the inability to utilize iron despite normal stores
     - Diagnosis: ↓Fe ↑Ferritin ↓TIBC. Can be microcytic or normocytic
     - Treatment: Treat underlying disease
2. **Normocytic (MCV 80–100 fL)**
   - Iron deficiency: Can be normocytic in early stages. See information above.
   - Anemia of chronic inflammation: Can be microcytic or normocytic. See information above.
   - Decreased bone marrow RBC production: Bone marrow suppression can be due to medications, alcohol, toxins, etc. Also hematopoiesis is suppressed in low erythropoietin states (e.g., CKD, endocrine disorders).
   - Aplastic anemia: Idiopathic, radiation, viral, medications. Diagnosis: Pancytopenia, hypoplastic bone marrow.
   - Bone marrow invasion: Malignancy (e.g., MDS, myelofibrosis, multiple myeloma), deposition diseases (e.g., amyloidosis). Diagnosis: Pancytopenia with tear drop shaped RBCs, bone marrow biopsy.
3. **Macrocytic (MCV >100 fL)**
   - Megaloblastic: Hypersegmented neutrophils
     - <u>Folate deficiency</u> (↓folate, ↑homocysteine)
       - The body typically has a 3-month store of folate. Folate is in fruits/veggies and flour is usually supplemented with folate in the United States, so it is uncommon for patients to become folate deficient unless they are experiencing extreme food insecurity.
       - Treatment: Oral folate replacement
     - <u>Vitamin B12 deficiency</u> (↓B12, ↑homocysteine, ↑methylmalonic acid)
       - The body typically has a 3-yr store of vitamin B12. B12 is in meat/fish. It is more common for patients to be B12 deficient than folate deficient, especially if vegan.
       - Differential diagnosis: Low B12 dietary intake, pernicious anemia (autoimmune destruction of parietal cells), decreased gut absorption (gastrectomy, Crohn's, celiac)
       - Treatment: Intramuscular B12 shots monthly vs. oral supplementation daily
   - Non-megaloblastic:
     - Liver disease (more lipoproteins), hypo/hyperthyroidism, alcohol use, medications (e.g., methotrexate, hydroxyurea, antiretrovirals), reticulocytosis, MDS, multiple myeloma

Anemia due to blood loss or increased RBC destruction
Elevated reticulocyte index (>2%); if due to hemolysis: ↑LDH, ↑Indirect bilirubin, ↓Haptoglobin. Think of three buckets: Blood loss, "bad RBC," and "bad world."
1. **Blood Loss:** GI bleed, retroperitoneal bleed
2. **"Bad RBC":** Hemolytic anemia due to intrinsic RBC defects – hemoglobinopathy or enzyme deficiency
   <u>Hemoglobinopathies</u>:
   - Thalassemia:
     - Pathophysiology: Inherited blood disorder characterized by decreased hemoglobin production. There are two main types, alpha and beta thalassemia. Either alpha globin or beta globin genes are missing, causing an abnormal ratio of α–β chains. The unpaired chains precipitate, causing destruction of RBC precursors in the bone marrow and leading to intravascular hemolysis.
       - <u>Alpha thalassemia</u>: There are 4 α-globin genes
         - Clinical features: Clinical phenotype depends on the number of α globin genes that are lost. 1 gene lost = silent (asymptomatic); 2 genes lost = thalassemia trait; 3 genes lost = HbH significant anemia; 4 genes lost = hydrops fetalis (incompatible with live birth)

- Beta thalassemia: There are 2 β-globin genes
  - β-minor: Typically causes mild anemia; no treatment needed
  - β-major: Typically causes severe anemia; often associated with extramedullary hematopoiesis (skull spike, hepatosplenomegaly), risk aplastic crisis
- Diagnosis: Microcytic anemia ($\downarrow\downarrow$MCV 60–75 fL), MCV/RBC<13 (Mentzer index), normal iron studies, target cells on smear. Diagnosis with hemoglobin electrophoresis.
- Treatment: RBC transfusions; hydroxyurea (induces HbF)

- Sickle cell anemia:
  - Pathophysiology: Autosomal recessive genetic disorder; HbS replaces HbA. HbS sickles when low oxygen → hemolysis and microvascular occlusion. Symptoms may start as early as age 6 months when HgF is replaced with HgS.
  - Clinical features:
    - Hemolytic anemia, pigmented gallstones, extramedullary hematopoiesis (hepatosplenomegaly), aplastic crisis with parvo B19 infection, increased risk of infection with encapsulated organisms due to functional asplenia (e.g., *Salmonella* osteomyelitis)
    - Vasoocclusion: Pain crisis, dactylitis (painful swelling of the hands, more common in children), acute chest syndrome, avascular necrosis, priapism, stroke, renal papillary necrosis with painless hematuria
  - Diagnosis: Sickle cells on smear, hemoglobin electrophoresis
  - Treatment:
    - Early vaccination for *H. influenzae, S. pneumoniae, N. meningitidis*
    - Folic acid supplement, hydroxyurea
    - Treat pain adequately
    - If concern for acute chest syndrome or stroke: Consult hematology, consider exchange transfusion

- Hemoglobin C disease:
  - Pathophysiology: Beta-globin chain mutation. Heterozygous = benign carrier state. Homozygous = mild hemolysis and mild to moderate anemia.
  - Diagnosis: ↑MCV. No sickling. Smear: Target cells.

RBC Membrane Defects:

- Hereditary spherocytosis:
  - Pathophysiology: Autosomal dominant mutation in spectrin which disrupts the vertical connections between the RBC membrane and the cytoskeleton
  - Clinical features: Hemolytic anemia, jaundice, splenomegaly, bilirubin gallstones, risk of aplastic crisis
  - Diagnosis: Osmotic fragility test. Smear: Spherocytes.
  - Treatment: Splenectomy
- Hereditary elliptocytosis:
  - Pathophysiology: Disruption of the horizontal connections between the RBC membrane and the cytoskeleton
  - Clinical features: Spectrum of asymptomatic to severe hemolytic anemia
  - Diagnosis: Elliptocytes on smear
  - Treatment: No treatment needed typically
- Paroxysmal nocturnal hemoglobinuria (PNH):
  - Pathophysiology: PIGA mutation (on X chromosome), which encodes an enzyme essential for the synthesis of glycosylphosphatidylinositol (GPI) anchors
  - Clinical features: May present as hemolytic anemia, aplastic anemia, or thrombus (e.g., Budd-Chiari)
  - Diagnosis: Flow cytometry of CD55/59 or FLAER for GPI anchor.
  - Treatment: Bone marrow transplant, eculizumab or ravulizumab (monoclonal antibody that inhibits complement activation), +/– glucocorticoids (limited evidence)
- G6PD deficiency:
  - Pathophysiology: X-linked recessive disorder; common in people of Mediterranean descent. ↓ATP so RBC is susceptible to oxidative stress. Can be triggered by medications (TMP/SMX, dapsone, sulfa), infection, fava beans.
  - Clinical features: 2–4 days after oxidative stress, develop back pain, jaundice, dark urine
  - Diagnosis: Smear with Heinz bodies, bite cells. G6PD levels often normal during hemolytic episode (cells with low G6PD levels already hemolyzed) → repeat labs 3 months after attack.
  - Treatment: Hydrate, stop causative agent
- Pyruvate kinase deficiency:
  - Pathophysiology: Autosomal recessive disorder. ↓ATP → Stiff RBC → Splenic trap.
  - Clinical features: Hemolytic anemia
  - Treatment: Folic acid, splenectomy

3. **"Bad World":** Hemolytic Anemia Due to Factors External to RBC
   - Autoimmune Hemolytic Anemia (AIHA): Auto-antibodies coat RBC surface and lead to hemolysis. Always evaluate for an underlying cause that has resulted in secondary AIHA.
     - Diagnosis: Direct antiglobulin test (DAT, aka a Coombs test) to detect auto-antibodies
     - **IgG = warm.** IgG binds RBC in body (warm) causing extravascular hemolysis.
       - Causes: SLE, CLL, medications
       - Treatment: Prednisone, folic acid, IVIG, splenectomy
     - **IgM = cold.** IgM binds RBCs in extremities (cold) causing intravascular hemolysis. Peripheral sludge: Cyanosis, pain, gangrene.
       - Causes: Mycoplasma pneumonia, mononucleosis, medications
       - Treatment: RBC transfusions if needed, avoid cold, consider rituximab or eculizumab (no steroids or splenectomy)
   - Mechanical:
     - Prosthetic heart valve
     - Microangiopathic hemolytic anemia (MAHA)
       - Terminology: Thrombotic microangiopathy (TMA) describes specific pathological lesions in which abnormalities in the arteriole and capillary vessel walls lead to microvascular thrombosis. Not all MAHA is caused by TMA, but most TMAs cause MAHA.
       - Pathophysiology: Non-immune (Coombs negative) hemolysis resulting from intravascular abnormalities or mechanical shear (i.e., prosthetic heart valve)
       - Diagnosis: Smear with schistocytes, helmet cells, negative DAT
   - Other: Medications, burns, toxins (snake bite, brown recluse spider), infections (*Malaria, Clostridium, Babesia*)

Polycythemia
   - Definition: High hemoglobin (Hbg >16.5 g/dL in men, Hbg >16 g/dL in women)
   - Clinical features: "Ruddy" complexion, hyperviscosity (if severe, can cause chest pain, headache, blurred vision, parasthesias, thrombosis)
   - Diagnosis: Check EPO level to differentiate primary vs. secondary
   - Differential diagnosis:
     - Primary (normal EPO): Polycythemia vera (see myeloproliferative neoplasms)
     - Secondary (↑EPO):
       - Chronic hypoxia (body responds to increase oxygen carrying capacity by producing more RBCs): COPD, OSA, heart failure, carbon monoxide exposure
       - Tumor-associated: Some tumors can produce EPO (e.g., RCC, HCC)
   - Treatment: Treat underlying cause

Platelet Disorders

There are <u>quantitative platelet disorders</u> (the number of platelets is too low or too high) and <u>qualitative platelet disorders</u> (the number of platelets is adequate, but they don't function properly).

Quantitative Platelet Disorders
Thrombocytopenia
   - Definition: Low number of platelets (<150K/µl)
   - Symptoms: Easy bruising or bleeding (e.g., mucosal bleeding such as gingiva or nasal mucosa, heavy menses, petechiae)
   - Work-up:
     - Get a peripheral blood smear:
       - Rule out pseudothrombocytopenia (platelet clumping), which can occur in the blood tube when the anticoagulant EDTA is present, causing a spuriously low platelet count. Evaluate by looking for platelet clumping on the blood smear. Resend platelets in a heparin or sodium citrate tube if needed.
       - Giant platelets can be falsely counted by the automated cell counter as WBCs or RBCs. Large platelets can occur with inherited platelet disorders.
     - Take a thorough history:
       - History of easy bleeding or bruising?
       - Systemic symptoms – fever, headache, abdominal pain, hematuria, diarrhea? These symptoms can occur with HUS or TTP.
       - Medications? In the hospital, consider heparin products, antibiotics, immunosuppressants.
       - History of autoimmune conditions? A history of autoimmune conditions makes ITP more likely.
     - Also check PT, PTT, reticulocyte count, fibrinogen, LDH, TSH, HIV, HCV, and other labs guided by the disease entity suspected

- Etiologies of thrombocytopenia: Consider three buckets:
  - **Decreased production:** Think about processes that cause bone marrow suppression or infiltration. Often multiple cell lines down!
    - Aplastic anemia, MDS, leukemia, Fanconi syndrome, infiltrative disorders
    - Medications/toxins: Alcohol, chemotherapeutic agents, chloramphenicol, benzene, radiation
    - Infections: Parvovirus, EBV, CMV, HCV, HIV
    - Nutritional deficiencies: B12 or folate deficiency
  - **Increased destruction:** Divide causes by immune-mediated or non-immune mediated. Also see additional details about these conditions in the section below.
    - Immune-mediated
      - Primary: ITP
      - Secondary: HIT, other medications (antibiotics, H2 blockers), infections, lupus, APS, lymphoprolifera-tive disease
    - Non-immune-mediated
      - Microangiopathic hemolytic anemia (MAHA): HUS, TTP, DIC, scleroderma renal crisis
      - HELLP
      - Mechanical: CVVH
  - **Sequestration/dilutional**
    - Hepatosplenomegaly: Cirrhosis and portal HTN can sequester 90% of platelets
    - Massive transfusion: 10U pRBCs decrease platelets by 50%

Additional Details about the Platelet Destructive Processes

Immune Thrombocytopenic Purpura (ITP)
- Pathophysiology: Anti-platelet antibodies → Splenic macrophages consume platelet/Ab complex
- Clinical features: Petechiae, purpura, bleeding; NO splenomegaly
- Diagnosis:
  - Isolated thrombocytopenia (platelets <20K/μl but rest of counts normal)
  - Smear typically has large platelets and NO schistocytes! Megakaryocytes are present in the bone marrow.
  - Diagnosis of exclusion: No antibody test. Must rule out other causes first (medication-induced, HIV, HCV, *H. pylori*, etc.). Do not usually have to do a bone marrow biopsy in younger patients, but must consider in older patients.
- Treatment:
  - 1st line: Dexamethasone (40 mg x 4 days) vs. prednisone 1mg/kg/day with slow taper. IVIG 1g/kg ×2 doses may be used with steroids if a rapid platelet count rise is needed.
  - 2nd line: Rituximab, TPO agonists (romiplostim); consider splenectomy if refractory

Hemolytic Uremic Syndrome (HUS)
- Pathophysiology: Endothelial damage caused by medications or Shiga toxin–mediated bloody diarrhea (*Ecoli* O157:H7, Shigella)
- Clinical features:
  - Three classic features: 1) Microangiopathic hemolytic anemia (MAHA); 2) Thrombocytopenia; 3) Renal failure
  - HUS is clinically similar to TTP, but more likely to have renal failure and less likely to have neurologic symptoms
- Diagnosis: Smear with schistocytes. Positive Shiga-toxin/EHEC test confirms STEC-HUS. Complement gene mutation panel evaluates for atypical (complement-mediated) HUS.
- Treatment: Supportive care; consider plasma exchange ("plex") and eculizumab for atypical HUS

Thrombotic Thrombocytopenic Purpura (TTP)
- Pathophysiology: Deficiency in the protease ADAMTS-13 (congenital defect or acquired autoantibody), which usually cleaves vWF. The uncleaved vWF clump and bind to platelets, leading to microvascular occlusion and thrombocytopenia.
- Clinical features: Same as HUS + fever + neurologic symptoms (seizures, altered mental status). Patients with TTP are less likely to have renal dysfunction than those with HUS.
- Diagnosis: Blood smear with schistocytes. Then this is a clinical diagnosis – start treatment right away! PLASMIC score can be helpful, but neither sensitive nor specific. Order ADAMTS-13 but don't wait for the result to initiate treatment.
- Treatment: Immediate plasmapheresis ("plex")! TTP is 90% fatal without therapy. Do NOT give platelets – can precipitate further hemolysis!

Heparin-Induced Thrombocytopenia (HIT)

Type 1 (non-immune mediated)

- Clinical features: Drop in platelets that occurs 1–4 days post-heparin, platelets decreased but still >100K/µl
- Treatment: Can continue heparin; does not change clinical management

Type 2 (immune mediated)

- Clinical features: 5–10 days post-heparin (higher risk with unfractionated heparin than LMWH). Caused by an antibody to platelet factor 4-heparin complex, which causes the platelets to clump/clot. Platelet count falls by >50%. Can cause DVT, PE, stroke, and necrotic skin lesions at the heparin injection site.
- Diagnosis: Calculate "4T score" to help predict risk (see online calculators). If 4T score is ≥4, send HIT assay.
- Treatment: Moderate/high risk: Hold heparin products and start alternative anticoagulation (e.g., argatroban, bivalirudin, fondaparinux) right away – do not wait for HIT assay to return to switch anticoagulants! Do NOT give platelets.

Disseminated Intravascular Coagulation (DIC)

- Definition: Mixed platelet/coagulation disorder. See section below.

Thrombocytosis

- Definition: High number of platelets (platelets >450K/µl)
- Etiologies:
  - Reactive (most cases): Extrinsic to megakaryocyte
    - Differential diagnosis: Iron deficiency, blood loss, post-splenectomy, infection, rebound thrombocytosis, iBD, malignancy
    - Treatment: Treat underlying problem, do not give aspirin
  - Autonomous: Clonal process involving megakaryocyte or precursor
    - Differential diagnosis: Myeloproliferative diseases – polycythemia vera (PV), essential thrombocythemia (ET), CML
    - Treatment: Treat by disease state. If thrombosis, hemorrhage (due to acquired vWD), or symptoms of stasis, consider aspirin, hydroxyurea, thrombocytopheresis/plateletpheresis.

Qualitative Platelet Disorders

- Definition: Normal platelet count but abnormal platelet function (i.e., normal platelet number but bleeding time is elevated)
- Etiologies:
  - Von Willebrand Disease (vWD): Mixed platelet/coagulation disorder
    - Pathophysiology: Defect or absence in vWF, which helps platelets aggregate when functioning appropriately. vWF is also a carrier for factor VIII.
    - Clinical features: Prolonged PTT, mucocutaneous bleeding, heavy menstrual or post-partum bleeding
  - Bernard-Soulier:
    - Pathophysiology: Autosomal recessive disorder. ↓GpIb defect in platelet to vWF adhesion.
    - Clinical features: Blood smear – platelets abnormally large, platelet count mildly low. Clinically, patients have bleeding out of proportion to their platelet number (which is often normal)
  - Glanzmann's thrombasthenia:
    - Pathophysiology: Autosomal recessive disorder. ↓GpIIb/IIIa defect in platelet-to-platelet aggregation.
    - Clinical features: Normal platelet count, no platelet clumping, mucocutaneous bleeding
  - Acquired: Medications (ASA, NSAIDs, antibiotics), uremia (toxins affect vWF/XIII), liver disease, bone marrow disorders, dysproteinemias (multiple myeloma), antiplatelet antibodies, cardiopulmonary bypass (partial degranulation of platelets)
- Treatment: Platelet transfusions, DDAVP

Peripheral Eosinophilia and Hypereosinophilia Syndromes
- Definition
  - <u>Eosinophilia</u>: Absolute eosinophil count >500/µl (500–1500/µl more likely due to atopic disease)
  - <u>Hypereosinophilia</u>: Severe eosinophilia >1500/µl; worry especially if >5000/µl since risk of end organ damage increases (e.g., eosinophilic dermatitis, myocarditis, hepatitis)
- Etiologies:
  - Neoplasms:
    - Monoclonal: Primary hypereosinophilic syndrome (can check for mutations like PDGFRB, PDGFRA, FGFR-1, AEL, and CEL, which cause a monoclonal eosinophil proliferation)
    - Polyclonal: T-cell lymphoma, Hodgkin's lymphoma, some solid organ malignancies cause reactive eosinophilia (e.g., cervical cancer, ovarian cancer, SCC, gastric and colon cancer, urothelial cancer)
  - Allergies, which includes asthma and drug-induced eosinophilia (including DRESS)
  - Adrenal insufficiency
  - Connective tissue diseases: Eosinophilic granulomatosis with polyangiitis (eGPA) and rheumatoid arthritis
  - Parasites
    - Lymphatic filiariasis, toxocara, trichinosis and strongyloides can all cause an eosinophil count >5000/µl. Only multicellular parasites cause eosinophilia.
    - Other infections may also cause lower degrees of eosinophilia (e.g., ABPA, cocci, HIV)
  - Organ-restricted hypereosinophilic conditions (e.g., eosinophilic fasciitis, eosinophilic cellulitis, etc.) can cause peripheral eosinophilia

Coagulation Disorders
- Definition: Elevated prothrombin time (PT) and/or partial thromboplastin time (PTT) with normal platelet count and bleeding time
- Differential diagnosis for coagulation disorders:
  - <u>Prolonged PT, normal PTT</u>: Factor VII deficiency or inhibitor, DIC, liver disease, vitamin K deficiency, warfarin
  - <u>Normal PT, prolonged PTT</u>: Deficiency of factors VIII, IX, or XI, Von Willebrand Disease (vWD, if severe, which can result in low levels of factor VIII), heparin exposure
  - <u>Prolonged PT and PTT</u>: Deficiency of factors V, X, II, or fibrinogen, severe liver disease, DIC, vitamin K deficiency, heparin overdose. If low fibrinogen is causing PT/PTT elevation, correcting fibrinogen should correct the PT/PTT as well.
  - <u>Normal PT and PTT</u>: Platelet dysfunction (acquired or congenital), vWD (if mild and factor VIII level not too low), scurvy, Ehlers-Danlos, hereditary hemorrhagic telangiectasia, deficiency of factor XII
  - Note: Since there is some crosstalk between the PT and PTT pathways, disease states that elevate one of these coagulation markers may elevate the other somewhat as well.

Hemophilia A/B
- Pathophysiology: X-linked recessive disorder (more common in males)
  - Hemophilia A = factor VIII deficiency (more common)
  - Hemophilia B = factor IX deficiency
- Clinical features: Cannot distinguish hemophilia A and B clinically. Common symptoms: 1) Hemarthrosis – bleeding into muscles/joints, 2) Intracranial or retroperitoneal hematoma, 3) Hematuria, hemospermia.
- Diagnosis: ↑PTT, normal PT. Factor activity assays (VIII, IX) are abnormal. Normal bleeding time (unlike vWF). Mixing studies correct PTT (as opposed to disorders due to inhibitors, such as lupus anticoagulant, that do not correct with mixing).
- Treatment:
  - Replace missing factor. Note that over time, patients can form autoantibodies to factor.
  - Hemophilia A <u>only</u>: DDAVP can be used to treat mild disease (leads to a 2–4-fold factor VIII increase)

Vitamin K deficiency
- Pathophysiology: Vitamin K comes from diet (leafy green vegetables) and gut flora. Taking antibiotics can kill gut flora and decrease vitamin K. Can also have malabsorption of vitamin K with IBD or other malabsorptive conditions.
- Clinical features: Increased bleeding; initially ↑PT (factor VII has the shortest half-life) then ↑PTT
- Treatment: Vitamin K replacement (10 mg PO/SQ ×3 days). If severe bleeding: IV vitamin K or FFP.

Coagulopathy of liver disease
- Pathophysiology: Liver failure → 1) ↓Synthesis of clotting factors, 2) Cholestasis = ↓vitamin K absorption, 3) Hypersplenism, portal hypertension → sequestration of platelets → thrombocytopenia
- Clinical features: Abnormal bleeding (e.g., GI bleed), ↑PT ↑PTT
  - To distinguish between liver failure, DIC, and vitamin K/warfarin overdose, check factors V, VII, VIII:
    - DIC = all low
    - Liver failure = normal factor VIII (synthesized by all endothelial cells, not just the liver)
    - Vitamin K/warfarin overdose = normal factor V (not vitamin K-dependent)
- Treatment: FFP, try giving vitamin K in case the patient is vitamin K deficient, platelet transfusions if thrombocytopenic, cryoprecipitate if hypofibrinogenemic

Mixed Platelet/Coagulation Disorders

Disseminated intravascular coagulation (DIC)
- Pathophysiology: Tissue factor release (e.g., gram negative sepsis, obstetric complications, APML, trauma) or other procoagulant (e.g., cancer). Tissue factor activates coagulation and fibrinolysis, causing platelet consumption, and leading to both bleeding and clotting.
- Clinical features: Can have both bleeding AND clotting
  - Bleeding – superficial purpura, GI or intracranial bleed, oozing from incisions
  - Clotting – stroke, DVT/PE
- Diagnosis: ↓fibrinogen (used up from clotting; a normal level rules out DIC), ↑D-dimer, ↓platelets, ↓factor V/VIII, ↑bleeding time, ↑PTT/PT, schistocytes on blood smear
- Treatment: Treat underlying condition; supportive care with FFP, platelets, cryoprecipitate

Von Willebrand's disease (vWD)
- Pathophysiology: Autosomal dominant disorder – vWF deficiency
  - vWF: Involved in platelet aggregation, binds to and stabilizes factor VIII (deficiency leads to ↓VIII levels)
  - Types: 1) Quantitative problem (low vWF levels), 2) Qualitative problem with vWF, 3) Absent vWF
- Clinical features: Family history of bleeding, cutaneous and mucosal bleeding, menorrhagia
- Diagnosis: ↑Bleeding time, ↑PTT (↓VIII), normal platelet count, ↓vWF antigen, ↓vWF activity (ristocetin cofactor assay, measures affinity of vWF binding to GP1b), ↓factor VIII activity in severe disease
- Treatment: DDAVP (desmopressin) releases vWF in endothelium (type I); vWF concentrate; factor VIII concentrate after trauma or for Type 3. Avoid ASA/NSAIDs.

Thrombotic Disorders

Inherited hypercoagulable states
- Factor V Leiden: Autosomal dominant disorder, but heterozygotes have an increased risk of thrombosis (avoid OCPs). Mutated form of Factor V lacks cleavage site for deactivation by Protein C.
- Prothrombin G20201A: Point mutation in the 3' untranslated region of prothrombin so ↑prothrombin → ↑thrombin → ↑thrombus risk
- Protein C/S deficiency: Autosomal dominant disorder. Normally, protein C and S inactivate factor V, VIII. Can cause increased risk of warfarin skin necrosis.
- Anti-thrombin (AT) deficiency: Autosomal dominant disorder. AT normally inactivates thrombin and factors II, VII, IX–XII.
- Antiphospholipid syndrome (APLS): Associated with SLE. Autoantibody against protein bound to phospholipids.
  - Clinical features: Venous and <u>arterial</u> clots, placental thrombosis (pregnancy loss), stroke, ↑PTT (antibodies interfere with the assay)
  - Diagnosis: Sapporo criteria – at least 1 lab abnormality + 1 clinical abnormality
    - Laboratory criteria (must confirm on two or more occasions, >12 weeks apart):
      - Anticardiolipin antibodies (IgG or IgM)
      - Anti-ß2-glycoprotein I antibodies (IgG or IgM)
      - Lupus anticoagulant
    - Clinical features:
      - Vascular thrombosis
      - Pregnancy morbidity
  - Treatment: Lifelong anticoagulation with warfarin (DOACs inferior in APLS), heparin during pregnancy

Secondary hypercoagulable states
- Differential diagnosis: Malignancy, myeloproliferative disorders, oral contraceptive pills (OCPs), immobilization, trauma, nephrotic syndrome, HIT, DIC

DISEASES & PATHOPHYSIOLOGY: MALIGNANT HEMATOLOGY

Oncologic Emergencies

Tumor lysis syndrome (TLS)

- Pathophysiology: When initiating treatment for a malignancy with a large tumor burden or high cell turnover rate, rapid cell lysis can occur, releasing intracellular contents (potassium, phosphorus, and nucleic acids that break down into uric acid) into the systemic circulation. This can lead to kidney injury (uric acid is a renal vasoconstrictor and deposits in the tubules) and electrolyte abnormalities.
- Symptoms: Nausea, vomiting, symptoms of hyperkalemia (arrhythmias), hypocalcemia (seizures), renal failure
- Diagnosis: ↑uric acid, ↑phos, ↑K^+, ↓Ca^{2+} (due to calcium-binding by phosphorus)
- Prophylaxis/treatment:
  - Hydration: Aggressive IVF to maintain urine output 80–100 cc/hr to improve excretion of uric acid and phosphorus
  - Uric Acid: For high risk cases, give rasburicase before treatment, then start allopurinol. For intermediate risk cases, start allopurinol before treatment. Add rasburicase before or during treatment if uric acid ≥ 8 mg/dL (consult heme/onc before starting). Allopurinol decreases the efficacy of rasburicase, so wait to give allopurinol until after rasburicase normalizes the uric acid level if possible.
  - Electrolyte management: Treat hyperkalemia, give phosphate binders. Do not replete calcium unless necessary for symptoms, particularly if phosphate is high as it can worsen renal damage.

Disseminated intravascular coagulation (DIC)

- Diagnosis: ↓fibrinogen, ↑D-dimer, ↓platelets, ↑aPTT/PT, schistocytes on smear
- Treatment: Supportive care, transfuse blood products as needed, treat underlying cause

Hyperviscosity syndrome/leukostasis

- Pathophysiology: Increased viscosity of blood due to increased protein or increased cellularity
  - Hyperproteinemia from monoclonal gammopathies (most common Waldenström; IgM is large and sticky)
  - High WBC from leukemia/lymphoma can cause leukostasis, which has a seven day mortality of 20–40%. The disease type and "stickiness" of the WBCs determine the level at which the WBC count becomes dangerous:
    - AML (>50–100K/µl)
    - ALL (>100–150K/µl)
    - CML (>200–250K/µl)
    - CLL (>400–500K/µl)
- Clinical features: Fever, chest pain, shortness of breath, blurry vision, headache, AMS, priapism
- Diagnosis: WBC, SPEP, light chains, BMP, LFTs, TLS/DIC labs
- Treatment: Aggressive hydration. Call hematology.
  - Hyperproteinemia → Plasmapheresis
  - Hyperleukocytosis → Leukapheresis +/− cytoreduction (hydroxyurea). Avoid RBC and platelet transfusions. Start chemotherapy ASAP.

Neutropenic fever

- Definition: Single oral temperature ≥38.3°C (101°F) or ≥38°C (100.4°F) for ≥1hr + absolute neutrophil count (ANC) <500/µl _or_ predicted nadir <500/µl within 48 hrs based on trend (IDSA Guidelines)
- Source of infection:
  - Most often from gut translocation due to breakdown of GI barrier after receiving chemotherapy. However, a pathogen is isolated in only 20–30% of cases (Freifeld et. al. _Clinical Infectious Diseases_ 2011).
  - Most common pathogens: GNRs, GPCs (line infections and mucositis), fungal (more common if prolonged neutropenia, TPN, or prolonged broad-spectrum antibiotics)
- Diagnosis:
  - Examine mouth to evaluate for mucositis, lines for signs of infection, skin to evaluate for infection, abdominal exam (do not perform a digital rectal exam in neutropenic patients)
  - Labs: CBC with differential, CMP, blood cultures ×2 (1 peripheral, 1 from central line/port if present), UA/UCx, sputum cx, respiratory viral panel/flu/COVID-19 PCR, C.diff testing if diarrhea
  - Imaging: CXR, low threshold for CT C/A/P and/or CT face/sinus if localizing symptoms

- Treatment:
  - Follow institution-specific guidelines if present. Also see Infectious Diseases Chapter 8.
  - <u>Empiric antibiotics</u>: Gram negative coverage (with pseudomonal coverage) +/– gram positive coverage (<u>only if</u> signs of line infection, pneumonia, or severe mucositis) +/– anaerobic coverage (if GI symptoms). Consider fungal coverage if febrile ×96 hours despite appropriate antibacterial coverage.
    - Example regimen: Cefepime +/– Vancomycin +/– Metronidazole
    - Duration: If pathogen identified, treat as appropriate. If no pathogen identified, stop antibiotics 48 hours after last recorded fever AND once ANC >500/µl. If ANC remains <500/µl, continue antibiotics until afebrile ×5–7 days.
  - Site specific considerations:
    - Typhlitis or neutropenic enterocolitis: Infection of the terminal ileum. Mortality rate has been reported as high as 50%. Make patient NPO and add anaerobic coverage to pseudomonal coverage (i.e., cefepime + metronidazole <u>or</u> pip/tazo <u>or</u> meropenem).
    - Sinusitis: Patients with prolonged neutropenia, on prolonged broad-spectrum antibiotics, or on TPN are at risk for aspergillus and mucor, and thus micafungin/caspofungin +/– amphotericin should be considered in consultation with ID to cover for invasive fungal infection

Leukemias

- Malignant hematology overview: Within malignant hematology, there are three broad categories of disease: 1) Leukemias, 2) Lymphomas, and 3) Multiple Myeloma
- Organizational framework for leukemias and disorders of the myeloid lineage: See Table 7.2

Acute Leukemia Basics

- Definition:
  - Leukemia: ≥20% blasts in the bone marrow OR periphery, OR characteristic chromosomal abnormality (e.g., 8:21)
  - Note: You usually cannot tell AML vs. ALL from the smear alone; must get flow and/or cell markers (unless you see Auer rods, which only occur in myeloid cells)
- Pearls:
  - Acute leukemia is an emergency at initial presentation – evaluate for leukostasis, TLS, DIC
  - With aggressive, high-intensity therapy, many patients can be cured
- Epidemiology:
  - AML: Most common adult acute leukemia, average age 65–70 yr
  - ALL: More common in children, although can also occur in adults
- Clinical features: Fevers, headaches, weakness, bleeding, bone pain (expansion of medullary cavity), abdominal pain (splenic enlargement)

TABLE 7.2 · Classifications of Acute and Chronic Leukemias		
	Myeloid Lineage	**Lymphoid Lineage**
Acute leukemia	Acute Myelogenous Leukemia (AML) Median age: 65–70 yr (most common acute leukemia in adults, 80%) Acute Promyelocytic Leukemia (APML) *Subtype of AML, similar age of onset and presentation	Acute Lymphoid Leukemia (ALL) Median age: Bimodal (children <6 yr, adults >60 yr) Most common cancer in children
Chronic leukemia	Chronic Myelogenous Leukemia (CML) Median age: 50 yr	Chronic Lymphoid Leukemia (CLL) Median age: 70 yr (more common M>F) Most common leukemia in adults (in Western countries)
Other subtypes	Myelodysplastic Syndrome (MDS) Myeloproliferative neoplasms	Prolymphocytic Leukemia Large Granular Lymphocyte Leukemia Hairy Cell Leukemia

- Diagnosis:
  - Labs: CBC with differential, CMP, LFTs, Ca^{2+}/Mg^{2+}/Phos, PT, PTT, fibrinogen, uric acid
    - Critical to look for early evidence of DIC and TLS
    - APML in particular is associated with DIC
  - Blood smear: See BLASTS (round blue cells with high nuclear-to-cytoplasmic ratio, open chromatin, visible nucleoli, larger than a RBC)
    - Look for Auer rods (only seen in AML, see Figure 7.4)
  - Peripheral flow cytometry: Can help differentiate AML, ALL, APML, etc.
  - Bone marrow evaluation (aspirate, core biopsy, flow cytometry, cytogenetics, DNA extraction)

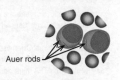

FIGURE 7.4: Auer rods. Auer rods (or Auer bodies) are large, crystalline cytoplasmic inclusion bodies sometimes observed in acute myeloid leukemias.

- Pre-treatment workup:
  - TTE (baseline, because many of the chemotherapy agents can cause cardiotoxicity)
  - HIV, hepatitis serologies, quantiferon gold, CMV IgG
  - Type and screen
  - UA +/– urine pregnancy (if needed)
- Evaluate for oncologic emergencies: Neutropenic fever, TLS, DIC, leukostasis

Acute Leukemia Subtypes

Acute myeloid leukemia (AML)

- Pathophysiology: Malignant transformation of myeloid precursor cells
- Epidemiology:
  - Median age at diagnosis is 65 yr
  - Risk factors: Radiation, toxins (benzenes, alkylating agents), Down syndrome
- Clinical features: Often patients are quite ill at the time of diagnosis. 1) Functional neutropenia (fevers, infection), 2) Thrombocytopenia (bruising), 3) Anemia (weakness), 4) Expansion of medullary cavity (bone pain), 5) Infiltration of skin, soft tissue, CNS
- Diagnosis: Requires more than 20% blasts in bone marrow or periphery, except in cases of certain chromosomal abnormalities
- Treatment: Usually a combination of chemotherapy +/– allogeneic stem cell transplant (Figure 7.5)
  - Chemotherapy = induction with "7+3" (7 days cytarabine, 3 days anthracyclines; Figure 7.5)
    - After 7+3, repeat bone marrow biopsy on day 14. If bone marrow has no blasts, continue to consolidation therapy. If not, repeat induction.
    - Consolidation therapy aims to maintain remission until the patient can receive a stem cell transplant, if eligible
  - Allogenic stem cell transplant: 15–25% treatment-related mortality, but possibility of cure

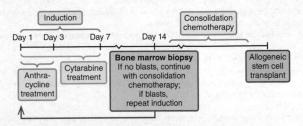

FIGURE 7.5: Induction and consolidation chemotherapy prior to allogeneic stem cell transplant. Shown is an example induction and consolidation chemotherapy plan prior to allogenic stem cell transplant. Induction and consolidation regimens vary based on the type of malignancy. Typically, a bone marrow biopsy is done prior to starting treatment (day 0) and is repeated after induction chemotherapy on day 14. If there is still evidence of residual disease on the day 14 bone marrow biopsy, then repeat induction chemotherapy is considered. Alternatively, if there is no evidence of residual disease, then patients can proceed with consolidation chemotherapy. Allogenic stem cell transplant is performed after consolidation chemotherapy is completed.

HEMATOLOGY AND ONCOLOGY

Acute promyelocytic leukemia (APML; subtype of AML)
- Pathophysiology: Caused by (15;17) chromosome translocation, which disturbs the retinoic acid receptor
- Clinical features: Often associated with severe DIC – must diagnose quickly because DIC can become severe. Smear: Atypical promyelocytes, +Auer rods.
- Treatment: ATRA (high-dose vitamin A) and arsenic.
  - Complications of ATRA:
    - Differentiation syndrome: Differentiation of blasts results in a profound inflammatory response, which causes SIRS, pulmonary edema, and AKI. Give steroid prophylaxis with ATRA; if differentiation syndrome occurs, then treat with high-dose steroids.
    - Hyperleukocytosis: See oncologic emergencies above
    - Pseudotumor cerebri: Hold ATRA; achieve pain control, consider steroids/diuretics

Acute lymphocytic leukemia (ALL)
- Epidemiology: Occurs in both children (2–5 yr) and adults (>60 yr). Outcomes are much better in children.
- Pathogenesis: Arises from mutations in hematopoietic progenitor cells. Some cases are BCR-ABL driven. Cases are uncommonly associated with genetic predispositions or exposure to radiation/chemotherapy.
- Clinical features: Lymphadenopathy, hepatomegaly, splenomegaly, bone pain; anterior mediastinal mass commonly occurs with T-ALL.
- Treatment:
  - Tends to involve "sanctuary sites" like CNS and testicles, so prophylactic intrathecal chemotherapy administered
  - If BCR-ABL present (Philadelphia chromosome-positive or Ph+ ALL), can treat with targeted agents
  - Induction chemotherapy +/– allogeneic stem cell transplant:
    - Common adult regimens: Hyper-CVAD (cyclophosphamide, vincristine, doxorubicin (Adriamycin), dexamethasone)
  - Chimeric antigen receptor (CAR) T cells: See treatment section. Target CD19 for B cell ALL

Chronic Leukemia Subtypes
Chronic myeloid leukemia (CML)
- Epidemiology: Common in older adults (median age 64 yr); risk factor = ionizing radiation
- Pathophysiology: Philadelphia chromosome: 9;22 chromosome translocation results in the fusion of BCR-ABL, which causes an activated tyrosine kinase
- Diagnosis: Elevated WBC, bone marrow biopsy to rule out AML/blast phase; quantitative PCR and FISH for BCR-ABL
- Clinical features:
  - Chronic phase (<15% blasts): Most patients in the United States diagnosed in the chronic phase based on abnormal labs or mild symptoms (fatigue, early satiety due to hepatosplenomegaly). Tyrosine kinase inhibitors (TKIs) work well for this phase. Progression to advanced phase typically occurs after >5 yr of disease.
  - Advanced phases: Accelerated phase (15–30% blasts), Blast crisis (>30% blasts – myeloid or lymphoid). These phases do not respond as well to TKIs; consider allogeneic stem cell transplant. Median survival without transplant is 6 months.
- Treatment: Tyrosine kinase inhibitors (TKIs). First approved was imatinib (Gleevec). Now multiple TKIs approved (i.e., dasatinib, nilotinib, bosutinib). Also consider allogeneic stem cell transplant if accelerated phase or blast crisis.

Chronic lymphocytic leukemia (CLL)
- Pathophysiology: Typically, elderly patients in 70s, M>F. Monoclonal proliferation of B cells (CD5/20+) that are mature but defective.
- Clinical features:
  - Patients often asymptomatic (diagnosed incidentally on CBC) or they may have bulky painless lymphadenopathy, splenomegaly, respiratory or skin infection (from hypogammaglobulinemia – can't make plasma cells)
  - Richter transformation: CLL can transform into diffuse large B cell lymphoma
- Diagnosis: Elevated WBC, but kappa or lambda restricted – demonstrated on flow cytometry. Smear with smudge cells (fragile leukocytes that break on slide). If patients develop pancytopenia = poor prognosis.
- Treatment: Can often observe until progressive symptoms; targeted therapies are used when treatment is indicated (e.g., ibrutinib, venetoclax). Early vaccination is very important as these patients have progressive immunocompromise and most often die from infection.

Other Subtypes/Precursors of Leukemia

Hairy cell leukemia

- Pathophysiology: Rare, indolent B-cell leukemia. Median age of diagnosis 50–55 yr.
- Clinical features: Palpable splenomegaly, cytopenias, fatigue
- Diagnosis: Lymphocytes with fine, hair-like, irregular projections and +tartrate-resistant acid phosphatase (TRAP) stain. Bone marrow may become fibrotic – dry tap.
- Treatment: Cladribine

Myelodysplastic syndrome (MDS)

- Pathophysiology: Age >50 yr. Elderly marrow "fails." Risk factors: Radiation, toxins (benzenes, alkylating agents). On spectrum of AML, but < 20% blasts. Can progress to AML, so requires monitoring.
- Clinical features: May be diagnosed incidentally on CBC or can lead to progressive anemia.
- Diagnosis:
  - Myeloblasts in peripheral blood/marrow <20% *and*
  - Dysplastic bone marrow (Pseudo-Pelger-Huet anomaly [Pince Nez], sideroblasts) *and*
  - Anemia, thrombocytopenia
- Prognosis: Use IPSS-R scoring system (Greenberg et. al. *Blood* 2012). Based on blood counts, blast percentage, and cytogenetics. Correlates with survival and risk of AML progression, which can help in treatment selection.
- Treatment: Usually can monitor unless patients develop symptomatic anemia or thrombocytopenia (i.e., recurrent bleeding), or recurrent infections in the setting of ANC <500/μl
  - <u>Supportive care</u>: Vitamin B6, B12, folate given high cell turnover. Transfuse pRBCs and platelets as needed.
  - <u>Low-intensity therapy</u>: Hematopoietic growth factor (erythropoietin), hypomethylating agents (azacitidine or decitabine), lenalidomide if patients have an isolated deletion of chromosome 5 [del(5q)]
  - <u>High intensity therapy</u>: Intensive combination chemotherapy + allogeneic stem cell transplant

Myeloproliferative Neoplasms

Clonal expansion of one or more myeloid lineage(s).

Polycythemia vera (PV)

- Pathophysiology: Median age of onset 60–65 yr. Abnormal hematopoietic stem cell (HSC) – constitutively active JAK2 receptor, cells proliferate without EPO stimulation:↑RBC, ↓EPO.
- Clinical features: **4 Hs**:
  - **H**yperviscosity of blood: "Ruddy complexion," headache, dizziness, blurry vision, thrombosis, DVT/PE, CVA, MI, hepatic or portal vein thrombosis
  - **H**ypervolemia and hypertension
  - **H**istamine: Pruritus particularly after bathing, peptic ulcers
  - **H**yperuricemia: ↑cell turnover, hepatosplenomegaly, gout
- Diagnosis: JAK2 mutation panel, consider bone marrow biopsy
  - PV: ↑RBCs (Hct >50%, Hgb >16.5 g/dL in males and >16 g/dL in females), ↓EPO. Also may have ↑WBC, ↑platelets, ↑B12. Almost 100% of patients have a JAK2 mutation.
  - Rule out secondary polycythemia: ↑RBCs ↑EPO (see section on polycythemia)
- Treatment: Repeated phlebotomy to lower Hct <45%, hydroxyurea, ASA, consider allopurinol if hyperuricemia; 2nd line ruxolitinib if patient has JAK2 mutation and is refractory to hydroxyurea. Must monitor for transformation to MDS/AML.

Essential thrombocythemia (ET)

- Pathophysiology: Overproduction of platelets by the megakaryocytes in the bone marrow. JAK2 mutation present in 40–50% of cases.
- Clinical features: Increased bleeding (from acquired vWF disorder) or thrombosis (CVA)
- Diagnosis: ↑Platelets (>450K/μl), leukocytosis may also be present. Rule out reactive thrombocytosis secondary to infection, inflammation, etc. Must not meet criteria for another myeloproliferative disorder (e.g., PV).
- Treatment: High risk patients (age >60 yr, >1 million plt/μl, history of thrombosis): Hydroxyurea and low-dose aspirin

Primary myelofibrosis

- Pathophysiology: Megakaryocytes make excess PDGF which causes bone marrow fibrosis. 50% of patients have a JAK2 mutation.
- Clinical features: Extramedullary hematopoiesis → splenomegaly (abdominal pain, early satiety), B symptoms. Risk of infection, thrombosis, bleeding.
- Diagnosis: ↓RBCs, +tear-drop–shaped erythrocytes. Bone marrow biopsy with reticulin or collagen fibrosis.
- Treatment: Hydroxyurea and ruxolitinib (JAK2 inhibitor). Allogeneic stem cell transplant indicated for patients <60 yr. Avoid splenectomy.

Lymphomas

- Organizational framework for lymphomas: See Table 7.3. Lymphoma may be Hodgkin's or Non-Hodgkin's. Follicular lymphoma is the prototypical indolent Non-Hodgkin's lymphoma subtype and diffuse large B-cell lymphoma (DLBCL) is the prototypical aggressive Non-Hodgkin's lymphoma subtype.

Hodgkin Lymphoma (HL)

- Epidemiology: Bimodal age of onset: 15–30 yr or >50 yr. Risk factors: HIV, EBV, immunosuppression.
- Clinical features: Asymptomatic lymphadenopathy or mediastinal mass, B-symptoms in ~40% of cases (fever, night sweats, weight loss)
- Diagnosis: Excisional lymph node biopsy. On pathology, typically see Reed-Sternberg cells
- Treatment: Common regimens:
  - Stage I–II: ABVD (doxorubicin (Adriamycin), bleomycin, vinblastine, dacarbazine) +/– radiation therapy
  - Stage II–V: ABVD + BEACOPP (bleomycin, etoposide, doxorubicin (Adriamycin), cyclophosphamide, Oncovin (vincristine), procarbazine, prednisone)
  - Refractory/relapsed: Chemotherapy + auto-SCT + brentuximab (Anti-CD30) for maintenance
- Long-term complications: Secondary malignancies, cardiac disease if radiation to the mediastinum
- Diagnosis:
  - Biopsy: Ideally get an excisional biopsy, but if not, then a core biopsy can suffice. FNA is rarely sufficient. A larger amount of tissue allows the hematopathologist to identify whether a lymphoma has retained nodal architecture (e.g., follicular lymphoma) or has a diffuse architecture (DLBCL, mantle cell lymphoma, small lymphocytic lymphoma, etc.).
  - Immunohistochemistry: Stains for specific surface markers to help identify the cell origin
  - FISH or PCR for chromosomal rearrangements may suggest specific types of lymphoma:
    - t(11;14) specific for mantle cell lymphoma
    - t(14;18) can be seen in both follicular lymphoma and DLBCL
    - Dual t(8;14) and t(14;18) rearrangement involving MYC and BCL2 in a high-grade lymphoma = chemotherapy-resistant phenotype, or "double hit" requiring more aggressive therapy
- Staging:
  - Both the histologic lymphoma subtype and the stage are crucial to determine the correct treatment
  - CT chest/abd/pelvis, PET/CT for most. Consider bone marrow biopsy, but not always needed.
  - LP should be performed for all patients with Burkitt lymphoma and considered for high-grade lymphomas to determine the need for CNS prophylaxis
    - Use the CNS International Prognostic Index (CNS-IPI) to determine need for LP (if score 3+): 1) Age >60 yr; 2) Elevated LDH; 3) ECOG >1; 4) Stage III/IV disease; 5) Extranodal involvement
  - At diagnosis also obtain: TTE (pre-treatment with anthracyclines), PFTs (if plan for bleomycin), CBC with differential, CMP, HIV, hepatitis serologies, quant iferon gold/PPD, LDH, uric acid
- Treatment:
  - Initial diagnostic and staging for NHL and HL are similar. However, they have distinct historical and clinical approaches, so are treated differently.
  - ABVD – doxorubicin (Adriamycin), bleomycin, vinblastine, dacarbazine

TABLE 7.3 · Classification of Lymphomas		
Hodgkin Lymphoma (HL)	**Non-Hodgkin Lymphoma (NHL)**	
Hodgkin Lymphoma	Indolent subtypes: • Follicular Lymphoma (FL) • Marginal zone lymphoma • Lymphoplasmacytic Lymphoma (LPL, includes Waldenström macroglobulinemia) • Small Lymphocytic Lymphoma (SLL) • Mycosis fungoides	Aggressive subtypes: • Diffuse Large B-cell Lymphoma (DLBCL) • Primary Mediastinal B-Cell Lymphoma • Mantle Cell Lymphoma • Lymphoblastic Lymphoma • Burkitt Lymphoma • Primary CNS Lymphoma • Lymphomas-Associated with Immunodeficiency • T- and NK-Cell Lymphomas

Non-Hodgkin's Lymphoma (NHL)
- Risk factors: HIV, immunosuppression, EBV/HTLV-1 infection, *H. pylori* (MALT lymphoma), autoimmune conditions
- Clinical features: Bulky lymphadenopathy (painless, firm, mobile), hepatosplenomegaly; B symptoms less common than with Hodgkin's lymphoma, hepatosplenomegaly
- NHL Subtypes:
  - See Table 7.3 – generally divided into indolent and aggressive subtypes
    - Follicular lymphoma is the most common indolent NHL (see details below)
    - Diffuse large B cell lymphoma (DLBCL) is the most common aggressive NHL (see details below)

Follicular lymphoma (FL)
- Epidemiology: Most common indolent NHL
- Clinical features: Typically, indolent course. However, it is incurable and can relapse despite prolonged remission. Life expectancy 12–15 yr from time of diagnosis.
- Treatment:
  - <u>For asymptomatic FL</u>: Typically, observe if low tumor burden, particularly in elderly patients. Watchful waiting vs. up-front treatment with rituximab does not affect overall survival. However, in some patients initial treatment with rituximab may improve quality of life and postpone cytotoxic chemotherapy.
  - <u>For symptomatic FL</u>: Consider treatment with anti-CD20 therapy (rituximab) if more lymph node involvement, splenomegaly, pleural effusions, systemic symptoms, large tumor causing organ dysfunction, etc. If severe disease, can consider cytotoxic chemotherapy with R-CHOP.
  - <u>Relapsed disease</u>: Restage, many treatment approaches
- Transformation: It is possible for FL to transform to a more aggressive lymphoma
  - All low-grade lymphomas can transform, but most literature focuses on FL. Risk of transformation to aggressive lymphoma (typically DLBCL) is 1–2% per year, with a lifetime risk of 30%.

Diffuse large B-cell lymphoma (DLBCL)
- Epidemiology: Most common aggressive NHL
- Clinical features: Lymphadenopathy; up to 40% present with disease in extranodal locations, most commonly in the GI tract, but also can involve the CNS, lungs, GU tract, and reproductive tract
- Morphology: Diffuse effacement of the normal lymph node architecture by intermediate to large-sized cells. Significant genetic heterogeneity.
- Treatment: R-CHOP or R-EPOCH chemotherapy
  - R-CHOP: Rituximab, cyclophosphamide, doxorubicin hydrochloride, vincristine (Oncovin), prednisone
  - R-EPOCH: Rituximab, etoposide, prednisone, vincristine (Oncovin), cyclophosphamide, doxorubicin hydrochloride
  - CNS prophylaxis is needed for patients with DLBCL who have high-risk features and for all patients with Burkitt's, lymphoblastic lymphoma, or HIV-associated aggressive lymphomas

HEMATOLOGY AND ONCOLOGY

Plasma Cell Disorders

A framework for plasma cell disorders:

- Spectrum of disease: See Figure 7.6
  - Monoclonal gammopathy of uncertain significance (MGUS) (asymptomatic)
  - Smoldering multiple myeloma (asymptomatic): <3g/dL M-spike or 10% plasma cells on bone marrow biopsy
  - Active multiple myeloma
  - Plasma cell leukemia
  - Amyloidosis: Some clones make light chains that are amyloidogenic – can occur with any of the four above

Monoclonal gammopathy of undetermined significance (MGUS)

- Pathophysiology: Asymptomatic pre-malignant plasma cell proliferation that typically occurs in elderly patients. See increase in serum protein with M-spike on SPEP, but no other associated symptoms. Fewer than 20% of patients with MGUS develop multiple myeloma (MM), but almost all patients with MM have preceding MGUS.
- Diagnostic criteria:
  - Serum monoclonal Ig protein (M-spike) <3 g
  - Bone marrow clonal plasma cells <10%
  - No end organ damage (i.e., no CRAB criteria)
- Work-up:
  - CBC, CMP, Mg^{2+}, phosphorus, LDH, total immunoglobulins (IgA, IgG, IgM)

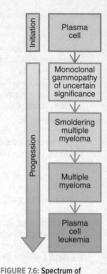

  - Serum protein electrophoresis (SPEP) – *quantifies* a monoclonal abnormal protein (M-spike)
  - Immunofixation (IFE) – *classifies* the abnormal protein
  - Serum free light chain (sFLC) – Detects LOW levels of free light chains in serum, so it can pick up lighter proteins. Note: In CKD, increased K:L ratio up to 3 can be normal due to ↓clearance of FLC
  - UA, urine spot protein/Cr.
  - 24hr UPEP – *quantifies* urine M protein, UIFE – *classifies* abnormal protein, urine free light chains (Bence Jones protein)
  - Beta-2-microglobulin: Strong prognostic value but non-specific
  - Skeletal survey (long bones, skull) to rule out lytic lesions suggesting multiple myeloma. Alternatively, can consider low dose whole body CT scan or MRIs.
- Treatment: None needed, observation. Monitoring depends on risk factors (Ig type, M-spike, light chains).

Multiple myeloma (MM)

- Pathophysiology: Malignant proliferation of a single plasma cell line that makes a monoclonal immunoglobulin – most often large amounts <u>IgG or IgA</u>
- Clinical features: Often patients in 60s with fractures or bone pain
  - Diagnostic criteria = **SLiM-CRAB**
    - **S**ixty percent plasma cells on bone marrow biopsy
    - Serum Free **Li**ght chain ratio >100
    - **M**RI with >1 focal lesion (plasmacytoma)
    - Hyper**C**alcemia (>10.5 mg/dL)
    - **R**enal insufficiency (immunoglobulins precipitate in renal tubules → Bence Jones protein, Cr >2mg/dL without an alternative diagnosis)
    - **A**nemia (Hgb<10 g/dL without an alternative diagnosis)
    - **B**ony disease ("punched out" lytic bone lesions or osteoporosis). Bone pain most common presenting symptom.
  - Other clinical features:
    - Amyloidosis: Kappa chain accumulation → carpal tunnel syndrome
    - Infection: Lack of immunoglobulin diversity can lead to increased risk of infection

TABLE 7.4 · R-ISS Staging for Multiple Myeloma: Criteria and Prognosis

R-ISS Stage	Diagnostic Criteria	5-Year Overall Survival	5-Year Progression-Free Survival
I	B2M<3.5 mg/L and serum albumin ≥3.5 g/dL, normal LDH, standard risk chromosomal abnormalities	82%	55%
II	Not stage I or III	62%	36%
III	B2M ≥5.5 mg/L + LDH above normal limits and/or detection of high risk chromosomal abnormal —del(17p), t(4;14), or t(14;16)	43%	29%

Abbreviations: Revised International Prognostic Scoring (R-ISS); beta-2 microglobulin (B2M); lactase dehydrogenase (LDH)
Source: Scoring system from Greenberg et. al. Blood 2012.

- Diagnosis: Need labs (SPEP, SFLC), imaging (usually PET/CT), and bone marrow biopsy
  - Serum monoclonal protein present (M-spike >3g)
  - Bone marrow clonal plasma cells >10%
  - End organ damage present (i.e., SLiM-CRAB)
  - Other common findings:↑ESR, ↑serum protein. Smear: RBC = Rouleaux ("stacks of RBCs" – RBCs stick together due to increased plasma proteins)
- Staging: Revised-International Staging System (R-ISS): Uses Beta-2-microglobulin, albumin, LDH, and chromosomal abnormalities to predict overall and progression-free survival at 5 yr. See Table 7.4.
- Treatment: Typically, chemotherapy followed by autologous stem cell transplant
  - Classes of therapy:
    - Proteasome inhibitors: Bortezomib, carfilzomib
    - Immunomodulatory agents: Lenalidomide
    - Monoclonal Antibody: Daratumumab (anti-CD38 targeting MM cells)
  - Common regimens:
    - Hyper CD (cyclophosphamide + dexamethasone) – commonly used for rapid reduction in patients with a high disease burden
    - RVD: lenalidomide (Revlimid), bortezomib (Velcade), dexamethasone
    - KRD: carfilzomid (Kyprolis), lenalidomide (Revlimid), dexamethasone
    - Daratumumab, lenalidomide, dexamethasone

Waldenström macroglobulinemia
- Pathophysiology: Malignant clonal proliferation of IgM producing plasmacytoid lymphocytes
- Clinical features: Similar to MM, but IgM protein is larger and "stickier," so it causes more symptoms of hyperviscosity syndrome (up to 30% of patients). Cold cryoglobulinemia in 10% of patients.
- Treatment: Plasmapheresis may be needed to emergently manage hyperviscosity. Treatment usually includes rituximab.

AL amyloidosis
- Pathophysiology: Immunoglobulin light chain amyloid from malignant clonal proliferation of plasma cells (e.g., MM, Waldenström). The proteins deposit in tissues and cause end organ damage.
- Clinical features: Nephrotic syndrome, restrictive cardiomyopathy, neuropathy
- Diagnosis: Biopsy (often fat pad biopsy) to look for deposition of amyloid protein. SPEP will show an M-spike and serum free light chains will show an abnormal sFLC ratio.
- Treatment: Treat underlying plasma cell disorder. Consider autologous stem cell transplant.

Other Malignant Hematologic Conditions
Hemophagocytic lymphohistiocytosis (HLH)
- Pathophysiology: Excess immune activation, inflammation, and tissue destruction that can be life threatening. Can be idiopathic or provoked by a viral trigger or malignancy.
- Clinical features: Fever, splenomegaly, cytopenias, mental status changes
- Diagnosis: 5 of the 8 criteria: Fever ≥38.5°C, splenomegaly, bicytopenia, ↑triglycerides or ↓fibrinogen, hemophagocytosis seen on pathology review, ↓natural killer cell activity, ferritin >500 ng/mL, ↑soluble IL-2 receptor.
- Treatment: Treat underlying cause. Give steroids. If acutely ill or decompensating, consider HLH-specific therapy based on the HLH-94 regimen (etoposide, dexamethasone, +/− intrathecal therapy)

KEY MEDICATIONS & INTERVENTIONS

Transfusion Medicine

Standard testing

- ABO typing: Determine A/B antigens present on RBCs (blood type A, B, AB, or O)
- Rh(D) typing: Tests for D antigen on RBCs (e.g., A+ vs. A−)
- Type and screen: Tests for unexpected antibodies in patient plasma that might react with transfused product and cause hemolysis. Must be done q72 hrs.
- Type and cross: Final confirmation test that is performed by mixing the patient's plasma and the donor's RBCs. Performed when transfusion is imminent/very likely.

Antibody testing

- Direct antiglobulin test (DAT or Coombs): Tests for auto-antibodies on the patient's RBCs
  - Mix patient's RBCs + Coomb's reagent (anti-IgG, anti-C3)
- Indirect Coombs: Tests for antibodies in the patient's plasma
  - Mix patient's plasma + donor RBCs and Coomb's reagent

Apheresis (separation of blood)

- Plasmapheresis: Removes high molecular weight proteins from plasma (i.e., antibodies). Used in TTP, hyperviscosity syndrome, cryoglobulinemia, myasthenia gravis, Guillain-Barré syndrome, anti-GBM, some ANCA vasculidities.
- Cytapheresis: Removes cellular components (i.e., leukapheresis: removes WBCs in acute leukemia)

Complications of transfusion

- Hypocalcemia: Citrate used to preserve pRBCs chelates calcium
- Volume overload: Blood products stay mostly intravascular, so 250 cc of pRBCs (1 unit) is equivalent to 1000 cc normal saline. Rapid increase in intravascular volume can lead to circulatory overload and increased hydrostatic pressure, which can worsen active bleeding.

Special preparations of blood

- Leukoreduced: WBCs filtered out
  - Decreased risk of febrile reaction in patients with prior febrile non-hemolytic transfusion reactions
  - Decreased risk of HLA/RBC alloimmunization in patients who are chronically transfused (i.e., patients with hematologic malignancies, transplant candidates)
- CMV reduced-risk: Requires CMV-negative donor or leukocyte reduction to remove mononuclear cells; prevents CMV transmission in CMV-negative recipients of bone/organ transplant, pregnant women, HIV+ patients
- Irradiated: Prevents donor T-cells from attacking host marrow
  - Used to prevent TA-GVHD in 1st degree–related donors for heme malignancy, bone marrow transplant (not solid tumor transplant or HIV+)
- Washed: Removes anti-IgA antibodies and plasma proteins
  - Prevents anaphylaxis in severe IgA deficiency

Types of blood products

- Packed red blood cells (pRBCs): 1 unit = 250cc, expect to increase Hgb by 1 g/dL
  - Transfusion time: 60–240 min
  - Transfusion goal: Depends on patient-specific factors
    - Goal: Hgb >7 g/dL in most patients
    - Goal: Hgb >8 g/dL in stable CAD and ACS
- Platelets: 1 pheresis (6-pk) = 300 cc, expect to increase platelet by 30K/μl
  - Transfusion time: 30–60 min
  - Pooled platelets = platelets removed from whole blood donation from many donors
  - Apheresis = platelets from a single donor
  - Transfusion goal: Depends on patient-specific factors
    - Goal: Plt >10K/μl prophylaxis against spontaneous bleeding in most patients
    - Goal: Plt >50K/μl if major bleed
- Fresh frozen plasma (FFP): 1U = 250 cc, contains all coagulation factors
  - Transfusion time: 30–60 min
  - Half-life <7 hrs
  - INR of FFP is ~1.6 (cannot decrease INR less than this with FFP transfusion)

- Cryoprecipitate: 10U = 150 cc, contains fibrinogen, fibronectin, factor XIII, VIII, vWF
  - Transfusion time: 30–60 min
  - Indications: Bleeding, low fibrinogen (e.g., DIC, massive transfusion)
  - Fibrinogen replacement: 0.2 bag/kg provides 100 mg/dL fibrinogen
    - If fibrinogen 50–100 mg/dL, give 10 U
    - If fibrinogen 0–50 mg/dL, give 20 U
  - Half-life 3–5 days
- Coagulation factors:
  - Plasma derived or recombinant factors VIII and IX (used in hemophilia)
  - Recombinant factor VIIa (Novo-seven)
  - Prothrombin Complex Concentrate (PCC, KCentra): 4-factor (contains factor II, VII, IX, X)
- Albumin: 5% (iso-oncotic) vs. 25% (hyper-oncotic)
  - All bottles contain 12.5g albumin + 154 mEq Na^+ (isotonic)
  - Approved uses for albumin: cirrhosis + HRS, cirrhosis + SBP, cirrhosis after large volume paracentesis ($\geq$4L fluid removed)

Transfusion reactions

TABLE 7.5 · Transfusion Reactions: Clinical Presentations and Management

Reaction (onset)	Presentation	Management
Urticaria/Hives (any time)	Localized or diffuse hives and redness. Can occur at any time during transfusion. Due to IgE mediated sensitivity to donor plasma.	Stop transfusion, give diphenhydramine. Can restart transfusion if symptoms resolve. Consider giving washed blood products in the future.
Anaphylaxis (sec/min)	Rapid onset shock, angioedema, urticaria, respiratory distress. IgA deficient individuals are at risk.	Stop transfusion, give IM epinephrine. Future transfusions should be IgA-deficient plasma, washed RBCs.
Primary hypotensive reaction (min)	Transient hypotension in a patient who is on an ACE inhibitor within minutes because of bradykinin in blood	Stop transfusion. Avoid ACE inhibitors prior to transfusions in the future.
Acute hemolytic reaction (<1hr)	Fever, flank pain, hemoglobinuria (cola-colored urine): Renal failure, DIC, pink plasma Dx: Hgb in urine, +DAT	Fluids +/– diuretic, aiming for goal urine output >100 cc/hr
Bacterial sepsis (min-hrs)	Contaminated blood products (platelets most common) → Fevers, chills, septic shock, DIC Dx: Blood cultures AND cultures of blood product	Antibiotics, quarantine all other similar products
Febrile non-hemolytic transfusion reaction (1–6 hrs)	Most common transfusion reaction. Stored blood contains cytokines → inflammation when transfused.	Stop transfusion, give anti-pyretic, give leukoreduced blood in the future
Transfusion-Related Acute Lung Injury (TRALI) (1–6 hrs)	Fever, hypoxia, hypotension, normal JVP. Respiratory distress and pulmonary edema due to donor anti-leukocyte antibody to host granulocytes. Risk greatest FFP>Plt>RBC.	Provide supplemental oxygen, consider intubation if needed. Alert the blood bank so that the donor cannot donate blood again in the future.
Transfusion-Associated Circulatory Overload (TACO) (1–6 hrs)	Cardiogenic edema, SOB, HTN. Increased risk with higher volume of blood products received. Dx: BNP, CXR	Oxygen, diuretics, slower transfusion rate
Delayed hemolytic reaction (2–10 days)	Mild fever and hemolytic anemia with flu-like illness Dx: + DAT, hemolysis labs	Supportive care

HEMATOLOGY AND ONCOLOGY

Anticoagulation

TABLE 7.6 · Parenteral and Oral Anticoagulants			
Route	**Agent**	**Dosing / Monitoring**	**Reversal**
Parenteral	**Unfractionated Heparin** Binds & activates ATIII → inactivates Xa & IIa Half-life: 60–90 min	ACS: PTT goal 60–80 VTE: PTT goal 70–100 DVT ppx (with renal dysfunction): 5000U SQ Q8–12 (no monitoring for SQ)	• Protamine: 1mg per 100U heparin
	Low-molecular weight heparin (enoxaparin / Lovenox) Binds & activates ATIII → inactivates Xa>>IIa Half-life: 4.5–7 hrs	VTE: 1mg/kg SQ BID vs. 1.5 mg/ kg QD DVT ppx: 40U SQ QD (30U QD if CrCl<60) No need for monitoring	• Protamine
	Fondaparinux (Arixtra) Binds & activates ATIII → inactivates Xa only Half-life: 17–21 hrs	VTE: Weight-based daily dosing DVT ppx (h/o HIT): 2.5 mg SQ daily Anti-Xa level for monitoring	• No reversal agent
	Argatroban Direct IIa inhibitor Half-life: 45 min	VTE (h/o HIT): 0.2–1 mcg/kg/min PTT monitoring	• No reversal agent
	Bivalirudin (Angiomax) Direct thrombin inhibitor Half-life: 25 min	VTE (h/o HIT): 0.15–0.2 mg/kg/hr PTT monitoring	• No reversal agent
Oral	**Warfarin (Coumadin)** Vitamin K antagonist – inhibits vitamin K-dependent carboxylation of Factor II, VII, IX, X, Protein C and S Half-life: 40 hr	*Dosing variable depending on goal INR* MI with LV thrombus: Goal INR 2–3 Non-valvular Afib: Goal INR 2–3 VTE: Goal INR 2–3 APLS: Goal INR 2–3 Mechanical valves: Goal INR 2.5–3.5 (varies by valve type and comorbidities)	• Vitamin K • Fresh Frozen Plasma (FFP) • Prothrombin concentrate complex (Kcentra; $$)
	Dabigatran (Pradaxa) Direct thrombin (IIa) inhibitor Half-life: 12–17h *Renal Excretion: 80–85%*	Non-valvular Afib: 150 mg PO BID if GFR >30, 75 mg PO BID if GFR 15–30 VTE: 150 mg PO BID after 5-day heparin bridge DVT ppx: 220 mg PO QD	• Idarucizumab: Monoclonal antibody that binds directly to dabigatran and neutralizes AC effect (onset of action = minutes; $$$) • PCC ($$)
	Rivaroxaban (Xarelto) Direct Xa inhibitor (xa in name denotes Xa inhibitor) Half-life: 5–13 hr *Renal Excretion: 35%*	Non-valvular Afib: 20 mg PO daily if GFR >30, 15 mg PO daily if GFR 15–30 VTE: 15 mg PO BID × 21 days, then 20 mg QD	• Andexanet (recombinant factor Xa; $$$) • FFP • PCC ($$) Notes: • Xa inhibitors should *NOT* be used in patients with severe renal dysfunction, APLS, or mechanical heart valves. • Rivaroxaban is the only DOAC studied in VTE for BMI >40.

(Continued)

HEMATOLOGY AND ONCOLOGY

TABLE 7.6 · Parenteral and Oral Anticoagulants (*Continued*)			
Route	Agent	Dosing / Monitoring	Reversal
	Apixaban (Eliquis) Direct Xa inhibitor Half-life: 8–15 hr *Renal Excretion: 25%*	Non-valvular Afib: 5mg PO BID if GFR >30 2.5mg PO BID if: GFR 15–30, Wt <60kg, age>80 yr VTE: 10 mg PO BID ×7d, then 5mg PO BID×x6 mos, then 2.5 mg PO BID >6 mos	See reversal for rivaroxaban above
	Edoxaban (Savaysa, Lixiana) Direct Xa inhibitor Half-life: 6–11 hr *Renal Excretion: 35%*	Non-valvular Afib: 60 mg PO QD 30 mg PO QD if CrCl 15–50 or <60 kg VTE: 60 mg PO QD (after 5-day heparin bridge) 30 mg PO QD if CrCl 30–50 or <60 kg	

Abbreviations: ACS = acute coronary syndrome, VTE = venous thromboembolism, DVT = deep vein thrombosis, CrCl = creatinine clearance, MI = myocardial infarction, LV = left ventricular, APLS = anti-phospholipid antibody syndrome, GFR = glomerular filtration rate, DOAC = direct oral anticoagulant. Adapted from: Hakoum MB et. al. Anticoagulation for the initial treatment of venous thromboembolism in people with cancer. Cochrane Database Syst Rev. 2018.

Chemotherapy, Targeted Therapy, and Immunotherapy
See Oncology treatment section at the end of this chapter.

Chimeric-Antigen Receptor (CAR)-T cell therapy
- Mechanism: T cells are collected from the patient and genetically modified with a chimeric antigen receptor (CAR) to direct the T-cells against the tumor cells.
- Indications:
  - B-cell ALL, NHL: CAR directed against CD19
  - Multiple myeloma: CAR directed against BCMA (B-cell maturation antigen; a cell surface TNF receptor)
- Toxicities:
  - Cytokine Release Syndrome (CRS):
    - Pathophysiology: Systemic inflammatory response due to cytokine release after CAR-T therapy
    - Clinical features: Fever, fatigue, headache, rash, myalgias, diarrhea. Can have very high fevers (104°F) and can progress to SIRS with hypotension and multi-organ failure. Confusion, lethargy, and even seizures/cerebral edema can occur 2–5 days after onset of CRS and can be progressive. CRS occurs in approximately 25–50% of patients who receive CAR-T cell therapy for B-ALL; less common for patients who receive CAR-T cell therapy for multiple myeloma.
    - Diagnosis: ↑CRP and ferritin, dramatic elevation of IL-6. Degree of IL-6 elevation is associated with severity of CRS. See American Society for Transplantation and Cellular Therapy guidelines for grading severity.
    - Treatment: Supportive care to manage SIRS. For severe CRS, consider steroids and/or tocilizumab (monoclonal antibody against IL-6) in consultation with the heme/onc team.
  - Neurotoxicity:
    - Pathophysiology: Not well understood, also thought to be related to cytokine release after CAR-T therapy. Also called ICANS (immune effector cell-associated neurotoxicity syndrome) or CRES (cytokine release encephalopathy syndrome).
    - Clinical features: Wide range of symptoms including headache, tremor, expressive aphasia, impaired attention, seizures, cerebral edema. Usually occurs 4–5 days after CAR-T infusion. Can occur independently of CRS.
    - Treatment: Steroids are the mainstay of treatment. Should discuss with heme/onc team.

Stem Cell Transplant Basics

- Types of hematopoietic stem cells (HSCs):
  - <u>Autologous</u>: Transplant of patient's own HSCs to "rescue" the bone marrow after high intensity chemotherapy
    - Uses: Multiple myeloma, some lymphomas, germ cell tumors
  - <u>Allogeneic</u>: Transplant of donor (non-self) HSCs to replace the bone marrow after high-intensity chemotherapy AND for graft vs. tumor effect
    - Uses: AML, ALL, CML, CLL
- Sources of cells:
  - Peripheral blood stem cells: The donor is given a growth factor (e.g., G-CSF, GM-CSF) to mobilize HSCs from the bone marrow and then peripheral blood is collected. Less invasive, lower risk for the donor.
  - Bone marrow: Bone marrow aspirated from the iliac crests
  - Umbilical cord: Umbilical cord blood has a high number of HSCs. However, there is only a limited amount of blood if engraftment fails.
- Matching for allogeneic transplant:
  - For allogeneic transplants, where non-self cells are given to a patient, donors are tested by HLA matching. There are 12 HLA alleles that are tested with a "12/12" match being the best match.
  - Potential donors:
    - Identical twin: Ideal source as they will be a 12/12 match in addition to matching on other alleles and antigens not tested
    - Matched related donor (MRD): Ideally a sibling
    - Matched unrelated donor (MURD)
- Side effects: For autologous and identical twin allogeneic transplants, will not develop GVT or GVHD
  - <u>Graft vs. tumor</u>: Desired therapeutic side effect where the transplanted T-cells recognize the tumor cells as foreign and immunologically attack the tumor cells
  - <u>Graft vs. host disease (GVHD)</u>: Undesired side effect where the transplanted T-cells attack the host's cells, causing an autoimmune syndrome. Most common sites: Skin, liver, GI tract.
    - Acute: Within 100 days of transplant
    - Chronic: >3 months after transplant, but can occur at any time
    - Prophylaxis: Patients receive immunosuppressive medicines to prevent graft rejection and prevent GVHD, such as tacrolimus, sirolimus, mycophenolate, methotrexate, post-transplant cyclophosphamide
    - Treatment: Depends on the timing and severity of GVHD. Treatment usually includes increasing immunosuppressive regimens and steroids.

KEY CLINICAL TRIALS & PUBLICATIONS
Bridging Anticoagulation
- **Bleeding, recurrent venous thromboembolism, and mortality risks during warfarin interruption for invasive procedures.** *JAMA Int Med* 2015;175(7):1163–1168.
  - Retrospective cohort study that evaluated 1178 patients on warfarin who underwent procedures with or without bridging anticoagulation. There was no significant difference in the rate of recurrent VTE between the bridge and non-bridge therapy groups (0 vs. 3; p=0.56). No deaths occurred in either group but there was increased rate of bleeding in the bridging anticoagulation group.
- **Perioperative bridging anticoagulation in patients with atrial fibrillation.** *N Engl J Med* 2015;373(9):823–833.
  - Multicenter randomized, double-blinded placebo-controlled trial that randomized patients with atrial fibrillation on warfarin who underwent perioperative interruption to receive bridging anticoagulation therapy with low-molecular-weight heparin vs. placebo from 3 days before the procedure until 24 hours before the procedure and then for 5–10 days after the procedure. Forgoing bridging anticoagulation was non-inferior to perioperative bridging with low-molecular-weight heparin for the prevention of arterial thromboembolism and decreased the risk of major bleeding events.

Acute Myeloid Leukemia
- **Midostaurin plus chemotherapy for acute myeloid leukemia with a FLT3 mutation.** *N Engl J Med* 2017;377(5):454–464.
  - Multicenter randomized phase 3 clinical trial to determine whether the addition of midostaurin, an oral multitargeted kinase inhibitor that is active in patients with AML and a FLT3 mutation, to standard chemotherapy would prolong overall survival in this population. The addition of midostaurin increased overall survival and event free survival.
- **Final results of a phase III randomized trial of CPX-351 versus 7+3 in older patients with newly diagnosed high risk (secondary) AML.** *J Clin Onc* 2016;34(15 suppl):7000.
  - Multicenter randomized phase 3 clinical trial that randomized patients 60–75 yr of age with untreated AML and a history of prior cytotoxic treatment, antecedent MDS or CMML, or AML with MDS-related cytogenic abnormalities to receive CPX-351 or 7+3 (cytarabine and daunorubicin) induction therapy. CPX-351 (later named Vyxeos) significantly improved overall survival, event free survival, and response without an increase in 60-day mortality or adverse event frequency or severity. The authors concluded that CPX-351 should become standard of care for older patients with secondary AML.
- **Venetoclax combined with decitabine or azacitidine in treatment-naive, elderly patients with acute myeloid leukemia.** *Blood* 2019;133(1):7–17.
  - Phase Ib dose escalation and expansion study that evaluated the safety and efficacy of venetoclax combined with decitabine or azacitadine in patients 65 yr or older. This combination showed tolerable safety and favorable overall response rate in elderly patients, changing the way we treat older adults with AML.

Lymphoma
- **Bendamustine plus rituximab versus CHOP plus rituximab as first-line treatment for patients with indolent and mantle-cell lymphomas: An open-label, multicentre, randomised, phase 3 non-inferiority trial.** *The Lancet* 2013;381(9873):1203–1210.
  - Multicenter randomized phase 3 non-inferiority trial that randomized patients with previously untreated indolent and mantle-cell lymphomas to bendamustine plus rituximab versus R-CHOP (rituximab, cyclophosphamide, doxorubicin, vincristine, and prednisone). At median follow-up of 45 months, median progression free survival was significantly longer in the bendamustine plus rituximab group than the R-CHOP group (69.5 months vs. 31.5 months). Thus, bendamustine plus rituximab can be considered as a preferred first line treatment approach in patients with previously untreated indolent lymphomas.

Multiple Myeloma
- **Lenalidomide, bortezomib, and dexamethasone with transplantation for myeloma.** *N Engl J Med* 2017;376(14):1311–1320.
  - Multicenter randomized controlled phase 3 clinical trial where 700 patients with multiple myeloma were randomly assigned to receive induction therapy with three cycles of lenalidomide, bortezomib, and dexamethasone (RVD) and then consolidation therapy with either five additional cycles of RVD or high dose melphalan plus stem-cell transplantation followed by two additional cycles of RVD. Median progression free survival was significantly longer in the group that underwent transplantation than in the group that received RVD alone (50 months vs. 36 months), suggesting that stem cell transplantation is beneficial for these patients.

HEMATOLOGY AND ONCOLOGY

ONCOLOGY

ANATOMY & PHYSIOLOGY

- Pathophysiology: Genetic and environmental factors can cause normal cells to become malignant. Typically, a solid tumor grows locally first and then has the potential to spread to other organs (metastasize).

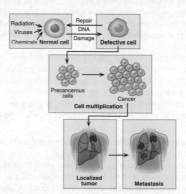

FIGURE 7.7: Agents that cause cancer and progression of normal cells to malignant cells.

DIAGNOSTICS

- Diagnosis is based on biopsy-proven diagnosis most of the time – "tissue is the issue"
  - Exceptions: Hepatocellular carcinoma (HCC), renal cell carcinoma (RCC), and glioblastoma can be diagnosed *without* biopsy via imaging
- General rules of thumb:
  - Biopsy distant metastasis. This provides the opportunity to diagnose the primary tumor type and confirm staging simultaneously.
  - More tissue is better, especially in the era of molecular testing.
  - Core biopsy is generally preferred over fine needle aspiration (FNA) (except FNA preferred for suspected head/neck carcinoma).
- Key resource: The National Comprehensive Cancer Network (NCCN.org) has guidelines on initial workup and staging by suspected cancer site. Trainees can register for a free account.

APPROACHES & CHIEF COMPLAINTS

General Approaches to Treating Cancer

Surgery, radiation, and medications

- Surgery (surgical oncology): Resecting the tumor +/– local lymph nodes
- Radiation therapy (radiation oncology): Can be external beam therapy or internal (e.g., brachytherapy)
- Medications (medical oncology):
  - <u>Chemotherapy</u>: Cytotoxic therapy that targets rapidly dividing cells
  - <u>Hormone Therapy</u>: Medications to suppress endogenous hormones that drive the growth of certain tumor types
  - <u>Targeted Therapy</u>: Medications that target specific genes and proteins that drive the growth of certain tumor types
  - <u>Immunotherapy</u>: Medications that activate the patient's own immune system to attack their cancer

Local vs. systemic treatment

- Local: Surgery, radiation. Sometimes sufficient for localized disease.
- Systemic: Medications (as above: chemotherapy, targeted therapy, immune therapy, hormone therapy). Goal is to treat cancer cells that may have spread throughout the body.

Timing/order of therapies

- Neoadjuvant: Treatment given *before* surgery to "shrink" the tumor to make it easier to resect and/or to better evaluate how the tumor responds to therapy before it is resected
- Adjuvant: Treatment given *after* surgery to kill any residual cancer cells and reduce recurrence risk
- Concurrent chemoradiation: When chemotherapy and radiation are given together; chemotherapy is usually radiosensizing.

DISEASES & PATHOPHYSIOLOGY

Oncologic Emergencies

Structural Emergencies

Increased intracranial pressure (ICP) from brain lesions

- Pathophysiology: Either primary brain tumor or metastasis causing vasogenic edema, leading to ↑ICP
- Symptoms: Headache, blurry vision, focal neurologic deficits, stroke
- Diagnosis: NCHCT vs. contrast MRI depending on urgency (MRI superior)
- Treatment: Mannitol, steroids, emergent neurosurgical intervention or radiation. Call neurosurgery and radiation oncology.

Neoplastic epidural spinal cord compression

- Pathophysiology: Compression of spinal cord from lesions in vertebral bones >> paraspinal mass extending locally into epidural space. Annual incidence is 3–5% among patients with metastatic cancer. ~50% cases from prostate, lung, and breast cancer.
- Symptoms: Back or SI joint pain, asymmetric leg weakness, saddle anesthesia, urinary retention, fecal incontinence (bowel/bladder problems are typically late findings)
- Diagnosis: Urgent MRI total spine with and without contrast
- Treatment: Call neurosurgery and radiation oncology ASAP. Start steroids (e.g., dexamethasone 10mg then 4mg q6) +/− emergent neurosurgical intervention or radiation.

Superior vena cava (SVC) syndrome

- Pathophysiology: Extrinsic compression of the SVC by a tumor or mediastinal lymph nodes that cause increased upper body venous pressure. Most common in NSCLC, small cell lung cancer, NHL.
- Symptoms: Sudden appearance of dilated veins on the chest = herald onset of SVC syndrome. Patients may also have facial swelling, "head fullness," SOB, blurry vision, hypotension (↓venous return to right atrium).
- Diagnosis: Imaging demonstrates SVC compression by tumor
- Treatment: If life-threatening symptoms (e.g., stridor, CNS symptoms) are present, consider endovascular stent, radiation, or rarely tumor resection. If no life-threatening symptoms are present, chemotherapy alone may be sufficient for chemotherapy-responsive tumors (e.g., SCLC, lymphoma). Anticoagulate if thrombus detected.

Metabolic Emergencies

Hypercalcemia of malignancy

- Pathophysiology: Multiple possible mechanisms
  - Tumor secretion of PTHrP (most common) – often SCC of lung, breast cancer, RCC
  - Osteolytic metastases, which cause increased bone turnover – commonly MM, breast cancer
  - Tumor production of 1,25-OH Vit D – Hodgkin's and NH lymphoma
- Symptoms: "Stones, groans, moans, psychiatric overtones" – kidney stones, nausea, vomiting, abdominal pain, bony pain, AMS
- Diagnosis: ↑Ca^{2+} level (corrected for albumin), dehydration (↑Cr, ↑Na^+)
- Treatment:
  - Aggressive hydration (200–300 mL/hr to maintain UOP of 100–150 ml/hr). Caution in heart failure and volume overload. Generally only use diuretics if there is concern for iatrogenic hypervolemia. Effect seen: Hours.
  - Calcitonin 4IU/kg Q6–12 hrs for up to 48 hrs (patients will develop tachyphylaxis after 48 hrs of therapy). Effect seen: Hours to days.
  - Bisphosphonate: Usually zoledronic acid. One-time dose, so full dose ok in renal dysfunction and no dental evaluation needed prior to treatment. Effect seen: 2–4 days.
  - Denosumab: Monoclonal antibody to RANK-ligand → blocks activation of osteoclasts, which promote bone breakdown and Ca^{2+} release. Generally, bisphosphonates are preferred over denosumab for acute treatment of hypercalcemia of malignancy. Effect seen: 4–10 days.

Neutropenic fever

- See details in the hematology section under oncologic emergencies

DIC and TLS

- Less common with solid than hematologic malignancies but can occur with solid tumor malignancies
- See details in the hematology section under oncologic emergencies

Breast Cancer

- Epidemiology: Most common cancer in women. Risk factors – older age, BRCA1 or 2 mutation, family history, menopause >55 yr, 1st birth >30 yr, nulliparity, smoking.
- Screening: USPSTF recommends screening mammogram every 2 yr for patients age 50–74 yr; for women age 40–49 yr the choice is an individual one.
- Clinical features: Breast mass, asymmetry, nipple inversion, edema/thickening of the skin (peau d'orange), axillary/supraclavicular mass
- Diagnosis: Mammogram and ultrasound, if mass identified get a core biopsy
- Treatment: Depends on receptor status and stage (see below)
- Prognosis:
  - Locally advanced disease (stage I–III): Goal is cure
  - Metastatic disease (stage IV): Not curable but treatable. Prognosis depends on receptor status and organs involved

Hormone-receptor positive (estrogen receptor [ER] and/or progesterone receptor [PR] +)

- Locally advanced hormone receptor positive disease (stage I, II, or III):
  - Locoregional disease control: Partial mastectomy (lumpectomy) vs. mastectomy with sentinel lymph node biopsy (SLNB) +/− radiation therapy
    * If patient undergoes partial mastectomy, typically perform post-operative radiation to that breast. Radiation can sometimes be omitted in early stage disease for elderly patients
    * Is SLNB positive, need axillary lymph node dissection or axillary radiation
  - Adjuvant endocrine therapy for 5-10 yr
    * Pre-menopausal women: Tamoxifen is typically first line, unless high risk disease and then consider ovarian suppression + aromatase inhibitor. Side effects of tamoxifen: VTE, hot flashes, increased risk endometrial cancer (need annual GYN screening)
    * Post menopausal women: Aromatase inhibitor (AI): Anastrazole, letrozole, exemestane. Side effects of AIs: Joint aches, decreased bone density, vaginal dryness, hot flashes
  - If high risk disease, also consider chemotherapy
    * Can use MammaPrint or OncotypeDX tumor testing to help identify patients who will derive the most benefit from chemotherapy. These tests are only validated for hormone receptor positive disease.
    * Chemotherapy:
      - **AC/T:** doxorubicin (Adriamycin) + cyclophosphamide, followed by paclitaxel (Taxol)
      - **TC:** docetaxel (Taxotere) + cyclophosphamide
- Metastatic hormone receptor positive disease (stage IV):
  - Typically endocrine therapy is first line. Often treat with multiple lines of endocrine therapy first before considering chemotherapy
  - CDK 4/6 inhibitors (palbociclib, ribociclib, abemaciclib) can be combined with aromatase inhibitors. Side effects: Lower ANC (although neutropenic fever less common), fatigue, GI side effects
  - If metastatic disease to bone: Also consider adding zolendronic acid or denosumab after dental clearance (risk osteonecrosis of the jaw)

HER2+

- Locally advanced HER2+ disease (stage I, II, III):
  - Consider neoadjuvant chemotherapy/HER2 targeted therapy prior to surgery
    * Common neoadjuvant regimen:
      - **TCHP:** docetaxel (Taxotere), carboplatin, trastuzumab (Herceptin or biosimilar), pertuzumab (Perjeta)
      - If the patient achieves a pathologic complete response (PCR) at the time of surgery, finish with 9 months of trastuzumab/pertuzumab. If PCR not achieved (i.e. there is residual disease at the time of surgery), consider adjuvant trastuzumab emtansine (TDM1) × 14 cycles
  - If ER+ or PR+ disease, 5–10 yr of adjuvant endocrine therapy is also recommended
- Metastatic HER2+ disease (stage IV):
  - Typical first line regimen is paclitaxel or docetaxel + trastuzumab/pertuzumab ×6–8 cycles. Then stop chemotherapy and continue trastuzumab/pertuzumab until disease progression

Triple negative breast cancer (TNBC) (ER-/PR-/HER2-)
- Locally advanced triple negative disease (stage I, II, III):
  - If triple negative disease and tumor >1.5cm, recommend neoadjuvant chemotherapy first. Common regimen: **AC/T** (doxorubicin (Adriamycin)/cyclophosphamide, followed by paclitaxel (Taxol)).
  - After neoadjuvant chemotherapy, proceed to surgery. If there is still residual disease at the time of surgery, consider adjuvant capecitabine (Xeloda) × 6–8 cycles
- Metastatic triple negative disease (stage IV):
  - Atezolizumab + paclitaxel first line for triple negative metastatic disease if PDL1+
  - Chemotherapy + immunotherapy if PDL1+

BRCA mutated breast cancer
- Epidemiology: BRCA1 and BRCA2 are the most common germline genetic mutations that increase the risk for breast cancer.
- Treatment:
  - See treatment regimens above depending on receptor type and stage
  - Of note, BRCA+ breast cancers respond well to PARP inhibitors (e.g., olaparib, talazoparib) and platinum-based chemotherapy
  - BRCA 1/2 mutations are also associated with other malignancies; discuss screening with genetic counseling team

Lung Cancer
- Epidemiology: Risk factors include smoking, asbestos exposure, older age, male gender.
- Screening: USPSTF recommends low-dose CT scan for patients 50–80 yr with 20+ pack year smoking history who are current smokers or quit within the last 15 yr.

Non-small cell lung cancer (NSCLC)
- Epidemiology: Approximately 85% of lung cancers
- Pathology: Adenocarcinoma (50–60%), squamous (25%), large cell (10%)
- Molecular drivers: KRAS, EGFR, BRAF, ALK, ROS1, RET, N-TREK, MET, HER2, PD-L1
- Staging: After diagnosis, get PET/CT (unless already known stage IV), MRI brain to evaluate for brain metastases, and molecular testing to evaluate for driver mutations if stage IV
- Treatment:
  - Stage I/II: Goal is cure. Surgical resection preferred if the patient is a surgical candidate. Adjuvant chemotherapy is usually not recommended for stage I disease, more controversial for stage II disease.
  - Stage III: Goal is cure. Typically surgery is recommended if the patient is a surgical candidate as well as adjuvant chemotherapy. If unresectable, chemoradiation followed by immunotherapy is standard.
  - Stage IV:
    - Not curable, but treatable
    - First, evaluate for driver mutations (targeted therapy) and PD-L1 status (immunotherapy)
    - Examples of driver mutations and possible targeted therapy:
      - EGFR mutation: Osimertinib
      - ALK mutation: Alectinib, brigatinib, ceritinib
    - If isolated brain metastases, consider surgical resection and/or radiation

Small cell lung cancer (SCLC)
- Epidemiology: Approximately 10–15% of lung cancers
- Pathology: Small round, blue cells. De-differentiated, aggressive.
- Clinical features: Cough, weight loss. Can cause paraneoplastic syndromes (e.g., SIADH)
- Staging: Staged as limited (hemithorax and regional nodes) or extensive (more widespread)
- Treatment:
  - If limited disease, consider radiation to the thorax
  - Chemotherapy + immunotherapy
  - Consider prophylactic cranial irradiation for all patients (limited or extensive) who have a complete or very good partial response after induction chemotherapy

Anterior Mediastinal Mass
- Anterior mediastinal mass: **4Ts**: **T**hymus, **T**eratoma/germ cell, (**T**errible) lymphoma, **T**hyroid
- Middle mediastinal mass: Lymph nodes, cysts
- Posterior mediastinal mass: Neurogenic tumors

Gastrointestinal Malignancies

Esophageal cancer

- Epidemiology:
  - <u>Squamous</u>: Top ⅓ esophagus. More common in Asia, Africa. Risk factors – alcohol, tobacco, diet (nitrosamines, hot tea), HPV, achalasia, Plummer-Vinson.
  - <u>Adenocarcinoma</u>: Bottom ⅓ esophagus. More common in the United States. Risk factors – GERD, Barrett esophagus, obesity, smoking.
- Clinical features: Solid food dysphagia is common
- Staging: CT C/A/P or PET/CT if not known to have stage IV disease
- Treatment:
  - If surgical candidate: Chemotherapy/radiation therapy then surgery
  - If not surgical candidate: Definitive chemotherapy/radiation therapy
  - Metastatic: Chemotherapy, add trastuzumab if HER2+

Gastric adenocarcinoma

- Pathophysiology: Adenocarcinomas, rare in the US, common in Japan (dietary exposures)
- Risk factors: Atrophic gastritis, gastric polyps, *H. pylori* (3–6×), pernicious anemia (3×), Menetrier's disease, preserved foods
- Pathology: Ulcerative, polypoid, superficial, linitis plastica (leather bottle)
- Clinical features: Abdominal pain, weight loss, anorexia, nausea/vomiting, anemia, melena. Common sites of metastasis: Krukenberg (ovary), Blumer's shelf (rectum), Sister Mary Joseph's node (periumbilical), Virchow's node (supraclavicular), Irish's node (left axillary adenopathy)
- Staging: CT C/A/P or PET/CT if not known to have stage IV disease
- Treatment: Surgical resection with wide margins (>5cm), chemotherapy, add trastuzumab if HER2+

Colorectal cancer (CRC)

- Epidemiology: Risk factors: Adenomatous polyps (villous, sessile worse), IBD (UC), family history (1st degree relative with CRC < 60 yr), diet (low fiber), genetic predispositions
  - <u>Hereditary nonpolyposis CRC (HNPCC)</u>:
    - Lynch I: Early onset CRC without preceding polyps
    - Lynch II: Same as Lynch I, but also with increased number of polyps, earlier recurrences, and risk of other cancers (e.g., GYN, skin, stomach, pancreas, brain, breast)
  - <u>Familial adenomatous polyposis (FAP)</u>: Autosomal dominant
  - <u>MYH-associated polpysis (MAP)</u>: Autosomal recessive. Need prophylactic colectomy.
  - <u>Gardner syndrome</u>: GI tract polyps plus osteomas, dental problems, benign soft tissue tumors, sebaceous cysts
  - <u>Turcot's syndrome</u>: Autosomal recessive. Higher risk of GI tract polyps, cerebellar medulloblastoma or GBM
  - <u>Peutz-Jeghers syndrome</u>: Single or multiple hamartomas, pigmented spots on lips/face/genitalia – low malignant potential. Increased risk for stomach, ovary, breast, cervical, lung, testicular cancer. Can cause intussusception, bleeds.
  - <u>Familial juvenile polyposis syndrome</u>: Rare, in childhood, only small risk CRC. Can remove colon if complicated by GI bleeding (vascular polyps).
- Screening: Start CRC screening at age 45–50 yr or 40 yr if positive family history. Options for screening: 1) Colonoscopy q10yr, 2) Flexible sigmoidoscopy q5yr with fecal occult blood test (FOBT) q3yr (USPSTF) or q1yr, 3) FOBT q1yr
- Clinical features: Melena, hematochezia, iron-deficiency anemia, occasionally obstruction
- Pathology: Mostly adenocarcinomas, less commonly carcinoid, lymphomas, Kaposi's sarcoma
- Staging: Colonoscopy, CT C/A/P, CEA, pelvic MRI for rectal primary, genetic testing (RAS, BRAF, MSI status)
- Treatment:
  - Confined to colon (stage I) or local invasion (stage II): Resection for cure
  - For rectal cancer: Neoadjuvant chemotherapy and radiation is often used
  - Metastatic to regional lymph nodes (stage III): Resection and adjuvant chemotherapy: 5-FU + oxaliplatin (FOLFOX) or 5-FU + irinotecan (FOLFIRI)
  - Distant metastases (stage IV): Resection of primary lesion for palliation (if needed) and chemotherapy (FOLFOX or FOLFIRI) or immunotherapy if MSI high
  - KRAS/NRAS mutation: Add EGFR inhibitor
  - MSI high tumors: Consider addition of checkpoint inhibitor
- Surveillance: Check CEA every 3–6 months. Follow-up CT abd/pelvis and CXR for 5 yr. Colonoscopy at 1 yr, then every 3 yr.

Pancreatic adenocarcinoma
- Epidemiology: Older patients, rare before age 40 yr. Location of the tumor within the pancreas: Head (75%), body (20%), tail (10%). Poor prognosis, with a 5 yr survival of only 5% of patients.
- Risk factors: Cigarette smoking, DM, chronic pancreatitis, alcohol use, BRCA 1 or 2 mutation
- Symptoms: Abdominal pain, jaundice, weight loss, recent mild diabetes, Courvoisier sign (palpable gallbladder due to distal bile duct compression) or Trousseau syndrome (migratory thrombophlebitis)
- Diagnosis:
  - Right upper quadrant ultrasound
  - CT abdomen/pelvis – consider CT pancreatic protocol
  - Endoscopic ultrasound (EUS) with biopsies (or ERCP if biliary obstruction)
  - Check CA 19-9
- Staging: CT chest or PET/CT if not already known to have stage IV disease
- Treatment: Surgical resection if possible and then concurrent chemotherapy/radiation therapy. If not resectable, chemotherapy and/or radiation

Pancreatic neuroendocrine tumors (PNET)
- Nonfunctional (75%): No hormone secretion, symptoms associated with mass – jaundice, abdominal pain
  - Genetic predisposition: MEN1 and VHL
- Functional (25%):
  - <u>Gastrinoma</u> (secrete gastrin, aka Zollinger-Ellison): Peptic ulcer disease, diarrhea, esophagitis. Associated with MEN1 syndrome. Treatment: PPI, resect tumor.
  - <u>Insulinoma</u> (secrete insulin): Hypoglycemia. Associated with MEN1 syndrome. Treatment: Resect tumor.
  - <u>VIPoma</u> (secrete vasoactive intestinal peptide): Watery diarrhea, hypokalemia, hypochlorhidria.
  - <u>Glucagonoma</u> (secrete glucagon): Dermatitis (necrolytic migratory erythema), diabetes, diarrhea, glossitis. Treatment: Resect tumor.
  - <u>Somatostatinoma</u> (secrete somatostatin): Triad of gallstones, diabetes, diarrhea
  - <u>GHRHoma</u> (secrete growth hormone releasing hormone): Acromegaly

Cholangiocarcinoma
- Definition: Tumor of intra/extrahepatic bile ducts, typically adenocarcinomas
- Risk factors: Primary sclerosing cholangitis (PSC) is a major risk factor in the United States. Other risk factors include UC, choledochal cysts, cirrhosis, viral hepatitis, liver flukes (*Clonorchis,* common in Asia)
- Clinical features: Abdominal pain, weight loss, obstructive jaundice
- Diagnosis: MRCP vs. EUS/ERCP with stenting and biopsy
- Staging: CT C/A/P with contrast
- Locations:
  - Proximal 1/3 common bile duct, aka Klaskin's tumor – poor prognosis
  - Distal extrahepatic – best prognosis
  - Intrahepatic – rare
- Treatment: Easier to resect distal bile duct tumors than proximal; can use stents to relieve obstruction; chemotherapy/immunotherapy

Hepatocellular carcinoma (HCC)
- Epidemiology: Risk factors – cirrhosis (but hepatitis B can proceed to HCC without cirrhosis), chemicals (aflatoxin, vinyl chloride, thorotrast), alcohol, tobacco, obesity, iron overload (hemochromatosis, chronic transfusions)
- Clinical features: Abdominal pain, weight loss, paraneoplastic syndromes possible (e.g., erythrocytosis, thrombocytosis, hypercalcemia, carcinoid)
- Diagnosis: Diagnose radiographically (quad phase CT). If imaging is convincing for HCC (LI-RADS 5), then can diagnose radiographically and do not need a biopsy. Check AFP level.
- Staging: CT C/A/P
- Treatment:
  - Localized disease: Surgical resection, radiofrequency ablation, transarterial chemoembolization, liver transplantation
  - Metastatic disease or no longer able to control with locoregional therapies above: Treat with a tyrosine kinase/VEGF inhibitor (sorafenib, lenvatinib) and/or immunotherapy

Genitourinary Malignancies

Renal cell carcinoma (RCC)

- Epidemiology: Median age at diagnosis 64 yr. Most cases sporadic. 2% associated with von Hippel-Lindau. Higher risk in males (M:F = 2:1). Risk factors: Cigarette smoking, dialysis, heavy metal exposure (cadmium), asbestos exposure, autosomal dominant polycystic kidney disease, obesity.
- Clinical features:
  - Hematuria, abd/flank pain or mass, weight loss, fever, anemia (due to ↓EPO production), paraneoplastic (rare – sometimes excess EPO production can cause polycythemia vera or exogenous PTHrP production can cause hypercalcemia). L-sided scrotal varices fail to empty when the patient is recumbent because the tumor obstructs the venous outflow.
  - Tumor thrombus renal vein/IVC → Hematologic spread to lung, liver, brain, bone
- Diagnosis: CT A/P or MRI +/– biopsy (RCC can often be radiographically diagnosed, does not always require biopsy)
- Treatment:
  - Surgical resection: Partial vs. radical nephrectomy (excision of kidney and adrenal gland)
  - Medical therapies: VEGF inhibitors (bevacizumab, sunitinib, pazopanib), mTOR inhibitors (temsirolimus and everolimus), immunotherapy (nivolumab or ipilimumab)

Bladder cancer

- Epidemiology: Median age at diagnosis 69 yr in men, 71 yr in women. 90% transitional cell carcinoma, local extension, likely to recur. Risk factors: Cigarette smoking, aniline/azo dyes, cyclophosphamide
- Clinical features: Painless hematuria, irritable bladder (dysuria, frequency)
- Diagnosis: Patients >40 yr with microscopic or gross hematuria should have a cystoscopy to evaluate for malignancy
- Treatment: Stage determined by depth of invasion
  - Non-muscle invasive disease: Transurethral resection of bladder tumor (TURBT) +/– intravesicular chemotherapy
    - Intra-vesicular immunotherapy with BCG: Live attenuated form of *Mycobacterium bovis* → generates local inflammatory response activating host immune system to respond to the tumor
  - Muscle invasive disease: Radical cystectomy +/– systemic neoadjuvant or adjuvant chemotherapy (usually with cisplatin), or bladder preservation therapy with concurrent chemotherapy/radiation

Prostate cancer

- Epidemiology: Median age at diagnosis 66 yr. Lifetime risk ~11%. Second most common cancer in men. Adenocarcinoma 95% of cases.
- Risk factors: Older age, high-fat diet, positive family history, pesticides, BRCA 1 or 2 mutation
- Screening: Controversial with limited evidence. USPSTF guidelines recommend prostate specific antigen (PSA) screening for men 55–69 yr *only* after shared decision making discussion. American Family Physicians (AFP) recommends against PSA screening.
- Clinical features:
  - Early: Often asymptomatic
  - Later: Obstructive symptoms with difficulty voiding, dysuria
  - Metastatic disease: Often presents with bone pain since bone metastases common
- Diagnosis: Digital rectal exam (DRE), PSA, transrectal ultrasound (TRUS) with biopsy if abnormal DRE, PSA >10 ng/mL or >0.75 ng/mL annual increase
- Staging: Gleason score – pathological grade incorporated into risk stratification. Higher risk disease needs CT A/P and bone scan.
- Treatment:
  - Low-risk: Active surveillance vs. radiation (external beam vs. brachytherapy) vs. prostatectomy
  - Intermediate to high risk: Prostatectomy or radiation +/– androgen deprivation therapy (ADT)
    - ADT: GnRH agonist (leuprolide – causes initial surge in testosterone, so must be paired with selective androgen receptor antagonist like bicalutamide) OR GnRH antagonist (degarelix, no testosterone surge)
    - Additional agents used in advanced disease:
      - Abiraterone: CYP17 inhibitor that blocks the synthesis of androgens (given with low-dose prednisone to counteract side effects of abiraterone→ cortisol decrease and mineralocorticoid excess)
      - Enzalutamide/apalutamide: Androgen receptor inhibitors

Testicular cancer
- Epidemiology: Most common in men 20–35 yr
- Risk factors: Cryptorchidism (surgical correction does not eliminate risk), Klinefelter's syndrome, infertility
  - <u>Germ cell</u>: 95%, highly curable
    - Seminomas (35%, slow growth, late invasion)
    - Nonseminomatous (65% – embryonal, choriocarcinoma, yolk sac, teratoma)
  - <u>Non-germ cell</u>: 5%, usually benign
    - Leydig: Secrete estrogen/androgens→ precocious puberty in children, gynecomastia
    - Sertoli: Usually benign
- Clinical features: Nodule or painless swelling of one testicle, rarely gynecomastia
- Diagnosis:
  - Scrotal ultrasound and serum tumor markers (AFP, β-hCG, LDH) → Radical inguinal orchiectomy for pathologic diagnosis
  - NO needle biopsy given concern for tumor seeding in the scrotal sac or metastatic spread into the inguinal lymph nodes
- Treatment: All receive orchiectomy (offer semen cryopreservation first if patient desires fertility). Check post-operative β-hCG and AFP.
  - Seminomas: Very sensitive to radiation. Chemotherapy – single-agent carboplatin or multi-agent chemotherapy if higher stage.
  - Non-seminomatous: Relatively radiation resistant. Consider retroperitoneal lymph node dissection and chemotherapy. Common regimen is BEP (<u>b</u>leomycin, <u>e</u>toposide, cisplatin) ×3–4 cycles.

GYN Malignancies
Ovarian cancer
- Epidemiology: Median age at diagnosis 63 yr, lifetime risk 1.3%. Risk factors: BRCA 1 or 2 mutation, older age, infertility, endometriosis, PCOS, cigarette smoking. Protective factors: OCPs, previous pregnancy, history of breastfeeding.
- Screening: No screening indicated; if high risk (e.g., ovarian cancer in first degree family member, BRCA mutation) can screen with CA-125, pelvic exams, and transvaginal ultrasounds, but little data
- Clinical features: Subacute presentation. Adnexal mass, ascites, early satiety, weight loss.
- Diagnosis: Transvaginal/abdominal ultrasound usually visualizes complex adnexal mass. Elevated CA-125. Pathologic diagnosis requires surgical exploration, as needle biopsy can rupture the mass and cause a worse prognosis.
- Treatment:
  - If surgical candidate: Exploratory-laparotomy for surgical excision +/– intraperitoneal chemotherapy (survival benefit in patients with small amounts of residual disease confined to the peritoneal cavity following surgery)
  - Adjuvant chemotherapy: Paclitaxel, carboplatin
  - Surgical debulking improves survival in metastatic disease
- Surveillance: Obtain CA-125 before surgery. Following CA-125 longitudinally post-surgery may help identify recurrence, but has not been shown to impact overall survival.

Cervical cancer
- Epidemiology: Median age at diagnosis 50 yr. Risk factors: HPV, immunosuppression, HIV, smoking
- Screening: Pap smear (every 3 yr for women age 21–29 yr, then every 5 yr with HPV co-testing for women age ≥30 yr)
- Clinical features: Abnormal vaginal bleeding (post-menopausal, post-coital, intermenstrual)
- Diagnosis: Pap smear cervical cytology, cervical biopsy and colposcopy
- Treatment:
  - Early (stage I): Loop electrosurgical excision procedure (LEEP) or cervical conization. After childbearing: Hysterectomy.
  - Advanced (stage III–IV): Concurrent chemotherapy/radiation therapy (cisplatin-based regimen) or chemotherapy alone for metastatic disease

Endometrial cancer
- Epidemiology: Median age at diagnosis 60 yr. Risk factors: Excess estrogen (e.g., obesity, postmenopausal estrogen without progesterone opposition), tamoxifen therapy, nulliparity, diabetes, Lynch syndrome
- Screening: No routine screening recommended
- Clinical features: Postmenopausal/irregular bleeding
- Diagnosis: Transvaginal ultrasound with thickened endometrial stripe → perform endometrial biopsy
- Treatment: Surgical resection of the uterus, cervix, and adnexa in early stages; later stages may require chemotherapy/radiation therapy

Melanoma

- Epidemiology: 5th most common cancer in the United States. Risk factors: Older age, sun exposure, fair complexion, red/blonde hair, high nevi count, immunosuppression.
- Clinical features: Atypical mole – **ABCDE** criteria (**A**symmetry, irregular **B**order, **C**olor variation, **D**iameter ≥6 mm, **E**volution)
- Diagnosis: Biopsy. Depth of invasion determines stage.
- Treatment:
  - Treatment depends on the stage:
    - Stage I/II: Wide local excision and sentinel lymph node biopsy is usually sufficient
    - Stage III: Surgery followed by adjuvant immunotherapy for 1 yr to reduce the risk of recurrence
    - Stage IV (metastatic): Recommend immunotherapy
  - Systemic therapy options:
    - Immunotherapy: Anti-PD1 monotherapy (pembrolizumab or nivolumab) vs. anti-PD1/anti-CTLA4 combination therapy (niviolumab + ipilimumab)
    - Targeted therapy: BRAF inhibitor (vemurafenib, dabrafenib, encorafenib) + MEK inhibitor (cobimetinib, trametinib, binimetinib) if patient has BRAF V600E mutation
  - Radiation: Can be used to treat symptomatic localized area of disease (e.g., brain metastases)

Head & Neck Malignancies

Thyroid cancer

- Diagnosis: Thyroid ultrasound and biopsy
- Risk factors: Older age, M>F, head/neck radiation, MEN2A/B (medullary thyroid cancer)
- Types of thyroid cancer:
  - <u>Papillary</u>: 85%. Diagnosis: More aggressive if BRAF-mutated. Treatment: Thyroid lobectomy or total thyroidectomy if >3cm. Adjuvant: TSH suppression therapy, radioiodine therapy for larger tumors, BRAF inhibition if indicated (metastatic disease).
  - <u>Follicular</u>: 12%. Malignant follicular cells invade through the fibrous capsule. Diagnosis: RAS mutation in 40% → more aggressive cancers. Treatment: Total thyroidectomy, post-operative iodine ablation.
  - <u>Medullary</u>: 1–2%. Malignant proliferation of parafollicular C cells. Elevated calcitonin → deposits as amyloid and stains with congo red. Diagnosis: Hypocalcemia, sometimes ↑calcitonin and CEA. Perform genetic testing for RET mutations and MEN2 syndrome. Treatment: Total thyroidectomy.
  - <u>Anaplastic</u>: 1%. Mortality nearly 100%; 90% of patients have invasion of local structures at time of diagnosis (e.g., larynx, trachea, esophagus), which may cause dysphagia, respiratory compromise. Treatment: Surgical resection if possible. If locally advanced inoperable disease, can give concurrent chemotherapy/radiation therapy. BRAF/MEK inhibition if BRAF V600E mutation present.

Sarcoma

Soft tissue sarcoma

- Epidemiology: Rare, heterogeneous tumor of mesenchymal origin. <1% of adult tumors. Most common soft tissue sarcoma = GI stromal tumor (GIST).
- Clinical features: Presents as gradually enlarging, painless mass. May have neuropathy or pain due to local compression. Common locations thigh/buttock/groin (46%) > torso (18%) > upper extremity or retroperitoneum (13% each).
- Diagnosis: Percutaneous core biopsy
- Staging: CT chest
- Treatment: Surgical excision if possible followed by radiation and chemotherapy (AIM = doxorubicin (**A**driamycin), **i**fosfamide, **m**esna). Consider neoadjuvant therapy for large tumors to shrink tumor before surgery. For metastatic disease, give chemotherapy and consider resection of metastatic sites if limited (metastasectomy).

Osteosarcoma

- Epidemiology: Rare bone tumor; many are secondary to other conditions in adults (e.g., Paget disease of bone)
- Clinical features: Localized bone pain; systemic symptoms are rare
- Diagnosis: MRI of suspected primary site, biopsy (open vs. core, coordinate location of biopsy with orthopedic surgeon)
- Staging: CT chest
- Treatment: Neoadjuvant chemotherapy (doxorubicin + cisplatin), surgical resection, and possibly radiation therapy. Chemotherapy for metastatic disease +/– metastasectomy.

Central Nervous System (CNS) Tumors

- Epidemiology:
  - In adults ≤30 yr, primary CNS tumors more common. See Table 7.7.
  - In adults >30 yr, brain metastases are more common (breast, lung, prostate, colorectal, melanoma)
- Clinical features: Small lesions can be asymptomatic. If symptomatic: Headache, signs of increased intracranial pressure (nausea/vomiting), new onset seizures, focal neurologic deficits.
- Diagnosis: MRI with contrast (much superior sensitivity than head CT). LP not typically needed unless concern for leptomeningeal disease (LMD). Tissue diagnosis via stereotactic biopsy vs. open surgery. Biopsy often not pursued for metastatic cancer with known primary site unless surgical resection is indicated for symptom-related reasons.
- Treatment: Glucocorticoids can reduce cerebral edema; then treatment depending on tumor type.

TABLE 7.7 · Primary Central Nervous System Tumors

Type of CNS tumor	Epidemiology	Imaging characteristics	Work-up / grading	Treatment
Low-grade gliomas	Most common primary CNS tumors in young adults	Can be well-circumscribed or more diffuse	WHO grade	• Maximal surgical resection +/− radiation therapy. • Can progress to high grade gliomas
Meningioma	Most common extra-axial tumor	Often have a "dural tail," helpful for diagnosis. Slow-growing, often incidentally noted.	WHO grade	• Small (<2cm), asymptomatic lesions can often be observed • If large or symptomatic, surgically resect if feasible • If too morbid to resect, consider radiation therapy
Primary CNS lymphoma	Biggest risk factor is HIV; associated with EBV in these patients.	CT: Hyperdense appearance MRI: Restricted water diffusion on diffusion-weighted sequences and homogeneous enhancement on post-contrast sequences	Avoid steroids prior to biopsy if possible – steroids are lympho-toxic and can make CNS lymphoma more difficult to diagnose.	• Not managed surgically • Highly sensitive to chemotherapy (high dose methotrexate) and radiation
Glioblastoma multiforme (GBM)	Most common in patients 50–70 yr. Grow rapidly, worst prognosis	Often identifiable on MRI, may cross the corpus collosum ("butterfly lesion")	Can often proceed to surgery without a biopsy if classic imaging findings	• Maximal safe surgical resection • Radiation +/− temozolomide (alkylating agent)

KEY MEDICATIONS & INTERVENTIONS

Chemotherapy

- Cell cycle non-specific phase: Activity not dependent upon the agent being available during a certain phase of the cell cycle. May administer over a shorter period of time, but may need higher drug concentration (peak). See gray box in Figure 7.8.
- Cell cycle–specific phase: Activity is primarily in one phase of the cell cycle. Often need to administer over a longer period of time. See green and blue boxes in Figure 7.8.

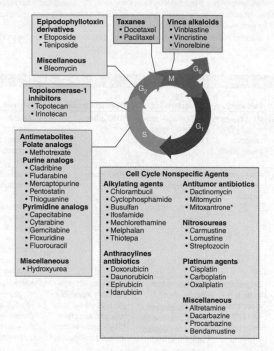

FIGURE 7.8: Cell cycle schematic and sensitivity to chemotherapeutic agents. The cell cycle is divided into several different phases, which can vary in length depending on the type and growth rate of the cell. The activity of different classes of chemotherapy agents are optimal at different phases of the cell cycle, whereas other types of chemotherapy are cell cycle non-specific. Shown above are examples of different chemotherapy classes and specific agents. *Mitoxantrone can be cell cycle specific at certain concentrations (e.g., primarily causes G2 arrest at lower concentrations but can cause both S and G2 arrest at higher concentrations).

Hormone Therapy

- Definition: Medications that suppress endogenous hormones that drive growth of certain tumor types (e.g., breast, prostate cancer)
- Examples:
  - Selective estrogen receptor modulators (SERMs): Tamoxifen used to treat hormone-receptor positive breast cancer
  - Aromatase inhibitors (AIs): Anastrozole, letrozole, exemestane. Used to treat hormone-receptor positive breast cancer
  - GnRH agonists: Leuprolide. Used for testosterone suppression in prostate cancer and ovarian suppression in breast cancer
  - GnRH antagonists: Degarelix
  - Selective androgen receptor antagonists: Flutamide, bicalutamide, enzalutamide, apalutamide
  - CYP17 inhibitors: Abiraterone blocks synthesis of androgens

Targeted Therapies

- Nomenclature:
  - Small molecule inhibitors end in "-inib"
  - Monoclonal antibodies end in "-mab"
- Tyrosine kinase inhibitors: Small molecule inhibitors, given orally
  - Imatinib (Gleevec), dasatinib: Bind to the inactive form of BCR-ABL and prevent activation. Used for treatment of CML.
  - Osimertinib, erlotinib: EGFR inhibitors used in NSCLC
  - Sorafenib, sunitinib: VEGF inhibitors used in HCC, RCC, thyroid
- Monoclonal antibodies: Given via infusion
  - Anti-HER2: Trastuzumab (Herceptin), pertuzumab (Perjeta) used in breast cancer. Trastuzumab also used in esophageal/gastric cancer.
  - Anti-CD20: Rituximab, targets B-cells, used in B-cell lymphomas
  - Anti-VEGF: Bevacizumab (Avastin), inhibits angiogenesis, used in colon cancer, RCC

Immunotherapy

- Mechanism: Checkpoint inhibitors enable the patient's own immune system to better target and destroy malignant cells by blocking the signals that turn the immune system off. In other words, they release the brakes on the immune response so that the immune system can more effectively fight malignancy (Figure 7.9).
- Indications: Approved for multiple types of cancer (e.g., melanoma, RCC, NSCLC, HCC, and now many more tumor types). PD-1 inhibitors are the first class of drugs with an FDA approval for a genetic pattern rather than an anatomical site (FDA approved for microsatellite instability [MSI]-high or mismatch repair deficient cancers and tumor mutational burden [TMB]-high cancers).
- Examples of checkpoint inhibitors by mechanism:
  - Anti-PD1
    - Nivolumab (Opdivo)
    - Pembrolizumab (Keytruda)
  - Anti-PD-L1
    - Atezolizumab (Tecentriq)
    - Avelumab (Bavencio)
    - Durvalumab (Imfinzi)
  - Anti-CTLA4
    - Ipilimumab (Yervoy)
- Side effects:
  - Immune-related adverse events (IRAEs): Autoimmune side effects due to excessive immune system activation
    - Most common: Thyroid disease, colitis, hepatitis, rashes
    - Less common but more serious: Hypophysitis, pneumonitis, myocarditis, myositis, neurologic autoimmune processes
  - Timing: IRAEs usually develop within the first few weeks to months after treatment initiation, but can occur at any time during or after treatment
  - Treatment: Depending on the grade of toxicity (See ASCO/NCCN guidelines), sometimes can treat through and other times need to stop immunotherapy and provide immunosuppression.

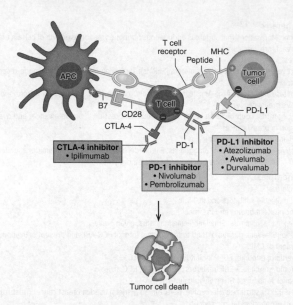

FIGURE 7.9: Mechanism of T cell activation and inhibition and the role of checkpoint inhibitor therapy. T cell activation is mediated by the interaction of the T cell receptor with the major histocompatibility complex (MHC) and the CD28 receptor with the B7 co-stimulatory molecule on the antigen presenting cell (APC). T cell inhibition is mediated by the interaction of PD-L1 and PD-1 as well as CTLA-4 and B7. Inhibitors of PD-1, PD-L1, and CTLA-4 prevent the inactivation of T cells, thus allowing the T cells to destroy the tumor cell more effectively. Activating interactions are noted with a (+) and inhibitory interactions are noted with a (−). Examples of check point inhibitors (CPIs) are listed above. Abbreviations: Antigen presenting cell (APC), major histocompatibility complex (MHC), programmed death receptor-1 (PD-1), programmed death receptor ligand-1 (PD-L1), cytotoxic T lymphocyte-associated protein 4 (CTLA-4).

KEY CLINICAL TRIALS & PUBLICATIONS

Breast Cancer

- **Extending aromatase-inhibitor adjuvant therapy to 10 yr.** *N Engl J Med* 2016;375:209–219.
  - Multicenter, double-blind, randomized placebo-controlled phase 3 clinical trial that randomized women with hormone-receptor positive early breast cancer to 5 yr of the aromatase inhibitor letrozole plus 5 yr of placebo vs. 10 yr of letrozole. Adjuvant aromatase inhibitor treatment for 10 yr resulted in significantly increased rates of disease-free survival and a lower incidence of contralateral breast cancer than those with placebo, but did not change overall survival.
- **Palbociclib and letrozole in advanced breast cancer.** *N Engl J Med* 2016;*375*(20):1925–1936.
  - Double-blind randomized phase 2 clinical trial that randomized 666 postmenopausal women with ER-positive, HER2-negative breast cancer, who had no prior treatment for advanced disease, to receive palbociclib (a small molecule cyclin-dependent kinase inhibitor) plus letrozole or placebo plus letrozole. The median progression-free survival was 24.8 months in the palbociclib–letrozole group, as compared with 14.5 months in the placebo–letrozole group.

Colon Cancer

- **Improved overall survival with oxaliplatin, fluorouracil, and leucovorin as adjuvant treatment in stage II or III colon cancer in the MOSAIC trial.** *J Clin Onc* 2009;27(19):3109–3116.
  - Multicenter, randomized phase 3 clinical trial that randomized patients with stage II and III colon to receive adjuvant 5-FU + leucovorin (LV5FU2) vs 5-FU+leucovorin+oxaliplatin (FOLFOX4). 5 yr disease-free survival (DFS) rates were 73.3% and 67.4% in the FOLFOX4 and LV5FU2 groups, respectively, and the addition of oxaliplatin to 5FU as adjuvant therapy also improved survival.

Esophageal Cancer

- **Preoperative chemoradiotherapy for esophageal or junctional cancer (CROSS trial).** *N Engl J Med* 2012;*366*(22), 2074–2084.
  - Multicenter randomized phase 3 clinical trial that randomized patients with resectable tumors to receive surgery alone or preoperative concurrent chemoradiation with weekly carboplatin/paclitaxel followed by surgery. Median overall survival was 49.4 months in the chemoradiation + surgery group versus 24.0 months in the surgery alone group.

Lung Cancer

- **Durvalumab after chemoradiotherapy in stage III non–small-cell lung cancer.** *N Engl J Med* 2017; 377(20):1919–1929.
  - Multicenter randomized phase 3 clinical trial that randomized patients with stage III non–small cell lung cancer (NSCLC) who underwent definitive chemoradiation to receive 1 yr of adjuvant therapy with the checkpoint inhibitor durvalumab vs. placebo. The addition of 1 yr of adjuvant durvalumab improved progression-free survival compared to placebo (16.8 vs. 5.6 months).
- **Pembrolizumab versus chemotherapy for PD-L1–positive non–small-cell lung cancer.** *N Engl J Med* 2016;375:1823–1833.
  - Multicenter, open-label phase 3 clinical trial that randomized patients with advanced NSCLC and PD-L1 expression of at least 50% of tumor cells and no sensitizing mutation of EGFR or ALK translocation to receive either pembrolizumab (at a fixed dose of 200 mg every 3 weeks) or the investigator's choice of platinum-based chemotherapy. Pembrolizumab treatment improved progression free survival (10.3 vs. 6.0 months) and was associated with fewer adverse events compared to platinum-based chemotherapy.
- **Osimertinib or platinum–pemetrexed in EGFR T790M–positive lung cancer.** *N Engl J Med* 2017;*376*(7):629–640.
  - Randomized, open-labeled, international phase 3 clinical trial that assigned 419 patients with T790M-positive advanced NSCLC, who had disease progression after first-line EGFR-TKI therapy to receive either the third generation EGFR-tyrosine kinase inhibitor osimertinib (80mg PO daily) or chemotherapy with IV pemetrexed and either carboplatin or cisplatin q3 weeks for up to six cycles. The median duration of progression-free survival was significantly longer with osimertinib than with pemetrexed plus platinum chemotherapy (10.1 months vs. 4.4 months, respectively).

Prostate Cancer

- **Chemohormonal therapy in metastatic hormone-sensitive prostate cancer.** *N Engl J Med* 2015;373(8):737–746.
  - Multicenter randomized phase 3 clinical trial that randomized patients with metastatic, hormone-sensitive prostate cancer to receive either androgen deprivation therapy (ADT) plus six cycles of docetaxel or ADT alone. At a median follow-up of 28.9 months, the median overall survival (OS) was 13.6 months longer with ADT plus docetaxel vs. ADT alone (57.6 months vs. 44.0 months).
- **Abiraterone for prostate cancer not previously treated with hormone therapy.** *N Engl J Med* 2017;377(4):338–351.
  - Multicenter randomized phase 3 clinical trial that randomized men with locally advanced or metastatic prostate cancer to receive ADT plus abiraterone and prednisolone vs. ADT alone. The addition of abiraterone was associated with significantly higher rates of overall and failure-free survival than ADT alone.

NOTES

Overview of Clinically Important Pathogens

TABLE 8.1 · Classification of Clinically Important Pathogens		
Type	**Classification**	**Clinically Important Examples**
Bacteria	Gram-positive:	
	Cocci	*Streptococcus* spp., *Staphylococcus* spp.
	Rods	*Bacillus* spp., *Clostridium* spp., *Listeria* spp.
	Gram-negative:	
	Cocci	*Neisseria* spp.
	Rods	*Escherichia coli, Klebsiella* spp., *Pseudomonas aeruginosa, Hemophilus* spp.
	Mycobacterium	*Mycobacterium tuberculosis*
	Spirochetes	*Treponema pallidum* (Syphilis), *Borrelia* spp., *Leptospira* spp.
	No cell wall	*Mycoplasma* spp.
Viruses	DNA viruses	Parvovirus, Papillomavirus (HPV), Adenovirus, Herpesvirus, Hepadnavirus (Hepatitis B)
	RNA viruses	Picornavirus, Hepevirus (Hepatitis E), Calicivirus (norovirus), Retrovirus (HIV), Orthomyxovirus (influenza), Coronavirus
Fungi	Yeasts	*Candida* spp., *Cryptococcus* spp.
	Dimorphics	*Coccidioides* spp., *Histoplasma* spp., *Blastomyces* spp., *Paracoccidioides* spp.
	Molds	*Aspergillus* spp., *Mucor* spp., *Rhizopus* spp.
Parasites	GI infections	*Giardia lamblia, Entamoeba histolytica, Cryptosporidium parvum*
	CNS infections	*Toxoplasma gondii, Naegleria fowleri*
	Hematologic infections	*Plasmodium* spp., *Babesia* spp.
	Sexually transmitted diseases	*Trichomonas vaginalis*
Helminths	Nematodes (roundworms)	*Enterobius vermicularis, Strongyloides stercoralis, Toxocara canis*
	Cestodes (tapeworms)	*Taenia solium, Echinococcus granulosus*
	Trematodes (flukes)	*Schistosoma* spp., *Clonorchis sinensis*

Adapted from: *Medical Microbiology & Immunology: A Guide to Clinical Infectious Diseases, 15e* Warren Levinson, Peter Chin-Hong, Elizabeth A. Joyce, Jesse Nussbaum, and Brian Schwartz (NY: McGraw-Hill Education, 2018).

Bacterial Infections

Gram-positive bacteria

TABLE 8.2 · Key Clinically Relevant Gram-Positive Bacteria

Gram-Positive		Organism	Clinical Symptoms/Key Associations
Cocci		Staphylococcus aureus	• Skin/soft tissue infections, septic arthritis, osteomyelitis, pneumonia, endocarditis, meningitis • Toxin-mediated: Toxic shock syndrome, scalded skin syndrome, food poisoning • Can be methicillin sensitive (MSSA) or methicillin resistant (MRSA). Culture and determine sensitivities. Cover for MRSA empirically up-front with IV vancomycin in hospitalized patients.
		Staphylococcus epidermidis	• Skin flora – can be a contaminant in culture or can be a true pathogen
		Streptococcus pneumoniae	• Meningitis, pneumonia, sinusitis, otitis media
		Streptococcus pyogenes (Group A strep)	• Skin/soft tissue infection, pharyngitis • Toxin-mediated: Toxic shock syndrome, scarlet fever, necrotizing fasciitis • Immune-mediated: Rheumatic fever, post-strep glomerulonephritis
		Streptococcus agalactiae (Group B strep)	• Meningitis, pneumonia, sepsis in babies
		Streptococcus bovis	• GI flora that can penetrate into the bloodstream and cause subacute bacterial endocarditis in the setting of colon cancer or IBD
		Enterococcus spp.	• UTI, biliary infection, subacute bacterial endocarditis • Infections associated with indwelling lines and catheters • Enterococcus faecium is often vancomycin resistant (VRE)
Rods	Spore-forming, aerobic	Bacillus cereus	• Pre-formed toxin that contaminates rice, causes diarrhea
		Bacillus anthracis	• Black painless ulcer, flu-like, lethal
	Spore-forming, anerobic	Clostridium tetani	• Wound gets infected, bacteria travels up neuron, can lead to spastic paralysis, trismus (lockjaw), risus sardonicus (spasm of facial muscles, appears like a grin)
		Clostridium botulinum	• Preformed toxin in canned food, leads to flaccid paralysis
		Clostridium perfringens	• Wound gets infected, can lead to muscle necrosis. Can also get food-borne disease that causes watery diarrhea
		Clostridium difficile	• Common nosocomial infection, but can also be acquired in the community • Watery diarrhea or, in severe cases, toxic megacolon
	Nonfilamentous non-spore forming	Corynebacterium diphtheria	• Diphtheria
		Listeria monocytogenes	• Poorly pasteurized milk/soft cheeses → penetrates GI track and causes gastroenteritis • Can cause meningitis in immunocompromised hosts and those over age 50 yr
	Filamentous non-spore forming	Actinomyces israelii	• Normally colonizes GI/GU tract, can infect intrauterine devices (IUDs), can cause abscesses
		Nocardia spp.	• Causes pulmonary infections and, less frequently, brain abscesses in immunocompromised hosts

Gram-negative bacteria

TABLE 8.3 · Key Clinically Relevant Gram-Negative Bacteria			
Gram-Negative		**Organism**	**Clinical Symptoms/Key Associations**
Cocci		*Neisseria gonorrhoeae*	· Sexually transmitted disease. Can cause vaginal discharge, pelvic inflammatory disease, septic arthritis, dermatitis, tenosynovitis, migratory polyarthritis, and Fitz-Hugh-Curtis syndrome (liver capsule inflammation from ascending GU infection)
		Neisseria meningitidis	· Meningitis
Rods	Facultative, straight	*Haemophilus influenzae*	· Encapsulated organism · Pneumonia, meningitis, otitis media, epiglottis
		Coxiella burnetti	· Flu-like illness, pneumonia, granulomatous hepatitis, culture-negative endocarditis
		Legionella pneumophilia	· Grows in water tanks, can cause severe pneumonia, GI symptoms, CNS symptoms. Can also cause hyponatremia, diarrhea, encephalopathy · Dx: Urine antigen test for legionella (only tests for certain, common serovars), culture on legionella specific media, or PCR
		Brucella	· Brucellosis; cheese, goat/cow exposure → fever, osteomyelitis, or endocarditis
		Bartonella henselae	· Cat scratch → regional lymph node enlargement, granulomas, fever · In patients with HIV, can cause a vascular proliferative form that has a similar morphology as Kaposi's sarcoma, known as bacillary angiomatosis
		Francisella tularensis	· Tularemia; Results from animal or rural exposure. Different forms of infection, including ulceroglandular (skin lesions and associated adenopathy), glandular (regional adenopathy), oropharyngeal (pharyngitis, neck swelling), pneumonic (fever, cough), typhoidal (systemic febrile illness without localizing features), among others
		Yersinia pestis	· Plague
		Escherichia coli	· Urinary tract infection, diarrhea (ETEC; EHEC – associated with HUS)
		Enterobacter	· Urinary tract infection, nosocomial infections
		Klebsiella	· Urinary tract infection, pneumonia, liver abscess
		Shigella	· Enterocolitis – diarrhea, can be bloody or watery
		Salmonella	· Enterocolitis – diarrhea, can be bloody. Can cause osteomyelitis in individuals with sickle cell disease. · *Salmonella typhi*: Can cause typhoid fever – high fever, headache, constipation > diarrhea, hepatosplenomegaly, and rash (rose spots)
		Proteus	· Urinary tract infection
	Facultative, curved	*Helicobacter pylori*	· Gastritis, peptic ulcer disease
		Campylobacter jejuni	· Enterocolitis – diarrhea, can be bloody
		Vibrio cholera	· Cholera, profuse watery diarrhea
	Aerobic	*Pseudomonas aeruginosa*	· Pneumonia, urinary tract infection, nosocomial infections
	Anerobic	*Bacteroides*	· Peritonitis

Other bacteria

TABLE 8.4 · Key Clinically Relevant Other Bacteria		
Class	**Organism**	**Clinical Symptoms/Key Associations**
Acid-fast	*Mycobacterium tuberculosis* (MTB)	• Primary tuberculosis: Lung disease or extra-pulmonary disease • Secondary tuberculosis: Reactivation in the upper lobes, extra-pulmonary TB (lymphadenitis, pleural TB, meningitis, vertebral osteomyelitis)
	Mycobacterium avium-intracellulare (MAC)	• Pneumonia, especially if pre-existing lung disease • Disseminated infection in patients with HIV and CD4 <50 cells/μL
	Mycobacterium leprae	• Skin and superficial nerves
Obligate intracellular parasites	*Rickettsia*	• Rocky Mountain spotted fever, typhus
	Chlamydia	• Sexually transmitted infection • Urethritis, psittacosis, lymphogranuloma venereum (LGV)

Spirochetes	*Treponema pallidum*	• Syphilis
		  - 1° – painless lesion (chancre) with firm, indurated rim
		  - 2° – disseminated phase with constitutional symptoms, rash that may involve the palms/soles
		  - 3° – gummas (granulomas); tabes dorsalis (dorsal column spinal cord – loss of pain/sensation/position sense), Argyll Robertson pupil; aortitis; Charcot joint
		  - Neurosyphilis/otosyphilis: Can occur any time after initial infection Symptoms include headache, vision changes, nausea, hearing loss. May have isolated eye symptoms with normal LP (this still warrants neurosyphilis treatment)

	Leptospira interrogans	• Leptospirosis – flu-like symptoms, jaundice, photophobia, conjunctivitis

	Borrelia burgdorferi	• Lyme disease. Transmitted by the *Ixodes* tick
		  - Early localized – erythema migrans ("bulls eye" rash), systemic symptoms
		  - Early disseminated – Bell's palsy, cardiac involvement
		  - Late – CNS involvement, arthritis

No cell wall	*Mycoplasma*	• Community acquired pneumonia

Viral Infections

DNA viruses

TABLE 8.5 • Key Clinically Relevant DNA Viruses

Virus Family	Envelope	Capsid Symmetry	DNA Structure	Clinically Important Viruses and Clinical Symptoms/Key Associations
Adenovirus	No	Icosahedral	DS linear	• **Adenovirus:** Pharyngitis, conjunctivitis (pink eye), UTIs
Parvovirus	No	Icosahedral	SS linear	• **Parvo B19 virus:** – Aplastic crisis in patients with sickle cell disease or those that are immunocompromised – Adult with RA-like symptoms and exposure to children – Fifth Disease in kids: "Slapped cheek rash", anemia – RBC destruction in fetus, which can lead to hydrops fetalis and fetal death
Papillomavirus	No	Icosahedral	DS circular	• **Human Papillomavirus (HPV):** Warts; can lead to cervical/anal squamous cell carcinoma
Herpesvirus	Yes	Icosahedral	DS linear	• **Herpes simplex virus (HSV)-1:** – Transmitted via respiratory secretions/saliva, and then can become latent in the trigeminal ganglia. – 1° Oral lesions (can also cause genital herpes) – 2° Reactivation: Cold sores, temporal lobe encephalitis, keratoconjunctivitis (inflammation of cornea), recurrent genital herpes • **Herpes simplex virus (HSV)-2:** – Most common cause of genital herpes. Transmitted during sexual contact with infected areas, usually when active lesions are present, but can also happen during asymptomatic periods – 1°: Painful genital ulcers, fever, tender inguinal adenopathy, or headache. Some are minimally symptomatic or asymptomatic. Symptoms last 2–3 weeks. – 2°: Recurrences of infection are often less severe than primary infections. Duration of symptoms is often shorter, as well (e.g., 10 days). • **VZV:** – Acquired through respiratory tract, and then can infect the dorsal root ganglion or trigeminal nerves – Primary = Chickenpox: Starts on trunk, and causes a vesicular and pruritic rash – Reactivation = Zoster (shingles): Usually in elderly or immunocompromised hosts – Lesion on side or tip of nose (Hutchinson's sign) warrants ophthalmologic evaluation for eye involvement (risk of retinal necrosis) – Increased risk of stroke (VZV vasculopathy) after shingles reactivation, especially if cranial nerve involvement

(Continued)

TABLE 8.5 • Key Clinically Relevant DNA Viruses *(Continued)*

Virus Family	Envelope	Capsid Symmetry	DNA Structure	Clinically Important Viruses and Clinical Symptoms/Key Associations

Herpesvirus (continued)	Yes	Icosahedral	DS linear	• **EBV:**
				  – **Mononucleosis:** Fever, cervical lymphadenopathy, hepatosplenomegaly, pharyngitis
				    • *Diagnosis:* May have positive heterophile antibody for EBV (no longer recommended by CDC given low sensitivity and specificity), serology, peripheral blood smear (large atypical lymphocytes)
				    • *Treatment:* Self-resolving (rest, fluids, avoid contact sports due to risk of splenic rupture)
				    • *Complications:* Thrombocytopenia/hemolytic anemia, hepatitis, HLH (rare), splenic rupture (rare), meningoencephalitis (rare)
				  – **Malignancies:** Burkitt's lymphoma, Hodgkin's lymphoma, nasopharyngeal carcinoma. Associated with latent stage
				• **CMV:**
				  – Immunocompetent: Mild mononucleosis-like syndrome (negative Heterophile antibody)
				  – Immunocompromised: Encephalitis, retinitis, esophagitis, colitis, hepatitis
				  – Maternal–fetal transmission: Mother usually asymptomatic; Baby: Hearing loss, seizures, rash characterized by cutaneous hemorrhage
				• **HHV-6: Roseola:** Infant with fever, seizures, rash (follows fever by several days)
				• **HHV-8:** Kaposi's sarcoma (patients with HIV), Multicentric Castleman's Disease (an HHV-8 associated lymphoproliferative disorder)

Polyomavirus	No	Icosahedral	DS circular	• **JC Virus:** Progressive multifocal leukoencephalopathy (PML) in patients with HIV • **BK Virus:** Typically occurs in transplant patients; commonly targets the kidney
Hepadnavirus	Yes	Icosahedral	DS partial circular	• **Hepatitis B virus (HBV)**
Poxvirus	Yes	Complex	DS linear	• **Smallpox:** Eradicated by live attenuated vaccine • **Molluscum contagiosum:** Umbilicated warts. Transmitted by direct skin-skin contact (e.g., wrestling)

RNA viruses

TABLE 8.6 · Key Clinically Relevant RNA Viruses				
Virus family	Envelope	Capsid Symmetry	RNA Structure	Clinically Important Viruses and Clinical Symptoms/Key Associations
Reovirus	No	Icosahedral	DS linear	· **Rotavirus:** Diarrhea
Picornavirus	No	Icosahedral	SS linear	· **Poliovirus:** Aseptic meningitis, flaccid paralysis · **Echovirus:** Aseptic meningitis · **Rhinovirus:** "Common cold" · **Coxsackievirus:** Hand-foot-mouth disease, myocarditis, encephalitis · **Hepatitis A Virus (HAV)**
Hepevirus	No	Icosahedral	SS linear	· **Hepatitis E Virus (HEV)**
Caliciviruses	No	Icosahedral	SS linear	· **Norovirus:** Viral gastroenteritis
Flaviviruses	Yes	Icosahedral	SS linear	· **Yellow fever:** Transmitted by the Aedes mosquito. Causes fever, nausea/vomiting, jaundice. · **Hepatitis C Virus (HCV)** · **Dengue:** Transmitted by the *Aedes* mosquito. Causes "breakbone" fever, joint aches. · **West Nile virus:** Transmitted by the *Culex* mosquito. Can cause fever, encephalitis, flaccid paralysis.
Togaviruses	Yes	Icosahedral	SS linear	· **Rubella:** Respiratory droplets. Causes post-auricular lymphadenopathy, rash, can be transmitted maternal–fetal. · **Eastern Equine Encephalitis** · **Western Equine Encephalitis**
Retroviruses	Yes	Icosahedral	SS linear	· **HIV** · **HTLV:** Can cause T-cell leukemia
Coronaviruses	Yes	Helical	SS linear	· **SARS-CoV-2 (COVID-19):** Novel coronavirus that causes fever, respiratory compromise, leukopenia
Orthomyxoviruses	Yes	Helical	SS linear	· **Influenza virus**
Paramyxoviruses	Yes	Helical	SS linear	· **Parainfluenza:** Croup, seal-like barking cough · **RSV:** Bronchiolitis, commonly causes wheezing in babies/toddlers · **Measles:** Cough, cold, conjunctivitis. Kolpik spots (red spots with blue-white center on buccal mucosa), then maculopapular rash including on palms/soles. Sequalae: Encephalitis years later with personality change, myoclonic jerks, blindness. · **Mumps:** Swollen neck/parotid glands (parotitis), orchitis (inflamed testes), pancreatitis
Rhabdoviruses	Yes	Helical	SS linear	· **Rabies:** Transmitted by bats, mammals; virus travels in retrograde fashion up nerve roots and causes fever, agitation, photophobia, hydrophobia. Can progress to paralysis and death.
Filoviruses	Yes	Helical	SS linear	· **Ebola hemorrhagic fever:** Often fatal. Initial syndrome includes abrupt onset febrile syndrome accompanied by malaise, headache, vomiting, and diarrhea. Patients may also have a diffuse, erythematous macular rash, and mucosal bleeding. Many progress to multi-organ failure and significant hemorrhage, with case fatality rates that approach 90%.

(Continued)

INFECTIOUS DISEASES

TABLE 8.6 · Key Clinically Relevant RNA Viruses (*Continued*)				
Virus family	**Envelope**	**Capsid Symmetry**	**RNA Structure**	**Clinically Important Viruses and Clinical Symptoms/Key Associations**
Arenaviruses	Yes	Helical	SS circular	• **Lymphocytic choriomeningitis virus (LCMV):** A rodent-borne virus transmitted to humans via exposure to secretions or excretions from infected animals. Patients develop a flu-like illness with headache and meningitis. WBC counts in CSF are often > 1,000 cells/μL. • **Lassa fever encephalitis:** Transmitted by rodents
Bunyaviruses	Yes	Helical	SS circular	• **Hantavirus:** Rodent feces in the Southwest US → hemorrhagic fever, pneumonia, respiratory failure, can cause death
Delta virus	Yes	Uncertain	SS circular	• **Hepatitis D virus (HDV):** Requires HBV for infection

Fungal Infections
Systemic fungal infections

TABLE 8.7 · Key Clinically Relevant Systemic Fungal Infections			
Genus	**Morphology in Tissue**	**Geographic Distribution**	**Clinical Information**
Coccidioides	Spherule	Southwestern US (CA, AZ), Latin America	• *Symptoms*: Typically starts as a pulmonary infection. Can disseminate to the bone, joints, meninges, skin. • *Diagnosis*: Serology (cocci immunodiffusion and complement fixation), culture, cocci antigen (in CNS) • *Treatment*: Fluconazole. If disseminated, IV liposomal amphotericin sometimes needed.
Histoplasmosis	Yeasts inside of macrophages	Mississippi/Ohio River Valley	• *Symptoms*: Cavitary lung lesions, granulomas in the liver and spleen, skin (wart-like microabscesses), bones (lytic lesions), prostate • *Diagnosis*: Histo urine antigen (in disseminated infection), serology (for localized pulmonary disease) • *Treatment*: Itraconazole; if severe, requires liposomal amphotericin B
Blastomyces	Yeasts with single broad-based buds	Southeastern US, Central America	• *Symptoms*: Inflammatory lung lesions, ulcerated skin lesions • *Diagnosis*: Visualize tissue with broad-based buds, antigen testing • *Treatment*: Itraconazole; if severe, requires liposomal amphotericin B
Paracoccidioides	Yeasts with multiple buds	Latin America	• *Symptoms*: Pneumonia or calcified lung mass, ulcerated oral mucosal lesions • *Diagnosis*: Culture • *Treatment*: Itraconazole; if severe, requires liposomal amphotericin B

Opportunistic fungal infections

	Morphology in	Geographic	
TABLE 8.8 • Key Clinically Relevant Opportunistic Fungal Infections			
Genus	**Tissue**	**Distribution**	**Clinical Features**

Candida	Yeast forms hyphae and pseudo hyphae	Worldwide	• *Symptoms*:
			  - <u>Vaginal</u>: "yeast infection" – thick cottage cheese–like vaginal discharge, itchy but not painful. Tx: Topical azole cream
			  - <u>UTI</u>: True UTI is rare, very common in catheterized patients, most often is asymptomatic candiduria
			  - <u>Mouth/oropharynx</u>: "thrush," thick white plaques, painless, check HIV. Tx: Clotrimazole 5×/day, nystatin mouth wash, fluconazole
			  - <u>Esophagitis</u>: White plaques that scrape off; Odynophagia. Tx: Fluconazole
			  - <u>Cutaneous</u>: Erythematous eroded patches with satellite lesions in folds of obese diabetic patients. Tx: Nystatin powder
			  - <u>Bacteremia</u>: Candidemia is *never* a contaminant; remove lines, GI exam. Tx: IV echinocandin pending speciation/sensitivities
			• *Diagnosis*: Clinical; KOH prep shows yeast, Germ test tube in animal serum shows pseudohyphae for *C albicans* and *C dubliniensis*, low pH

Crypto-coccus	Yeast with large capsule	Worldwide	• *Pathogenesis*: Pigeon droppings → inhale → hematogenous spread • *Risk factors*: HIV (CD4 <50 cells/μL), immunosuppressed patients • *Symptoms*: Pulmonary disease, meningitis with elevated opening pressure • *Diagnosis*: Serum cryptococcal antigen (CrAg), LP – detect cryptococcal antigen, often elevated opening pressure • *Treatment*: Fluconazole 6–12 mos (longer if HIV, treat until CD4 100 cells/μL for 3 mos). Amphotericin B + Flucytosine induction therapy if meningitis.

Aspergil-lus	Mold with narrow angle branching, septate hyphae	Worldwide	• *Symptoms*:
			  - <u>Allergic bronchopulmonary aspergillosis (ABPA)</u>: Type I hypersensitivity reaction; causes difficult to control asthma, eosinophilia, +IgE. Tx: Steroids, +/− azoles
			  - <u>Aspergilloma</u>: Fungus ball. Occurs in pre-existing pulmonary cyst (e.g., TB, bronchiectasis, sarcoid). Causes chronic cough, hemoptysis. Tx: May need surgical removal, +/− azoles
			  - <u>Invasive aspergillosis</u>: Invades lungs, sinuses, brain in immunocompromised pts (neutropenia, solid organ transplant, steroids). Tx: Voriconazole.
			• *Diagnosis*: Serum galactomannan is a polysaccharide in the Aspergillus cell wall; Beta-D-glucan is positive but not specific.

Mucor & Rhizopus	Mold with 90-degree angle branching, non-septate hyphae	Worldwide	• *Symptoms*: Invades blood vessels and causes a necrotic lesion, look for "reverse halo sign" on chest CT • *Treatment*: Liposomal amphotericin, surgical debridement

Parasitic Infections

Protozoa infections

Protozoa are single celled parasites under the parent category of parasites.

TABLE 8.9 · Key Clinically Relevant Protozoa		
Organism	**Transmission**	**Clinical Features**
GI Infections		
Giardia lamblia	Ingestion of cysts in water (e.g., while camping, hiking) or person-to-person (e.g., at daycare) → infects small intestine	Giardiasis: Foul-smelling fatty diarrhea
Entamoeba histolytica	Ingestion of cysts in water, especially in tropical locations → infects large intestine, liver	Invades GI tract → bloody diarrhea, ulcers, liver abscess, RUQ pain
Cryptosporidium parvum	Ingestion of cysts in water → infects GI tract	Diarrhea, can be particularly severe in immunocompromised patients
CNS Infections		
Toxoplasma gondii	Ingestion of cysts in poorly cooked pork, cat feces → CNS infection	Rim-enhancing brain lesion(s) Maternal–fetal transmission: Can cause chorioretinitis, hydrocephalus, intracranial calcification in infant
Naegleria fowleri	Swimming in a fresh water lake → CNS infection	Rapidly fatal meningoencephalitis
Trypanosoma brucei *Trypanosoma gambiense* *Trypanosoma rhodesiense*	Tsetse fly (painful bite)	African sleeping sickness: Enlarged lymph nodes (Winterbottom's sign), recurring fever, personality changes, somnolence, coma
Hematologic Infections		

Plasmodium
     P. vivax/ovale
     P. falciparum
     P. malariae
	Mosquito (*Anopheles*)	Malaria: Fever, anemia, splenomegaly

Babesia	*Ixodes* tick in the Northeastern US (same *B. burgdorferi*)	Babesiosis: Fever and hemolytic anemia, increased risk if asplenia. Most common transfusion-related infection.
Visceral Infections		
Trypanosoma cruzi	Reduviid bug (painless bite) in South America	Chagas' disease: Dilated cardiomyopathy, megacolon and megaesophagus, unilateral eye swelling at time of bite (Romaña's sign)
Leishmania donovani	Sandfly	Visceral leishmaniasis: Lesions on face and skin, round belly, spiking fevers, hepatosplenomegaly, pancytopenia
Sexually Transmitted Disease		
Trichomonas vaginalis	Sexual transmission	Vaginitis: Foul-smelling frothy yellow/green discharge

Helminthic infections

Helminth are multicellular worms under the parent category of parasites.

TABLE 8.10 · Key Clinically Relevant Helminthic Infections		
Organism	**Transmission**	**Clinical Features**
Nematodes (roundworms) – Intestinal		
Enterobius vermicularis (Pinworm)	Food contaminated with eggs	Intestinal infection with perianal itching in children (Scotch tape test)
Ascaris lumbricoides (Giant white roundworm)	Fecal–oral; eggs, and sometimes worms, visible in feces under the microscope	Eggs hatch in duodenum; migrate through the lungs and cause pneumonitis; then swallowed and mature in the GI tract; can also cause obstruction of the biliary or GI tract
Strongyloides stercoralis	Larvae in soil penetrate skin	Intestinal infection: Vomiting, diarrhea, anemia Disseminated infection: Pulmonary symptoms (ranging from cough to ARDS), cutaneous symptoms (rash on the thighs, buttocks or widespread purpura/petechiae), GI symptoms (abdominal pain, GI bleed, obstruction)
Ancylostoma duodenale Necator americanus (Hookworm)	Larvae in feces penetrate skin	Intestinal infection: Can cause microcytic anemia by sucking blood from intestinal walls
Nematodes (roundworms) – Tissue		
Dracunculus medinensis	Drinking water with copepods	Migrate down leg (painful), then cause skin inflammation/ulcers
Onchocerca volvulus	Female blackfly bite	Hyperpigmented skin, river blindness
Loa Loa	Deer fly, horse fly, mango fly	Swelling in skin, worm in conjunctiva
Wuchereria bancrofti	Female mosquito	Blocks lymphatic vessels; elephantitis
Toxocara canis	Food contaminated with eggs	Visceral larva migrans
Cestodes (Tapeworms)		
Taenia solium	Ingestion of larvae in under-cooked pork Central America, Southeast Asia	Larvae: Intestinal infection Eggs: Neurocysticercosis → brain cysts + seizures
Diphyllobothrium latum	Consumption of fresh water or raw fish. (Scandinavia, the former Soviet Union, and Japan)	Most patients are asymptomatic. The classic manifestation is vitamin B12 deficiency and megaloblastic anemia. This is due to the organisms' competition with the host for vitamin B12 absorption.
Echinococcus granulosus	Ingestion of eggs in dog feces	Cysts in liver: Anaphylaxis if antigens are released (surgeon should pre-inject ethanol to kill cysts before removal)
Trematodes (Flukes)		
Schistosoma S. haematobium S. mansoni	Snails are host; Penetrate skin → liver → bladder	"Swimmer's itch," fever. Eggs become lodged in the liver and spleen, evoking an immune response and leading to the development of hepatic granulomas and fibrosis in some patients *S. haematobium* – hematuria, bladder cancer *S. mansoni* – non-cirrhotic portal HTN
Clonorchis sinensis (Chinese Liver Fluke)	Undercooked fish, Southeast Asia	Biliary tract inflammation, which can cause recurrent pyogenic cholangitis, pigmented gallstones. Associated with cholangiocarcinoma.
Paragonimus westermani	Undercooked crab meat	Lung inflammation

APPROACHES & CHIEF COMPLAINTS

TABLE 8.11 · An Approach to Diagnosing and Treating Infectious Diseases	
Phase of Clinical Decision-making	**Approach**

Define the illness	Host:
	• Different individuals, depending on their age, exposure history, prior infections, and immune status, are at risk for different types of infections.
	• An understanding of the host allows us to better understand the organisms to which they are most susceptible.
	Tempo:
	• Different pathogens cause different tempos of illness. Labeling the illness tempo will help us determine with more precision which infections are more or less likely.
	• Generally, we can label the time course as acute (from hours/days to 1 week), subacute (weeks to months), and chronic (months to years).
	Clinical syndrome:
	• Define the clinical syndrome (e.g., pneumonia or cholangitis).
	Putting it together:
	• The first step in a suspected infection is to frame the patient based on these three features, for example:
	  - An individual with HIV and a CD4 112 cells/μL presents with subacute onset of fever and cough.
	  - An elderly person with hypertension presents with acute onset fever and cough.
	• While these two individuals have a similar clinical syndrome, the potential organisms that cause this syndrome vary based on the host (individual with HIV vs. elderly immunocompetent person) and tempo (weeks vs. days).

Select an empiric therapy	• Many infections have a high morbidity and mortality early in the course of illness when there is still diagnostic ambiguity. Therefore, we often start antimicrobial therapy prior to identifying the definitive pathogen(s). Most suspected infections that require hospitalization warrant empiric antibiotic therapy. • Based on the host, tempo, and clinical syndrome, generate a list of possible and probable pathogens, which guides empiric antibiotic therapy. • See Table 8.12 for empiric antibiotic regimens for commonly encountered infections.
Finalize the management plan	Targeted antibiotics and duration of therapy: • Targeted antibiotics depend on the antimicrobial susceptibilities of the identified organism(s) • The duration of therapy depends on the type of infection Source control: Source control is a key step in controlling any infection. Niduses for ongoing infection include: • Indwelling catheters • Infected fluid pockets (e.g., an abscess or effusion) • Obstructed organs (e.g., pyelonephritis with an obstructing stone or cholangitis)

TABLE 8.12 • Empiric Antibiotic Regimens for Hospitalized Immunocompetent Patients

Clinical Syndrome	Common Pathogen(s)	Possible Empiric Antibiotic Regimen* (all are required unless indicated with OR or +/−)	Comments
Meningitis (community onset, age <50 yr and no immuno-compromising condition)	**Bacteria:** • *Streptococcus pneumoniae* • *Neisseria meningitidis* • Group B Streptococcus • *Hemophilus influenzae* **Viruses:** • HSV1 • VZV	• vancomycin • ceftriaxone (2 g IV q12hr) • +/− acyclovir (if HSV encephalitis is suspected) • +/− adjunctive corticosteroids (dexamethasone 0.15 mg/kg q6hr)	• Perform a lumbar puncture (LP) to confirm the diagnosis • Do not delay empiric antibiotics if the LP is delayed • Immunocompromising conditions include HIV, solid organ or bone marrow transplant, neutropenia, immunosuppressive therapy, etc. • Both antibiotics and antivirals are used in some cases where there is overlap of meningitis and encephalitis symptoms (e.g., neck stiffness, headache, *and* profound confusion) • Vancomycin is used in acute bacterial meningitis to empirically cover ceftriaxone-resistant *S. pneumoniae*. Note that ceftriaxone dosing is higher to achieve adequate CNS penetration • Add coverage for *Listeria monocytogenes* with ampicillin for patients >50 yr or immunocompromised patients • If *S. pneumoniae* meningitis is suspected, give dexamethasone 10 mg PO/IV q6hr ×4 days prior to initial dose of antibiotics (decreases mortality and rate of hearing loss or other neurologic complications)
Meningitis (age >50 yr or immuno-compromising condition)	See above, plus: • *Listeria monocytogenes* • Gram-negative rods (e.g., *E. coli*)	• vancomycin • ceftriaxone (2g IV q12hr) • ampicillin (2g IV q4hr) • +/− acyclovir (if HSV encephalitis is suspected) • +/− adjunctive corticosteroids (dexamethasone 0.15 mg/kg q6hr)	

(Continued)

INFECTIOUS DISEASES

TABLE 8.12 · Empiric Antibiotic Regimens for Hospitalized Immunocompetent Patients (*Continued*)

Clinical Syndrome	Common Pathogen(s)	Possible Empiric Antibiotic Regimen* (all are required unless indicated with OR or +/–)	Comments

Community Acquired Pneumonia (CAP)	**Common pathogens:**
	• *S. pneumoniae*
	• *Mycoplasma pneumoniae*
	• *Chlamydia pneumoniae*
	• *H. influenzae*
	• *Legionella pneumophilia*
	• *Klebsiella pneumoniae*
	
	Respiratory viruses:
	• Influenza
	• RSV
	• Rhinovirus
	• Sars-cov-2
	
	Other pathogens to consider:
	• *S. aureus*
	• *Pseudomonas aeruginosa*
		Immunocompetent patient admitted to the medical ward:
		• ceftriaxone (1 g IV daily) OR cefepime (if risk factors for *P. aeruginosa*)
		• doxycycline (100 mg PO/IV q12hr) OR azithromycin (500 mg PO/IV daily)
		
		Immunocompetent patient admitted to the ICU:
		• vancomycin
		• ceftriaxone (1g IV daily) OR cefepime (if risk factors for *P. aeruginosa*)
		• azithromycin (500 mg IV daily)
			• Empirically treat with or broaden to vancomycin (to cover MRSA pneumonia), and cefepime (to add pseudomonal coverage) if the patient has risk factors or is severely ill/clinically worsening after 48–72 hours of therapy.
			• Risk factors for CAP from *P. aeruginosa*:
			  - Structural lung disease (e.g., bronchiectasis)
			  - Prior respiratory isolation of *P. aeruginosa*
			  - Recent hospitalization and receipt of IV antibiotics in the last 90 days
			• Risk factors for CAP from MRSA:
			  - Necrotizing pneumonia
			  - Co-existing empyema
			  - Known colonization or prior infection with MRSA
			  - Post-influenza pneumonia
			  - Injection drug use
			  - HIV/AIDS
			• Get influenza testing and give oseltamivir during flu season until testing returns.
			• Consider viral panel testing to evaluate for other respiratory viral pathogens including COVID-19 in those who are critically ill or immunocompromised.
			• Anaerobic coverage (e.g., with metronidazole) is only needed in: pulmonary abscesses, necrotizing pneumonia, empyema. It is NOT needed for suspected aspiration pneumonia.

Hospital-Acquired Pneumonia/ Ventilator Associated Pneumonia	• *P. aeruginosa*
	• *Klebsiella* spp.
	• *E. coli*
	• *Enterobacter* spp.
	• Multidrug-resistant Gram-negative rods (e.g., ESBL-producing organisms)
	• *S. aureus*
		• vancomycin
		• cefepime OR piperacillin-tazobactam
		• +/– a 2nd Gram-negative agent (e.g., ciprofloxacin). See comments.
			• Double cover for Gram-negative organisms in patients who are critically ill with risk factors for multidrug-resistant organisms such as:
			  - Septic shock
			  - Development of pneumonia >5 days after hospitalization
			  - ARDS
			  - Renal replacement therapy

(Continued)

TABLE 8.12 · Empiric Antibiotic Regimens for Hospitalized Immunocompetent Patients (Continued)			
Clinical Syndrome	Common Pathogen(s)	Possible Empiric Antibiotic Regimen* (all are required unless indicated with OR or +/–)	Comments
Spontaneous bacterial peritonitis (SBP)	· E. coli · Klebsiella spp. · Streptococci spp.	· ceftriaxone (1g IV daily)	· Sample peritoneal fluid and obtain gram stain
Secondary bacterial peritonitis; intra-abdominal abscess	· E. coli · Klebsiella spp. · B. fragilis · Streptococcus spp.	· ertapenem (1 g IV daily) OR piperacillin/tazobactam (3.375 g IV q6hr–4.5g IV q6hr) · +/– vancomycin (if critically ill)	· Secondary bacterial peritonitis is often polymicrobial · Identification of secondary bacterial peritonitis should prompt evaluation for a bowel perforation

Urinary Tract Infections	· E. coli far and away the most common cause	**Asymptomatic bacteriuria:** No treatment needed unless special scenarios (see comments)
		
		Pyelonephritis:
		· ceftriaxone (1g IV daily) OR ertapenem (if risk factors for ESBL-producing organisms)
			· Do not need to treat asymptomatic bacteriuria in most cases (exceptions: pregnant woman, kidney transplant within 1 month, patients undergoing urologic procedures that will cause mucosal bleeding)
			· Ceftriaxone provides adequate Gram-negative coverage for most community acquired genitourinary (GU) infections. Check prior culture data if available to see if the patient has previously been infected with multidrug-resistant organisms such as ESBL and consider broader antibiotics if needed
			· For hospital-associated UTIs, consider broader Gram-negative coverage with ertapenem, cefepime, or piperacillin/tazobactam
			· Other risk factors for ESBL-producing organisms include those who:
			  - Recently completed a course of antibiotics with a fluoroquinolone, broad-spectrum beta-lactam, or trimethoprim sulfamethoxazole
			  - Traveled to areas with high-rates of antimicrobial resistance (e.g., India, Mexico, Spain, or Israel)
			  - Traveled to the areas listed above and received a course of antibiotics during that travel (e.g., for travel-associated diarrhea)

Endocarditis	· S. aureus · Streptococcus spp.	· vancomycin · ceftriaxone (2g IV daily)	· Get transthoracic echo (TTE); if inconclusive, get transesophageal echo (TEE) · Obtain 3 sets of blood cultures on initial evaluation if clinical suspicion for endocarditis is present

(Continued)

INFECTIOUS DISEASES

TABLE 8.12 · Empiric Antibiotic Regimens for Hospitalized Immunocompetent Patients (Continued)

Clinical Syndrome	Common Pathogen(s)	Possible Empiric Antibiotic Regimen* (all are required unless indicated with OR or +/−)	Comments
Bloodstream infections	• S. aureus • Streptococcus spp. • E. coli • Klebsiella spp. • Candida spp.	**Gram-positive cocci:** • vancomycin **Gram-negative rods:** • ceftriaxone OR piperacillin-tazobactam OR cefepime OR carbapenem (e.g., ertapenem) **Yeast:** • echinocandin (e.g., caspofungin)	• Consult ID for all cases of S. aureus bacteremia • Treat cases of S. lugdunensis bacteremia as S. aureus • Ceftriaxone can be used as empiric therapy for GNR bacteremia in most cases • Patients with hospital-acquired infections or prior infections with P. aeruginosa can be empirically treated with an anti-pseudomonal beta-lactam (e.g., piperacillin-tazobactam or cefepime) • Individuals with prior infections with ESBL-producing organisms can be empirically treated with a carbapenem (e.g., ertapenem) • Candidemia warrants an ID consult, ophthalmology consult (to evaluate for endophthalmitis), and, if possible, removal of any indwelling central catheters
Cellulitis: Non-purulent and purulent (e.g., presence of abscess or pustules)	• S. aureus • Strep spp.	**Non-purulent SSTI:** • cefazolin (1–2 mg IV q8hr) **Purulent SSTI:** • vancomycin	• Vancomycin covers Gram-positive bacteria, including MRSA • In cases of non-purulent cellulitis that do not improve after 72 hours of therapy, consider imaging to rule out abscess, which would require source control and drainage • If drainable abscess is present, perform incision and drainage (I&D). Clinical trials support the use of antibiotics after I&D, though most patients will be cured with or without antibiotics after I&D.
Necrotizing fasciitis	• S. aureus • Group A strep • Anaerobes • Gram-negative rods	• vancomycin • ertapenem (1 g IV daily) OR piperacillin/tazobactam (3.375 g IV q6hr to 4.5 g IV q6hr) • clindamycin	• Emergent surgical and ID consult • Clindamycin used for anti-toxin effect • In addition to antimicrobials, treatment requires surgical debridement
Septic arthritis	• S. aureus • Streptococci spp. • N. gonorrhoeae • Enterobacteriaceae (rarely)	• vancomycin • ceftriaxone (2 g IV qD) OR cefepime (2 g IV 8 hrs if risk factors for P. aeruginosa)	• Sample the joint fluid to confirm the diagnosis of septic arthritis and get a gram stain to guide therapy

(Continued)

TABLE 8.12 · Empiric Antibiotic Regimens for Hospitalized Immunocompetent Patients (*Continued*)

Clinical Syndrome	Common Pathogen(s)	Possible Empiric Antibiotic Regimen* (all are required unless indicated with OR or +/−)	Comments
Osteomyelitis	• Presumed hematogenous source – *S. aureus*	• vancomycin • ceftriaxone (2g IV q12hr)	• Consider obtaining a bone biopsy to determine the causative pathogen prior to initiation of antimicrobial therapy if the patient is clinically stable
	• If vascular insufficiency or diabetic foot ulcer, also consider *P. aeruginosa* and anaerobic coverage	• vancomycin • piperacillin/tazobactam **OR** ceftriaxone (1g IV daily) • metronidazole (500 mg IV q8 hr)	• If the patient has a diabetic foot ulcer, vascular insufficiency, or hardware, add Gram-negative coverage. Other organisms are possible so consider an ID consult, especially if hardware microbial infection
Severe sepsis with unclear source	• Not yet determined	• vancomycin • ertapenem (1g IV daily) **OR** piperacillin/tazobactam (3.375 g IV q6 hr to 4.5 g IV q6 hr) **OR** cefepime (2 g IV q8 hr)	• First attempt history, physical exam, labs, and imaging to try to identify a source • If the source is still unclear and the patient has sepsis or septic shock requiring inpatient admission, provide broad empiric anti-microbial coverage with Gram-positive and Gram-negative coverage • Choice of empiric Gram-negative coverage depends on the severity of illness, patient factors, and suspected source. For example, consider whether the patient needs pseudomonal coverage, ESBL coverage, CNS penetration, etc.

*The above recommendations provide general guidelines for immunocompetent hospitalized patients, but antimicrobial regimens should be tailored for the individual patient and clinical context. Each antibiotic listed with a separate bullet is recommended in combination with the others, unless stated with "OR" or "+/−". Antibiotics are color-coded as follows: red = mainly Gram-positive coverage, blue = mainly Gram-negative coverage, green = atypical or anerobic coverage, brown = anaerobic coverage, purple = anti-viral coverage, and orange = anti-fungal coverage. The dosing above is listed for patients with normal renal and hepatic function; adjust as needed if organ dysfunction is present.

INFECTIOUS DISEASES

Principles of Antibiotic Selection and Infection Management

- Start antibiotics early: Early antibiotics in sepsis decrease mortality
- Cultures before antibiotics: Whenever possible, obtain blood cultures and easily-accessible organ-specific cultures (e.g., sputum culture/urine culture) prior to starting antibiotics
- Antibiotics before invasive procedures: In an acutely ill patient, do not delay antibiotics for time-intensive culture sampling (e.g., lumbar puncture, paracentesis, thoracentesis, intra-abdominal abscess drainage, etc.)
- Use prior microbiology data: Prior microbiology data can help you understand the organisms with which a patient has previously been infected and the antibiotic susceptibilities of these organisms
- Immunocompromised patients: Consider a broader differential diagnosis and broader empiric antibiotic/antiviral/antifungal coverage for immunocompromised patients
- Obtain source control ASAP: Consider removing and/or draining potential contained sources of infection, including indwelling catheters, hardware (e.g., prosthetic joints or cardiac devices), or effusions and abscesses
- Use cultures to guide antibiotic choice: As culture data returns, use culture data and susceptibilities to narrow antibiotics. Keep local antibiotic resistance patterns in mind

Primary Fever Syndromes

Fever

- Definition: A regulated elevation in core body temperature, usually defined as $\geq 38.3°C$, as part of the body's inflammatory response
- Differential diagnosis: Infectious, autoimmune/inflammatory conditions, malignancy, drug reactions, transfusion reactions, deep venous thrombosis (DVT)
- Workup and management: See Table 8.13

Fever of unknown origin (FUO)

- Definitions:
  - **Classic FUO**: 1) Fever >38.3°C, 2) Continuing 3 weeks in duration, 3) No diagnosis despite a thorough evaluation (3 days inpatient or three outpatient visits)
  - **Nosocomial FUO**: Fever >38.3°C starting after a patient is hospitalized, lasting for 3 or more days, with an unclear source of fever despite a thorough evaluation
  - **Neutropenic FUO**: Fever >38.3°C on multiple occasions in a patient with an absolute neutrophil count (ANC) >500 cells/μL (or expected to fall to that level in 1–2 days). Also see Hematology/Oncology Chapter 7
  - **HIV-associated FUO**: Fever >38.3°C (100.9°F) on multiple occasions over more than 4 weeks (or more than 3 days for hospitalized patients with HIV)
- Differential diagnosis: See Table 8.14
- Workup:
  - History: Localizing symptoms, sick contacts, travel history, exposures, systemic symptoms
  - Physical exam
  - Labs and imaging:
    - The initial workup should focus on key features identified in the history and physical
    - Focus on organ systems with localizing symptoms (e.g., chest imaging in those with pulmonary symptoms, a transthoracic echocardiogram in those with a new murmur, etc.)
    - Consider the following diagnostic tests: CBC with diff, CMP, urinalysis and urine culture, blood cultures (3 sets), HIV Ag/Ab, ESR, CRP, latent TB testing, ANA, RF, SPEP, CXR and/or CT chest, CT of the abdomen and pelvis. Consider testing for viral (e.g., EBV, CMV) and atypical pathogens (e.g., Q fever, *Bartonella*, *Brucella*) if the patient has risk factors and a compatible syndrome
  - Advanced diagnostics: If the above diagnostic workup is unrevealing, consider FDG-PET (now preferred over indium-111-labeled leukocyte scanning)

TABLE 8.13 · Steps in Evaluation of a Fever	
Step	**Diagnostic and Management Tips**
1. Evaluate for signs of sepsis	**SIRS Criteria:** Two or more criteria = SIRS • Temperature >38.0°C • Heart rate >90 beats/min • Respiratory rate >20 breaths/min or $PaCO_2$ <32 mmHg • White blood count (WBC) >12,000 cells/µL or <4000/mm³ **qSOFA Score:** A score of >2 raises concern for an infection causing life-threatening organ dysfunction • Respiratory rate ≥22 breaths/min • Altered mental status • Systolic blood pressures ≤100 mmHg Note: The absence of fever does not rule out infection. Many patients, such as the elderly or immunocompromised, may not have the immune response necessary to mount a fever. Furthermore, interventions in the intensive care unit, such as CRRT or ECMO, lower the core body temperature and may mask the development of a fever.
2. Review localizing signs and symptoms	A thorough history and physical exam can help identify a possible infectious source: • Cough or sputum production may suggest a respiratory tract infection • Dysuria, urinary urgency, or flank pain may suggest a urinary tract infection • An erythematous or painful lower extremity may suggest a skin or soft tissue infection • Diarrhea or abdominal pain may suggest a gastrointestinal infection • Rigors may suggest bacteremia
3. Perform diagnostic evaluation	Localizing signs and symptoms in step 2 can help target your diagnostic workup. Send two sets of blood cultures in any patient with a suspected severe infection causing sepsis. In patients with a clear localizing source of infection, the work-up should focus on the affected organ system (e.g., chest X-ray in a patient with suspected pneumonia). In patients with no clear localizing symptoms, the following studies can help localize a potential infection: • Urinalysis and urine culture to evaluate for urinary tract infections • A chest X-ray to evaluate for pneumonia. • CT scan of the abdomen/pelvis with or without IV contrast
4. Treat sepsis or any suspected infection	Core principles of sepsis management include: • Volume resuscitation with at least 30 mL/kg of fluids within the first 3 hours • Supporting a mean arterial blood pressure of >65 mmHg using fluids and, when necessary, vasopressors • Administration of empiric antibiotic therapy within one hour of identifying sepsis
5. If the initial infectious work-up is unrevealing, consider other sources of infection and non-infectious causes of fever	Sometimes, no clear infectious source is identified. Possible causes include: • An overlooked source of infection in the primary evaluation (e.g., a subtle consolidation on CXR) • Antibiotic administration interfered with the accuracy of certain tests (e.g., antibiotics before blood cultures) • There is an indolent or difficult to diagnose infection (e.g. an organism that cannot be isolated with standard cultures) • There is a non-infectious cause of fever (rheumatologic, oncologic, drug fever, VTE, etc.) In these situations, there are multiple diagnostic pathways to pursue in parallel: • Re-evaluate for common causes of infection (e.g., UTI, PNA, SSTI) • Consider noninfectious causes of fever, listed above • Consider more indolent infections (e.g., epidural abscess, osteomyelitis, endocarditis, etc.) based on any potential localizing findings • Consider viral or atypical pathogens

INFECTIOUS DISEASES

TABLE 8.14 · Common Etiologies of Fever of Unknown Origin (FUO) in Adults
Infections
• Tuberculosis (often extrapulmonary [e.g., lymph nodes] or disseminated)
• Cytomegalovirus
• Epstein-Barr virus
• Endocarditis (often culture-negative)
• Occult abscesses (abdominal, perinephric, prostatic, dental, etc.)
• Osteomyelitis
• Sinusitis
• Zoonotic infections (Q-Fever, bartonellosis, brucellosis, etc.)
Systemic Inflammatory/Rheumatologic Diseases
• Systemic lupus erythematosus
• Adult Still's Disease
• Giant cell arteritis
• Other vasculitides (Takayasu's arteritis, granulomatosis with polyangiitis [GPA])
• Rheumatoid arthritis
• Sarcoidosis
• Inflammatory bowel disease
• Thyroiditis
Neoplasms
• Lymphomas
• Leukemias
• Multiple myeloma
• Solid tumors (e.g., breast, lung, colorectal, kidney, liver, etc.)
• Castleman's disease
Other
• Drug fevers
• Thromboembolic disease
• Hematomas
• Hereditary fever disorders (e.g., familial Mediterranean fever)

Febrile neutropenia (FN)
- Definition: Fever and neutropenia
  - Fever: Defined as a single oral temperature of $\geq 38.3°C$ (101.0°F) or a temperature of 38.0°C (100.4°F) for over 1 hour
  - Neutropenia: Definition varies, often absolute neutrophil count (ANC) $<1000/\mu L$ or sometimes defined as ANC $<500/\mu L$
- Pathogenesis:
  - Cytotoxic chemotherapy nonspecifically targets rapidly proliferating cells, including myelopoietic stem cells, resulting in decreased cell counts, including decreased absolute neutrophil count
  - Other conditions that cause bone marrow suppression (infections, medications, autoimmune conditions, fibrotic conditions, etc.) can also result in neutropenia
  - Cytotoxic chemotherapy can also destroy rapidly proliferating gastrointestinal mucosal cells, resulting in decreased integrity of the gastrointestinal mucosa. This results in an increased frequency of bacterial translocation across the gut barrier and, as a result, bacteremia, which is the most common cause of infection in patients with FN
- Pathogens:
  - Bacterial infections: Most common cause of FN
  - Fungal infections: Most invasive fungal infections that cause FN are due to *Candida* spp., which develop after translocation across the gut barrier, and *Aspergillus* spp., which develop after inhalation of spores
  - Viral: Human herpesviruses are the most common viral pathogens to cause FN. These include herpes simplex viruses (HSV) 1 and 2, herpes zoster, Epstein Barr virus (EBV), or cytomegalovirus (CMV)

- Diagnostics: History, physical exam, labs, pan-culture
- Treatment:
  - Many institutions have institution-specific guidelines, which should be followed if present
  - Various national guidelines help risk stratify patients that can be treated as outpatients vs. those that should be hospitalized (see IDSA, NCCN, and/or MASCC Risk Index)
    - For those patients deemed safe for <u>outpatient management</u>: Oral antibiotic regimens should include anti-pseudomonal coverage with a fluoroquinolone. Potential regimens include (adjust for renal dysfunction if needed):
      - Levofloxacin 750 mg orally once daily
      - Ciprofloxacin 500 mg orally twice daily + amoxicillin-clavulanate (500 mg/125 mg orally three times daily or 1000 mg/250 mg orally twice daily)
    - For those patients who warrant <u>inpatient management</u>: IV antibiotics that include anti-pseudomonal coverage should be administered immediately. Potential therapeutic regimens include (adjust for renal/hepatic dysfunction if needed):
      - Cefepime 2 g IV q8 hr
      - Meropenem 1 g IV q8 hr
      - Piperacillin-tazobactam 4.5 g IV q6 hr
      - Consider addition of Gram-positive coverage and fungal coverage pending patient risk factors and clinical stability.
        - Indications for Gram-positive coverage (e.g., vancomycin) include shock, pulmonary infection, indwelling central venous catheters, skin and soft-tissue infections
        - Indications for fungal coverage (e.g., an echinocandin or liposomal amphotericin B) include shock or persistent fevers for 4+ days with no source identified

Fever in a "returning traveler"
- Approach:
  - When considering travel-related fevers, consider **geography** and **incubation period** to narrow the differential diagnosis
  - It is important to note that a patient can have a fever due to their travel OR independent of it
  - Thus, alongside travel-dependent fevers, it is important to consider the usual, travel-independent categories of fever, including infectious (e.g., CAP, UTI, etc.) and non-infectious (e.g., malignancy, rheumatologic, medications/toxins, etc.)
- History:
  - Travel history (destination, urban/rural, vaccinations and malaria prophylaxis)
  - Exposures (animals, bites, water, diet, tattoos, sexual contact)
  - Timing (incubation period)
- Pathogens to consider by geography:
  - Caribbean, Central America, and South America: Chikungunya, dengue, malaria, zika, typhoid and paratyphoid fever (in South America)
  - South-Central Asia and Southeast Asia: Dengue, malaria, and typhoid and paratyphoid fever (in South-Central Asia)
  - Sub-Saharan Africa: Dengue, malaria, tickborne rickettsial infections, schistosomiasis
- Infections with an incubation period <21 days:
  - Bacterial: Typhoid, non-typhoidal salmonellosis, leptospirosis, meningococcemia, rickettsial diseases
  - Viral: Zika, dengue, chikungunya, EBV (mononucleosis), West Nile virus (WNV), Japanese encephalitis, yellow fever
  - Parasitic: Malaria
- Infections with an incubation period >21 days:
  - Bacterial: Q-fever
  - Mycobacterial: Tuberculosis
  - Viral: Viral hepatitis (e.g., hepatitis A, hepatitis E), acute HIV, rabies
  - Fungal: Endemic fungi (check prevalence by region)
  - Parasitic: Leishmaniasis

DISEASES & PATHOPHYSIOLOGY

Because diagnostic and therapeutic decisions in infectious diseases are heavily informed by a patient's clinical syndrome, they are included with each specific disease.

Central Nervous System Infections

Meningitis

- Note: Meningitis and encephalitis are two distinct clinical entities, each with their own list of causative organisms. However, in practice the distinction may be blurred as these syndromes can share clinical features
- Clinical features:
  - Classic triad: 1) Fever, 2) Nuchal rigidity, 3) Altered mental status, although less than 50% of patients have all three symptoms
  - Physical exam: The diagnostic utility of these tests are quite poor and they have limited negative predictive values. In other words, the absence of positive findings for any of the following tests does not meaningfully decrease the probability of meningitis and encephalitis
    - Kernig's sign: Inability to fully extend knees when patient is supine with hips flexed
    - Brudzinski's sign: Flexion of legs/thighs that is brought on by passive flexion of neck
    - Jolt test: Painful to turn head side-to-side
    - Rashes:
      - *N. meningitides*: Maculopapular rash with petechiae/purpura (~50% of patients will have a rash on presentation)
      - HSV: Vesicular lesions (may be present, but their absence in a patient with encephalitis does not decrease the likelihood of HSV encephalitis)
      - VZV: Vesicular lesions (encephalitis may develop weeks before or weeks after the onset of rash)
- Pathogens:
  - Bacteria:
    - Neonates: *Group B strep, E.coli, L. monocytogenes*
    - Children >3 months: *N. meningitidis, S. pneumoniae, H. influenzae*
    - Adults: *S. pneumoniae* (>70% cases), *N. meningitis* (12%), *Group B strep* (7%), *H. influenzae* (6%)
    - Elderly/immunocompromised: *L. monocytogenes* (<5%)
  - Viruses: Enterovirus, HSV-2, VZV, HIV, mumps, arbovirus (West Nile virus, St. Louis encephalitis virus)
  - Other pathogens: *Mycobacterium tuberculosis*, syphilis, *Cryptococcus* spp., *Coccidioides* spp.
- Diagnosis: Lumbar puncture (LP)
  - Ensure there are no other contraindications to LP (e.g., a deteriorating level of consciousness, anti-coagulation, epidural abscess)
  - Perform non-contrast head CT (NCHCT) prior to LP if new focal neurologic deficits, altered mental status, age >60 yr, immunocompromised, concern for increased intracranial pressure (papilledema, vomiting), seizures, known brain metastases
  - Obtain blood cultures prior to antibiotics, but do not delay empiric antibiotics while waiting for head imaging or LP
  - The following studies should be sent from the CSF:
    - Cell count and differential
    - Gram stain and bacterial culture
    - Glucose concentration (check simultaneous serum glucose to evaluate the ratio of CSF:serum glucose)
    - Protein concentration
    - More advanced diagnostic tests can be sent depending on the concern for specific pathogens (E.g., viral PCR testing, fungal testing, metagenomic next generation sequencing, universal PCR testing)
  - Typical CSF profiles for CNS conditions: See Table 8.15
- Treatment: See Table 8.16
- Prevention:
  - Vaccinate all individuals 65+ yr and immunocompromised patients for *S. pneumoniae*
  - Vaccinate all asplenic patient for *S. pneumoniae, N. meningitidis, H. influenzae*

TABLE 8.15 · Typical CSF Profiles of CNS conditions			
Condition	**Cell Count and Differential (cells/µL)**	**Glucose (mg/dL)**	**Protein (mg/dL)**
Normal	0–5	45–80	18–58
Bacterial meningitis	>500 (PMN predominant)	<40	>200
TB meningitis	5–1000 (lymph predominant)	<10	>400
Viral meningitis	100–1000 (lymph predominant)	45–80	50–200
Guillain-Barré	0–5	45–80	45–1000

Encephalitis
- Clinical features:
  - Encephalopathy, seizures, altered mental status
  - HSV1 infects the temporal lobe, causing aphasia, olfactory hallucinations, personality changes
- Pathogens:
  - Viral: HSV1, HSV2, VZV, arbovirus (eastern equine encephalitis, West Nile virus, St. Louis encephalitis virus), enterovirus, measles, mumps, EBV, CMV
  - Parasitic: Toxoplasmosis
  - Non-infectious: Autoimmune encephalitis (e.g., anti-NMDA receptor antibody often associated with ovarian teratomas), T-cell lymphoma
- Diagnosis: NCHCT then LP. MRI brain: Increased T2 flair in frontotemporal region if HSV1.
- Treatment: Often supportive. See Table 8.16 for empiric therapy. If CMV encephalitis, use IV ganciclovir

TABLE 8.16 · Empiric Therapy for Suspected Acute Meningitis and Encephalitis in Adults		
Host Characteristics	**Organisms to Cover with Empiric Therapy**	**Empiric Regimen[b]**
Adult patient <50 yr and without an immunocompromising condition[a]	**Bacteria:** • *Streptococcus pneumoniae (most common organism)* • *Neisseria meningitidis* • *Group B Streptococcus* • *Hemophilus influenzae* **Viruses:** • HSV1 • VZV • See full ddx in chapter text above	vancomycin[c] + ceftriaxone (2g IV q12 hr) & acyclovir (if concerned for encephalitis) & adjunctive corticosteroids (dexamethasone 0.15 mg/kg q6h ×4 days)[e]
Adult patient >50 yr or with an immunocompromising condition[a]	**Bacteria:** • *Streptococcus pneumoniae* (most common organism) • *Neisseria meningitidis* • *Group B Streptococcus* • *Hemophilus influenzae* • *Listeria monocytogenes* • Gram-negative rods (e.g., *E. coli)* **Viruses:** • HSV1 • VZV • See full ddx in chapter text above	vancomycin[c] + ceftriaxone (2g IV q12h) + ampicillin[d] (2 g IV q4h) & acyclovir (if concerned for encephalitis) & adjunctive corticosteroids (dexamethasone 0.15 mg/kg q6h ×4 days)[e]

[a] Immuncompromising conditions include HIV, solid organ or bone marrow transplant, neutropenia, immunosuppressive therapy, etc.

[b] Both antibiotics and antivirals may be used in suspected acute meningitis or encephalitis because of the overlap in the clinical features and types of organisms that can cause each syndrome

[c] Vancomycin is used in acute bacterial meningitis to empirically cover ceftriaxone-resistant *S. pneumoniae*

[d] Ampicillin is used to cover *Listeria monocytogenes*

[e] First dose of steroids should be given before antibiotics and continued only if *S. pneumoniae* is suspected (based on CSF gram stain or culture results)

Brain abscess
- Pathophysiology: Complication of otitis media, sinusitis, odontogenic infection, post-surgical infection
- Clinical features: Often non-specific features, including fever, headache, and/or focal neurologic deficits. Classic triad of all three is present in only ~20% of cases.
- Pathogens: *Streptococcus* spp. and *Staphylococcus* spp. are the most frequent organisms. Often polymicrobial infections (~40%) that contain both aerobic and anaerobic organisms.
- Diagnosis: Brain MRI. Needle aspiration and surgical excision are possible options for making a microbiologic diagnosis of the causative organism(s).
- Treatment:
  - Empiric antibiotics: vancomycin + ceftriaxone 2 g IV q12 hrs + metronidazole 500 mg IV/PO q8 hr
  - Immediate neurosurgical evaluation for consideration of neurosurgical excision or drainage
  - Consider adjunctive glucocorticoids if mass effect seen on imaging, but neurosurgical consultation should be used to make this decision

Spinal epidural abscess
- Pathophysiology: Bacteria can spread from infected vertebrae or nearby soft tissues, or via hematogenous spread
- Clinical features:
  - Presentation is often slow and insidious with symptoms lasting weeks to months, but can be more acute with aggressive organisms like *S. aureus*
  - Back pain is the most common symptom. Fever is variably present. ~50% of patients have a neurologic symptom (e.g., radiculopathy, motor or sensory dysfunction), which often develop later in the disease course.
- Pathogens: *Streptococcus* spp. and *Staphylococcus* spp.
- Diagnosis: Spinal MRI
- Treatment:
  - Empiric antibiotics with vancomycin IV + ceftriaxone IV 2 g q12 hr. Ceftriaxone can be substituted for an anti-pseudomonal beta-lactam, such as cefepime 2 g IV q8 hr.
  - Immediate neurosurgical evaluation and consideration of surgical drainage

Pulmonary Infections
Community acquired pneumonia (CAP)
- Definition: An acute pulmonary infection that develops outside of the hospital or within the first 48 hours of admission
- Pathophysiology:
  - Organisms that colonize the nasopharynx make their way to the lungs via microaspiration
  - Once in the lung, poor mucociliary clearance and the organism's virulence factors allow replication and establishment of infection
  - The body's immune response to the organisms creates the clinical features of pneumonia
- Clinical features: Cough, shortness of breath, fever. Patients who meet the following criteria can be classified as having severe CAP (relevant for some diagnostic tests, see Table 8.17)
- Pathogens:
  - Typical bacteria:
    - *S. pneumoniae*: Historically the most common cause of CAP; rates are decreasing due to use of the pneumococcal vaccines in the United States
    - *H. influenzae*: Especially prominent in those with underlying lung disease
    - *M. catarrhalis*
  - Atypical bacteria:
    - *M. pneumoniae*: Transmitted with high frequency via close contact
    - *C. pneumoniae* and *C. psittaci*
    - *Legionella spp*: Outbreaks are associated with exposure to aerosols, including those from air conditioners, showers, spas, and fountains; also associated with travel
  - Other clinically relevant bacteria:
    - *S. aureus*:
      - CAP from *S. aureus* includes both MSSA and MRSA isolates
      - Preceding influenza is a risk factor for *S. aureus* pneumonia
      - CAP from MRSA often causes a severe pneumonia, and is most commonly seen in patients with:
        - Necrotizing pneumonia or co-existing empyema
        - Known colonization or prior infection with MRSA
        - Recent broad-spectrum antibiotic use
        - Post-influenza pneumonia, injection drug use, HIV/AIDS

- Gram-negative rods
  - *Pseudomonas aeruginosa*: Relatively uncommon cause of CAP. Specific risk factors for community-acquired *P. aeruginosa* infections include:
    - Structural lung disease (e.g., bronchiectasis or cystic fibrosis)
    - Recent broad-spectrum antibiotic use
    - Severe immunocompromise (e.g., HIV, solid organ of hematopoietic stem cell transplant, neutropenia, immunosuppressive therapy)
    - Frequent COPD exacerbations requiring glucocorticoid and/or antibiotic use
  - *K. pneumoniae*: Most common in patients with underlying lung disease or heavy alcohol use
- Viruses: There is increasing evidence to suggest viruses are a common cause of CAP, either as the sole pathogen or with a bacterial infection. Notable viruses include:
  - Influenza A/B
  - Respiratory syncytial virus (RSV)
  - Parainfluenza viruses (especially in immunocompromised adults)
  - Rhinovirus (frequently isolated, though there is conflicting evidence on whether it is a true pathogen or a bystander organism)
  - Human metapneumovirus
  - Coronavirus (including SARS-CoV-2 of the COVID-19 outbreak)
- Diagnosis:
  - CXR and/or chest CT showing a focal consolidation with a compatible clinical syndrome suggesting pneumonia
  - Obtain blood cultures, sputum Gram stain, and sputum culture in patients with severe CAP (see Table 8.17), immunocompromised hosts, patients being empirically treated for MRSA or *P. aeruginosa*
  - Obtain a nasopharyngeal (NP) swab for influenza PCR testing in all patients with suspected CAP during influenza season
    - In critically ill patients, obtain both upper and lower NP swab and do not stop empiric anti-viral therapy until the lower respiratory specimen is negative. This is because some patients may stop shedding influenza virus form the upper airways but not the lower airways, leading to a false-negative upper airway NP swab.

TABLE 8.17 · Criteria to Define Severe Community Acquired Pneumonia (CAP)	
Severe CAP is defined as the presence of one or more major criteria OR 3 or more minor criteria	
Major Criteria	• Septic shock requiring vasopressors • Respiratory failure requiring mechanical ventilation
Minor Criteria	• Respiratory rate $\geq$30 breaths/min • PaO_2/FiO_2 $\leq$250 • Multilobar infiltrates • Confusion/encephalopathy • BUN $\geq$20 mg/dL • Leukopenia (WBC <4000 cells/μL) from infection alone • Thrombocytopenia (Plt <100K cells/μL) • Hypothermia (Temperature <36°C) • Hypotension requiring fluid resuscitation

Source: Metlay et al., *Am J Respir Crit Care Med* 2019;200(7):345–67.

- Treatment:
  - <u>CAP that can be managed in the outpatient setting</u>:
    - No recent antibiotics/comorbidities: PO amoxicillin, doxycycline, or azithromycin
    - If recent antibiotics, more severe case, and/or notable medical comorbidities (e.g., chronic lung disease, CKD, chronic liver disease, alcohol use disorder, cardiac disease):
      - [PO amoxicillin/clavulanate or cefpodoxime or cefuroxime] AND [PO doxycycline or azithromycin] OR
      - A respiratory fluoroquinolone (e.g., PO levofloxacin or moxifloxacin)
  - <u>CAP requiring hospital admission to the general medical floor</u>: ceftriaxone + [azithromycin or clarithromycin] + empiric oseltamivir during flu season until influenza testing returns
  - <u>Severe CAP, requiring ICU admission</u>: vancomycin + [ceftriaxone or cefepime (if *P. aeruginosa* coverage needed)] + azithromycin + empiric oseltamivir during flu season until influenza testing returns
    - When empiric MRSA coverage is started (e.g., vancomycin) can use a negative MRSA swab to narrow antibiotics. A negative MRSA nasal swab has a ~95% negative predictive value for MRSA pneumonia
  - <u>Duration of therapy</u>:
    - Five days of antibiotics is appropriate for most patients
    - Treatment duration can be extended in those with a delayed response to therapy
    - Patients with *S. aureus* or *Pseudomonas* should be treated for at least 7 days

Hospital-acquired pneumonia (HAP) & ventilator-acquired pneumonia (VAP)
- Definitions:
  - <u>Hospital-acquired pneumonia (HAP)</u>: Pneumonia diagnosed >48 hrs after hospital admission and not present at hospital admission
  - <u>Ventilator-associated pneumonia (VAP)</u>: Pneumonia diagnosed >48 hrs after intubation
- Pathogens:
  - Gram-negative rods: *P. aeruginosa*, *Klebsiella* spp., *E. coli*, *Enterobacter* spp. There is an increased risk for multidrug-resistant Gram-negative rods, as well (e.g., ESBL-producing organisms)
  - Gram-positive cocci: *S. aureus*
- Clinical Features: Similar to CAP, the clinical features of HAP/VAP include the presence of new systemic signs of infection (e.g., fever, leukocytosis) + suggestion of a new pulmonary process (including a new lung infiltrate on chest imaging, purulent sputum production, and new or worsening hypoxemia)
- Diagnosis: Obtain the following for any patient suspected for HAP/VAP:
  - Sputum cultures from either produced sputum or endotracheal or endobronchial sampling, such as a tracheal aspirate
  - Peripheral blood cultures
  - MRSA nasal swab
  - Chest imaging (CXR or CT chest)
- Treatment:
  - <u>Empiric therapy for HAP/VAP should include</u>:
    - Coverage of MRSA, such as with vancomycin
    - Coverage of *P. aeruginosa* and Gram-negative rods, such as with piperacillin-tazobactam or cefepime
    - Consider whether ESBL coverage and/or a second agent for Gram-negative organisms (e.g., ciprofloxacin) is needed for critically-ill patients
  - <u>Duration of therapy</u>:
    - Seven days is an effective duration of therapy for most patients
    - Complications such as bacteremia, lung abscess or complicated pleural effusions may warrant longer courses

Parapneumonic effusions
- Definition: Pleural effusions that develop in the setting of and adjacent to pneumonia, representing a common complication of pneumonia
- Pathogens: Pyogenic bacterial infections with Gram-positive organisms are most common, including:
  - *S. pneumoniae*
  - Viridians streptococci, including members of the *S. anginosus* group
  - *S. aureus* (most common cause of hospital-acquired parapneumonic effusions)
  - Anaerobic oral flora, such as *Fusobacterium* spp., *Prevotella* spp., *Peptostreptococcus* spp., and *Bacteroides* spp.
- Clinical features: Similar to pneumonia. Dullness to percussion on exam may increase suspicion
- Diagnosis:
  - Parapneumonic effusions are often found on imaging (CXR, CT, bedside ultrasound)
  - Characterization of a parapneumonic effusion relies on pleural fluid analysis: See Table 8.18
- Treatment: See Table 8.18

TABLE 8.18 · Parapneumonic Effusions: Diagnosis and Management		
Type of Parapneumonic Effusion	**Features**	**Management**
Uncomplicated parapneumonic effusion	• Free-flowing, without loculations • Pleural fluid analysis will be exudative by Light's criteria and sterile • pH and glucose levels will be normal	• **Antibiotics:** Antibiotic selection is the same as that for the underlying pneumonia (e.g., CAP or HAP/VAP) • **Drainage:** Not indicated, can be managed with antibiotics alone
Complicated parapneumonic effusion	• Often see loculations on imaging • Exudative on Light's criteria • Have one of the following: pH <7.2, pleural fluid glucose <40 mg/dL, and/or a Gram stain or culture that reveals organism growth	• **Antibiotics:** Antibiotic coverage should include anaerobic organisms (e.g., metronidazole, beta-lactam plus beta-lactamase inhibitors, such as ampicillin-sulbactam or piperacillin-tazobactam, or a carbapenem, such as ertapenem or meropenem). Duration is long, often 4–6 weeks for complicated parapneumonic effusions and empyema
Empyema	• Shares the characteristics of a complicated parapneumonic effusion with the addition of frank pus seen on pleural fluid sampling	• **Drainage:** A complicated parapneumonic effusion or empyema should be drained with a chest tube as soon as possible

Pneumocystis jirovecii pneumonia (PJP, aka PCP)
- Risk factors:
  - HIV (CD4 <200 cells/μL)
  - Cancer, solid organ transplant, or bone marrow transplant
  - Rheumatologic disease (granulomatosis with polyangiitis [GPA] has intrinsic risk)
  - Patients on chronic steroids (prednisone ≥20 mg for 20+ days, or the equivalent)
- Clinical features:
  - In HIV-infected patients, there is often a gradual onset of fever, cough, and dyspnea over days to weeks
  - In non-HIV-infected patients, symptoms may be more aggressive and abrupt in onset
- Diagnosis:
  - Bronchoscopy is gold standard. Can also check beta-D glucan, LDH. Test characteristics differ in patients with HIV versus non-HIV infected patients
  - Can often perform testing on induced sputum samples that can make the diagnosis if positive. If negative, bronchoscopy should be performed
  - Treat empirically while awaiting bronchoscopy, as organisms will be present for up to 2 weeks on BAL microscopy

- Treatment:
  - High-dose trimethoprim-sulfamethoxazole: 15–20 mg/kg of trimethoprim divided in 3–4 daily doses for 21 days
  - Add adjunctive glucocorticoids if: A-a gradient >35 mmHg or PaO_2< 70 mmHg
  - Steroids are not well studied for non-HIV-infected patients but are generally recommended
- Prophylaxis: Bactrim (alternatives include dapsone, atovaquone, inhaled pentamidine). Prophylaxis is indicated in the following scenarios:
  - Patients with HIV and a CD4 count <200 cells/μL
  - Individuals with another immunocompromising condition (e.g., autoimmune disease, hematologic malignancy, or another immunocompromising medication) treated with glucocorticoids at a dose >20 mg prednisone for 20 days or more ("20/20" rule)
  - Patients with acute lymphocytic leukemia
  - Allogenic stem cell transplant recipients and most autologous stem cell transplant recipients
  - Solid organ transplant recipients
  - Patients with certain primary immunodeficiencies (e.g., severe CVID, hyper IgM syndrome)

Influenza

- Virus: Influenza, commonly known as the flu, is caused by an influenza virus. Three of the four types of influenza viruses infect humans: A, B, and C
- Clinical features: Spread by respiratory droplet. Symptoms include fevers, chills, cough, and malaise. Can also be asymptomatic
- Diagnosis: CXR: Normal or alveolar pattern. Check influenza PCR
- Treatment: Oseltamivir, supportive care

Severe acute respiratory syndrome coronavirus 2 (SARS-CoV-2)

- Virus:
  - Coronaviruses are a family of viruses that can cause mild illnesses such as the common cold or more severe illness such as severe acute respiratory syndrome (SARS) and Middle East respiratory syndrome (MERS). In 2019, a new coronavirus was identified as the cause of a disease outbreak and subsequently caused a global pandemic.
  - The severe acute respiratory syndrome coronavirus 2 (SARS-CoV-2) is the name of the virus, which causes the disease known as coronavirus disease 2019 (COVID-19)
- Clinical features: Spread mainly by respiratory droplets. Causes cough, fever, shortness of breath, muscle aches, gastrointestinal symptoms, loss of smell, and leukopenia. Can be asymptomatic in ~40% of cases
- Diagnosis: Molecular tests are the main method of diagnosis, although rapid antigen tests may be used in certain situations
- Treatment:
  - Supportive care is the mainstay of therapy
  - Remdesivir in hospitalized patients with lower respiratory tract disease: 200 mg IV ×1 then 100 mg IV q24h for 4 additional days. May consider extending treatment to 10 days on a case-by-case basis (e.g., if the patient is intubated and not responding to the initial course).
  - Dexamethasone 6 mg IV or PO for up to 10 days (or until hospital discharge, whichever comes first) can be given to patients undergoing mechanical ventilation, non-invasive ventilation, high-flow nasal cannula, or supplemental oxygen (e.g., ≥ 3–4 L of nasal cannula or whose trajectory suggests increasing severity of disease). Dexamethasone is not needed if patients are not hypoxic.
  - Clinical trials are underway to determine the benefit of other therapeutic interventions
- Prevention: Several highly effective and safe vaccines are now available.

Mycobacterium tuberculosis (MTB)
- Subtypes: See Table 8.19
- Diagnosis:
  - Screening for latent TB (LTBI): PPD (consider to be positive if >15mm and no risk factors, >10mm and medium risk factors, >5mm and high risk factors) or interferon gamma release assay (IGRA) for latent TB infection. The results of these tests are <u>not</u> useful to evaluate for active infection
  - CXR or CT chest for pulmonary TB
  - CT imaging of the suspected area for extra-pulmonary TB
  - Core biopsy (or excisional if high suspicion and core biopsy negative) to diagnose TB lymphadenitis. Ultrasound of an infected lymph nodes may show necrotizing lymphadenopathy
  - Sputum AFB cultures and TB PCR
- Treatment:
  - <u>Latent TB (LTBI)</u>: First rule out active TB, then treat with rifampin ×4 mo OR isoniazid/rifapentine ×3 mo OR isoniazid ×9 mo
  - <u>Active TB</u>: RIPE therapy (<u>r</u>ifampin, <u>i</u>soniazid (INH), <u>p</u>yrazinamide, <u>e</u>thambutol)
    - All patients treated with isoniazid should also be treated with pyridoxine to prevent peripheral neuropathy
    - If the patient is <u>smear positive</u> at the time of diagnosis, they are no longer infectious when all of the following conditions are met: 1) Adequate TB treatment ×2 wks, 2) Improvement of symptoms, 3) Three consecutive negative AFB smears

TABLE 8.19 · Subtypes of Tuberculosis	
Subtypes of Tuberculosis	**Clinical Features**
Primary TB	• Bacilli are inhaled; some bacteria are ingested by alveolar macrophages but surviving ones form granulomas • Asymptomatic unless weak immune system, then can have progressive primary TB • CXR: Ghon's complex: calcified primary focus with associated lymph nodes; if fibrosis is present, it is known as Ranke's complex
Secondary (reactivation) TB	• If host immunity is weak, TB reactivation may occur at the apical/posterior portion of the lung • Symptomatic: Fever, night sweats, weight loss, malaise, cough (either dry or productive) • CXR: Infiltrates in the upper lobe or superior segment of the lower lobes (due to higher O_2 content) with cavitation, centrilobular nodules

Extrapulmonary TB	• TB can spread via hematogenous or lymphatic spread to almost any organ:
	  - Lymph nodes are most common
	  - Adrenal glands, GU tract, and bones can also be seen
	  - Pleural effusions from TB are considered extrapulmonary TB

Miliary TB	• Hematogenous spread of tuberculosis • CXR: Diffuse reticulonodular infiltrate • CT Chest: Innumerable, randomly distributed nodules

Non-tuberculous mycobacteria (NTM)
- Pathogens:
  - *M. avium* (MAC): Most common NTM infection that often occurs in middle-age men with underlying lung disease OR female non-smokers. Patients present with subacute-chronic cough +/− weight loss
  - *M. kansasii*: Second most common NTM infection. Risk factors for infection include COPD, HIV, and hematologic malignancy. Patients typically have symptoms similar to those with TB. CXR: May show a fibrocavitary lesion (thin-wall)
  - *M. abscessus, M. fortuitum, M. chelonae*: Can cause disease in those with underlying lung disease and/or immunosuppression
- Diagnosis: CXR or chest CT, AFB cultures, PCRs
- Treatment: Regimens vary, see IDSA guidelines or others

Intra-Abdominal Infections
Peritonitis/intra-abdominal abscess
- Pathogenesis: Disruption of or inflammation in the GI tract may allow normal bowel flora to enter the abdominal cavity and cause frank peritonitis and/or the development of intra-abdominal abscesses
- Pathogens:
  - These infections are almost always polymicrobial
  - Colonic organisms are the predominant pathogens, which include: *E. coli, Klebsiella* spp., *Proteus* spp., *Enterobacter* spp., *Enterococcus* spp., anaerobic organisms, such as *B. fragilis*
- Clinical features:
  - Abdominal pain, nausea, vomiting, or bloating +/− fever, tachycardia, hypotension. Some patients may appear relatively stable, while others may have florid shock
  - Patients age 65+ yr, immunocompromised, or those on chronic steroids may have especially occult presentations of severe intra-abdominal infections with less pronounced pain
- Diagnosis:
  - If unstable, consult general surgery to determine the need for immediate surgical intervention vs. whether to first obtain diagnostic imaging studies (typically CT abdomen/pelvis with contrast)
- Treatment:
  - <u>Procedural interventions</u>: Surgical intervention or percutaneous drainage are key aspects of management for complicated intra-abdominal infection. Consult general surgery and/or interventional radiology. Obtain cultures from drained material to guide antimicrobial management
  - <u>Antibiotic therapy</u>:
    - Start antibiotics ASAP to cover enteric Gram-positive, Gram-negative, and anerobic organisms
    - Patients with certain risk factors are considered high-risk (age >70 yr, diffuse peritonitis, severe sepsis, immunocompromising conditions, health care–acquired infections) and warrant coverage of multidrug-resistant (MDR) organisms
    - Regimens include:
      - <u>Low-risk community acquired infections</u>:
        - Ertapenem
        - Ciprofloxacin or ceftriaxone + metronidazole
      - <u>High-risk community acquired infections or hospital-acquired infections</u>:
        - Piperacillin-tazobactam
        - Meropenem
        - Cefepime + metronidazole

Clostridium difficile
- Pathophysiology:
  - *C. difficile* colitis can occur as a result of either community-acquired or nosocomial infections
  - Not all strains of *C. difficile* cause infection; only toxin producing strains cause diarrhea and colitis.
  - Risk factors for *C. difficile* infection include:
    - Recent antibiotic use (commonly implicated antibiotics include clindamycin, fluoroquinolones, and cephalosporins)
    - Age ≥65 yr
    - Suppression of gastric acid with PPIs or H2-blockers is also associated with an increased risk of *C. difficile* infection, though the exact mechanism for this is unknown
- Clinical features:
  - Range from mild diarrheal illness to a severe, fulminant, and potentially fatal colitis
  - Criteria for severe *C. difficile* infection:
    - More frequent diarrhea and more severe abdominal pain
    - Very high leukocytosis, often ≥15K cells/μL
    - Hypotension and lactic acidosis due to hypovolemia and sepsis
    - AKI with Cr ≥1.5 mg/dL
    - Colonic ileus with little to no diarrhea, which is known as "toxic megacolon"
- Diagnosis:
  - Perform *C. difficile* stool testing in patients with a diarrheal illness (e.g., ≥3 watery stools in a day) and no alternative reason to have loose stools (e.g., laxative use)
  - Consider CT abdomen/pelvis if concern for severe or fulminant disease

- Treatment:
  - <u>First-line treatment</u>: Vancomycin 125 mg PO QID ×10 days or fidaxomicin 200 mg PO BID ×10 days. Add metronidazole 500 mg IV TID only if fulminant disease.
  - <u>Recurrent disease</u>: Defined by resolution of symptoms with therapy followed by return of symptoms within 2 months of treatment completion. Requires longer course of antibiotics.

Genitourinary (GU) Infections

Asymptomatic bacteriuria

- Definition: Bacterial growth in a properly collected urine culture specimen from a patient *without* symptoms of inflammation of the GU system, such as urinary urgency, frequency, dysuria, or flank pain
- Management:
  - Does not warrant treatment in most individuals because there is a low risk for progression to a UTI
  - Three populations who warrant treatment of asymptomatic bacteriuria include:
    - <u>Pregnant individuals</u>: Asymptomatic bacteriuria confers worse outcomes in pregnancy, including preterm birth, perinatal mortality, and low fetal birth weight
    - <u>Renal transplant recipients</u>: Treatment of asymptomatic bacteriuria is indicated within one month of renal transplant, as these patients are at higher risk for symptomatic UTI and acute graft rejection
    - <u>Patients undergoing a urologic procedure expected to cause mucosal bleeding</u>: Untreated bacteriuria prior to a urologic intervention is associated with increased rates of infectious complications

Simple cystitis

- Definition: An infection of the urinary tract <u>without</u> signs or symptoms that suggest extension beyond the bladder and lower urinary tract, such as:
  - Temperature ≥100.0°F or 37.8°C
  - Signs and symptoms of systemic illness, such as rigors, chills, or significant malaise
  - Flank pain or costovertebral angle tenderness
  - Perineal or pelvic pain in men (which can suggest prostatitis)
- Pathophysiology: Simple cystitis arises from ascent of bacteria (usually intestinal flora) that gain access to the urinary tract
- Pathogens: *E. coli* (80%), *S. saprophyticus*, *Klebsiella* spp., *Enterococcus* spp., *Proteus* spp., *Pseudomonas aeruginosa*, *Enterobacter* spp., Group B strep
- Clinical features: Symptoms of lower urinary tract inflammation, such as, urinary frequency or urgency, dysuria, suprapubic pain
- Diagnosis:
  - Urinalysis (UA): A urinalysis that demonstrates pyuria is required, but not sufficient, for diagnosis of a urinary tract infection. Pyuria is also very common in asymptomatic bacteriuria, so pyuria is <u>not</u> equivalent to a UTI. The absence of pyuria strongly suggests against a UTI. The urinalysis may demonstrate:
    - Leukocyte esterase, which reflects the presence of WBCs in the urine
    - Nitrites, which reflect the presence of Gram-negative organisms of the Enterobacteriaceae family
    - WBCs seen on microscopic analysis of urine (>10/hpf = pyuria)
  - Urine culture: Assists with identifying the causative organism and tailored antibiotic therapy
- Treatment:
  - First-line options include:
    - Nitrofurantoin 100 mg BID for 5 days
    - Trimethoprim-sulfamethoxazole 1 DS tablet BID for 3 days
  - Alternative agents (e.g., because of intolerance or allergies):
    - Amoxicillin-clavulanate 500 mg BID for 5–7 days
    - Cefpodoxime 100 mg BID for 5–7 days
    - Cephalexin 500 mg PO QID for 5–7 days

Pyelonephritis
- Pathophysiology: Arises when ascending infections extend beyond the bladder and enter the upper urinary tract (e.g., the ureters and kidneys)
- Microbiology:
  - Gram-negative: *E.coli, Klebsiella* spp., *Enterobacter* spp., *Pseudomonas aeruginosa*
  - Gram-positive: *Enterococcus faecalis, S. aureus* (suggests descending UTI from a bloodstream infection)
- Clinical features: Flank pain, costovertebral angle (CVA) tenderness, signs of systemic illness (fevers, chills, rigors)
- Diagnosis:
  - Clinical features suggestive of pyelonephritis $+$ pyuria and/or bacteriuria is sufficient to make the diagnosis of pyelonephritis
  - Urinalysis and urine culture; false negative UA/UCx can occur with obstructing kidney stones
  - Blood cultures: Pyelonephritis can lead to bloodstream infections. Obtain blood cultures in patients with severe sepsis, septic shock, or other symptoms of bacteremia (e.g., rigors)
  - Imaging is not necessary in all patients with pyelonephritis, but consider ordering a renal ultrasound or CT abdomen/pelvis in the following situations:
    - Severely ill patients (e.g., severe sepsis or septic shock)
    - Persistent illness despite 48–72 hours of appropriate antibiotic therapy in order to rule out renal abscess, urinary tract obstruction, and prostatitis
    - Suspected urinary tract obstruction (e.g., progressive oliguria, worsening renal function, known nephrolithiasis)
- Treatment:
  - <u>Outpatients</u>: Oral antibiotic regimens such as PO ciprofloxacin, levofloxacin, trimethoprim-sulfamethoxazole, cefpodoxime, or cephalexin
  - <u>Inpatients</u>:
    - If low risk for multidrug-resistant organisms and not critically ill: ceftriaxone 1 g IV daily
    - Review prior urine cultures to see if the patient has had prior UTIs with *P. aeruginosa* or ESBL-producing organisms; consider a prior antibiotic regimen if the patient has a history of multidrug-resistant organisms
    - Also consider a broader empiric antibiotic regimen if the patient is critically ill

Catheter-associated UTI (CAUTI)
- Epidemiology: CAUTIs are the most common health care-acquired infection
- Microbiology: Similar to other UTIs with the addition of *Candida* spp.
- Clinical features: Symptoms are often non-specific; can cause dysuria and abdominal pain
- Diagnosis:
  - Pyuria and bacteriuria ($\geq 10^5$ CFU/mL) or funguria in a patient with an indwelling urinary catheter AND
  - Systemic findings suggestive of an infection (e.g., fever, leukocytosis) or findings that localize to the urinary tract (e.g., flank pain, suprapubic pain) AND
  - Exclusion of an alternative source of infection (e.g., skin and soft tissue infection, bacteremia, pneumonia)
- Treatment: Antibiotics, remove urinary catheter as soon as possible

Prostatitis
- Pathogens: Gram-negative rods: *E.coli, Klebsiella* spp., *Proteus* spp., *Pseudomonas aeruginosa, Enterobacter* spp.

Acute bacterial prostatitis:
- Pathophysiology: Pathogens gain entrance to the prostate via the urethra
- Clinical features: Patients are typically acutely ill with high fevers, chills, dysuria, urgency, frequency, as well as pelvic or perineal pain (most localizing feature to the prostate)
- Diagnosis: Digital rectal exam will reveal a boggy, exquisitely tender prostate. Urinalysis may show profound pyuria with sheets of WBCs on microscopy. Urine culture is almost always positive.
- Treatment:
  - Mild illness: Outpatient management with empiric trimethoprim-sulfamethoxazole 1 DS tablet BID or ciprofloxacin 500 mg BID
  - Severe illness: Admit to the hospital and treat with IV ciprofloxacin or ceftriaxone. Carbapenems (e.g., ertapenem 1 g IV daily) may be used in those with risk-factors for multidrug-resistant organisms or previously cultured ESBL-producing organisms
  - Narrow antibiotics based on culture results
  - Duration of antibiotics: 2–6 weeks depending on severity of illness
- Complications:
  - Some patients will develop bacteremia or a prostatic abscess, or they will go on to develop chronic bacterial prostatitis
  - In patients who fail to improve despite initial antibiotic therapy, obtain a CT of the abdomen/pelvis with IV contrast to evaluate for a prostatic abscess, which may require procedural drainage

Chronic bacterial prostatitis:
- Pathophysiology: Similar to acute prostatitis, with chronic bacterial prostatitis arising from incomplete treatment
- Clinical features: More common than acute bacterial prostatitis. Occurs in men age 40–70 yr. These patients are often asymptomatic or only mildly ill. Patients often have symptoms of recurrent urinary tract infections, and the same organism is frequently isolated from urine culture. Dull back, scrotal, perineal, or suprapubic pain may be present
- Diagnosis: More difficult to diagnose than acute bacterial prostatitis. Diagnostic standard is finding bacteria at a higher concentration in prostatic fluid compared to urinary tract specimens, but testing is insensitive, so the diagnosis can also be presumed and treatment can be empiric
- Treatment: Prolonged antibiotics (4 weeks). Fluoroquinolones or trimethoprim-sulfamethoxazole both achieve excellent concentrations in prostatic tissue

Infective Endocarditis
- Pathogens:
  - Culture-positive endocarditis: Gram-positive cocci are the most common organisms to cause infective endocarditis (IE): *Staphylococcus aureus* (the most common cause), coagulase-negative staphylococci, *Streptococcus* spp., such as viridans streptococci, and *Enterococcus* spp
  - Culture-negative endocarditis:
    - The HACEK organisms were traditionally considered the predominant pathogens in culture-negative endocarditis. However, improved culture techniques have made them more easily identifiable on blood cultures
      - **HACEK** organisms = **H**emophilus spp., **A**ggregatibacter spp., **C**ardiobacterium hominis, **E**ikenella corrodens, and **K**ingella spp
    - *Coxiella burnetii* and *Bartonella* spp. are now the most common causes of true culture-negative endocarditis, in addition to non-infective causes of endocarditis (e.g., marantic endocarditis)
    - The most common reason for "culture-negative" endocarditis is that antibiotics were given prior to blood culture collection
  - Prosthetic valve endocarditis:
    - The differential diagnosis for the organisms that cause prosthetic valve endocarditis depends on the time after valve replacement that the infection develops:
      - 0–1 yr after surgery: *S. aureus* and coagulase negative staphylococci are most common
      - ≥1 yr after surgery: Pathogens similar to native valve endocarditis

- Risk factors:
  - Age >60 yr
  - Injection drug use (IDU): Carries high risk for bacteremia, which occurs when bacteria enter the venous system and seed the right side of the heart first (usually the tricuspid valve). Also IDU can cause direct valve damage by exposing valves to the particulate matter present in the injected material, increasing the risk of IE.
  - Poor dentition and/or dental infection: Oral flora can translocate and seed cardiac valves
  - Structural heart disease (e.g., valvular heart disease): Structural abnormalities of cardiac valves allow bacteria to attach more easily
- Clinical features:
  - Fever (most common symptom of IE) and inflammatory symptoms (chills, weight loss, myalgias)
  - A new cardiac murmur (present in ~70% of cases)
  - <u>Left-sided endocarditis</u>: Can cause embolic phenomena from the **left heart → systemic circulation**
    - Left-sided septic emboli to any organ: Brain, spleen, kidneys, and bone/joints
    - Splinter hemorrhages (microemboli visible in the nail beds)
    - Janeway lesions: Painless, erythematous macules that are usually seen on the palms and soles. These are microabscesses from septic emboli.
    - Osler nodes: Painful nodules on the fingers pads. Due to vasculitis or septic emboli.
  - <u>Right-sided endocarditis</u>: Can cause embolic phenomenon from the **right heart → lungs**
    - Cough, pleuritic pain, shortness of breath
    - Septic pulmonary emboli, which present as diffuse, peripheral, randomly distributed pulmonary nodules that may have cavitation. Pulmonary infarcts or abscesses may also develop
    - Can rarely see findings associated with left-sided IE as well
- Diagnosis:
  - Collect at least three sets of blood cultures prior to the administration of antibiotics
  - Transthoracic echocardiography (TTE) should be performed in all patients. If negative TTE, obtain transesophageal echocardiogram (TEE) which is more sensitive. TEE is also preferred to evaluate for vegetations in patients with prosthetic valves and when there is concern for perivalvular abscess
  - Also consider: ECG to evaluate for emerging heart block, CXR or CT chest to evaluate for pulmonary complications, CT abdomen/pelvis to evaluate for metastatic foci of infection
  - A diagnosis can be made based on the <u>modified Duke criteria</u> (See Table 8.20). Specifically:
    - Any pathologic criteria OR
    - Two major criteria; one major and three minor criteria; five minor criteria

TABLE 8.20 · Modified Duke's Criteria for Diagnosing Native-Valve Infective Endocarditis

<u>Pathologic Criteria</u>
- Histologic evidence of active endocarditis on sampling of a vegetation or endocardial abscess
- Culture or histology of a valvular vegetation or endocardial abscess that shows microorganisms

<u>Major Criteria</u>
Positive blood cultures that meet one of the following criteria:
- Two blood cultures positive with organisms that typically cause endocarditis (e.g., *viridans streptococci*, *S. aureus*, *S. bovis*, HACEK organisms, or enterococci without a primary source)
- Persistently positive blood cultures, defined as:
  - Two cultures drawn more than 12 hours apart with typical endocarditis organisms or
  - Three or a majority of at least four sets of positive blood cultures with organisms that may be common skin contaminants (with first and last culture drawn at least one hour apart)
- Single positive blood culture for *Coxiella burnetii* or phase I IgG titer >1:800

Echocardiographic findings of IE, including:
- Vegetation
- Abscess
- Dehisced prosthetic valve
- A new valvular regurgitation

<u>Minor Criteria</u>
- Fever
- Risk factors (e.g., injection drug use, valvular heart disease)
- Embolic phenomena (e.g., septic emboli, Janeway lesions)
- Immunologic phenomena (e.g., Osler nodes, Janeway lesions, glomerulonephritis)
- Positive blood cultures that do not meet major criteria

Source: Adapted from Baddour et al., *Circulation* 2015:132(15):1435–1486.

TABLE 8.21 · Surgical Indications for Infectious Endocarditis by Valve Type		
Left-Sided Native Valve Endocarditis	**Right-Sided Native Valve Endocarditis**	**Prosthetic Valve Endocarditis**
• Patients with heart failure • Patients with fungal endocarditis or endocarditis from multidrug-resistant organisms • Persistent infection (e.g., persistent bacteremia or fever >5–7 days) despite effective therapy • Complicated infections including paravalvular abscess, heart block, or fistula formation • Recurrent emboli or enlarging vegetation despite appropriate antibiotics • Large vegetations >1 cm in size, especially if associated with severe valvular regurgitation	• Vegetations >2 cm in size • Persistent or recurrent septic pulmonary emboli • Severe tricuspid regurgitation not responsive to therapy • Heart failure not responsive to medical therapy	• Heart failure • Heart block, valvular abscess, or destructive infection (e.g., fistula) • Fungal endocarditis or endocarditis from multidrug-resistant organisms • Vegetation >1 cm in size • Persistent bacteremia clearly from endocarditis for >5–7 days despite appropriate antibiotics

- Treatment:
  - Antibiotic therapy:
    - Native-valve endocarditis: Empiric vancomycin IV + ceftriaxone 2 g IV daily, then narrow antibiotics based on culture results for 4–6 weeks total duration
    - Prosthetic valve endocarditis: Empiric vancomycin IV + an antipseudomonal cephalosporin (e.g., cefepime) +/− gentamicin and rifampin (not always required empirically, decisions should be made in consultation with ID), narrow based on culture results for 6 weeks total duration in most cases
  - Valve replacement:
    - Some patients will require valve replacement to control the infection and prevent severe hemodynamic complications that develop as a consequence of extensive valvular damage
    - Consult cardiothoracic surgery. The decision for valve surgery is up to the consulting surgeon, but general indications for valve replacement are shown in Table 8.21.

Bloodstream Infections

- Pathophysiology: A bloodstream infection can arise from:
  - An endovascular source of infection (e.g., endocarditis or septic thrombophlebitis)
  - As a complication of another organ infection (e.g., *E. coli* bacteremia due to pyelonephritis)
  - As a result of direct blood stream innoculation (e.g., as a complication of a central line infection or intravenous drug use)
- Risk factors:
  - Any risk factor for severe infection portends an increased risk for bacteremia
  - The presence of any indwelling device increases the risk for bacteremia, such as indwelling central venous catheters (e.g., a central line) or hemodialysis catheters
  - Certain infections carry an increased risk for bacteremia (e.g., pyelonephritis, cholangitis, pyogenic liver abscess, severe HAP or VAP, severe SSTI)
- Pathogens: Can be Gram-positive, Gram-negative, or fungal. Common organisms include:
  - Gram-positive: *S. aureus, S. pneumoniae* (often as a complication of *S. pneumoniae* pneumonia), viridans streptococci, *Enterococcus* spp., *S. lugdunensis*
  - Gram-negative: *E. coli, K. pneumoniae, P. aeruginosa, Enterobacter* spp.
  - Fungi: Most often *Candida* spp., particularly common in immunocompromised or critically ill patients
- Clinical features: Rigors suggest a bloodstream infection. Other clinical features are non-specific (e.g., fevers, malaise, etc.)
- Diagnosis: Blood cultures ×2. Of note, the presence of a positive blood culture does not always mean that there is a clinically significant blood stream infection (See Table 8.22).

TABLE 8.22 · Interpretation of Positive Blood Cultures		
Organisms that should always be considered clinically significant on blood cultures	**Organisms that are often clinically significant but occasionally a contaminant**	**Organisms that are often contaminants**
• *S. aureus* • *S. lugdunensis* • *S. pneumoniae* • Group A streptococcus • *P. aeruginosa* • *E. coli* • *Klebsiella pneumoniae* • *Candida* spp.	• *Enterococcus* spp. • Viridans streptococci	• Coagulase negative staphylococci (except *S. lugdunensis*) • *Corynebacterium* spp.
<u>Management:</u> • Any patient with blood cultures (either a single or multiple) that grow one of the above organisms should be started on treatment and further evaluated for the source of the bloodstream infection	<u>Management:</u> • 2/2 positive blood cultures with one of these organisms likely represents true bacteremia. • 1/2 positive blood cultures may reflect true bacteremia or contamination depending on the patient's clinical status and the suspicion for a bloodstream infection.	<u>Management:</u> • In some situations, particularly in immunocompromised hosts, positive blood cultures with these organisms may represent a true infection.

- Treatment:
  - <u>Source control</u>: Remove central venous catheters if possible, drain any fluid collection(s) if present, order a TTE in all cases of *S. aureus* bacteremia or if suspicion for endocarditis
  - <u>Empiric antibiotic therapy</u>:
    • <u>Gram-positive cocci</u>: Vancomycin
    • <u>Gram-negative rods</u>: Ceftriaxone IV 2 g daily (or consider broader Gram-negative coverage if risk factors for *P. aeruginosa* or ESBL infection). For intra-abdominal infection, empyema, or necrotizing SSTI, ensure you have anaerobic coverage by adding metronidazole to ceftriaxone or cefepime or using piperacillin-tazobactam or a carbapenem.
    • <u>*Candida* spp.</u>: An echinocandin
  - <u>Targeted antibiotic therapy and duration of treatment</u>:
    • Targeted antibiotic therapy will depend on the antimicrobial susceptibilities
    • Duration of therapy depends on the source of the infection and the organism isolated
    • Gram-positive organisms: Endocarditis and *S. aureus* bacteremia are often treated for 4–6 weeks. Other Gram-positive organisms such as *S. pneumoniae* or viridans streptococci are often treated for 10–14 days.
    • Gram-negative rods are often treated for 7–14 days. Patients with uncomplicated Gram-negative rod bacteremia can be transitioned to oral therapy after initial clinical improvement if antibiotic susceptibilities allow. Most data is with an oral fluoroquinolone, although emerging data suggests oral beta lactams can also be used in certain clinical situations.
  - <u>Special considerations for bacteremia with certain organisms</u>:
    • *S. aureus*
      - Consult ID for all cases due to improved mortality with ID involvement
      - Obtain a TTE for all cases of *S. aureus* bacteremia. If TTE negative, TEE may be necessary depending on the clinical suspicion for endocarditis.
    • *S. lugdunensis*
      - Obtain a TTE and consult ID as this can cause a very aggressive infection with multiple metastatic foci (this organism should be treated similarly to *S. aureus*)
    • *Candida* spp.
      - Consult ID for all cases
      - Consult ophthalmology to evaluate for endophthalmitis
      - Remove any central venous catheters; it may be okay to leave a central venous catheter in place if there is a clear GI source of candidemia (e.g., chemotherapy induced mucositis), but this should be discussed with an infectious disease consultant discuss with ID

Skin and Soft Tissue Infections (SSTIs)

Non-purulent and purulent cellulitis

- Pathophysiology: Cellulitis is an infection of the deeper layers of the dermis. It can be non-purulent or purulent (e.g., associated with pustules or a skin abscess)
- Pathogens: Gram-positive cocci, including:
  - Non-purulent cellulitis: Beta-hemolytic streptococci, especially group A streptococci (e.g., *S. pyogenes*)
  - Purulent cellulitis or abscess: *S. aureus*, including MRSA
- Clinical features:
  - Unilateral warmth, tenderness, and erythema, often of a distal extremity. Bilateral involvement is rare.
  - Fever, chills, or other systemic manifestations can be present.
  - Abscess: Features of cellulitis + a focal collection of pus within the subcutaneous tissue
- Diagnosis: Cellulitis is a clinical diagnosis! No diagnostic tests are typically needed, but consider the following if the clinical picture is unclear and/or the patient is critically ill:
  - Advanced imaging (e.g., CT with contrast) of an affected extremity if there is concern for a necrotizing skin and soft tissue infection or abscess
  - Blood cultures in cases where there are notable systemic symptoms (e.g., fevers, rigors)
  - Gram stain and culture of purulent fluid after incision and drainage of an abscess
  - Superficial wound cultures are <u>not</u> useful in isolating organisms as they are often polymicrobial and do not reliably distinguish the causative organism from normal skin flora
  - A skin biopsy may be helpful in cases that do not respond to appropriate therapy, in immunocompromised patients, and/or when the diagnosis of cellulitis is uncertain
- Treatment:
  - **Non-purulent cellulitis:** Beta-hemolytic streptococci is the most common pathogen; MRSA is rarely implicated in non-purulent cellulitis (exceptions: penetrating trauma or MRSA colonization)
    - Outpatient therapy:
      - Cephalexin 500 mg PO QID (preferred) or clindamycin 300 mg PO TID (alternative)
      - Duration of therapy: 5 days. If the patient is not responding to initial therapy after 72 hours, obtain imaging to rule out an underlying abscess, expand antibiotic coverage to include MRSA coverage, and consider alternative diagnoses.
    - Inpatient therapy:
      - Cefazolin 1 g IV q8 h. If not responding, broaden to vancomycin IV. Can narrow to a PO antibiotic when improving.
      - Duration of therapy: Typically 5 days. If the patient is not responding to therapy, obtain imaging to rule out an underlying abscess, expand antibiotic coverage to include MRSA coverage (e.g., IV vancomycin), consider alternative diagnoses, and consider consulting ID and/or dermatology.
  - **Purulent cellulitis:** Almost always caused by *S. aureus*, and often MRSA
    - Outpatient therapy:
      - If a drainable abscess is present: Patient should undergo incision and drainage (I&D). Clinical trials support the use of antibiotics after I&D, but many patients will improve without them, so the decision should be made on a case-by-case basis based on the risk and benefits for each individual patient
      - If no abscess is present: Treat with empiric PO antibiotics that have MRSA coverage, such as:
        - Trimethoprim-sulfamethoxazole 1 DS Tabs BID or
        - Doxycycline 100 mg BID or
        - Clindamycin 300 mg PO TID (alternative agent)
      - Duration of therapy: 5 days. If the patient is not responding to initial therapy, obtain imaging to rule out an underlying abscess, consider inpatient admission for IV antibiotics, and consider alternative diagnoses.
    - Inpatient therapy:
      - IV vancomycin (preferred). Alternatives: IV daptomycin or linezolid. If the patient is responding to initial therapy, switch to a PO antibiotic (see options above).
      - Duration of therapy: Typically 5 days from the start of vancomycin. If the patient is not responding to initial therapy, obtain imaging to rule out an underlying abscess, consider alternative diagnoses, and consider consulting ID and/or dermatology.

Necrotizing fasciitis
- Pathophysiology:
  - Necrotizing fasciitis is an aggressive, morbid, and limb- and life-threatening infection within the deep layers of the skin
  - Type 1 = Polymicrobial. Often both aerobic organisms (e.g., *E. coli, Klebsiella* spp.) and anaerobic organisms (*Bacteroides* spp., *Clostridium* spp., *or Peptostreptococcus* spp.).
  - Type II = Monomicrobial. Group A strep (GAS) is the most common, less often beta-hemolytic *streptococci* or others
- Clinical features:
  - Physical exam: Erythema (often more purple), pain out of proportion to degree of skin findings (e.g., "pain out of proportion to exam"), crepitus (because of subcutaneous gas production)
  - Labs: Non-specific, but can have leukocytosis, hyponatremia, elevated inflammatory markers
- Diagnosis:
  - Necrotizing fasciitis is a <u>clinical diagnosis</u>. Consult general surgery <u>immediately</u> if you suspect necrotizing SSTI
  - Imaging can be helpful to further risk-stratify (look for soft tissue gas, although not a sensitive finding), but should not delay surgical consultation
  - Clinical prediction tools: No reliable tools. The LRINEC score has previously been described and used but it has not demonstrated reliable sensitivity in follow-up studies
- Treatment:
  - Empiric antibiotics should be started right away, but are ineffective alone. Possible empiric antibiotic regimen = vancomycin + ertapenem or piperacillin-tazobactam + clindamycin (because of its antitoxin effect and the Eagle effect, where it is more effective than PCN at high inoculation states)
  - Emergent surgical debridement. Mortality approaches 100% without surgery.

Bite-related infections
- Pathogens: Consider pathogens in the animal's mouth and pathogens on the patient's skin:
  - Oral flora of canines and felines includes *Pasteurella* spp., *Capnocytophaga canimorsus* (especially in dogs), as well as *Staphylococcus* spp. and *Streptococcus* spp.
  - Cat bites are more morbid than dog bites and become infected more frequently (>80% of cat bites compared to ~5% of dog bites) because their teeth can penetrate more deeply
  - The human oral flora includes *Staphylococcus* spp. and *Streptococcus* spp. as well as anaerobic organisms including *Eikenella corrodens, Peptostreptococcus* spp., *Fusobacterium* spp., and *Prevotella* spp.
  - The majority of bite-related infections are polymicrobial
- Treatment:
  - Antibiotic prophylaxis with amoxicillin-clavulanate 875 mg PO BID should be administered for 3–5 days in patients with any of the following: Laceration requiring stiches, bite wounds on the hand/face/genitals, underlying immunocompromise or advanced liver disease, edema of the infected area, a deep puncture, and/or a vascular graft near the bite site
  - Consider surgical consultation if deep space infection, infection of the hand or face, underlying immunocompromise, crepitus on physical exam, and/or persistent signs of infection despite antibiotics
  - Ensure tetanus vaccination is up-to-date
  - Consider need for rabies post-exposure prophylaxis in dog and raccoon bites. Consult ID and contact the local health department

Bone/Joint Infections

Osteomyelitis
- Types of osteomyelitis and pathogenesis:
  - <u>Hematogenous osteomyelitis</u>: Develops in the setting of bacteremia (e.g., endocarditis or another endovascular infection). *S. aureus* is the most common pathogen.
  - <u>Vertebral osteomyelitis</u>: Develops due to hematogenous spread, local tissue invasion (e.g., from a psoas abscess), or direct inoculation after a procedure. *S. aureus* is the most common pathogen, along with *Streptococcus* spp., Gram-negative rods, and *Mycobacterium* spp. (Pott disease = TB osteomyelitis of the spine).
  - <u>Non-hematogenous osteomyelitis</u>: Develops in the setting of poor wound healing, such as diabetic foot ulcers and sacral decubitus ulcers, followed by direct inoculation from the skin and soft tissue to the exposed bone. Common skin flora, in addition to Gram-negative organisms (including *P. aeruginosa*) are the most common pathogens.

- Symptoms:
  - Dull pain over the site of the infected bone, often develops gradually
  - Symptoms of local infection (e.g., erythema, warmth, swelling, or tenderness) or systemic infection and bacteremia (e.g., fevers, rigors) may be present
- Diagnostic tests:
  - Labs: Usually non-specific, and can include leukocytosis and an elevated ESR and CRP
  - Blood cultures: Obtain in all patients prior to antibiotic administration. Blood cultures are most often positive in patients with hematogenous osteomyelitis.
  - Imaging: MRI is the most sensitive imaging modality. X-ray can be useful in patients with long-standing symptoms but is not helpful in detecting early infection. CT with contrast can detect cortical irregularities but is less sensitive than MRI.
- Establishing the diagnosis: There are two ways to make a diagnosis of osteomyelitis:
  - Definitive diagnosis with bone biopsy. In general, open bone biopsy (such as during debridement) has a higher diagnostic yield than needle biopsy
  - An inferred diagnosis with a combination of clinical features (e.g., imaging findings, positive blood cultures)
- Treatment:
  - Antibiotic therapy: Empiric therapy with vancomycin + ceftriaxone 2 g IV daily or cefepime 2 g IV q8 hr if *P. aeruginosa* coverage is needed. Narrow antibiotics based on culture sensitivities. Typical duration is 6 weeks.
  - Surgical intervention: Bone debridement is sometimes needed, especially if bone necrosis is present. Consult an orthopedic surgeon (or a neurosurgeon in the case of vertebral osteomyelitis) to determine the need for debridement.

Septic arthritis

- Pathogenesis:
  - <u>Hematogenous seeding</u>: Septic arthritis most commonly develops as a result of hematogenous seeding of the synovial membrane, which then extends into the joint space
  - <u>Direct inoculation</u>: Less often, septic arthritis develops via local spread from contiguous tissues. This occurs in situations such as a bite wound or joint space procedure (e.g., arthroscopy or intra-articular injection)
- Risk factors: Rheumatoid arthritis (RA) or other conditions that cause joint pathology (e.g., osteoarthritis)
- Pathogens:
  - *S. aureus*: Most common cause of septic arthritis, especially in patients with a prosthetic joint or RA
  - *Neisseria gonorrhoeae*: Most common cause of septic arthritis in young, previously healthy adults
  - *Streptococcus* spp.: Patients with functional or true asplenia are at increased risk
  - Gram-negative organisms (e.g., *P. aeruginosa*): Immunocompromised patients are at highest risk
  - *Mycobacterium* spp.: Patients with underlying immunocompromise or TB risk factors
- Clinical features: Red, hot, swollen, and tender joint with extreme pain with either passive or active range of motion. A joint effusion is also often present. Fever may be absent, especially in older adults.
- Diagnosis: Arthrocentesis and synovial fluid analysis. Consider the following studies:
  - <u>Synovial fluid WBC count</u>: The likelihood of septic arthritis is directly related to the WBC count
    - A synovial fluid WBC count >50K cells/μL, and especially >100K cells/μL, suggests septic arthritis. The differential is often neutrophil-predominant. Crystal arthritis (e.g., an acute gout flare) can have a similarly high WBC count and commonly mimics septic arthritis
    - A synovial fluid WBC count <20K cells/μL suggests against septic arthritis
  - <u>Synovial fluid Gram stain</u>: A positive Gram stain confirms the diagnosis of septic arthritis, but is only positive in 50% of cases; therefore a negative Gram stain does not rule out septic arthritis
  - <u>Synovial fluid culture</u>: In cases of non-gonococcal septic arthritis, the synovial fluid culture is positive over 60% of the time
  - <u>Crystals</u>: The presence of crystals in synovial fluid suggests crystal arthritis. Of note, patients with crystal arthropathy (e.g., underlying gout or pseudogout) can *also* develop concurrent septic arthritis; the presence of crystals on arthrocentesis does not exclude septic arthritis
- Treatment:
  - Empiric antibiotic therapy:
    - Vancomycin + ceftriaxone 2 g IV daily (no *P. aeruginosa* coverage)
    - Vancomycin + cefepime 2 g IV q8hr (for *P. aeruginosa* coverage)
    - Narrow based on culture results. Duration 2–4 weeks.
  - Joint drainage: Surgical joint washout is the cornerstone of management to adequately control the infection. Consult orthopedic surgery for surgical decision making.

Systemic Fungal Infections

- Pathogens:
  - See Tables 8.7 and 8.8 for organisms that cause systemic and opportunistic fungal infections
- Diagnostic tests to evaluate for fungal infections:
  - **1,3-Beta-D-glucan (BDG):** Tests for a cell-wall polysaccharide that is present in most, but not all, fungi. It is 75–85% sensitive and specific for a fungal infection.
    - Relevant fungi for which it tests include:
      - *Candida*
      - *Aspergillus*
      - *Pneumocystis*
      - *Histoplasma*
      - *Coccidioides*
    - It does <u>not</u> detect mucormycosis (e.g., *Rhizopus* spp. and *Mucor* spp.), *Cryptococcus* spp., and *Blastomyces* spp.
    - False positives can occur with administration of IVIG, albumin, and some hemodialysis filters
  - **Galactomannan:** Tests for a specific component of the cell wall in *Aspergillus*. Sensitivity of ~70% in serum. More sensitive on BAL samples (~80%). Rarely, false positives can occur in patients receiving TPN. Piperacillin/tazobactam causes false positives, but less commonly now due to new formulations of the antibiotic
  - **Cryptococcal antigen (CrAg):** Tests for an antigen associated with *Cryptococcus*. The serum test is useful in patients with HIV/AIDS and CD4 counts <100 cells/µL.
    - If serum CrAg is negative, there is a very low likelihood that the patient has cryptococcal meningitis (especially in HIV, may not be as sensitive in other types of immunocompromise)
    - If serum CrAg is positive, get an LP to rule out cryptococcal meningitis in all patients
    - If LP demonstrates crypto meningitis, treatment includes induction therapy with amphotericin B + flucytosine, followed by consolidation and maintenance therapy with fluconazole once repeat LP demonstrates clearance of the organism from CSF
  - *Histoplasma* **antigen:** Tests for an antigen associated with histoplasmosis. Can be tested off of serum or urine; >90% sensitivity (urine) and 80% sensitivity (serum). Urine *Histoplasma* antigen is very sensitive for disseminated histoplasmosis in HIV infection.
  - **Cocci immunofixation and complement fixation:** Used to evaluate for coccidioidomycosis. Different sensitivity/specificity for these tests in blood vs. CSF.
- Treatment: Antifungal agents – see Table 8.24

Sexually Transmitted Infections (STIs)

Chlamydia & gonorrhea

- Pathogens: *Chlamydia trachomatis* & *Neisseria gonorrhoeae*. Most common bacterial STIs
- Clinical features: Purulent urethral discharge, scrotal pain or pelvic pain, dysuria, intermenstrual bleeding
- Diagnosis:
  - Vaginal or urinary nucleic acid amplification test (NAAT)
  - Obtain pharyngeal and/or rectal swabs for NAAT in patients with a history of oral sex or receptive anal intercourse
- Treatment:
  - Chlamydia: Azithromycin (1000 mg oral dose) alone
  - Gonorrhea: ceftriaxone 250 mg IM ×1 + 1000 mg azithromycin
  - Sexual partners should be referred for evaluation and presumptive therapy

Disseminated gonococcal infection (DGI)

- Pathophysiology: A systemic infection caused by *N. gonorrhoeae* that develops when genital infection spreads to the blood stream
- Clinical features: There are two classic clinical syndromes of DGI:
  - Tenosynovitis, dermatitis, and polyarthralgias. A pustular or vesiculopustular rash is present in about ~75% of cases, but the absence of a rash does not rule out DGI.
  - Acute, purulent arthritis of one or multiple joints. Common joints = wrists, knees, ankles.
- Diagnosis:
  - Blood cultures may return positive for *N. gonorrhoeae*
  - Positive NAAT testing of mucosal sites (genitals, rectum, or oropharynx)
  - Synovial fluid analysis (in patients with an acute arthritis)
- Treatment:
  - Ceftriaxone 1 g IV daily in all patients + azithromycin 1 g PO ×1 +/− surgical joint drainage in patients with an acute arthritis who are not responding to therapy

Herpes simplex virus (HSV)
- Subtypes:
  - HSV-1 (oropharynx or genital ulcers): Adults are often asymptomatic with HSV-1 primary infection, but the virus can remain dormant in the trigeminal ganglia and later reactivate to cause lesions near the mouth/lips (grouped vesicles on an erythematous base). Treatment: Acyclovir.
  - HSV-2 (recurrent genital ulcers): *Painful* genital ulcers, prodrome burning/pruritus, lymphadenopathy. Treatment: Acyclovir (chronic suppressive therapy if ≥6 outbreaks/yr or to prevent transmission to a seronegative partner, or episodic therapy for those with fewer outbreaks)
- Complications:
  - Disseminated HSV: Can cause encephalitis, meningitis, keratitis, and chorioretinitis, typically in immunocompromised individuals
  - Ocular disease: HSV-1 or HSV-2 can cause keratitis, blepharitis, keratoconjunctivitis
  - Herpetic whitlow: HSV-1 or HSV-2 on the hand, which causes a throbbing pain in the distal pulp space
- Diagnosis: PCR (most sensitive, if available) or viral culture

Syphilis (*T. pallidum* spirochete)
- Microbiology & pathogenesis:
  - A slender spirochete with rotary-type movements. Can be seen with darkfield microscopy.
  - Transmission of syphilis occurs due to direct contact with an open lesion (chancre or condyloma lata) infected with organisms during intercourse or other physical or sexual contact.
  - During initial infection, two paradoxical events happen:
    - The host immune response controls the local infection, leading to resolution of the chancre. During this time, antibodies to *T. pallidum* develop and the infection can progress into its latent, asymptomatic phase.
    - However, even with local control of the infection and resolution of the chancre, the spirochetes disseminate widely throughout the body, which can lead to the systemic manifestations of secondary and tertiary syphilis.
- Phases:
  - **Primary:** Painless ulcerated lesion with raised and indurated edges. Often accompanied by regional lymphadenopathy. It usually resolves spontaneously within two weeks, with or without treatment.
  - **Secondary:** A syndrome characterized by systemic symptoms (e.g., fevers, chills, malaise) and multiple potential manifestations, including:
    - Rash: A diffuse macular rash of the trunk, extremities, palms, and soles. The absence of palm and sole involvement does not decrease the likelihood of syphilis
    - Mucous patches: White, erosive lesions of the oral mucosa or tongue
    - Condyloma lata: Raised lesions that can arise in the perineal or oral areas
    - Alopecia: Patchy, scattered, "moth-eaten" alopecia. It is often irreversible
  - **Latent:** Asymptomatic phase of infection between symptomatic phases. Patients will have positive syphilis tests.
    - Early latent syphilis: Infection known to occur in the last 12 months.
    - Late latent syphilis: Infection occurred at an unknown time or >12 months ago.
  - **Tertiary:** Late manifestations of untreated syphilis. Rare in the antibiotic era, but still present given rising rates of syphilis worldwide. Primarily affects the cardiac and neurologic systems.
    - Cardiovascular manifestations include a large vessel vasculitis that can cause aortitis or aortopathy (e.g., aortic insufficiency)
    - Neurologic manifestations include:
      - General paresis: A dementia syndrome characterized by memory deficits and eventual psychosis
      - Tabes dorsalis: Disease of the posterior columns of the spinal cord, which causes lancinating pains of the extremities, back or face, sensory ataxia, and pupillary defects (Argyll-Robertson pupil, which does not react to light but accommodates when light is shown in the contralateral eye)
  - Neurosyphilis: Can develop at any phase of disease because the spirochetes quickly disseminate after initial inoculation. Symptoms include meningitis, uveitis (ocular syphilis), hearing loss or tinnitus (otosyphilis), and, rarely, a CNS vasculitis.

INFECTIOUS DISEASES

- Diagnosis:
  - Direct visualization with darkfield microscopy after samples from skin lesions with high organism burden (chancre, mucous patch, or condyloma lata)
  - Serologic testing, which uses:
    - Non-treponemal tests: These monitor disease activity but are not specific to syphilis. Non-treponemal test titers wane with time or treatment. Non-treponemal tests include:
      - Rapid plasma reagin (RPR)
      - Venereal Disease Research Laboratory (VDRL)
    - Treponemal test: These test for antibodies to *T. pallidum*. They will remain positive even after treatment. Treponemal tests include:
      - Fluorescent treponemal antibody absorption (FTA-ABS)
      - *T. pallidum* particle agglutination assay (TPPA)
      - *T. pallidum* enzyme immunoassay (TP-EIA)
      - Chemiluminescence immunoassay (CIA)
- Interpretation of serologic tests: Serologic tests for syphilis include an algorithm that starts with either a treponemal (reverse algorithm) or non-treponemal test (traditional algorithm). The interpretation of the test results depend on the testing algorithm used.
- Diagnosis of neurosyphilis: Positive CSF analysis for neurosyphilis or symptoms consistent with ocular or otosyphilis
- Treatment:
  - Primary, secondary, early latent: Penicillin G 2.4 million units IM ×1 dose
  - Tertiary or late latent: Penicillin G 2.4 million units IM once weekly ×3 weeks
  - Neuro: Penicillin G 3–4 million units IV q4 hours ×10–14 days
  - For all: See IDSA guidelines and follow post-treatment monitoring recommendations

Chancroid (*H. ducreyi*)
- Clinical features: <u>Painful</u> genital ulcer(s) with a ragged border and unilateral painful inguinal lymphadenopathy (buboes) that occurs at the same time as the ulcer(s)
- Diagnosis: No serologic tests available; rule out syphilis and HSV-2
- Treatment: Azithromycin (oral, one dose) OR ceftriaxone (IM, one dose)

Lymphogranuloma venereum (*C. trachomatis*)
- Clinical features: <u>Painless</u> anal or genital lesion(s) that often go unnoticed. This is followed by tender lymphadenopathy weeks later. The third phase is a genital/anal/rectal syndrome with pelvic lymphadenopathy, diarrhea, proctitis, and, in severe cases, abscesses or fistulas.
- Diagnosis: *C. trachomatis* NAAT (urine, rectal), antibody testing (LGV is caused by serovars L1–L3)
- Treatment: Doxycycline 100 mg PO BID ×21 days

Genital warts (HPV 6 and 11)
- Clinical features: <u>Painless</u> flesh-colored, exophytic lesions
- Treatment: Podophyllin, TCA, cryotherapy, surgery. Treatment of genital warts does not prevent HPV transmission.

HIV/AIDS

- Pathogenesis: See Figure 8.1. The 4 main steps in HIV infection include:
  - Viral entry: The HIV virus enters host cells by binding its gp120 viral envelope protein to the CD4 protein on the host's CD4+ T cell surface. gp120 then interacts with a second surface protein, a chemokine receptor, and then the gp41 protein mediates fusion of the viral envelope with the host's CD4+ T-cell membrane, allowing the virion core to enter the cytoplasm.
    - Medications that impact this step include the <u>entry/fusion inhibitors</u>:
      - Enfuvirtide: Binds to the viral envelope protein GP41 to prevent <u>fusion</u>
      - Maraviroc: Binds to the chemokine co-receptor 5 (CCR5) to prevent <u>entry</u>
      - Ibalizumab: Binds to the domain 2 of CD4+ T cells, to prevent <u>entry</u>
  - Transcription of the viral RNA into double stranded DNA by the reverse transcriptase: Once in the cytoplasm, the virus's reverse transcriptase transcribes the HIV RNA genome into double-stranded DNA.
    - Medications that impact this step include the <u>NRTIs and NNRTIs</u>:
      - NRTIs include lamivudine, tenofovir alafenamide (TAF), tenofovir disoproxil fumarate (TDF), emtricitabine, and abacavir
      - NNRTIs include efavirenz, rilpivirine, etravirine, doravirine, and nevirapine
  - Integration of the viral DNA with the host DNA: The double-stranded DNA then migrates into the nucleus and integrates into the host DNA via a virus-encoded integrase.
    - Medications that block this step are <u>integrase inhibitors</u>: Dolutegravir, raltegravir, bictegravir
  - Cleavage of the viral RNA into large polyproteins by proteases: The viral mRNA is then transcribed by the host RNA polymerase, translated, and then cleaved by proteases into several large polyproteins.
    - Medications that impact this step include the <u>protease inhibitors</u>, ritonavir and atazanavir
- Transmission: HIV infection occurs via sexual intercourse (oral, vaginal, or anal), exposure to infected blood (injection drug use, or, rarely, needlestick), or perinatal transmission

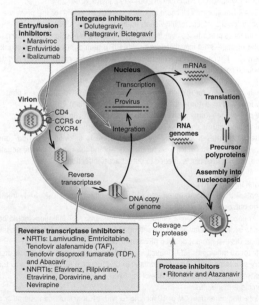

FIGURE 8.1: Life cycle of the HIV virus and mechanisms of anti-retroviral medications. Shown are the steps of the HIV life cycle and relevant medications that act on each step of viral replication.

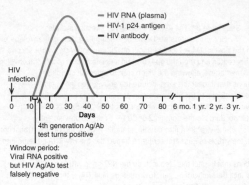

FIGURE 8.2: Changes in serum markers of HIV infection during the early phase of HIV infection in untreated patients.

- Stages: These stages of HIV infections are based on the CDC's updated staging system:
  - Stage 0: If the individual had a negative HIV test within 6 months (180 days) of the diagnosis of HIV infection, they are classified as Stage 0, which reflects early infection. The criteria for Stage 0 supersede criteria for other stages and individuals diagnosed at stage 0 remain stage 0 for the first 180 days after diagnosis.
  - Stage 1: CD4 T-lymphocyte cell count ≥500 cells/µL or ≥26%*
  - Stage 2: CD4 T-lymphocyte cell count of 200–499 cells/µL or 14–25%*
  - Stage 3: CD4 T-lymphocyte cell count of <200 cells/µL or <14%* or the presence of any Stage-3 defining opportunistic infection.# Individuals in this stage have AIDS.
    *Cell count takes precedence over %. Use the % only if the absolute count is missing.
    #Examples of stage-3 defining illnesses include PJP pneumonia, esophageal candidiasis, TB infection of any site, Kaposi sarcoma, CMV retinitis, extrapulmonary cryptococcosis, extrapulmonary or disseminated coccidioidomycosis or histoplasmosis
- Diagnosis:
  - There are three markers for HIV infection, and each turns positive at different phases (Figure 8.2):
    - The HIV RNA viral load (turns positive ~10 days after infection)
    - The HIV p24 antigen (turns positive ~15–20 days after infection)
    - The HIV antibody (turns positive ~20–30 days after infection)
  - These differential times to positivity means that there is a "window period" during which the fourth-generation HIV test (which tests for the p24 Ag and the HIV Ab) can be negative. During this time period, the HIV RNA test is needed to detect acute infection
- Treatment:
  - Antiretroviral therapy (ART):
    - All patients with HIV should be offered ART at the time of diagnosis. Early treatment improves long-term outcomes and retention in care.
    - In certain patients with specific opportunistic infections, ART initiation should be delayed. The decision to initiate or delay ART in the setting of OIs should be made with the assistance of an ID consultant. OIs that prompt delayed ART start include:
      - Cryptococcal meningitis (CM): Induction of ART may precipitate immune reconstitution inflammatory syndrome (IRIS). This can be fatal in cryptococcal meningitis due to the inflammatory response of IRIS in the closed space of the CNS.
      - Tuberculous meningitis
      - CNS infection other than CM or TB meningitis with evidence of brain edema or mass effect
      - CMV retinitis
      - Patients who are intubated or hypotensive as a result of non-CNS or non-ocular OI or bacterial infection
- Vaccinations in individuals with HIV: Regular and strict adherence to vaccination schedules is a key component of HIV management. See IDSA and CDC guidelines.
- Opportunistic infections & prophylaxis: Table 8.23 reviews the different opportunistic infections in individuals living with HIV, as well as prophylaxis regimens for each infection

INFECTIOUS DISEASES

TABLE 8.23 · Opportunistic Infections and Prophylaxis Regimens in Individuals Living with HIV

CD4 Count	Opportunistic Infections & Specific Features	Prophylaxis Regimen

All CD4 Counts	· Tuberculosis
	  - All individuals with HIV are at increased risk for tuberculosis
	  - Screen for latent TB
	  - Have a low threshold to evaluate for primary or reactivation TB in patients with the appropriate clinical syndrome (e.g., pneumonia or lymphadenopathy)
		No specific prophylaxis regimen

CD4 Count ≤250 cells/μL	· Coccidioidomycosis
	  - Individuals with HIV living in regions where coccidioidomycosis is endemic are at increased for asymptomatic and symptomatic infection
	  - Test annually for IgG and IgM antibodies to *Coccidiodes* spp.
		· Fluconazole 400 mg daily if the patient has positive cocci serology and no signs or symptoms of active disease
		· Stop prophylaxis when the CD4 count is >250 cells/μL for at least 6 months and the HIV viral load is undetectable

CD4 count ≤200 cells/μL	· Pneumocystis Pneumonia (PCP)
	  - PCP is an often indolent, progressive respiratory disease in patients with HIV/AIDS
	  - Clinical manifestations: Fever, cough and dyspnea
	  - Imaging: Diffuse infiltrates or ground glass opacities
		· Trimethoprim-sulfamethoxazole:
		  - 1DS tab daily (most commonly used regimen)
		  - 1SS tab daily
		  - 1DS tab 3× weekly
		· Dapsone:
		  - 100 mg daily
		· Atovaquone:
		  - 1500 mg daily with food

CD4 count ≤150 cells/μL	· Histoplasmosis
	  - In areas where histoplasmosis is endemic (e.g., certain parts of South America or French Guiana) prophylaxis may be administered
	  - In general, does not warrant prophylactic therapy
		· Itraconazole until the CD4 count is >150 cells/μL for 6 months after starting ART

CD4 count ≤100 cells/μL	· Toxoplasmosis
	  - Can cause a ring-enhancing CNS lesion in individuals with CD4 counts ≤100 cells/μL
		· Trimethoprim-sulfamethoxazole:
		  - 1DS tab daily (most common regimen)
		  - 1SS tab daily
		  - 1DS tab 3× weekly
		· Atovaquone
		  - 1500 mg daily with food
		· If TMP-SMX or atovaquone cannot be used:
		  - Dapsone 50 mg PO qD + pyrimethamine 50 or 75 mg + leucovorin 25 mg

	· Cryptococcus
	  - Can cause pulmonary, skin and soft tissue, or CNS infections
	  - Cryptococcal meningitis is an opportunistic infection that warrants delaying ART initiation (use serum cryptococcal antigen to screen. If positive, the patient needs an LP to rule out cryptococcal meningitis)
		- Preventative therapy is not recommended
		- Patients treated for active disease often remain on maintenance therapy (200 mg fluconazole daily) until the CD4 count rises above 100 cells/μL while on ART with a sustained undetectable viral load for least 3 months after at least 1 yr of maintenance therapy

CD4 count ≤50 cells/μL	· Mycobacterium avium complex (MAC)
	  - Localized infection that often causes lymphadenitis or, rarely, subcutaneous nodules, osteomyelitis, or pulmonary disease
	  - Disseminated infection can cause fever, night sweats, lymphadenopathy, abdominal pain, and diarrhea
	  - Lab abnormalities: May have an isolated elevated alkaline-phosphatase
		· No longer necessary if the patient is starting ART (low risk of infection after ART treatment, prophylaxis may precipitate macrolide resistance)

Source: Adapted from recommendations from the Centers for Disease Control and Prevention, the National Institutes of Health, and the HIV Medicine Association of the Infectious Diseases Society of America.

- HIV Prevention:
  - **Post-exposure prophylaxis (PEP):** This approach to HIV prevention can be used in individuals who had a high-risk exposure to HIV (e.g., receptive or penetrative vaginal or anal intercourse without condom use or percutaneous exposure to blood). Obtain a baseline HIV test and start therapy with tenofovir disoproxil fumarate/emtricitabine + dolutegravir or raltegravir.
  - **Pre-exposure prophylaxis (PrEP):** This approach to HIV prevention is used for certain populations who have a high risk of HIV exposure, and thus take an antiretroviral medication daily to reduce the risk of getting HIV if they are exposed to the virus. See CDC guidelines for indications for PrEP, recommended testing prior to starting PrEP, possible regimens, and monitoring recommendations.

Tick-Borne Illnesses
Lyme disease

- Etiology: *Borrelia burgdorferi* spirochete is spread by the *Ixodidae scapularis* tick in the Northeastern United States, Northern Midwest.
- Stages:
  - <u>Stage 1</u>: Early localized (1–4 wks) – single erythema migrans target-shaped skin lesion
  - <u>Stage 2</u>: Early disseminated infection (weeks-months) – multiple erythema migrans skin lesions, fever, headache, heart block/myocarditis, cranial nerve palsy, meningitis
  - <u>Stage 3</u>: Late infection (mo-yr later) – oligoarticular arthritis, encephalopathy or encephalomyelitis
  - <u>Post-Lyme disease syndrome</u>: There is no biologic evidence for "chronic Lyme" infection and there is no benefit to antibiotics for this syndrome
- Diagnosis: Two tier testing with ELISA and Western blot confirmation
- Treatment: PO doxycycline; use IV ceftriaxone for more severe stage 2 and 3 disease (e.g., meningitis)

Other tick-borne illnesses

- Ehrlichiosis: Bacterial illness transmitted by the Lone Star tick. Can cause leukopenia, thrombocytopenia, and rash (less common). Treatment: Doxycycline
- Anaplasmosis: Bacteria transmitted by the *Ixodes* tick (same tick that transmits the Lyme spirochete and babesiosis – so can get co-infection!). Causes fever, rash. Treatment: Doxycycline
- Babesiosis: Parasite transmitted by the *Ixodes* tick. Can cause hemolytic anemia, jaundice, hemoglobinuria, renal failure. Typically, the patient does not have a rash (unlike other tick-borne illnesses). Patients are at particular risk if they are asplenic. Diagnosis: Smear with intra-erythrocytic parasites that look like a Maltese cross. Treatment: Atovaquone + azithromycin OR quinine + clindamycin if severe infection
- Rocky Mountain Spotted Fever: Bacteria transmitted by the *Dermacentor* tick. Can cause fever, nausea/vomiting, and then a rash that starts on the palms and soles and spreads to the rest of the body. Can also cause, interstitial pneumonitis, elevated LFTs, thrombocytopenia. Treatment: Doxycycline

KEY MEDICATIONS & INTERVENTIONS

Antibiotics

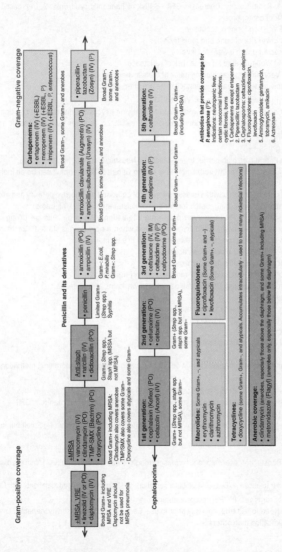

FIGURE 8.3: **Antibiotic coverage map.** This image depicts a simplified way to visually organize antibiotic coverage. See also Tables 8.11, 8.12 and "Principles of antibiotic selection and infection management" at the beginning of this chapter. For each drug, the generic name is listed first and then the trade name follows in parentheses for some drugs. Antibiotics with stronger Gram-positive (Gram+) coverage are positioned on the left of the figure in red and antibiotics with stronger Gram-negative (Gram–) coverage are positioned on the right of the figure in blue. The further left or right an antibiotic is positioned generally reflects broader Gram-positive or Gram-negative coverage respectively. At the bottom, antibiotics with atypical coverage are in green boxes and those with anaerobic coverage are in a brown box. Please note that this is a simplified way to depict the relative coverage of antibiotics, as many of these antibiotics cover multiple classes of organisms with some caveats listed in the figure below each box. Please refer to other resources for a more complete overview of antibiotic sensitivities.

Abbreviations: (P) indicates antibiotics that cover *Pseudomonas aeruginosa* (also see text in the bottom right of the figure), +MRSA indicates antibiotics that cover methicillin-resistant *Staphylococcus aureus*; +VRE indicates antibiotics that cover vancomycin-resistant *enterococcus*; +ESBL indicates antibiotics that cover extended-spectrum beta lactamase producing bacteria; IV, intravenous; PO, per os.

Antiretroviral Therapy (ART)

Antiretroviral therapies are listed here, with select pros (+) and cons (−) indicated.

Nucleoside reverse transcriptase inhibitors (NRTI)

- Abacavir: (−) Risk hypersensitivity − must rule out HLA-B*5701 mutation first.
- Tenofovir: (−) 1. Renal toxicity: Decreases GFR → Risk of Fanconi's syndrome. 2. Decreased bone density and risk of osteoporosis.
  - TAF and TDF are two forms of tenofovir
    - TAF has a lower risk of bone and renal toxicities
    - TDF is associated with lower lipid levels
- Lamivudine: (+) Well-tolerated (−) Higher risk of resistance
- Emtricitabine: Very similar to lamivudine (think of them as being equivalent)
  ** Abacavir/lamivudine and tenofovir/emtricitabine are often paired.

Nonnucleoside reverse transcriptase inhibitors (NNRTI)

- Efavirenz: (−) Can cause bad dreams, worsening of underlying psychiatric disorders and suicidality
- Rilpivirine: (+) Better tolerated (−) Higher likelihood of resistance, requires food and gastric acid for absorption (can't use with a PPI)

Protease inhibitors (PI)

- Darunavir: (+) Potent (i.e., high barrier to resistance) (−) Nausea, diarrhea, hyperlipidemia
- Atazanavir: Causes an indirect hyperbilirubinemia due to Gilbert's. Not harmful; can be an indication of medication compliance.
  - Boosters: PIs are often given with a booster (ritonavir of cobicistat) to improve potency and allow for less frequent and lower dosing. Both ritonavir and cobicistat are CYP450 inhibitors.
  - Drug–drug interactions: PIs have many drug–drug interactions. When patients are taking a PI, it is worth discussing any dosing modifications needed when a new drug is started. Common drug classes with drug-drug interactions in the setting of PI use include:
    - Acid reducers (PPIs, H2 blockers, antacids)
    - Alpha-blockers (e.g., tamsulosin, prazosin, etc.)
    - Anti-mycobacterial, macrolides, anti-fungals, and anti-malarials
    - Anti-coagulants (including DOACs, dabigatran, and warfarin), anti-platelets
    - Anti-convulsants
    - Anti-depressants, anxiolytics, and anti-psychotics
    - Anti-arrhythmics (e.g., amiodarone), beta-blockers
    - HCV treatment
    - Hormonal agents, including oral contraceptives
    - Statins
    - Opioids and medications used to treat opioid use disorder (e.g., buprenorphine, methadone)

Integrase inhibitors

- Elvitegravir: (−) Lower barrier to resistance than dolutegravir
- Dolutegravir: (+) Difficult to become resistance (−) Small bump in Cr, but no change in GFR
- Raltegravir: (−) BID dosing makes compliance more challenging
- Bictegravir: (+) High barrier to resistance, fewer side effects than dolutegravir (−) Small bump in Cr, similar to dolutegravir

Pharmacokinetic boosters

- Ritonavir: (+) Boosts protease inhibitors, increases trough so can be dosed daily (−) Nausea, diarrhea, hyperlipidemia
- Cobicistat: Similar to above (−) Decreases tubular secretion, so should not be used in patients with CKD

C-C chemokine receptor type 5 (CCR5) receptor antagonist

- Maraviroc: (−) Need to test tropism assay prior to use. Can cause hypersensitivity, hepatitis. Overall a less potent medication than others

Fusion inhibitors (not 1st line)
- Enfuvirtide: (–) Injectable, very common to get injection site reactions

Common starting ARV regimens
- Biktarvy = Bictegravir/tenofovir alafenamide/emtricitabine
- Descovy + Tivicay = Tenofovir alafenamide/emtricitabine + dolutegravir (TAF/FTC + DTG)
- Truvada + Tivicay = Tenofovir disoproxil fumarate/emtricitabine + dolutegravir (TDF/FTC + DTG)
- Raltegravir + (emtricitabine or lamivudine) + (TAF or TDF)
- Triumeq = Dolutegravir-abacavir-lamivudine (DTG/ABC/3TC)
  - Only use in patients confirmed to be HLA-B*5701 negative given the adverse reaction associated with ABC in HLA-B*5701 positive individuals
- Dovato = Dolutegravir/lamivudine (DTG/3TC)
  - This regimen cannot be used when: 1) HIV RNA > 500,000 copies/mL, 2) there is HBV co-infection, or 3) ART is going to be started before HIV resistance testing for reverse transcriptase or HBV testing are available

Antifungal Therapies
First-line treatments for invasive fungal infections
- Anti-fungal agents: See Table 8.24 for antifungal therapies and spectrums of their coverage
- Invasive candidiasis (e.g., candidemia): Initiate echinocandins are 1st line for invasive candidiasis
  - Can transition to fluconazole for some species (e.g., *C. albicans*)
  - *C. krusei* is intrinsically resistant to fluconazole
  - If *Candida* spp. cultured from bloodstream, consult ID and also consult ophthalmology to evaluate for endophthalmitis
- Concern for angioinvasive fungal infection:
  - Suspect mucormycosis: Initiate empiric amphotericin B
  - Suspect invasive *Aspergillus*: Initiate empiric voriconazole

TABLE 8.24 • Spectrum of Coverage for Antifungal Agents

		Fluconazole	Itraconazole	Isavuconazole	Voriconazole	Posaconazole	Amphotericin B	Echinocandin
Dimorphic	Histoplasmosis		X	X	X	X	X	
	Blastomycosis		X	X	X	X	X	
	Coccidioidomycosis	X	X	X	X	X	X	
Yeasts	C. albicans	X	X	X	X	X	X	X
	C. galbrata			X	X	X	X	X
	C. parapsilosis	X	X	X	X	X	X	X
	C. krusei			X	X	X	X	X
	Cryptococcus neoformans	X	X	X	X	X	X	
Molds	Aspergillus fumigatus		X	X	X	X	X	
	Fusarium spp.			X	X	X	X	
	Scedosporium spp.			X	X	X		
	Mucormycosis			+/-		+/-	X	
		Useful for most C. albicans isolates		Similar to voriconazole but with increased activity against mucor	First line empiric therapy if Aspergillus suspected, but not mucor	Similar to voriconazole but with increased activity against mucor	Broadest of the anti-fungals with coverage that includes Aspergillus and mucor	Use for empiric broad spectrum coverage of invasive candidiasis prior to speciation

KEY CLINICAL TRIALS & PUBLICATIONS
Fever of Unknown Origin
- **Fever and fever of unknown origin: Review, recent advances, and lingering dogma.** *Open Forum Infect Dis* 2020;7(5): ofaa132.
  - A review article that integrates new data on fever of unknown origin (FUO) into the clinical approach and diagnosis and considers how this new data should influence clinical decision making and definitions of FUO.

Neutropenic Fever
- **[Guideline] Clinical practice guideline for the use of antimicrobial agents in neutropenic patients with cancer: 2010 update by the infectious diseases society of America.** *Clin Infect Dis* 2011;52(4):e56–93.
  - This clinical practice guideline from the IDSA is intended to guide the use of antimicrobial agents in patients with cancer who develop fever in the setting of chemotherapy-induced neutropenia. It includes the risk stratification algorithm to determine which patients are at high- and low-risk of complications.
- **[Guideline] Outpatient management of fever and neutropenia in adults treated for malignancy: American society of clinical oncology and infectious diseases society of America clinical practice guideline update summary**. *J Oncol Pract* 2018;14(4):250–255.
  - This guideline seeks to answer questions around which patients with fever and neutropenia can be managed as outpatients. It also includes recommendations on the basic workup of febrile neutropenia.
- **Antimicrobial-resistant Gram-negative bacteria in febrile neutropenic patients with cancer: Current epidemiology and clinical impact.** *Curr Opin Infect Dis* 2014;27(2):200–210.
  - A review that examines recent trends in epidemiology and antimicrobial resistance in Gram-negative infections in neutropenic cancer patients. It pays particular attention to the impact of antimicrobial resistance on the outcomes of severe infections caused by these organisms.

Fever in a Returning Traveler
- **Approach to Fever in the Returning Traveler.** *N Engl J Med* 2017;376(6):548–560.
  - This review focuses on epidemiologic features of infections in traveling patients and offers an approach to life-threatening and highly transmissible infectious diseases that commonly impact travelers. It includes key information on geography, incubation period, and transmission of clinically relevant infections in travelers.

CNS Infections
- **Corticosteroids for acute bacterial meningitis.** *Cochrane Database Syst Rev* 2015;2015(9): CD004405.
  - A systematic review of 25 randomized trials that included data from 4121 patients and examined outcomes and adverse effects of corticosteroid use for acute bacterial meningitis. Corticosteroids significantly reduced hearing loss and neurological sequelae but did not reduce overall mortality. This review supports the use of corticosteroids in patients with bacterial meningitis.
- **Computed tomography of the head before lumbar puncture in adults with suspected meningitis.** *N Engl J Med* 2001;345(24):1727–1733.
  - A prospective cohort study of 301 adults with suspected meningitis. Clinical features associated with an abnormal finding on CT of the head were an age of at least 60 yr, immunocompromise, a history of CNS disease, and a history of seizure within a week of presentation. The following neurologic abnormalities were also associated with abnormal imaging: An abnormal level of consciousness, an inability to answer two consecutive questions correctly or to follow two consecutive commands, gaze palsy, abnormal visual fields, focal deficits, and abnormal language (e.g., aphasia). This study supports the idea that clinical features can be used to identify those who need CT imaging of the head before lumbar puncture.
- **How do I perform a lumbar puncture and analyze the results to diagnose bacterial meningitis?** *JAMA* 2006;296(16):2012–2022.
  - A systematic review that includes evidence about test accuracy of CSF analysis in adult patients with suspected bacterial meningitis. It demonstrated that a CSF: Blood glucose ratio of 0.4 or less and a CSF WBC count of 500 cells/μL or higher significantly increase the likelihood of bacterial meningitis.

INFECTIOUS DISEASES

Pneumonia

- **[Guideline] Diagnosis and treatment of adults with community-acquired pneumonia. An official clinical practice guideline of the american thoracic society and infectious diseases society of America.** *Am J Respir Crit Care Med* 2019;200(7):e45–e67.
  - This guideline provides evidence-based clinical practice guidelines on the management of adult patients with community-acquired pneumonia. Key items include antimicrobial regimens based on risk factors for certain pathogens and the site of care, as well as updates on the use of specific diagnostics tests (e.g., blood cultures, sputum cultures, and procalcitonin levels).
- **[Guideline] Management of adults with hospital-acquired and ventilator-associated pneumonia: 2016 clinical practice guidelines by the infectious diseases society of America and the american thoracic society.** *Clin Infect Dis* 2016;63(5):e61–e111.
  - This guideline discusses the diagnosis and management of patients with hospital-acquired pneumonia (HAP) and ventilator-associated pneumonia (VAP). It also includes the rationale behind the removal of the previously used category of healthcare-associated pneumonia (HCAP).
- **Short-course versus prolonged-course antibiotic therapy for hospital-acquired pneumonia in critically ill adults.** *Cochrane Database Syst Rev* 2011;(10):CD007577.
  - A systematic review of eight studies that included 1,703 patients and concluded that a short course of antibiotics (7 or 8 days) may be more appropriate than a prolonged course (10–15 days) for HAP/VAP given a decreased rate of recurrence and no difference in other negative outcomes.

Influenza

- **Diagnosis of influenza in intensive care units: Lower respiratory tract samples are better than nose-throat swabs.** *Am J Respir Crit Care Med* 2012;186(9):929–930.
  - This brief communication to the editor includes important data on the frequency of discordant upper and lower respiratory tract specimens tested for influenza via PCR methods. This supports the idea that critically ill patients with negative upper respiratory tract specimens should also undergo testing of lower respiratory tract specimens (e.g., endotracheal aspirate) for ongoing presence of influenza virus.

Tuberculosis

- **One Month of Rifapentine plus Isoniazid to Prevent HIV-Related Tuberculosis.** *N Engl J Med* 2019; 380(11):1001–1011.
  - This randomized, open-label, noninferiority trial evaluated the efficacy and safety of a 1-month regimen if rifapentine plus isoniazid compared with 9 months of isoniazid alone in HIV-infected individuals. The 1-month regimen was not inferior to 9 months of isoniazid alone and was associated with high treatment completion rates. This study has led to the use of a new, short treatment regimen for latent tuberculosis infection in individuals with HIV.

Clostridium difficile

- **[Guideline] Clinical practice guidelines for *Clostridium difficile* infection in adults and children: 2017 update by the infectious diseases society of America (IDSA) and society for healthcare epidemiology of America (SHEA).** *Clin Infect Dis* 2018; 66(7):987–994.
  - This clinical practice guideline update includes substantial changes in the management of *C. difficile* infection, as well as updates on diagnosis, infection prevention, and environmental management strategies for healthcare facilities.

GU Infections

- **[Guideline] International clinical practice guidelines for the treatment of acute uncomplicated cystitis and pyelonephritis in women: A 2010 update by the Infectious Diseases Society of America and the European Society for Microbiology and Infectious Diseases.** *Clin Infect Dis* 2011;52(5):e103–120.
  - This clinical guideline update focuses on the treatment of urinary tract infections in non-pregnant women and includes recommendations on empiric antimicrobial regimens based on antimicrobial resistance patterns.
- **[Guideline] Diagnosis, prevention, and treatment of catheter-associated urinary tract infection in adults: 2009 international clinical practice guidelines from the infectious diseases society of America.** *Clin Infect Dis* 2010;50(5):625–663.
  - This clinical guideline update reflects the most recent recommendations from the IDSA on the diagnosis, prevention, and management of individuals with catheter-associated urinary tract infections (CA-UTI).

- **[Guideline] Clinical Practice Guideline for the Management of Asymptomatic Bacteriuria: 2019 Update by the Infectious Diseases Society of America.** *Clin Infect Dis* 2019;68(10):e83–e110.
  - This clinical guideline reflects the most recent recommendations from the IDSA on the management of asymptomatic bacteriuria, including adult populations that were not previously addressed, such as solid organ transplant recipients. In addition, it reviews the interpretation of non-localizing symptoms (e.g., confusion) in patients with otherwise asymptomatic bacteriuria.

Endocarditis

- **[Guideline] Infective endocarditis in adults: Diagnosis, antimicrobial therapy, and management of complications: A scientific statement for healthcare professionals from the American heart association.** *Circulation.* 2015;132(15):1435–1486.
  - This clinical guideline update on infective endocarditis includes key changes to the diagnosis and management of infective endocarditis, including the addition of specific criteria for *Coxiella burnetii* testing as a major criterion for diagnosis of infective endocarditis and the removal of minor echocardiographic criteria.
- **Comprehensive diagnostic strategy for blood culture-negative endocarditis: A prospective study of 819 new cases**. *Clin Infect Dis.* 2010;51(2):131–140.
  - This prospective, multimodal study incorporated serological, molecular, and histopathological assays to investigate 819 cases of culture-negative endocarditis (CNE). This study highlighted the major role of zoonotic agents in cases of CNE, including *Bartonella* and *Coxiella* spp., as well as the previously underappreciated prevalence of noninfectious diseases. This study contributed to the evidence that shifted the evaluation of CNE from HACEK organisms towards zoonotic organisms and noninfectious processes.

S. aureus Bacteremia

- **Impact of routine infectious diseases service consultation on the evaluation, management, and outcomes of *Staphylococcus aureus* bacteremia.** *Clin Infect Dis* 2008;46(7):1000–1008.
  - This study compared evaluation, management, and outcomes of cases of *S. aureus* bacteremia (SAB) before and after an institution mandated consultation with infectious diseases for all cases of SAB. It demonstrated the landmark finding that infectious diseases consultation decreases rates of treatment failure, increased adherence to guideline-directed care, and improved the diagnosis of endocarditis and metastatic foci of infection.
- **Impact of infectious disease consultation on quality of care, mortality, and length of stay in *Staphylococcus aureus* bacteremia: Results from a large multicenter cohort study.** *Clin Infect Dis* 2015;60(10):1451–1461.
  - A retrospective cohort study that examined consecutive cases of SAB from six academic and community hospitals and compared those with and without infectious diseases consultation. Outcomes included quality measures of management (e.g., echocardiography, repeat blood cultures, removal of infectious foci, and antibiotic therapy), in-hospital mortality, and length of stay. ID consultation was associated with better quality measures, reduced in-hospital mortality, and decreased length of stay.
- **[Guideline] Clinical practice guidelines by the infectious diseases society of America for the treatment of methicillin-resistant *Staphylococcus aureus* infections in adults and children**. *Clin Infect Dis* 2011;52(3):e18–55.
  - This comprehensive clinical practice guideline includes recommendations from the IDSA on the management of multiple types of MRSA infections, including skin and soft tissue infection, endocarditis, bacteremia, CNS infections, and bone and joint infections. It also discusses treatment failure and emerging resistance patterns in MRSA (e.g., reduced vancomycin susceptibility).

Gram-Negative Bacteremia

- **Seven versus 14 days of antibiotic therapy for uncomplicated Gram-negative bacteremia: A noninferiority randomized controlled trial.** *Clin Infect Dis* 2019;9(7):1091–1098.
  - This is a randomized, multicenter, open-label, noninferiority trial that evaluated 7 vs. 14 days of antibiotics for Gram-negative bacteremia in patients who were afebrile and hemodynamically stable for 48 hours without an uncontrolled focus of infection. 7 days was not inferior to 14 days based on all-cause mortality. This study supports the practice change towards shorter courses of antibiotics for uncomplicated Gram-negative bacteremia.

- **Association of 30-day mortality with oral step-down vs continued intravenous therapy in patients hospitalized with Enterobacteriaceae bacteremia.** *JAMA Intern Med* 2019;179(3):316–323.
  - This retrospective multicenter cohort study included 4967 unique propensity score-matched patients hospitalized with monomicrobial Enterobacteriaceae bacteremia. It compared patients treated with oral step-down therapy within the first 5 days of treatment with those treated with continuous intravenous antibiotics. 30-day mortality was not different among the groups, which suggests that oral step-down therapy may be effective in patients with adequate source control and clinical response to initial therapy. It's important to note that most patients received either a quinolone or trimethoprim-sulfamethoxazole. Oral beta-lactams were not thoroughly evaluated.

Invasive Candidiasis

- **[Guideline] Clinical practice guideline for the management of candidiasis: 2016 update by the infectious diseases society of America.** *Clin Infect Dis* 2016;62(4):e1–50.
  - This clinical practice guideline includes recommendations on the diagnosis, management, and prevention of invasive candidiasis. It covers important topics, such as treatment considerations in neutropenic patients, management of central venous catheters in patients with candidemia, empiric therapy in cases of suspected invasive candidiasis, and best-practices for management of *Candida* spp. isolated from the respiratory and urinary tract.

Skin and Soft Tissue Infections

- **[Guideline] Practice guidelines for the diagnosis and management of skin and soft tissue infections: 2014 update by the infectious diseases society of America.** *Clin Infect Dis* 2014; 59(2):147–159.
  - This clinical practice guideline includes recommendations from the IDSA on the management of a variety of skin and soft tissue infections, including those in immunocompromised hosts. It was updated to be aligned with the recommendations of the management of infections from MRSA.
- **A placebo-controlled trial of antibiotics for smaller skin abscesses.** *N Engl J Med* 2017; 376(26):2545–2555.
  - This multicenter, prospective, double-blind, randomized controlled trial that evaluated outcomes of patients who did and did not receive antibiotics after I&D of skin abscesses 5cm or smaller. Administration of antibiotics (TMP-SMX or clindamycin) led to higher cure rates compared to those who received placebo. It's worth noting that most patients in the placebo group also recovered (81.7% and 83.1% in treatment groups vs. 68.9% in placebo group). This suggests that antibiotics after I&D improves short-term outcomes, though the benefits of this approach must be weighed against the risks of antibiotics.

Sexually Transmitted Diseases

- **[Guideline] Sexually transmitted diseases treatment guidelines, 2015.** *MMWR Recomm Rep.* 2015;64(RR-03):1–137.
  - This comprehensive clinical practice guideline covers the diagnosis and management of nearly all sexually transmitted infections and reflects the CDC's most recent recommendations on the topic.

HIV/AIDS

- **[Guideline] Panel on Antiretroviral Guidelines for Adults and Adolescents. Guidelines for the Use of Antiretroviral Agents in Adults and Adolescents with HIV. Department of Health and Human Services.**
  - These guidelines reflect the current knowledge regarding the use of ARV drugs for the treatment of HIV. It includes recommended regimens for starting antiretroviral therapy, managing patients who experience treatment failure, considerations in those with coinfections, as well as drug-drug interactions and other safety considerations.
- **[Guideline] Guidelines for the Prevention and Treatment of Opportunistic Infections in HIV-infected Adults and Adolescents: Recommendations from the Centers for Disease Control and Prevention, the National Institutes of Health, and the HIV Medicine Association of the Infectious Diseases Society of America.**
  - This clinical practice guideline covers the treatment and prevention of nearly all opportunistic infections for which individuals with HIV are at risk. It is the most comprehensive resource for opportunistic infections in those living with HIV in the United States.

NOTES

NOTES

Rheumatology

9

Axial and Appendicular Skeleton

The skeletal system is divided into the axial skeleton and the appendicular skeleton (Figure 9.1):

- <u>Axial skeleton</u>: Forms the central axis of the body and includes the bones of the skull, ossicles of the middle ear, hyoid bone of the throat, vertebral column, and thoracic cage (i.e., the rib cage)
- <u>Appendicular skeleton</u>: Consists of the bones of the pectoral limbs, pelvic limb, and pelvic girdle

Synovial Joint Anatomy

- Joint capsule ("articular capsule"): Envelope surrounding a synovial joint that connects to the periosteum (Figure 9.2). Each capsule has two layers: 1) An outer fibrous layer, 2) An inner membrane lined by synovium
- Synovial fluid: Viscous fluid secreted by synovial cells that lubricates the joint
- Articular cartilage: Thin layer of hyaline cartilage, composed of type II collagen, proteoglycans, and water, that covers the articulating surface of each bone
- Enthesis: The site at which tendons or ligaments insert into the bone

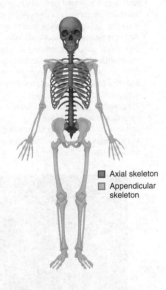

■ Axial skeleton
□ Appendicular skeleton

FIGURE 9.1: The axial and appendicular skeleton.

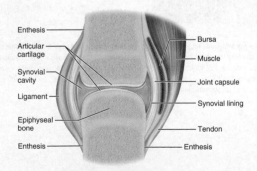

Enthesis
Articular cartilage
Synovial cavity
Ligament
Epiphyseal bone
Enthesis

Bursa
Muscle
Joint capsule
Synovial lining
Tendon
Enthesis

FIGURE 9.2: The anatomy of a synovial joint.

DIAGNOSTICS

Diagnostic Reasoning in Rheumatology

- Most rheumatologic diseases are diagnosed "clinically" – e.g., a rheumatologist weighs the exam findings, labs, imaging and/or tissue biopsy results and makes a (sometimes tentative) diagnosis based on the strength of concordance between these findings and a given disease entity.
- Classification criteria: Diagnostic criteria exist to ensure homogeneity of patients with rheumatologic diseases who enroll in clinical trials. Therefore, these criteria are biased in favor of specificity and NOT intended to diagnose rheumatic diseases.

Approach to Reading a Hand X-Ray

- Alignment: Misaligned joints can help suggest specific pathologies. For example, ulnar deviation of the metacarpophalangeal joints (MCPs) is suggestive of rhematoid arthritis (RA).
- Bone density: Lucency can be used to assess bone density; denser regions of bone are brighter on x-ray. When the lucency of juxta-articular bone is similar to that of the central metacarpal, there is said to be periarticular osteopenia, which is an early pathologic change in RA. Conversely, subchondral sclerosis (increased brightness of the juxta-articular bone) is suggestive of osteoarthritis (OA).
- Cortical edges: Erosions appear as interruptions in the smooth contour of the peri-articular cortex and raise concern for the inflammatory arthropathies or erosive OA. Osteophytes appear as irregular outgrowths of bone and suggest OA.
- Joint spaces: Joint space narrowing suggests arthritis, but does not distinguish inflammatory from non-inflammatory pathology.
- Soft tissues: The triangular fibrocartilage sits between the ulna and the carpal bones and is a good site to assess for chondrocalcinosis (i.e., calcium pyrophosphate crystal build-up, commonly due to pseudogout).

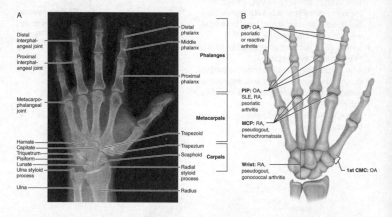

FIGURE 9.3: **Hand x-ray and joints typically affected by rheumatologic and non-rheumatologic diseases.**
A) Hand x-ray with anatomy labeled. B) Joints in the hand and differential diagnosis of rheumatologic and non-rheumatologic conditions that typically affect these joints. Abbreviations: CMC, carpometacarpal joint; DIP, distal interphalangeal joint; MCP, metacarpophalangeal joint; OA, osteoarthritis; PIP, proximal interphalangeal joint; RA, rheumatoid arthritis; SLE, systemic lupus erythematosus.

APPROACHES & CHIEF COMPLAINTS

Diagnostic Approach to Joint Pain

(1) Consider non-articular mimics of joint pain
- Articular structures: Synovium, synovial fluid, articular cartilage, intraarticular ligaments, joint capsule, and juxtaarticular bone
- Non- or peri-articular structures: Extraarticular ligaments, tendons, bursae, muscle, fascia, bone, nerve, and overlying skin

(2) Characterize the joint pain
- Temporality: Acute versus chronic
  - **Acute**: <6 weeks
  - **Chronic**: >6 weeks
- Inflammation: Inflammatory or non-inflammatory; assess for inflammatory features:
  - History: Morning stiffness lasting >30–60 min
  - Exam: "Rubor, calor, tumor" – Peri-articular erythema, warmth and joint swelling
  - Labs: Elevated ESR and/or CRP, synovial fluid WBC >2K cells/μL
- Number of joints involved: Mono-, oligo-, and polyarthritis
  - **Monoarthritis**: Single joint
  - **Oligoarthritis**: 2–4 joints
  - **Polyarthritis**: ≥5 joints

(3) Analyze synovial fluid

Synovial fluid analysis is particularly critical in patients with acute monoarthritis.
- Cell count:
  - **WBC <2K cells/μL**: Noninflammatory
    - Bloody: Trauma, coagulopathy, tumor
    - Non-bloody: OA, avascular necrosis, Charcot arthropathy (peripheral neuropathy resulting in unwitting pathologic joint trauma typically in the feet and ankles)
  - **WBC 2–10K cells/μL**: Inflammatory arthritis, gout, and pseudogout
  - **WBC >20K cells/μL**: Very high concern for infectious arthritis; gout and pseudogout are also possible, but orthopedic surgical consultation for consideration of washout is essential
- Crystals:
  - **Monosodium urate**: Needle-shaped, negatively birefringent crystals (yellow when parallel to the microscope polarization axis). Suggestive of gout in the setting of acute monoarthritis.
  - **Calcium pyrophosphate dihydrate**: Rhomboid crystals with weak positive birefringence (blue when parallel to the polarization axis). Suggestive of pseudogout in the setting of acute monoarthritis.

TABLE 9.1 · Differential Diagnosis for Joint Pain Based on Clinical Characteristics

	Inflammatory	Non-Inflammatory
Acute	• **Mono:** Gout, pseudogout, septic arthritis, gonococcal arthritis • **Oligo:** Disseminated gonococcal infection, rheumatic fever, acute leukemia • **Poly:** HIV, HBV, HCV, parvovirus B19, chikungunya, rubella, acute leukemia	• **Mono:** Bony/ligamentous trauma, hemarthrosis, osteonecrosis/AVN (hip, knee) • **Oligo:** Sickle vaso-occlusive crises • **Poly:** Type II hyperlipoproteinemia (migratory, episodic polyarthritis)
Chronic	• **Mono:** Borrelia (Lyme), mycobacterial, fungal • **Oligo:** Axial spondyloarthritis, peripheral spondyloarthritis (e.g., reactive arthritis, IBD-associated arthritis), sarcoidosis (esp. knee), AAV, Whipple's disease • **Poly:** RA, PsA, CTDs (SLE, Sjögren's, SSc, PM/DM, MCTD), CPPD, pseudo-RA	• **Mono:** OA (knee/hip), primary bone tumor, bony metastases • **Oligo:** OA (hand/knee/hip), DISH, infiltrative diseases (amyloid arthropathy, hemochromatosis, Wilson's disease) • **Poly:** CPPD pseudo-OA, infiltrative diseases (amyloid arthropathy, hemochromatosis, Wilson's disease)

Abbreviations: Mono, monoarthritis; Oligio, oligoarthritis; Poly, polyarthritis; OA, osteoarthritis; RA, rheumatoid arthritis; PsA, psoriatic arthritis; AAV, ANCA-associated vasculitis; PM, polymyositis; DM, dermatomyositis; MCTD, mixed connective tissue disease; SLE, systemic lupus erythematosus; SSc, systemic sclerosis; CPPD, calcium pyrophosphate deposition; AVN, avascular necrosis; DISH, diffuse idiopathic skeletal hyperostosis; HIV, human immunodeficiency virus; HBV, hepatitis B virus; HCV, hepatitis C virus

Rheumatologic Differential Diagnosis for Common Clinical Syndromes

TABLE 9.2 · Rheumatologic Differential Diagnosis for Common Clinical Syndromes		
Clinical syndrome	**Rheumatologic differential diagnosis**	**Labs/diagnostics to consider**
Fever of unknown origin (FUO)	GCA/PMR, AOSD, SLE, RA, PsA, SpA, PAN, AAV, cryoglobulinemic vasculitis, HSP, periodic fever syndromes	ESR, CRP, ANA, Rf, ANCA, Cryos
Pulmonary HTN	SSc (limited > diffuse), MCTD, SLE, PM/DM	ANA, anti-Scl-70, anti-centromere, anti-RNA Pol III, anti-U1RNP
Diffuse alveolar hemorrhage	AAV, Goodpasture's, SLE, APLS	ANCA, anti-GBM, ANA, C3/C4
Interstitial lung disease	SSc, MCTD, DM/PM, anti-synthetase syndrome, SLE (rare)	ANA, dsDNA, anti-Sm, anti-U1RNP, anti-Ro/La, ANCA, ± myositis panel
Cavitary pulmonary lesions	AAV	ANCA, anti-GBM
Pleuritis/ Pericarditis	SLE, RA, MCTD, DM/PM, AAV, Sjögren's, PAN	ANA, anti-dsDNA, anti-Sm, anti-U1RNP, anti-Ro/La, Rf, anti-CCP, ANCA
AKI/ Glomerulonephritis	SLE (GN or nephrotic), AAV (GN/RPGN), SRC, Sjögren's (RTA/TIN), PAN (renal infarcts), HSP (GN), Goodpasture's (GN), cryoglobulinemic vasculitis (GN)	ANA, anti-Ro/La (RTA/TIN), anti-dsDNA, C3/C4, anti-RNA Pol III (SRC), anti-Scl-70 (SRC), ANCA, anti-GBM, Cryos
Mononeuritis Multiplex	AAV, RA, PAN, Sjögren's, cryoglobulinemic vasculitis, sarcoidosis, SLE	ANA, anti-Ro/La, ANCA, Cryos, Rf, anti-CCP, HCV, HBV
Uveitis	• Anterior: AS, ReA, IBD • Posterior: GPA • Anterior or posterior: Sarcoidosis, Behçet's, syphilis (not rheumatologic but common)	CXR, RPR, ANCA, HLA-B27
Venous AND Arterial Thrombosis	APLS, Behçet's	Lupus anticoagulant testing, anti-β2-GP1, anti-cardiolipin
Erythema Nodosum	Sarcoidosis, Behçet's (notable for ulceration), relapsing polychondritis	CXR
Cutaneous Leukocytoclastic Vasculitis (LCV)	AAV (including drug-induced, e.g., levamisole), IgA vasculitis, cryoglobulinemic vasculitis, hypocomplementemic urticarial vasculitis; many cases of LCV are ultimately idiopathic.	ANCA, C3, C4, Cryos, HCV, Rf, ANA
Livedo Reticularis/ Retiform Purpura	APLS, GPA, EGPA, PAN, cryoglobulinemic vasculitis, rheumatoid vasculitis	Lupus anticoagulant testing, anti-β2-GP1, anti-cardiolipin, ANCA, Cryos, Rf, CCP
Sweet Syndrome	RA, Behçet's, relapsing polychondritis	Rf, CCP

Abbreviations: <u>Rheumatologic conditions</u>: GCA, giant cell arteritis; PMR, polymyalgia rheumatica; AOSD, Adult-onset Still's disease; SLE, systemic lupus erythematosus; RA, rheumatoid arthritis; PsA, psoriatic arthritis; SpA, spondyloarthritis; PAN, polyarteritis nodosa; HSP, Henoch Schönlein purpura; SSc, systemic sclerosis; MCTD, mixed connective tissue disease; PM, polymyositis; DM, dermatomyositis; AAV, ANCA-associated vasculitis; APLS, antiphospholipid syndrome; GN, glomerulonephritis; RPGN, rapidly progressive glomerulonephritis; AKI, acute kidney injury; RTA, renal tubular acidosis; TIN, tubulointerstitial nephritis; LCV, leukocytoclastic vasculitis; GPA, granulomatosis with polyangiitis; EGPA, eosinophilic granulomatosis with polyangiitis; SRC, scleroderma renal crisis. <u>Labs</u>: ESR, erythrocyte sedimentation rate; CRP, c-reactive protein; ANA, antinuclear antibodies; Rf, rheumatoid factor; ANCA, anti-neutrophil cytoplasmic antibody; cryos, cryoglobulins; anti-GBM, anti-glomerular basement membrane; HCV, hepatitis C virus; CCP, cyclic citrullinated peptide.

DISEASES & PATHOPHYSIOLOGY

ANA-Associated Connective Tissue Disorders

- Rheumatologic conditions associated with a +ANA:
  1. Systemic lupus erythematosus (SLE)
  2. Systemic sclerosis (SSc)
  3. Myositis (often ANA-negative; ~50% of dermatomyositis/polymyositis cases are ANA-positive)
  4. Mixed connective tissue disease (MCTD)
  5. Primary Sjögren's
- ANA Testing Pearls:
  - Antinuclear antibodies (ANA) are autoantibodies that bind to the contents of the cell nucleus. The ANA test detects the ANA autoantibodies that are present in the patient's serum.
  - ANA can be elevated in many disorders including autoimmune conditions, infection, and malignancy. 20% of healthy women have a positive ANA. Therefore, it is non-specific and should only be sent if clinical suspicion is high for one of the disorders above.
  - The level of autoantibody is reported as a titer, which is the highest dilution of the serum at which the autoantibodies are still detectable (e.g., 1:640 is more dilute than 1:80, suggesting more autoantibodies are present in the 1:640 sample). The probability of autoimmunity increases with higher ANA titers:
    - ANA ≥1:80 required by EULAR/ACR SLE classification criteria
    - ANA ≥1:640 → 95.8% specific for SLE
  - If an ELISA-based ANA test is negative but clinical suspicion for CTD high, ask the lab to carry out an immunofluorescence (IF)-microscopy-based ANA test, which is more specific.

TABLE 9.3 · Test Characteristics & Clinical Associations for ANA & Sub-Serologies

Antibody (anti-X)	Target Antigen	Prevalence	Clinical Associations
ANA	Various (see below)	95% in SLE 95% in SSc >80% Sjögren's >50% PM/DM	Non-specific, best screening test for SLE
dsDNA	dsDNA	70% in SLE	95% specific for SLE. Titer tracks with disease activity in most patients. Associated with nephritis risk.
Sm	Various proteins that bind to small non-coding RNAs	25% in SLE	99% specific for SLE
U1RNP		40% in SLE	MCTD (see below)
Ro (SS-A)		30% in SLE 30–70% Sjögren's	Annular subacute cutaneous lupus rash; congenital heart block. Seen in primary Sjögren's > RA-associated seconodary Sjögren's.
La (SS-B)		10% in SLE 25–40% Sjögren's	Rarely seen in the absence of Anti-Ro. Lower risk of nephritis.
Histone	Chromatin-associated histones	95% in drug-induced lupus 50–70% in SLE	Drug-induced lupus associated with procainamide, hydralazine, isoniazid
Centromere	Chromosomal kinetochore proteins	15% in SSc 60% in CREST	Limited cutaneous SSc
Scl70	Topoisomerase-I	40% in SSc	Diffuse cutaneous SSc + ILD
RNA-Pol-III	RNA-Pol-III	4–20% in SSc	Paraneoplastic SSc (+ test should trigger malignancy work-up), positive in 60% of patients with scleroderma renal crisis
Mi-2	Helicase	15–20% in DM	DM with fulminant skin > muscle involvement, excellent treatment response, ↓risk of associated malignancy
PM-Scl	Nucleolar exosome complex	4–12% of SSc	PM-SSc overlap syndrome with ILD, nonerosive arthritis, Raynaud's, mechanic's hands

Systemic lupus erythematosus (SLE)
- Pathogenesis:
  - Decreased clearance and increased responsiveness to self-nucleic acids → excessive IFNα production by innate immune cells (especially plasmacytoid dendritic cells) → inappropriate activation of autoreactive B cells → autoantibody production, immune complex deposition in skin, glomeruli, joints, and other tissues
- Epidemiology:
  - 90% of affected patients are women of childbearing age (F:M = 1:1 before adolescence, 9:1 after)
  - US prevalence: 100 per 100,000 white women, 400 per 100,000 black women
- Clinical features: Features in the **2019 EULAR/ACR SLE Classification Criteria** are noted in red (# points)
  - **Constitutional**: Fever (**2**); fatigue; weight loss
  - **MSK**: Arthralgias/myalgias (95% prevalence); inflammatory polyarthritis of the hands/wrists/knees (**6**; 60% prevalence). Jaccoud arthropathy (reducible finger swan neck deformities)
  - **Derm**: Acute cutaneous lupus (**6**; e.g., malar "butterfly" rash); discoid lesions (**4**); subacute cutaneous lupus lesions (**4**); oral ulcers (**2**); non-scarring alopecia (**2**); Raynaud's; photosensitivity
  - **Heme**: Leukopenia (**3**); thrombocytopenia (**4**); autoimmune hemolysis (**4**); APLS (antiphospholipid antibodies and clinical thrombosis); 7× risk non-Hodgkin's lymphoma
  - **CNS**: Acute confusional state (**2**); psychosis (**3**); seizures (**5**); transverse myelitis
  - **Cardiac**: Acute pericarditis (**6**); pericardial effusion (**5**); myocarditis; Libman-Sacks endocarditis; 3–10× risk of ASCVD
  - **Pulm**: Pleural effusion (**5**; 30–50% lifetime prevalence); chronic ILD; acute lupus pneumonitis; DAH (high DLCO); shrinking lung syndrome
  - **Renal**: Proteinuria ≥0.5 g/24 hrs (**4**; 30–50% lifetime prevalence); Class II or V nephritis (**8**); Class III or IV nephritis (**10**). +Anti-dsDNA is associated with an increased risk of lupus nephritis.
  - **GI**: Hepatitis, peritonitis, mesenteric vasculitis (all rare)
  - **Autoantibodies/hypocomplementemia**: Antiphospholipid antibodies (**2**; may be lupus anticoagulant, anti-cardiolipin, or anti-β2GP1; IgG, IgM or IgA); ↓C3 (**3**), ↓C4 (**3**), both (**4**); anti-dsDNA OR anti-Smith antibody (**6**)
- Notable syndromes:
  - Drug-induced lupus
    - Arthritis/arthralgias, serositis, and rash. Notably, <u>no</u> CNS or renal involvement.
    - Culprit medications:
      - Associated with +anti-histone (95%): hydralazine, procainamide, isoniazid
      - Associated with +anti-dsDNA: minocycline, penicillamine, TNFi
      - Other: HCTZ, ACEi, chlorpromazine
  - Discoid lupus erythematosus (DLE)
    - Cutaneous plaques with central hypopigmentation and peripheral hyperpigmentation
    - Pearl: Most patients with DLE do NOT have <u>systemic</u> lupus symptoms
- Diagnosis:
  - 2019 EULAR/ACR Classification Criteria: For patients with **ANA ≥1:80**, score the clinical features in red above. Only count the highest weighted criteria in each category and do not count features better explained by another disease process. Patients with a score ≥10 are classified as having SLE.
  - Caveat about classification criteria: Clinician diagnosis is still the gold standard! These classification criteria are more specific than sensitive; intended to ensure homogeneity of clinical trial patients, not as diagnostic criteria.

  Clinical reasoning pearl: Lupus flare or infection?
  - Favors lupus flare: Predominant ESR elevation, normal CRP; no fever; C3/C4 below the patient's baseline; dsDNA above the patient's baseline; leukopenia; thrombocytopenia
  - Favors infection: Concomitant ESR and CRP elevation; fever; C3/C4 at baseline; dsDNA at baseline; leukocytosis; thrombocytosis (including relative thrombocytosis above the patient's normal platelet baseline)
- Serial disease assessment:
  - Each clinic visit: CBC with differential, BMP, ESR, CRP, C3/C4, UA, UPCR, anti-dsDNA

- Treatment:
  - Non-organ threatening disease:
    - Start hydroxychloroquine (Plaquenil) for all patients regardless of disease activity unless contraindications
      - Reduces flare frequency and incidence of renal disease, and it is also effective for arthritis/arthralgias and skin disease
      - Need annual ophthalmologic exams while taking
    - Arthritis: Low-dose prednisone can be helpful
    - Arthralgias: Limited evidence to guide sequence of therapy
    - Skin disease: Depending on the severity of skin disease involvement, start with sunscreen/hydroxychloroquine → topicals (steroids, tacrolimus) → mycophenolate → belimumab
  - Moderate organ-threatening disease: Profound cytopenias, acute CNS lupus with seizures, DAH, myocarditis
    - Prednisone 1 mg/kg OR methylprednisolone 1 g IV daily ×3–5 days followed by prednisone taper
    - IVIG may be effective for SLE-related ITP
  - Severe organ-threatening disease: Proliferative class III/IV nephritis
    - See Table 9.4 for features and management of lupus nephritis

Class	Histopathology	Management
I (Minimal Mesangial)	LM appearance normal; immune complexes visible in the mesangium by IF or EM	• Best prognosis • Monitor proteinuria • ACEi/ARB, blood pressure control, sodium bicarb and phosphate binder if needed
II (Mesangial Proliferative)	Mesangial proliferation visible on LM	
III (Focal Proliferative)	Thickened capillary loops on LM, <50% of glomeruli affected. Subendothelial immune complexes seen on EM. Lesions scored as active or chronic.	• Worst prognosis If lesions are active on biopsy, treat with: • 1 g IV methylprednisolone daily ×3–5 days, then prednisone taper over weeks • Mycophenolate 2–3 g daily ×6 months. Non-inferior to cyclophosphamide (*JASN* 2009;20:1103) with lower risk of infection, alopecia, and amenorrhea (*New Engl J Med* 2005;353:2219 and *J Rheum* 2011;38:69).
IV (Diffuse Proliferative)	Thickened capillary loops on LM, >50% of glomeruli affected. Subendothelial immune complexes seen on EM. Lesions scored as active or chronic.	
V (Membranous)	Subepithelial immune complex deposition with GBM thickening. Commonly manifests with nephrotic range proteinuria.	• Moderately poor prognosis owing to extrarenal effects of nephrotic syndrome • Due to risks from proteinuria (including long term risk of renal dysfunction), treatment approach is usually similar to class III/IV
VI (Advanced Sclerosing)	>90% globally sclerotic glomeruli. Final common outcome of other classes.	• Poor prognosis, often advanced CKD/peri-dialysis • Not responsive to immunosuppression • ACEi/ARB if GFR/serum potassium allow, blood pressure control, sodium bicarb and phosphate binder if needed

TABLE 9.4 • Features and Management of Lupus Nephritis

Abbreviations: LM, light microscopy; IF, immunofluorescence microscopy; EM, electron microscopy.

Systemic sclerosis (SSc)

- Pathogenesis: Poorly understood confluence of 1) microvasculopathy, 2) fibrosis, and 3) humoral autoimmunity
- Epidemiology: Prevalence 275 cases per 1 million; SLE is ten times more common than SSc
- Clinical features: Features in the **2013 EULAR/ACR SSc Classification Criteria** are noted in red (# points)
  - **Derm:** Skin thickening of the hands (**9** points if proximal and **4** points if distal to the MCPs; finger skin thickening is called sclerodactyly, best seen as loss of skin wrinkles between the finger joints); puffy fingers/non-pitting edema (**2**); facial skin tightening; telangiectasias (**2**, often facial); calcinosis. Skin involvement is typically most severe over the first 18–24 months, then improves with or without therapy.
  - **Vascular:** Raynaud's phenomenon (**3**, present in 95% of SSc patients), nail-fold capillary disease (**2**, reduced density of nailfold capillaries), fingertip ulcers or pitting scars (**2** or **3**, respectively)
  - **Pulm:** ILD (**2**, especially in diffuse SSc), WHO Group I pulmonary HTN (**2**, especially in limited SSc)
  - **Cardiac:** Arrhythmias, HFpEF, rarely myocarditis
  - **GI:** Reduced oral aperture, GERD, gastric antral vascular ectasia (GAVE, a.k.a. "watermelon stomach", usually heralded by iron deficiency anemia), colonic pseudo-obstruction (Ogilvie's), SIBO
  - **Renal:** Scleroderma renal crisis (SRC)
    - Can be conceptualized as "Raynaud's of the kidneys": Narrowing of renal arterioles leads to hypoperfusion of the juxtaglomerular apparatus and consequent excess renin production
    - Presents with hypertensive emergency (may have retinopathy, PRES), proteinuric AKI and MAHA
    - SRC is the presenting manifestation in ~20% of patients with SSc
    - 60% of patients are Anti-RNA-Pol-III+
  - **MSK:** Inflammatory non-erosive polyarthritis of the hands and wrists, involving the DIPs
  - **Autoantibodies:** Anti-Scl70 (**3**), anti-centromere (**3**), anti-RNA-pol-III (**3**). Max points from auto-Ab = 3.
- Limited vs. diffuse disease: These terms refer ONLY to the extent of skin involvement – both can feature organ fibrosis and vasculopathy (Table 9.6)
- Diagnosis: Clinical diagnosis, but score ≥9 on 2013 EULAR/ACR SSc Classification Criteria is highly specific
- Treatment: Treatments are tailored to the involved organ system(s):
  - **Derm:** Mycophenylate if severely symptomatic and early in disease course (e.g., <1 yr as symptoms often improve without treatment within 2 yr)
  - **ILD:** Mycophenylate is the treatment of choice depending on ILD severity. Lung transplantation may be considered.
  - **Pulmonary HTN:** Monotherapy with an endothelin receptor antagonist (e.g., ambrisentan) or PDE inhibitor (e.g., tadalafil) for patients with WHO functional class I symptoms; combination therapy with ERA and PDEi for patients with WHO class II and III symptoms. Consider evaluation for lung transplantation.
  - **Myocarditis:** Glucocorticoids
  - **Scleroderma renal crisis:** Titrate ACEi to max dose (captopril PO or enalaprilat IV), then add CCB (amlodipine PO or nicardipine IV). Do not reduce MAP by more than 20 mmHg in the first 24 hrs, goal is normotension within 72 hrs. No role for immunosuppression.

TABLE 9.5 · Comparison of Limited and Diffuse Systemic Sclerosis (SSc)			
Feature	Limited	Diffuse	SSc Sine Scleroderma
Extent of skin involvement	Skin distal to knees and elbows only	Skin proximal to knees elbows, including trunk	None
Proportion of SSc patients	70%	20%	10%
Associated auto-ab	Anti-Centromere	Anti-Scl70	Most similar to limited
Raynaud's	99%	98%	
Digital ulcers	50%	25%	
Esophageal disease	90%	80%	
ILD	35%	65%	
Pulmonary HTN	15%	15%	
Myopathy	11%	23%	
Renal crisis	2%	15%	

Inflammatory and non-inflammatory myopathies
- Differential diagnosis for inflammatory myopathies: Dermatomyositis (DM), polymyositis (PM), immune-mediated necrotizing myositis (IMNM), and inclusion body myositis (IBM). See Table 9.6.
- Differential diagnosis for non-inflammatory myopathies:
  - Endocrine: Hypothyroid myopathy, glucocorticoid-related myopathy (Cushing's or exogenous steroids)
  - Medication/toxin-induced myopathies: Alcohol, cocaine, NRTI (AZT in particular), colchicine, gemcitabine, statins
  - Inherited myopathies: Glycogen storage diseases, disorders of muscle lipid export (e.g., carnitine transporter deficiency), mitochondrial myopathies (impairment in oxidative phosphorylation, e.g., MERRF), Duchenne/Becker muscular dystrophy, Limb-Girdle muscular dystrophy
- Distinguishing inflammatory vs. non-inflammatory myopathies: Clinical features of the myopathy can provide clues. See Table 9.7

TABLE 9.6 · Inflammatory Myopothies

	Dermatomyositis (DM)	Polymyositis (PM)	Immune-Mediated Necrotizing Myositis (IMNM)	Inclusion Body Myositis (IBM)
Epidemiology	Prevalence 9–14 per 100,000			Prevalence 51–70 cases per million
Pathogenesis	Immune-complex & complement-mediated damage to endomysial capillaries → ischemic injury to outer fascicular fibers	CD8+ T cell mediated muscle destruction	Unknown; statins or natural statin-like compounds may ↑HMGCR expression → loss of tolerance	Combination of CD8+ T cell mediated myocyte damage and abnormal proteostasis
Auto-antibodies & Clinical Correlations	**DM-Specific** **Mi-2** – Skin > muscle involvement, treatment-responsive **MDA5** – Often amyopathic; ILD in 70%; rapidly progressive **TIF1** – Malignancy in 78%	**DM + PM** **tRNA synthetases*** – ILD in 70% of Jo-1+ **NXP2** – Associated with calcinosis and malignancy **SAE** – Associated with dysphagia	**HMGCR** – ~65% associated with preceding statin exposure (in US cohort) **SRP** – Treatment refractory	**cN1A** – 33% of IBM
Clinical Features	Symmetric proximal muscle weakness (i.e., deltoids, hip flexors, neck flexors), with possible upper esophageal dysphagia can occur. Facial muscles spared. Progresses over months for DM/PM or weeks for IMNM			Proximal, distal, and facial muscle weakness; dysphagia; onset over years
	CK up to 50× ULN (median peak 700 U/L) **Derm:** Photosensitive erythematous/violaceous rash over joints and sun-exposed areas · Heliotrope rash: Over eyelids · V sign: Over anterosuperior chest · Gottron papules/rash: Papules/macules with fine scale over MCP/PIPs or knees (rash only) **Amyopathic DM:** CK/strength within normal limits for ≥ 6 months	CK up to 50× ULN No cutaneous manifestations **Anti-Synthetase Syndrome (DM, PM, SSc, MCTD):** Constellation of ILD, mechanic's hands (fissuring lateral aspect/tip of index fingers), Raynaud's, non-erosive peripheral arthritis occurring in patients with autoantibodies to one or more tRNA synthetase*	CK up to 50× ULN (median peak 4700 U/L) Extramuscular manifestations are rare Ab-negative cases are associated with malignancy	CK up to 10× ULN Median time to wheelchair-dependence = 14 yr (*Brain* 2011;134:3176) Life expectancy overall unaffected

(*Continued*)

TABLE 9.6 · Inflammatory Myopothies (*Continued*)				
	Dermatomyositis	**Polymyositis**	**Immune-Mediated Necrotizing Myositis**	**Inclusion Body Myositis**
Diagnosis	No biopsy required if +Gottron papules/rash since these are highly specific. Otherwise, typical biopsy findings: perifascicular atrophy on muscle biopsy (specific for DM), +/− complement deposition on endomysial capillaries	Biopsy required. Diagnosis of exclusion after ruling out non-inflam myopathies, DM, IMNM, IBM. Typical biopsy findings: CD8+ T cell infiltrate and myofiber MHC-I expression	No biopsy required if +SRP/HMGCR. Otherwise, typical biopsy findings: necrosis, myophagocytosis, regeneration and ↑Mφ ↑pDC ↓lymph	Biopsy required. Typical biopsy findings: CD8+ T cell infiltrate and myofiber MHC-I expression + myofiber vacuolization
Evaluation	MRI to identify inflamed muscle. High resolution chest CT if anti-MDA5+, anti-synthetase+, or dyspnea/cough. Age-appropriate cancer screening, consider CT C/A/P.		Age-appropriate cancer screening, CT C/A/P if ab-neg	MRI to guide biopsy
Treatment	• Glucocorticoids 1 mg/kg for 4–6 wks, taper over 2–3 months as strength/CK improve • For suspected IMNM or rapidly progressive DM/PM: Start with 1g IV methylprednisolone for 3–5 days, then oral prednisone taper • If responsive to glucocorticoids: Add methotrexate, azathioprine, or mycophenolate mofetil for glucocorticoid sparing agent • If suboptimal steroid response or suspected IMNM, consider IVIG 2 g/kg over 2–5 days, then monthly • Exercise/PT are critical for regaining strength			Not responsive to immunosuppression Exercise, PT, hand OT, speech and language pathology

*Anti-Synthetase Abs: Jo-1 (His), Ha (Tyr), PL7 (Thr), PL12 (Ala), OJ (Ile), Zo (Phe), KS (Asn), EJ (Gly)

TABLE 9.7 · Inflammatory vs. Non-Inflammatory Myopathies			
	Favors Inflammatory Myopathy	**Non-specific**	**Favors Non-inflammatory Myopathy**
History	↓Strength over weeks to months	–	• ↓Strength over years • Exercise-induced cramping • Family history of similar symptoms (inflammatory myopathies are not hereditary) • Culprit medications, substance use
Exam	Gottron sign/papules or heliotrope rash (suggests DM → NO need for muscle biopsy)	–	–
Muscle Biopsy	Perifascicular atrophy → specific for DM	Endomysial/perimysial/perivascular lymphocyte infiltrate (seen in IBM, Duchenne/Becker muscular dystrophy, Limb-Girdle muscular dystrophy)	–
Treatment Response	Rapid ↑strength with glucocorticoids	↓CK with glucocorticoids	–

Mixed connective tissue disease (MCTD)
- Pathogenesis: Not known in detail, presumably similar to constituent diseases SLE, SSc, and myositis
- Epidemiology: Rare (exact prevalence not described); F:M = 4:1
- Diagnosis: MCTD is an overlap syndrome in which patients satisfy classification criteria for $\geq$2 of SLE, SSc, and DM/PM, AND have high titer anti-U1-RNP autoantibodies. See Table 9.8 for disambiguation from Overlap Syndrome and Undifferentiated Connective Tissue Disease.
- Clinical features:
  - **Vascular:** Raynaud's, pulmonary hypertension. Vascular manifestations are common and are the main driver of mortality.
  - **Other:** Arthritis, puffy fingers, sclerodactyly, serositis, esophageal dysmotility, myositis, ILD. Renal disease is uncommon.
- Treatment: Targeted toward organ-system-specific manifestations; see SLE/SSc/myositis sections

TABLE 9.8 · Comparison of MCTD, UCTD, and Overlap Syndromes		
Diagnostic Label	**# of distinct classification criteria met (SLE, SSc, DM/PM)**	**Anti-U1-RNP**
Mixed Connective Tissue Disease (MCTD)	$\geq$2	Positive
Overlap Syndrome	$\geq$2	Negative
Undifferentiated Connective Tissue Disease (UCTD)	0*	Negative

*May have a few clinical features associated with SLE, SSc, or DM/PM, but not satisfying classification criteria for any specific CTD

Sjögren's syndrome
- Pathogenesis: Autoimmune destruction of the lacrimal and salivary glands; unclear underlying mechanism but increased risk associated with specific HLA alleles implicates cell-mediated autoimmunity.
- Epidemiology: Prevalence of 0.3–1 in 1000 worldwide. F:M = 9:1
- Clinical features:
  - Glandular manifestations:
    - Severe dry eye (may cause corneal ulceration)
    - Dry mouth (may cause dental caries, result in malnutrition)
  - Extraglandular manifestations:
    - **Constitutional:** Fatigue
    - **Derm:** Xerosis; cutaneous leukocytoclastic vasculitis (small vessel, 30% of these cases associated with cryoglobulins); subacute cutaneous lupus rash (annular photosensitive lesions) associated with anti-Ro antibodies
    - **Articular:** Inflammatory polyarthritis resembling RA except non-erosive
    - **Pulm:** 5–9% overall incidence including bronchiolitis obliterans, ILD
    - **Renal:** 5–6% overall incidence including type 1 RTA, interstitial nephritis, immune-complex GN
    - **Vascular:** Cryoglobulinemic vasculitis; Raynaud's phenomenon (16%)
    - **Neuro:** 8–27% overall incidence including CNS demyelinating lesions, myelopathy/transverse myelitis, cranial neuropathies, mononeuritis multiplex, distal symmetric polyneuropathy
    - **GI:** Primary biliary cholangitis; autoimmune hepatitis
    - **Heme:** Lymphoma (2% overall risk, 15–20-fold increase in risk of non-Hodgkin lymphoma, largely MALT lymphoma in the salivary glands with marginal-zone histology)
    - **Immunologic:** Cryoglobulinemia; positive Rf in ~50%
- Disease categories:
  - Primary Sjögren's: Not meeting criteria for another CTD or rheumatic disease
  - Secondary Sjögren's: Occurring in the context of another rheumatic disease, most commonly RA or SLE (10–30% prevalence in these groups), but also scleroderma, myositis

- Diagnosis:
  - **2017 EULAR/ACR Sjögren's classification criteria:** See Table 9.9
  - Description of special tests for Sjögren's:
    - Ocular fluorescein/lissamine staining: Performed by ophthalmology, scored 0–12
    - Schirmer test: Strip of filter paper applied to the conjunctiva, tear output saturates the length of the strip via capillary action. The total distance moistened is measured over 5 min. Normal is >5 mm.
  - Differential diagnosis for sicca symptoms:
    - Inflammatory and malignant diseases with tropism for parotid glands: Sarcoidosis, IgG4-related disease, GPA, lymphoma
    - Viral infections with tropism for parotid glands: Mumps, HCV, HIV
    - Medications: Anticholinergics, cannabinoids
- Treatment:
  - Eye care:
    - Artificial tears
    - Topical cyclosporine
    - Pilocarpine or cevimeline (muscarinic agonists) to stimulate tear production
  - Oral care:
    - Sugar-free candies to stimulate saliva flow
    - Meticulous oral hygiene and regular dental exams
    - Pilocarpine or cevimeline (muscarinic agonists) to stimulate saliva production
  - Extraglandular manifestations:
    - Arthritis: Methotrexate, hydroxychloroquine
    - Severe CNS disease (demyelinating disease, transverse myelitis): Cyclophosphamide + rituximab

TABLE 9.9 · Sjögren's Classification Criteria (2017 ACR/EULAR)	
Criterion: Sicca symptoms and $\geq$ 4 points below → classified as Sjögren's*	**Score**
Salivary gland biopsy with $\geq$1 focus of lymphocytic infiltrate/4 mm^2	3
Anti-Ro/SSA autoantibodies	3
Fluorescein/lissamine ocular staining score $\geq$5 (0–12) in at least one eye (determined by ophthalmologist)	1
Schirmer test $\leq$5 mm/5 min in at least one eye	1
Unstimulated whole saliva flow rate $\leq$0.1 mL/min	1

* **Exclusion criteria:** Prior head/neck radiation; active HCV infection; advanced HIV; sarcoidosis; amyloidosis; GVHD; IgG4-related disease

Arthridities

Osteoarthritis (OA)

- Pathogenesis: Progressive cartilage and meniscal degradation due to complex interplay of pathologic joint loading (due to obesity, joint malalignment, specific types of exercise or occupation, etc.) and dysregulated joint repair processes.
- Risk factors: Age >55 yr, female sex, obesity, acute or chronic joint injury
- Clinical features and diagnosis:
  - OA is a clinical diagnosis made in a patient with compatible risk factors, joint pain that is worse with activity and relieved by rest, and absence of inflammatory features (e.g., absence of morning stiffness, absence of constitutional symptoms).
  - Joint effusions may occur (particularly in the knees) but the WBC count will be <2K cells/μL.
  - Radiographic hallmarks include:
    - Joint space narrowing
    - Subchondral sclerosis (i.e., increased bone density deep to cartilage)
    - Subchondral cysts
    - Osteophytes
    - No erosions (with the exception of inflammatory (or "erosive") OA of the hand)
- OA clinical phenotypes:
  - Primary OA: Most common; no identifiable secondary cause. Typical joints = hands (especially 1st CMC, DIPs, PIPs), hips, knees, and cervical and lumbar spine. Involvement may be asymmetric.
  - Secondary OA: Disease of the synovial joints resulting from a predisposing condition
    - Local: Prior trauma (e.g., tibial plateau fracture), inflammatory/infectious arthritis or surgical intervention (e.g., ACL repair, meniscectomy) at the affected joint/joint space
    - Systemic/metabolic: Hemochromatosis (2nd and 3rd MCPs and CMCs), hyperparathyroidism (wrists, MCPs), CPPD (MCPs, wrists, knees, hips), neuropathic arthropathy (such as in DM2), or OA-like pathologic changes accompanying inflammatory arthritis (such as psoriatic arthritis)
- Inflammatory hand OA:
  - Associated with intermittent flares of swelling and redness of the affected joints (DIPs, PIPs) and erosions on hand X-ray
  - The erosions are characteristically found in the central joint space, as opposed to the marginal (peripheral) erosions seen in RA
  - Diffuse idiopathic skeletal hyperostosis (DISH): Characterized by calcification and ossification of the spinal ligaments and entheses, presenting with back pain and flowing osteophytes in the T spine on plain films (R side predominates in most cases)
- Treatments:
  - Joint offloading: Work with occupational therapy/physical therapy to identify appropriate assistive devices (e.g., cane) or orthotics (e.g., thumb brace for 1st CMC OA)
  - Exercise to strengthen periarticular muscles (potentially guided by physical therapy)
  - Systemic and intra-articular pharmacotherapy (analgesic, not disease-modifying):
    - NSAIDs
    - Duloxetine
    - Intraarticular glucocorticoids can be considered for knee and hip OA pain. Can be administered every 3 months (at which point pain relief effect tends to wane). No clear evidence of long-term harm with repeated injections, though one study showed an adverse effect on cartilage thickness (a finding that lacks any clear clinical correlate) (McAlindon et al. *JAMA* 2017).
  - Surgical therapy: Knee or hip joint replacement provides pain relief and improves function for patients who have failed conservative therapy

Rheumatoid arthritis (RA)

- **Pathogenesis:** Mucosal inflammation triggers loss of tolerance to self-antigens in susceptible hosts, culminating in autoimmune destruction of synovial tissue.
- **Epidemiology and risk factors:** 0.5–1% prevalence in the general population, F:M = ~3:1. Increased risk in patients with periodontal disease and those who smoke cigarettes.
- Clinical features:
  - Symptoms:
    - Typically AM stiffness that lasts one hour, improves with activity, and is aggravated by rest
  - Physical exam:
    - Inflammatory polyarthritis with a predilection for the MCPs, PIPs, and MTPs with sparing of the DIPs of the upper and lower extremities. Variable involvement of the wrists, elbows, shoulders, hips, knees, ankles, and C-spine (characteristically involves the C1–C2 articulation; T- and L-spine are typically spared). Involvement is symmetric but severity may be asymmetric.
    - Hand deformities: Ulnar deviation of MCP, Boutonniere deformities (contracture involving PIP flexion/DIP hyperextension), Swan-Neck deformity (contracture involving PIP hyperextension/DIP flexion)
  - Radiographic hallmarks (plain film):
    - Periarticular osteopenia (earliest finding), symmetric joint space narrowing, erosions (typically at the medial and lateral joint margins including the ulnar styloid), and alignment deformities including subluxation and ulnar deviation of the MCPs
  - Lab findings:
    - Rheumatoid factor (Rf; 50% patients have positive Rf in first 6 months; 75–85% by 2 yr)
    - Anti-cyclic citrullinated peptide (CCP) antibodies: More specific than Rf (sensitivity 70%, specificity 95%)
    - 10–20% of cases are seronegative (e.g., Rf-negative, anti-CCP-negative)
    - ESR and/or CRP is elevated in 75% of patients
  - Extra-articular manifestations:
    - **Derm:** Rheumatoid nodules (30% of patients) occurring at pressure points including the olecranon; neutrophilic dermatoses including pyoderma gangrenosum and Sweet syndrome; small vessel cutaneous vasculitis may occur in patients with a history of smoking and/or longstanding RA
    - **Cardiac:** Independent risk factor for CAD and CHF; pericarditis
    - **Pulm:** Air trapping reflecting small airway inflammation in 50%, clinically apparent ILD in 10%; bronchiolitis; bronchiectasis; pleuritis (typically complicated exudative effusion with low pH/low glucose); cricoarytenoid arthritis (rare complication, presents with hoarseness, dysphagia, and stridor)
    - **Eyes:** Sicca symptoms/secondary Sjögren's; episcleritis; scleritis; keratitis
    - **CNS:** Mononeuritis multiplex due to peripheral nerve entrapment; c-spine subluxation can lead to cervical myelopathy (rare)
    - **Heme:** Anemia of inflammation; Felty syndrome (rare autoimmune condition characterized by the triad of neutropenia, splenomegaly, and longstanding seropositive RA); increased risk of large B cell lymphomas

TABLE 9.10 • Rheumatoid Arthritis Classification Criteria (2010 ACR/EULAR)

Criterion: 6 points needed for classification as RA	Score
Joint involvement (must have ≥ 1 joint with clinical synovitis)	
1 large joint (shoulders, elbows, hips, knees, ankles)	0
2–10 large joints	1
1–3 small joints (MCPs, PIPs, wrists, 205 MTPs)	2
4–10 small joints	3
>10 small joints	5
Serology	
Negative Rf or anti-CCP antibodies	0
Low-positive Rf or anti-CCP antibodies (<3× ULN)	2
High-positive Rf or anti-CCP antibodies (>3× ULN)	3
Acute phase reactants	
Normal CRP and ESR	0
Abnormal CRP or ESR	1
Duration	
<6 wk	0
>6 wk	1

- Diagnosis: ACR/EULAR criteria: See Table 9.10.
- Symptom monitoring:
  - The Simplified Disease Activity Index (SDAI) incorporates tender and swollen joint counts, CRP level, and a clinician and patient-derived global assessment.
  - SDAI <3.3 defines remission according to the ACR/EULAR guidelines.
- Treatment:
  - <u>Methotrexate</u> is the first-line disease-modifying antirheumatic drug (DMARD)
    - Titrate to the maximum tolerated dose (up to 25 mg weekly) at 12-week intervals
    - At doses >15 mg weekly, consider subcutaneous dosing to improve bioavailability
    - Contraindications to methotrexate include liver disease, advanced CKD, and heavy alcohol use
    - Leflunomide can be used as first-line DMARD if there are contraindications to methotrexate use
    - 30–50% of paitents respond to methotrexate monotherapy
  - For patients who do not respond to methotrexate, consider adding:
    - Sulfasalazine and hydroxychloroquine
    - A TNF-α inhibitor
    - Rituximab
    - Tocilizumab
    - Tofacitinib
  - Additional considerations:
    - Prednisone 5–10 mg daily may be used to rapidly improve symptoms while awaiting therapeutic effect of disease modifying anti-rheumatic drugs (DMARDs)
    - Methotrexate/hydroxychloroquine/sulfasalazine combination therapy may have similar efficacy to methotrexate and TNF-α inhibitor
    - Patients with a very low SDAI score at diagnosis may be candidates for sulfasalazine or hydroxychloroquine monotherapy
  - Pregnancy:
    - Pre-existing RA improves during pregnancy in 2/3 of cases and has a stable or worsening course in the other 1/3.
    - Methotrexate and leflunomide are contraindicated in pregnancy
    - Hydroxychloroquine and sulfasalazine are safe in pregnancy

Spondyloarthritis (SpA)
Group of disorders with shared features of inflammatory arthritis with varying degrees of axial skeleton involvement, enthesitis (inflammation of tendon-bone insertion points), overt or subclinical intestinal inflammation, association with uveitis, and association with the HLA-B27 MHC allele.

Ankylosing spondylitis (AS)
- Pathogenesis:
  - Not fully elucidated but several hypotheses exist regarding the role of the HLA-B27 risk allele, including presentation of self-peptides to CD8+ T cells and pathologic formation of oligomers that activate NK cells
- Epidemiology:
  - Prevalence 0.9–1.4% in the United States, M:F = ~3:1.
  - Age of onset is typically between 20–30 yr
  - HLA-B27 genetics:
    - Overall prevalence of HLA-B27 in Northern Europeans is 6%
    - Prevalence of SpA (all categories) in HLA-B27+ individuals is 2–10%
    - HLA-B27 is present in 74–90% of patients with spondyloarthritis overall and 95% of patients with ankylosing spondylitis
- Definition:
  - Updated Assessment of Spondyloarthritis International Society (ASAS) nomenclature: Ankylosing spondylitis → <u>Axial spondyloarthritis +/− radiographic sacroiliitis</u> ("with radiographic sacroiliitis" is included only if the associated sacroiliitis is severe enough to be detected on plain film x-ray)

- Clinical features:
  - **Axial spine involvement:**
    - Begins with the sacroiliac (SI) joints in nearly all cases, presenting with pain localizing to the hip or buttock (as opposed to hip arthritis pain which typically localizes to the groin).
    - Initially MRI is the most sensitive imaging modality (detects subchondral marrow edema in the SI joints). As disease progresses, damage becomes visible on PA pelvic plain film (reveals erosive changes, joint space narrowing and eventual bone joining [aka ankylosis or syndesmophytosis]).
    - Following SI joint involvement, spinal involvement is typically next (causing inflammatory back pain with morning stiffness). Joint involvement usually then proceeds cranially in a continuous fashion without skip lesions.
    - End stage disease in the spine = ankylosis of the vertebral facet joints and heterotopic ossification of the anterior and posterior spinal ligaments, resulting in "bamboo spine" (occurs in 10–15% of patients).
  - **Peripheral articular/periarticular involvement:** Enthesitis may be seen at the achilles tendon or plantar fascia entheses; asymmetric oligoarthritis of the hips, knees, ankles, and shoulders; less commonly dactylitis of the toes
  - **Ocular:** Recurrent anterior uveitis (30% of patients)
  - **Cardiovascular:** Increased risk of CAD; aortitis may occur in <1% of patients
  - **Pulmonary:** Restrictive lung disease may occur due to fusion of the costovertebral joints
- Diagnosis:
  - ASAS Diagnostic Algorithm for Axial Spondyloarthritis: See Figure 9.4
- Treatment:
  - Continuous NSAIDs are first-line and can slow radiographic disease progression
  - TNF-α inhibitors are typically started in patients with persistent symptoms or radiographic progression on NSAIDS
  - Anti-IL-17a therapy with secukinumab or ixekizumab is recommended for patients with persistent symptoms after trial of one TNF-α inhibitor (e.g., without trying a different TNF-α inhibitor)
  - Intra-articular glucocorticoids can be helpful for SI joint pain
  - Methotrexate is NOT efficacious

IBD-associated arthritis
- Epidemiology: Occurs in 6–46% of patients with Crohn's and ulcerative colitis (UC); disease onset can occur any time in the course of IBD
- Definition: Updated ASAS nomenclature: IBD-associated arthritis → Peripheral spondyloarthritis with IBD
- Clinical features:
  - **Articular –** three clinical phenotypes:
    - Sacroiliitis/spondylitis: Most common (25% patients). 50–75% are HLA-B27 positive. Axial disease activity does not track with enteric disease activity. Patients may be asymptomatic.
    - Chronic inflammatory polyarthritis: Occurs in <5% of patients, typically involving the PIPs, MCPs, wrists, elbows, knees, shoulders and ankles. Does not track with IBD activity.
    - Acute oligo or polyarthritis: Occurs in 5% of patients, typically involves the knees and tracks with IBD activity (e.g., may co-occur with an IBD flare).
  - **Derm:** Pyoderma gangrenosum and erythema nodosum
  - **Ocular:** Anterior uveitis
- Treatment:
  - Non-biologic DMARDs sulfasalazine, azathioprine, 6-mercaptopurine and methotrexate are first-line
  - TNF-α inhibitors are useful in patients who have persistent symptoms on non-biologic DMARDs. Only select agents are effective for both bowel and joint manifestations: Infliximab, adalimumab, golimumab, certolizumab pegol (etanercept not effective)
  - NSAIDs are not recommended as they may worsen IBD

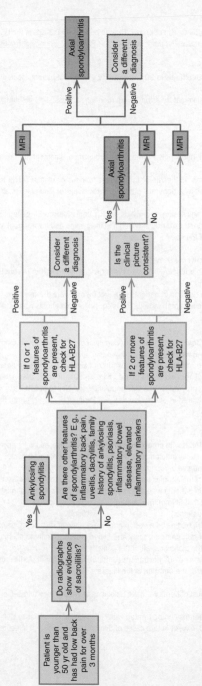

FIGURE 9.4: Algorithm for the diagnosis or exclusion of axial spondylarthritis. Adapted from Tuaurog et al. *New Engl J Med* 2016;374:2563.

Psoriatic arthritis

- Epidemiology: Occurs in 7–42% of patients with psoriasis. Overall prevalence 0.3–2% in the US
- Definition: Updated ASAS nomenclature: Psoriatic arthritis → Peripheral spondyloarthritis with psoriasis
- Clinical features:
  - Psoriasis precedes or co-occurs with arthritis in 90% of patients; in <10% of patients, joint disease can precede skin findings
  - **Clinical phenotypes** (all involve inflammatory arthritis with morning stiffness, +/−erosions)
    - Symmetric polyarthritis
    - Asymmetric oligoarthritis
    - DIP-predominant polyarthritis
    - Spondyloarthritis
    - Arthritis mutilans: End stage of hand polyarthritis with subluxation, ligamentous laxity, and telescoping of the phalanges
  - **Other peri-articular manifestations:** Enthesitis of the Achilles tendons or plantar fascia is common, as is dactylitis of the toes. Nail dystrophy/nail pitting is a risk factor for joint disease and DIP-predominant disease in particular.
  - **Axial spine involvement:** Unlike ankylosing spondylitis, which begins in the SI joints and proceeds cranially, axial disease in psoriatic arthritis may begin in the c-spine and involvement may be non-contiguous along the length of the spine
- Treatment:
  - Continuous NSAIDs for non-destructive/non-severe disease
  - Methotrexate is effective for pain in patients with non-severe disease who fail NSAIDs, but it does not impact radiographic progression
  - TNF-α inhibitors slow radiographic damage in patients with erosive or severe disease
  - Ustekinumab (anti-IL-12/23) and secukinumab (anti-IL-17a) is considered in patients who have failed two different TNF-α inhibitors

Reactive arthritis

- Pathogenesis: Preceding diarrhea (*Salmonella*, *Shigella*, *Campylobacter*, *Yersinia*) or *Chlamydia trachomatis*, followed by joint pain 2–6 weeks later. If sudden onset, rule-out HIV.
- Epidemiology: Prevalence of reactive arthritis after an episode of bacterial dysentery ranges from 2–33%. HLA-B27 is positive in 90% of *Yersinia*-related cases and 30–50% of cases associated with other pathogens (over-represented compared to HLA-B27 population prevalence of 6%)
- Definition: Updated ASAS nomenclature: Reactive arthritis → Peripheral spondyloarthritis with preceding infection
- Clinical features:
  - **Articular:**
    - Inflammatory non-erosive oligoarthritis with predilection for the knees, ankles, and wrists, occurring 2–3 weeks after an episode of bacterial inflammatory diarrhea (*Salmonella, Campylobacter, E. coli, Shigella, Yersinia*) or urethritis (*Chlamydia trachomatis* and *Ureaplasma urealyticum*)
    - 90% of cases involve enthesitis of the Achilles tendon and plantar fascia (i.e., plantar fasciitis)
    - Dactylitis is fairly common (40% in patients with disease triggered by *Chlamydia* urethritis)
    - Spine involvement is uncommon, but SI joint involvement may occur in up to 20%
  - **Ocular:** Sterile conjunctivitis (25% patients)
  - **Derm:** Keratoderma blenorrhagicum begins as a vesicular or waxy papular rash of the palms and soles and subsequently becomes erythematous, scaly and hyperkeratotic. Circinate balanitis is a serpiginous shallow ulceration on the glans or shaft of the penis
  - **Genitourinary:** In patients whose preceding infection was urethritis, a subsequent sterile urethritis, prostatitis, or cervicitis may persist for the duration of the illness
  - Treatment:
  - Continuous NSAIDS are first-line. Most patients will have resolution of symptoms within 3–6 months, obviating need for further therapy
  - Disease activity persisting >3–6 months can be treated with sulfasalazine or methotrexate
  - Antibiotics are not typically needed, except in rare cases of demonstrated persistent infections

Crystal-Induced Arthritis

Gout

- Pathogenesis:
  - Hyperuricemia above the uric acid saturation point of 6.8 mg/dL leads to crystal formation in the synovial fluid. This causes activation of the NLRP3 inflammasome in tissue macrophages/recruited monocytes, which leads to IL-1β production and PMN recruitment and ultimately results in acute joint swelling and pain.
  - Hyperuricemia can occur due to uric acid under-excretion (largely due to genetic variation in renal tubular urate handling, but also CKD, thiazide/loop diuretics, pyrazinamide/ethambutol) vs. less commonly by uric acid overproduction (inborn errors of purine metabolism, hematologic malignancies).

  Clinical features:
  - **Asymptomatic hyperuricemia:** Population prevalence of hyperuricemia is approximately 20%, but 95% remain asymptomatic with no treatment required
  - **Acute gouty arthritis:** Acute monoarticular swelling, erythema, warmth, and exquisite tenderness that peaks within 12–24 hrs of onset
    • Periarticular soft tissue involvement is common (bursitis, tenosynovitis, panniculitis) and can clinically mimic a skin and soft tissue infection
    • In men, the first gout attack typically occurs age 20–40 yr and >50% involve the 1st MTP. After years of disease, attacks may involve other joints (e.g., midfoot, ankles, knees, spine, or polyarticular)
    • In women, the first gout attack typically occurs after menopause
  - **Tophaceous gout:** After 10–20 yr of intermittent gout attacks and poorly controlled hyperuricemia, some patients develop tophi, which are conglomerates of uric acid crystals and inflammatory cells with a fibrous rind
    • Common locations of tophi include the extensor surfaces of the elbows, distal Achilles tendon, PIPs, and ear cartilage
    • Tophi may directly erode bone, cause functional impairment, or become superinfected, requiring debridement or amputation
- Diagnosis:
  - Perform arthrocentesis (removal of joint fluid for analysis):
    • Mandatory for larger joints (ankle, knee) to rule out infection with gram stain and culture (infection may co-exist with gout flare!). Arthrocentesis may not be feasible for midfoot or MTP flares, but localization to these sites increases the likelihood of gout
    • Diagnostic gold standard is detection of needle-shaped, negatively birefringent monosodium urate crystals in the synovial fluid
      - Negative birefringence: yellow when parallel to the polarizing axis
      - Synovial WBC >2K cells/μL and may be >100K cells/μL with PMN-predominance
  - Other lab findings:
    • ↑ESR/CRP (non-specific)
    • Checking serum uric acid is only sometimes useful; an elevated serum uric acid in a patient with acute monoarticular arthritis can support a diagnosis of gout, but serum uric acid may be low during an acute attack because inflammatory cytokines can reduce uric acid
- Treatment of acute flares:
  - **Colchicine**: 1.2 mg loading dose followed 1 hr later by 0.6 mg, continued daily until flare resolves. Most effective if started within 24 hrs of symptom onset. Avoid in patients with GFR <60 mL/min.
  - **Prednisone**: 0.5 mg/kg/day for 5 days (or longer if long-standing disease). Best for patients with CKD.
  - **NSAIDs**: Max dose NSAID (e.g., naproxen 500 mg BID) for 5–7 days. Avoid in patients with CKD, CHF, GIB risk). Potentially a good option for relatively healthy patients with first flare.
  - **IL-1β blockade – Anakinra**: Use for refractory flares in patients with long-standing disease and contraindications to and/or failure of other therapies used for acute flare management. Not used as maintenance therapy.
  - **Intra-articular glucocorticoids**: Consider as monotherapy for monoarticular flares, particularly in the 1st MTP. Avoid or proceed with caution if synovial culture is pending.
  - **Check serum uric acid 2 wks post-flare** to gauge steady-state level.

- Urate lowering therapy:
  - Indications: ≥2 attacks per year; CKD2 or higher; tophaceous disease; uric acid nephrolithiasis
  - Serum uric acid targets: No specific randomized controlled trials have studied the impact of different targets. ACR/EULAR recommends targeting uric acid <5mg/dL for patients with tophi and <6 mg/dL for others
  - Timing: Urate-lowering therapy may be started during an acute flare as long as the patient is also on appropriate systemic anti-inflammatory therapy
  - Auxiliary measures: Alcohol cessation, low purine diet (limit shellfish, red meat), avoid thiazide/loop diuretics/ASA if feasible
  - Medications:
    - **Xanthine oxidase inhibitors**: Prevent uric acid generation from upstream purine metabolites
      - **Allopurinol**: First-line therapy; start 100mg daily (or 50mg daily if CKD) and uptitrate to max dose of 800 mg/day. Check HLA-B5801 in patients of Asian descent, as this allele is associated with increased risk of severe cutaneous adverse reactions including DRESS and SJS-TEN
      - **Febuxostat**: 40–120 mg daily (40 mg febuxostat ~ 300 mg allopurinol)
    - **Uricosuric agents**: Promotes renal tubular uric acid excretion. Probenecid is the most widely available agent. These agents are less potent than xanthine oxidase inhibitors as a monotherapy but can be added if needed. Avoid in patients with CKD
    - **Pegloticase**: Recombinant uricase infused every two weeks. Indications = recurrent and/or tophaceous gout with intolerance to or failure of other therapies. 30–50% of patients develop anti-drug antibodies
    - **Anti-inflammatory prophylaxis during active uric acid lowering:** Colchicine 0.6 mg daily, low-dose NSAID (e.g., naproxen 250 mg BID), or low-dose prednisone (5 mg daily) should be provided to prevent flares during active titration of uric acid lowering therapy, and should be continued for 3 months after reaching the serum uric acid target (6 months in patients with tophi)

Calcium pyrophosphate deposition (CPPD) arthropathies
- Pathophysiology: Calcium pyrophosphate crystals accumulate in joints with age (~50% of patients age >80 yr have detectable chondrocalcinosis). Secondary chondrocalcinosis may develop in younger patients due to systemic metabolic disturbances (e.g., chronic hypomagnesemia, hypophosphatemia, hyperparathyroidism, or hemochromatosis).
- Clinical syndromes and diagnosis:
  - Asymptomatic chondrocalcinosis: Four most common locations in descending order are the knees, triangular fibrocartilage of the wrist (between ulna and carpals), pubic symphysis, and MCPs
  - Pseudo-gout: Acute monoarticular arthritis with synovial fluid showing presence of rhomboid-shaped, positively birefringent crystals on polarized light microscopic analysis (blue when parallel to the polarizing axis). Synovial WBC typically >2K cells/μL
  - "Pseudo-OA": Characterized by OA-like radiographic changes (e.g., joint space narrowing, subchondral sclerosis, subchondral cysts, osteophytosis) in joints with preceding or concurrent evidence of chondrocalcinosis, often accompanied by deformity out of proportion to the duration of arthritis (knees most common; valgus deformity is suggestive)
  - "Pseudo-RA": A rare entity characterized by inflammatory polyarthritis of the wrists and MCP joints with chondrocalcinosis that is typically non-erosive and does not meet criteria for RA (occasionally low-positive Rf)
- Treatment:
  - There is no therapy to dissolve CPP crystals
  - Pseudo-gout flares: Management similar to gout flare; prophylaxis with colchicine 0.3 mg daily or low-dose NSAIDs (e.g., naproxen 250 mg BID) is reasonable if ≥3 attacks per year
  - Pseudo-OA: Management similar to OA without chondrocalcinosis
  - Pseudo-RA: Low-dose daily colchicine or low-dose daily NSAIDs; serial clinical/radiographic/laboratory diagnostic reassessment as patients may ultimately prove to have true RA

Vasculitis
Definitions:
- Vasculitis: Vessels narrow and become occluded due to inflammation in the vessel wall and subsequent endothelial proliferation. Each disease state tends to have a tropism for either large, medium, or small vessels; small vessel vasculitis may be subclassified into 1) ANCA-associated and 2) immune-complex mediated.
- Vasculopathy: Vessels narrow and become occluded due to a thrombosis, septic embolism, or intravascular protein deposition. Examples include calciphylaxis, APLS, septic emboli in infective endocarditis, cryoglobulinemia (can cause vessel wall inflammation OR proteinaceous occlusion).

Large Vessel Vasculitis

Temporal arteritis/giant cell arteritis (GCA)

- Pathogenesis: Not fully elucidated; association with HLA-DRB*04 suggests cell-mediated autoimmunity resulting in granulomatous inflammation of vessel walls. Most commonly affects the major aortic branch vessels or secondary branch vessels (e.g., external carotid, subclavian, axillary, temporal).
- Epidemiology: Incidence of 10–20/100,000 individuals annually in the United States; F:M = 2:1
- Clinical features: Headache, scalp pain, jaw claudication. Ophthalmic artery involvement may present with amaurosis fugax and can cause blindness. 50% of patients with GCA also have PMR.
- Diagnosis:
  - New headache in an adult ≥50 yr with temporal artery tenderness, ESR ≥50 mm/hr (although normal ESR does not exclude the diagnosis), and temporal artery biopsy showing mononuclear cell infiltration of the vessel wall, potentially with giant multinucleated macrophages and granulomas.
  - Do not delay steroids to get biopsy! Diseased tissue remains abnormal for up to two weeks after treatment initiation.
- Treatment:
  - **Prednisone:** High-dose prednisone 1 mg/kg/day (started immediately without waiting for biopsy results) and ASA 81 mg daily. Followed by prolonged, slow steroid taper
  - **Tocilizumab:** Anti-IL-6 receptor monoclonal antibody, given weekly or biweekly. Tocilizumab + prednisone resulted in higher rate of glucocorticoid-free remission at 1 yr compared to prednisone alone (53–56% remission vs. 18%) (GiACTA study *New Engl J Med* 2017)

Takayasu's arteritis

- Pathogenesis: Histology of vascular lesions is similar to GCA, but typically involves larger vessels, most commonly the aorta followed by the subclavian, common carotid, renal, and pulmonary arteries
- Epidemiology: Prevalence is 40/million individuals in Japan and 4.7–8/million individuals elsewhere. Predominantly affects young women.
- Clinical features: Involvement of the subclavian arteries can cause limb claudication, absent or reduced brachial artery pulses, subclavian bruits, blood pressure discrepancies between arms. Carotid involvement can cause neck pain and tenderness to palpation on exam. ESR and CRP are typically elevated.
- Diagnosis: MR angiography demonstrates thoracic vessel stenoses and vessel wall inflammation
- Complications: Limb ischemia, aortic aneurysm, aortic regurgitation, stroke, renal artery stenosis with secondary hypertension
- Treatment: High-dose prednisone (1 mg/kg) with prolonged slow taper. May need surgery or angioplasty to recannulate stenosed vessels, but this should be deferred until resolution of active vessel inflammation.

Medium Vessel Vasculitis

Polyarteritis nodosa (PAN)

- Epidemiology: Incidence 3–4.5/100,000. Average age of onset 50 yr, M>F. Only 5% of cases are associated with HBV in the post-HBV vaccine era
- Clinical features:
  - **Neuro** (75–80%): Mononeuritis multiplex or distal symmetric polyneuropathy
  - **Constitutional** (65%): Fever, malaise, weight loss
  - **Cutaneous** (50–60%): Livedo reticularis (lace-like rash), nodules, necrotic ulcers of the lower extremities
  - **Renal** (40%): Can lead to hypertension, AKI/CKD if bilateral, hematuria, proteinuria
  - **GI** (35–40%): Acute or chronic mesenteric ischemia
- Diagnosis:
  - Diagnosis confirmed with biopsy of involved tissue (e.g., sural nerve) showing focal segmental pan-mural necrotizing inflammation
  - If there are no clear biopsy targets but GI or renal involvement is suspected, mesenteric or renal angiography can show a combination of aneurysms and stenoses at vessel branch points
  - Avoid renal biopsy given high risk of bleeding with aberrant vasculature
  - Inflammatory markers are typically elevated
- Treatment:
  - Prednisone and cyclophosphamide for severe non-HBV associated cases
  - Antivirals for HBV-related disease

Primary angiitis of the central nervous system (PACNS)
- Epidemiology: Incidence is 2.4/100,000 annually. Median age of onset is 50 yr
- Clinical features: Medium vessel vasculitis with isolated CNS involvement. Presents with triad of headache, cognitive impairment or altered mental status, and new or progressive focal neurologic deficits due to strokes
- Diagnosis: MRA or conventional angiography may show beading of CNS artery branches; the gold standard for diagnosis is a brain or leptomeningeal biopsy showing lymphocytic vessel wall inflammation
- Treatment: High-dose glucocorticoids and cyclophosphamide. Permanent disability commonly occurs due to strokes.

Kawasaki disease
- Clinical features:
  - Medium vessel vasculitis most common in children (80% of cases present prior to age 5 yr), typically Asian boys
  - Manifestations include high fevers, conjunctivitis, mucositis (strawberry tongue), non-suppurative cervical adenitis, truncal rash, and plamar/plantar erythema
  - Coronary aneurysms occur in 25% of cases
- Treatment:
  - IVIG and aspirin. Excellent prognosis
  - Coronary aneurysms may develop and cause CHF and/or need for CABG in adulthood

Small Vessel Vasculitis: ANCA-Associated Vasculitides (AAV)

Granulomatosis with polyangiitis (GPA, formerly Wegener's granulomatosis)
- Epidemiology: Incidence is 7–12/million individuals annually. Typical age of onset 45–60 yr.
- Diagnosis:
  - Most patients with systemic disease are <u>c-ANCA</u> and <u>anti-PR3</u> positive
  - Tissue biopsy showing pauci-immune necrotizing granulomatous vasculitis is gold standard
- Clinical features:
  - **ENT** (70–100%): Sinusitis, rhinorrhea, otitis media, chondritis of the ears and nose with saddle nose deformity, nasal septal perforation
  - **Pulm** (50–90%): Cavitary nodules, diffuse alveolar hemorrhage, tracheal subglottic stenosis
  - **Renal** (40–100%): Pauci-immune necrotizing glomerulonephritis
  - **Derm** (10–50%): Palpable purpura, nodules, pyoderma gangrenosum
  - **Neuro** (30%): Mononeuritis multiplex, distal symmetric polyneuropathy, pachymeningitis
  - **Ocular** (15–60%): Posterior uveitis, scleritis, episcleritis, retro-orbital pseudotumor, dacryoadenitis (lacrimal gland inflammation)
  - **Cardiac** ($<$10%): Pericarditis, myocarditis, conduction disorder
  - **GI** (5–10%): Ulceration
- Treatment:
  - <u>Systemic organ-threatening disease</u>:
    - Induction therapy: Pulse dose glucocorticoids (1 g per day $\times$ 3–5 days) followed by 1 mg/kg, then add rituximab or cyclophosphamide. Rituximab is non-inferior to cyclophosphamide for induction therapy in ANCA+ GPA and MPA (RAVE *New Engl J Med* 2010) and is associated with less infertility and alopecia.
    - Maintenance therapy: Rituximab for 12–24 months after remission, azathioprine, or methotrexate
  - <u>Limited upper airway disease</u>: Glucocorticoids plus methotrexate or rituximab

Microscopic polyangiitis (MPA)
- Epidemiology: Incidence is 2.7–94/million individuals annually. Average age of onset is 50–60 yr
- Diagnosis:
  - Small vessel vasculitis of the lungs (diffuse alveolar hemorrhage) and kidneys (crescentic RPGN)
  - 50–75% ANCA+ and generally <u>p-ANCA</u> and <u>anti-MPO</u> positive
  - Tissue biopsy is the gold standard and shows non-granulomatous necrotizing pauci-immune vasculitis (as opposed to granulomatous in GPA)
- Clinical features:
  - **Renal** (80–100%): Necrotizing glomerulonephritis
  - **Derm** (30–60%): Palpable purpura with histology showing leukocytoclastic vasculitis; livedo reticularis; nodules; necrotic skin ulcers
  - **Neuro** (30–70%): Mononeuritis multiplex; distal symmetric polyneuropathy; pachymeningitis
  - **Pulm** (25–55%): Diffuse alveolar hemorrhage, organizing pneumonia, ILD with radiographic phenotype of usual interstitial pneumonia (UIP)
  - **ENT** (10–30%): Sinusitis; sensorineural hearing loss
- Treatment: Similar to treatment of GPA

Eosinophilic granulomatosis with polyangiitis (EGPA, formerly Churg-Strauss syndrome)
- Epidemiology: Rarest ANCA-associated vasculitis; 0.1–2.66/million individuals annually
- Diagnosis:
  - Small vessel vasculitis that typically occurs in patients with preceeding adult-onset asthma and nasal polyps
  - 50% ANCA+ and usually p-ANCA and anti-MPO positive
  - Eosinophilia >1500 cells/µL often present
  - Diagnostic gold standard is biopsy of involved tissue (e.g., nerve) showing pauci-immune necrotizing granulomatous vasculitis with eosinophilic infiltration of vessel walls and tissues (eosinophilic infiltration distinguishes EGPA from MPA and GPA)
- Clinical features:
  - **Neuro** (70%): Mononeuritis multiplex or distal sensory polyneuropathy
  - **Pulm:** Most patients (95–100%) have preceding asthma that often improves during the vasculitic phase. Patients also may have migratory pulmonary consolidations similar to those seen with eosinophilic pneumonia during the vasculitis phase
  - **Cardiac** (20–40%): Pericarditis, endomyocarditis, conduction system disease, CHF
  - **Renal** (25%): Pauci-immune glomerulonephritis
- Treatment:
  - Glucocorticoids alone may be sufficient unless there is major organ involvement, in which case cyclophosphamide is indicated
  - Lowest mortality among all the ANCA-associated vasculitidies (5 yr survival 97%)

Small Vessel Vasculitis: Immune-Complex Mediated
Palpable purpura on exam, leukocytoclastic vasculitis on skin biopsy

Cryoglobulinemic vasculitis
- Pathogenesis: Immune complex-mediated small vessel vasculitis caused by Ig molecules that precipitate at temperatures lower than 37ºC, known as cryoglobulins. Types of cryoglobulins:
  - Type I – IgM rheumatoid factor associated with multiple myeloma
  - Type II and III – "Mixed cryoglobulinemia" because the precipitating antibodies are a mixture of polyclonal IgG and either:
    - Polyclonal IgM rheumatoid factor (Type II)
    - Monoclonal IgM rheumatoid factor (Type III)
- Diagnosis:
  - 90% of cases of mixed cryoglobulinemia are associated with HCV infection (test for HCV if cryos are identified!), but SLE and Sjögren's can also cause Type III
  - Additional lab findings include +Rf and very low C4
  - Pearl about sample collection: Must keep at >37°C to avoid premature precipitation and false negative result
- Clinical features:
  - **Derm** (70–90%): Palpable purpura, Raynaud's, ulcers, skin necrosis, livedo reticularis
  - **Neuro** (60%): Distal symmetric polyneuropathy
  - **Arthritis** (40%)
  - **Renal** (40%): Immune complex glomerulonephritis
- Treatment:
  - Treat HCV or control the underlying rheumatic disease (e.g., Sjögren's or SLE)
  - For organ-threatening disease such as acute renal failure, plasmapheresis or glucocorticoids plus rituximab or cyclophosphamide are options

IgA vasculitis (Henoch-Schönlein purpura, HSP)
- Epidemiology: Childhood vasculitis that rarely occurs in adults with incidence of 14/million individuals annually
- Clinical features: Often preceded by viral URI or strep pharyngitis. Main manifestations include small vessel luminal vasculitis causing abdominal pain, GIB (65%), arthritis and arthralgias (63%) and glomerulonephritis (40%).
- Diagnosis: Gold standard is skin biopsy with leukocytoclastic vasculitis and heavy IgA deposits, or renal biopsy showing IgA nephropathy
- Treatment:
  - Self-limited in children
  - Adults may require glucocorticoids and/or cyclophosphamide for severe organ-threatening disease

Hypersensitivity vascultiis
- Clinical features: A small vessel vasculitis with isolated cutaneous involvement (palpable purpura) triggered by exposure to a known or unknown antigen
- Diagnosis:
  - Skin biopsy shows leukocytoclastic vasculitis without IgA staining in the correct clinical context
  - Typically, the vasculitis will resolve 7–10 days after removal of the offending antigen. Persistent symptoms for more than a month should raise suspicion for the presence of an alternative diagnosis
- Treatment: Removal of the offending antigen

Other Rheumatologic Conditions

Polymyalgia rheumatica (PMR)
- Clinical features:
  - Syndrome of neck, shoulder, and hip girdle stiffness that is typically worse after immobility; associated with elevations in markers of systemic inflammation (e.g., ESR, CRP)
  - 50% of patients with GCA have PMR, and 20% of patients with PMR have GCA
- Diagnosis:
  - A diagnosis of exclusion made after ruling out myopathies (for myopathy, weakness > pain; for PMR, pain > weakness) or non-systemic periarticular syndromes, such as adhesive capsulitis
  - May be difficult to distinguish from seronegative RA as some patients have a distal polyarthritis; when present, erosive disease favors a diagnosis of RA
  - Improves briskly with prednisone 12.5–20 mg daily and failure to improve as expected with steroids should raise suspicion for the presence of an alternative diagnosis
- Treatment: Prednisone 20 mg/day and prolonged taper (often 1–2 yr)

Behçet syndrome
- Pathogenesis: Not fully elucidated; increased risk with HLA-B51 allele implicates cell-mediated autoimmunity (US cases tend not to be associated with this HLA type)
- Epidemiology: Incidence 1/100,000 individuals annually in the United States; 400/100,000 individuals annually in Turkey. Also relatively more prevalent in Iran, Saudi Arabia, Greece, Japan, Korea, and China, tracking with the distribution of the HLA-B51 allele. Age of onset typically 20–30 yr.
- Clinical features:
  - **Derm**: Recurrent genital and oral ulcers (the latter occur in nearly 100% of patients and are painful, unlike those that occur in SLE); erythema nodosum with ulceration; pseudofolliculitis/nodular cystic acne of the face and neck
  - **Vascular**: Vasculitis with potential small (retinal), medium (mesenteric) and large (pulmonary, carotid, aortic, iliac, femoral) vessel involvement; venous <u>and</u> arterial thrombi (potentially IVC thrombosis, dural venous sinus thrombosis, arterial thromboses, and aneurysms)
  - **GI**: Apthous ulcers of the ileum/cecum presenting with abdominal pain, anorexia, diarrhea, GI bleeding
  - **Articular**: Inflammatory oligoarthritis in ~50% of patients with large joint-predominance (knees most common); sacroiliitis
  - **Ocular**: Uveitis (anterior, posterior, or panuveitis); retinal vasculitis
  - **CNS**: Headache, altered mental status; CSF may show elevated protein and leukocytosis; cranial neuropathies including CN VIII
- Diagnosis: See Table 9.11
  - **Pathergy**: A skin prick is performed with a sterile needle, and the site is assessed 48 hr later. Patients who develop a pustule are deemed to have a positive test.
  - **DDx for recurrent oral ulcers**: HSV, HIV, Crohn's, nutritional deficiency (iron, zinc, folate, B1, B2, B6, B12), cyclic neutropenia, reactive arthritis, methotrexate

TABLE 9.11 · International Criteria for Behçet's Disease	
Criterion: ≥ 4 points needed for diagnosis*	**Score**
Oral ulcers	2
Genital ulcers	2
Pathergy	1
Skin lesions (pseudofolliculitis; skin ulcers; erythema nodosum)	1
Eye lesions (anterior uveitis; posterior uveitis; retinal vasculitis)	2
CNS lesions	1
Vascular lesions (arterial thrombosis; large vein thrombosis; phlebitis)	1

* Reference: *J Eur Acad Dermatol Venereol* 2014;28:338

- Treatment:
  - <u>Oral and genital ulcers</u>: Topical glucocorticoids for management of active lesions; colchicine for prevention of new genital lesions and erythema nodosum
  - <u>Arthritis</u>: Colchicine for acute flares; azathioprine or TNFα inhibitors for chronic arthritis
  - <u>Thrombotic events</u>: Anticoagulation, also consider immunosuppression with glucocorticoids
  - <u>Intestinal ulcer flares</u>: High-dose glucocorticoids (1 mg/kg) with subsequent mesalamine or azathioprine
  - <u>CNS disease</u>: High-dose glucocorticoids (1 mg/kg) with subsequent introduction of azathioprine

Relapsing polychondritis

- Pathogenesis: Not fully elucidated; involves episodic immune-mediated damage to cartilaginous tissues including the ears, nose, and proximal tracheobronchial tree
- Epidemiology: Incidence 3.5/million individuals annually, mean age at diagnosis 47 yr
- Disease categories:
  - Primary: No evidence of a separate underlying rheumatic or hematologic disease
  - Secondary (30%): Occurring in the context of GPA, RA, SLE, or myelodysplastic syndrome
- Clinical features:
  - **Inflammation of cartilaginous tissues:** Auricular chondritis (red/tender cartilaginous ear with sparing of the lobe, 90% patients), nasal cartilage inflammation which can cause septal perforation and saddle nose deformity
  - **Articular manifestations:** Episodic, migratory inflammatory oligoarthritis in ~70% patients, occurring contemporaneously with inflammation at other cartilaginous sites
  - **Airway disease:** Subglottic tracheal stenosis; bronchiectasis
- Diagnosis:
  - Clinical diagnosis typically made on the basis of auricular chondritis, saddle nose deformity, tracheobronchial involvement, and exclusion of other conditions
  - If atypical manifestations, auricular cartilage biopsy during flare reveals perichondrium inflammatory cell infiltration
- Differential diagnosis:
  - Ddx for auricular erythema: Otitis externa/auricular cellulitis
  - Ddx for nasal inflammation/saddle nose deformity: GPA, Crohn's, NK cell lymphoma, syphilis, leprosy, leishmaniasis
- Treatment:
  - Flares of cartilaginous inflammation (auricular or nasal chondritis): Glucocorticoids first-line
  - Tracheobronchial disease: Local glucocorticoid injections, stents for stenotic areas, CPAP

IgG4-related disease

- Pathogenesis: Not fully elucidated, but involves tissue infiltration with IgG4 plasma cells as well as copious lymphocytes, eosinophils, and dense fibrosis
- Epidemiology: Prevalence not yet described; M:F = ~3:1 for IgG4-related pancreatitis
- Clinical features:
  - **General patterns of disease:** Tumefactive fibrotic organ infiltration with predominant involvement of exocrine organs. Preceding atopic disease is common but typically less active
  - **Ocular:** "Orbital apex syndrome"/orbital pseudotumor causing proptosis
  - **Exocrine glands:** Autoimmune pancreatitis (presenting with abdominal pain and/or obstructive jaundice; serum IgG4 is often elevated but a biopsy is typically needed to rule out malignancy); sclerosing cholangitis; inflammation/enlargement of the submandibular, parotid, and lacrimal glands
  - **Endocrine glands:** Fibrosing thyroiditis, lymphocytic hypophysitis
  - **Vascular:** Ascending or descending aortitis (histopathologically may not be a true vasculitis)
  - **Retroperitoneum:** Retroperitoneal fibrosis and periaortitis
  - **Renal:** Tumefactive lesions occasionally mistaken for renal cell carcinoma; tubulointerstitial nephritis
  - **Neuro:** Pachymeningitis of the dura
- Diagnosis:
  - Made by biopsy of involved tissue, with key findings of >30 IgG4+ plasma cells per high power field and characteristic dense lymphoplasmacytic infiltrate and "storiform" fibrosis
  - Serum IgG4 is elevated in only 70–80% of patients
- Treatment:
  - Prednisone 0.5 mg/kg daily for 2–4 weeks, then tapered over 3–6 months
  - Mycophenolate, methotrexate, or azathioprine have been used as glucocorticoid-sparing remission-maintenance therapy, but have not been studied in clinical trials
  - Rituximab can be used for relapsed or refractory disease

Adult-onset Still's Disease (AOSD)
- Pathogenesis: Thought to be due to dysregulated innate immunity and thus it is an autoinflammatory rather than an autoimmune syndrome
- Diagnosis and clinical features:
  - Yamaguchi Criteria for Adult-onset Still's: See Table 9.12
  - Complications may include hemophagocytic lymphohistiocytosis (HLH), disseminated intravascular coagulation, and fulminant hepatitis
- Differential diagnosis:
  - Infectious:
    - Bacterial: Staphylococcal toxic shock syndrome; *Neisseria meningitidis* infection; secondary syphilis; rickettsial, anaplasma, or erlichia infection
    - Viral: Acute HIV; primary VZV or rarely zoster; EBV or CMV mononucleosis; parvovirus B19; dengue; chikungunya
  - Malignant: Cutaneous lymphoma or leukemia; paraneoplastic dermatoses (pemphigus; Sweet syndrome)
  - Autoimmune: SLE, dermatomyositis, MCTD
  - Drug: DIHS (formerly DRESS); SJS/TEN
- Treatment: DMARDs such as methotrexate are effective for arthritis; IL-1 inhibitors are effective for fevers and other manifestations

TABLE 9.12 • Yamaguchi Criteria for Adult Onset Still's Disease	
Criterion: 5 criteria including ≥2 major criteria needed for diagnosis*	Frequency
Major Criteria	
Daily spiking fever to ≥39°C	99%
Arthralgia/arthritis >2 weeks	85%
Non-pruritic salmon-colored macular/maculopapular rash on trunk/extremities	85%
Leukocytosis >10K/μL	90%
Minor Criteria	
Sore throat	66%
Lymphadenopathy and/or splenomegaly	65%
Elevated AST, ALT or LDH	70%
Negative ANA and Rf	–

*Must also exclude other causes of fever/rash; see differential diagnosis in the text

Sarcoidosis
- Pathogenesis: Incompletely characterized but thought to involve dysregulated activation of CD4+ T cells and formation of granulomas (nodular collections of epithelioid macrophages) in multiple tissues
- Clinical features:
  - **Pulm** (>90%): Bilateral hilar adenopathy, perilymphatic nodules, and ILD-related fibrotic changes (reticulation, honey-combing, traction bronchiectasis)
  - **Ocular** (20–30%): Uveitis – usually anterior but can also be posterior
  - **Cutaneous** (20–30%): Erythema nodosum; lupus pernio (facial rash involving violaceous plaques and nodules over the nose, nasal alae, malar areas, nasolabial folds, scalp, and hairline)
  - **Articular** (5%): Polyarticular (and rarely erosive) arthritis typically affecting the ankles, knees, and wrists; typically resolves in weeks to months without intervention
  - **Musculoskeletal**: Lytic bone lesions (10%), sarcoid myopathy (common but only symptomatic in 0.5–5% patients)
  - **Cardiac** (10%): Heart block/conduction system disease, ventricular arrythmias, dilated cardiomyopathy. Consider cardiac PET or cardiac MRI if suspicion for cardiac involvement.
  - **Neuro:** CN VII palsy most common, but CN II (optic neuritis), III, V, VIII and IX lesions can also occur. Aseptic meningitis and hypophysitis are less common manifestations.
  - **Exocrine glands:** Parotitis resulting in sicca symptoms
- Sarcoidosis sub-syndromes: These syndromes obviate the need for diagnostic biopsy in most cases
  - Asymptomatic bilateral hilar adenopathy (e.g., no fevers, night sweats, weight loss to suggest malignancy)
  - Löfgren syndrome: Constellation of bilateral hilar adenopathy, erythema nodosum, migratory polyarthralgias/arthritis. 95% specific for sarcoidosis and obviates the need for biopsy
  - Heerfordt syndrome (uveoparotid fever): Fever, uveitis, parotitis +/- CN VII palsy, associated with sicca symptoms

- Diagnosis: Biopsy of involved tissue (e.g., hilar lymph node, lung parenchyma) showing non-caseating granulomas (e.g., no central necrosis). Patients presenting with one of the sub-syndromes above may not require a biopsy unless diagnostic uncertainty is present.
- Treatment:
  - Generally, treat disease if symptomatic but can often just monitor if asymptomatic
  - Glucocorticoids (e.g., prednisone 20mg daily) for at least 8–12 months are the first-line therapy for symptomatic pulmonary and extrapulmonary disease
  - For patients who have persistent disease activity or intolerable side effects with glucocorticoids alone:
    - Methotrexate is effective for disease activity in multiple tissues
    - Hydroxychloroquine and doxycycline/minocycline are effective for cutaneous disease
    - TNFα inhibitors are used for patients with persistent disease activity despite non-biologic DMARD therapy

Fibromyalgia

- Pathogenesis: Thought to involve inappropriately strong or persistent sensory pain signals from neurons in the dorsal root ganglia and impairment of efferent adrenergic neurons that normally dampen pain sensation, causing allodynia and "temporal summation" of pain stimuli
- Epidemiology: Prevalence estimate 2–3% of population, F:M = 3:1
- Diagnosis and clinical features:
  - There are multiple screening tools; one of the most simple ones is from the American Pain Society and the FDA (*J Pain* 2019;20:611) and involves pain at $\geq$6 body sites as well as insomnia (Table 9.13)
  - Key differential diagnostic considerations include depression, hypothyroidism, or adrenal insufficiency, which should be excluded
  - Fibromyalgia often coexists with rheumatologic disease; thus, it is important to still pursue an appropriate workup in patients with clinical symptoms suggestive of an autoimmune disease
- Treatment:
  - Aerobic exercise in a graded fashion
  - Assess trauma history and treat co-morbid psychiatric disorders including anxiety, PTSD, substance use
  - Gabapentin, pregabalin, and TCAs may be effective for both pain and insomnia; cyclobenzaprine can be useful if muscle spasms are present

TABLE 9.13 · Fibromyalgia Diagnostic Criteria (2019 AAPT*)
Diagnosis made if all criteria met; may co-exist with other illnesses
Multi-site pain at $\geq$ 6 of 9 possible sites (head, L/R arm, chest, abdomen, upper/lower back, L/R leg)
Moderate sleep problems or fatigue
Sleep issues and pain have been present for $\geq$ 3 months

*AAPT = Analgesic, Anesthetic, and Addiction Clinical Trial Translations Innovations Opportunities and Networks (ACTTION)-APS Pain Taxonomy

Inherited Diseases of Connective Tissues
See Table 9.14

TABLE 9.14 · Inherited Connective Tissue Diseases

| | Ehlers-Danlos Syndrome | | | | Marfan Syndrome | Osteogenesis Imperfecta |
	Hypermobility	Classic	Kyphoscoliotic	Vascular		
Genetic Testing & Pathogenesis	70% heritable in twin study but likely not monogenic	*COL5A1; COL5A2* – Type V collagen mutations disrupt formation of Type I fibrils (bone, tendon, skin)	*PLOD1* – lysyl hydroxylase deficiency impairs crosslinking of multiple collagen types	*COL3A1* – dominant negative mutation in Type III collagen	*FBN1* – mutations result in fibrillin deficiency and hyperactive TGFβ signaling	*COL1A1* or *COL1A2* (most common) – mutations affect the quantity or structural integrity of Type I collagen
Inheritance	Autosomal dominant	Autosomal dominant	Autosomal recessive	Autosomal dominant	Autosomal dominant	Autosomal dominant or recessive
Clinical Findings						
Musculoskeletal	Joint hypermobility, joint instability; musculoskeletal pain; early OA	Hypermobility; joint dislocations; pes planus	Hypermobility; progressive scoliosis; marfanoid habitus	Hypermobility; joint dislocations	Hypermobility; tall stature; arachnodactyly; pectus excavatum; scoliosis	Pathologic fractures; short stature
Skin	Easy bruising; mild laxity	Smooth, velvety skin; easy bruising; hyperextensible	Easy bruising; hyperextensible	Easy bruising	Hyperextensible	–
Cardiovascular	No risk of organ rupture or dissection	Mitral/tricuspid valve prolapse; aortic root dilation (rare); arterial rupture (rare)	Medium-size artery rupture; mitral/tricuspid valve prolapse	Arterial rupture; aneurysm; dissection	Aortic aneurysm/ dissection; mitral valve prolapse	–
Other	–	Muscular hypotonia; delayed motor development	Muscular hypotonia; scleral fragility and risk of globe rupture; restrictive lung disease	Organ rupture (uterus, bowel, rarely spleen, liver); pneumothorax; gingival recession	Myopia in 60% patients; ectopia lentis; high arched palate; pneumothorax; blue sclerae	Blue sclerae; discolored (blue/gray or yellow/brown) teeth prone to breakage
Management	Joint protection; supportive care	Joint protection; TTE/ vascular monitoring; preconception counseling; PT; bracing	Joint protection; TTE/ vascular monitoring; preconception counseling	Joint protection; TTE/vascular monitoring; preconception counseling	Annual ophthalmic examination; periodic aortic arch imaging; β-blockers; joint protection; preconception counseling	Bisphosphonates; audiology assessments; joint and bone protection; dental evaluations

KEY MEDICATIONS & INTERVENTIONS

Anti-Inflammatory Agents

NSAIDS

- Mechanism: Decreased prostaglandin production and thus reduced prostaglandin-mediated capillary leakage and inflammatory cell recruitment. Most NSAIDs are non-selective inhibitors of both cyclooxygenase isoforms (COX1 and COX2).
- Clinical use: Analgesic only in most rheumatologic diseases
- Side effects: GI bleed, hypertension, hyperkalemia, AKI (ATN from inappropriate afferent arteriole constriction or tubulointerstitial nephritis)

Glucocorticoids

- Mechanism: Suppress antibody production by B cells; promote T cell apoptosis; inhibit inflammatory chemokine/cytokine production and antigen presentation by myeloid cells
- Clinical use: Rapid suppression of acute disease activity in RA, SLE, gout/pseudogout, inflammatory myopathies, PMR, etc. (1 mg/kg = common initial dose for organ-threatening rheumatologic disease)
  - PJP prophylaxis should be provided for all patients on $\geq$20 mg prednisone daily for $\geq$3 weeks
  - Prevention and treatment of glucocorticoid-induced osteoporosis:
    - All patients on $\geq$2.5 mg prednisone $\geq$3 months should take oral calcium and vitamin D supplementation
    - For patients >40 yr old on $\geq$2.5 mg prednisone $\geq$3 months: Check DEXA. If DEXA indicates moderate to high risk for fracture based on FRAX score, consider bisphosphonate therapy
- Side effects: Immunosuppression, osteoporosis, skin thinning, glaucoma, cataracts, weight gain, DM2, hypertension, mania/altered mental status, avascular necrosis, HPA axis suppression

Colchicine

- Mechanism: Impairs microtubule polymerization, and thus impairs neutrophil function
- Clinical use: Gout, pseudogout, familial Mediterranean fever, hypersensitivity vasculitis
- Side effects: Diarrhea, neuromuscular toxicity especially when co-administered with statins. Dose reduction needed for CKD

Non-Biologic Disease Modifying Antirheumatic Drugs (DMARDs)

- Definition: DMARDs comprise a group of otherwise unrelated medications that are used to treat rheumatoid arthritis and other rheumatic conditions. The term is used in contrast to NSAIDs and steroids.
- Medications: See Table 9.16

Biologic Disease-Modifying Antirheumatic Drugs (aka "Biologics" or Biologic DMARDs)

- Definition: DMARDs that work by targeting immune system pathways
- General principles of use:
  - Screen for chronic infections prior to starting biologic DMARD therapy: Tuberculosis (PPD or IGRA), HepB, HepC, HIV
  - Biologic DMARD administration: Subcutaneous medications can be self-administered; IV medications are administered at an infusion center
  - Lab monitoring: Check CBC/CMP q2–3 months to evaluate for cytopenias and check renal/hepatic function
  - Do not administer live vaccines while on biologics, including live influenza vaccine, Zostavax ($\rightarrow$ use Shingrix instead), yellow fever vaccine
  - Nomenclature: See Table 9.15 for structure-suffix relationships for therapeutic antibodies
- Medications: See Table 9.17

TABLE 9.15 · Structure-Suffix Relationship of Therapeutic Antibodies			
Suffix	**Structure**	**Description**	**Example**
-ximab	"Chimeric"	Fab = mouse Fc = human	Infliximab
-zumab	"Humanized"	CDRs = mouse Rest of antibody = human	Certolizumab
-mumab	"Human"	Fully human antibody*	Adalimumab
-cept	Receptor-IgG Fc fusion	Utilizes an endogenous binding partner to neutralize a cytokine or cell-surface molecule	Etanercept

*Generated by immunizing transgenic mice that have mouse VDJ locus replaced with human

TABLE 9.16 · Non-Biologic DMARDs

Medication	Mechanism of Action	Clinical Use	Monitoring
methotrexate	**Low dose:** ↑Extracellular adenosine concentration → inhibits lymphocyte proliferation **High dose:** Antifolate effect, antineoplastic	RA, psoriatic arthritis, SLE arthritis, reactive arthritis, DM/PM, vasculitis 7.5–25 mg PO or SQ weekly Take with folate 1 g/day Contraindicated with alcohol use (hepatotoxic) and ≥CKD3	Baseline: CXR, HepB/C screening, CBC, CMP Then CBC, CMP q2–3 mo
hydroxychloroquine (Plaquenil)	Uncertain; impairs acidification of endosomes resulting in impairment of toll-like receptor signaling and major histocompatability complex peptide loading	SLE; RA Safe for use in pregnancy	Baseline: CBC, CMP, retinal exam Annual retinal exam after 5 yr of therapy
sulfasalazine	Unknown; may involve perturbation of lymphocyte NFkB signaling and/or osteoclast RANK signaling	RA; psoriatic arthritis; IBD 500–1500 mg BID Safe for use in pregnancy	Baseline: CBC, CMP Then CBC, CMP q3–6mo
leflunomide	Inhibits pyrimidine synthesis (needed for lymphocyte proliferation)	RA 10–20 mg daily	Baseline: CBC, CMP, HepB/C screening Then CBC, CMP q2–3mo
azathioprine	Inhibits purine synthesis (needed for lymphocyte proliferation)	SLE; DM/PM; vasculitis; IBD 1–2 mg/kg daily for induction/maintenance TPMT deficiency increases risk of bone marrow suppression so avoid if TPMT activity = 0	Baseline: CBC, CMP Then CBC, CMP q3mo
cyclophosphamide	Alkylating agent; covalent crosslinking of DNA blocks DNA replication leading to cell death	Organ/life-threatening complications of SLE, DM, PM, and vasculitis PJP prophylaxis and reproductive counseling (contraception and fertility preservation)	CBC, CMP, UA q1–2 mo Return precautions and close monitoring for infection
mycophenolate mofetil	Active metabolite (mycophenolic acid) inhibits de novo purine synthesis, which is required for lymphocyte proliferation	SLE (esp. nephritis); vasculitis (maintenance therapy); DM/PM; SSc 1–1.5 g BID induction 0.5–1 g BID maintenance	Baseline: CBC, CMP Then CBC, CMP q3 mo
cyclosporine	Inhibits calcineurin, resulting in impaired T cell proliferation	SLE (class V nephritis); RA 100–200 mg BID, adjust to goal trough 150–250 mcg/L	Baseline: CBC, CMP Then CBC, CMP q2–3 mo
tofacitinib	Impairs T cell proliferation by inhibiting JAK-1 and JAK-3 kinases	RA 5 mg BID or 11 mg daily	Baseline: CBC, CMP, Lipids, PPD/IGRA Then CBC, CMP q2 mo Repeat lipids at 2 mo, then q6 mo
apremilast	Inhibits phosphodiesterase 4	Psoriatic arthritis 30 mg BID	Baseline: Weight, depression screening

TABLE 9.17 · Biologic DMARDs				
Agent	**Structure**	**Target**	**Clinical Use**	**Comments**
adalimumab	Humanized mAb	TNFα	RA; PsA; AS; IBD 40 mg SQ biweekly	Increased risk of bacterial/mycobacterial/fungal infections; skin cancer; drug induced lupus in 0.2% of patients Certolizumab safe in pregnancy If disease flares in patient on long term therapy, check for anti-drug anti-bodies
etanercept	Two p75 TNFα receptors + IgG Fc		RA; PsA; AS 50 mg weekly/25 mg biweekly SQ	
certolizumab pegol	Humanized Fab' attached to PEG		RA; PsA; AS 40 0 mg SQ biweekly ×3 Then 200 mg biweekly	
golimumab	Humanized mAb		RA; PsA; AS 50 mg SQ q4wk	
infliximab (Remicade)	Chimeric mAb		RA; PsA; AS; IBD 3 mg/kg IV wk 0, 2, 6 Then 3–10 mg/kg IV q4–8 wk	
abatacept	CTLA4 + IgG Fc fusion	CD80/CD86; blocks T-cell costimulation	RA IV: 500–1000 mg on wk 0, 2, 4 → monthly thereafter SQ: 125 mg weekly	Trend towards less infections, but increased risk respiratory infection/COPD exacerbation
rituximab	Chimeric mAb	CD20 on naïve/memory B cells	RA; AAV; occasionally SLE (off-label); IgG4RD 1g IV d0, d14, then q24 wk	Infusion reaction in 20–30% of patients with first dose Can cause transient or persistent ↓IgG
tocilizumab	Humanized mAb	IL-6 receptor	RA; JIA; Castleman disease; GCA IV: 4–8 mg/kg monthly SQ: 162 mg q1–2 wk	Side effects include ↑transaminases, HLD, cytopenias, risk of bowel perforation (avoid if history of diverticulitis)
belimumab	Human mAb	BLyS/BAFF	SLE IV: 10 mg/kg 0, 2, 4 → monthly thereafter SQ: 200 mg weekly	Used for skin disease or arthritis uncontrolled with prednisone or non-biologic DMARDs
ustekinumab	Human mAb	IL-12/IL-23	Psoriasis; PsA 45–90 mg SQ wk 0, 4 → then q12 wk	Useful in patients who fail two different TNF-α inhibitors
secukinumab	Human mAb	IL-17a	PsA; AS 150 mg SQ weekly ×5 → monthly	
anakinra	Recombinant version of endogenous IL-1 receptor antagonist	IL-1β receptor	CAPS; AOSD (off-label); acute gouty arthritis (off-label) 100 mg SQ daily	Reversible neutropenia can develop

KEY CLINICAL TRIALS & PUBLICATIONS

Rheumatoid Arthritis

- **Methotrexate and mortality in patients with rheumatoid arthritis: a prospective study**. *Lancet* 2002;359:1173–7.
  - Prospective observational study that demonstrated a 60% decrease in all-cause mortality and a 70% decrease in cardiovascular mortality among adults with RA treated with methotrexate compared to other DMARDS or prednisone. Decreased all-cause and CV mortality was not seen for sulfasalazine or hydroxychloroquine. This study underscores the notion that systemic inflammation in RA contributes to cardiovascular mortality and that methotrexate ameliorates this.
- **The Tight COntrol for Rheumatoid Arthritis (TICORA) Study**. *Lancet* 2004;364:263–269.
  - Single-blind randomized controlled trial evaluating monthly visits with DMARD titration (MTX, SSZ, HCQ) to a goal disease activity score <2.4 versus q3 mo visits with titration per usual care. Patients in the "intensive management" group had higher rates of remission (65% vs. 16%) at 18 months. This study supported a "treat-to-target" approach using a disease activity score (DAS28 in this case) to guide therapy escalation.

Systemic Lupus Erythematosus (SLE)

- **A randomized study of the effect of withdrawing hydroxychloroquine sulfate in systemic lupus erythematosus**. *New Engl J Med* 1991;324:150–154.
  - Small, double-blind randomized controlled trial that randomized patients to either continue hydroxychloroquine therapy or to replace hydroxychloroquine with placebo for 24 weeks. The relative risk of clinical flare was 2.5x higher in the placebo arm than the hydroxychloroquine. This demonstrated that patients with quiescent SLE on hydroxychloroquine were less likely to have a clinical flare-up if they were maintained on the drug.
- **Mycophenolate mofetil versus cyclophosphamide for induction treatment of lupus nephritis**. *J Am Soc Nephrol* 2009;20:1103–1112.
  - Randomized, single-blind study comparing IV cyclophosphamide 0.5–1 g/m2 monthly) to PO mycophenolate (3 g/d) for treatment of class III and IV lupus nephritis. Mycophenolate was non-inferior to cyclophosphamide for achieving the primary outcome of decrease in UPCR and stabilization in serum creatinine at 24 weeks. Prior studies established less infections, alopecia, and amenorrhea with mycophenolate compared to cyclophosphamide (*New Engl J Med* 2005;353:2219 and *J Rheum* 2011;38:69).
- **Development of autoantibodies before the clinical onset of systemic lupus erythematosus**. *New Engl J Med* 2003;349:1526–1533.
  - Retrospective study of 130 armed forces personnel who provided serum on enlistment and biennially thereafter, showing that autoantibodies including ANA and dsDNA develop years before SLE diagnosis (mean of 3 yr vs. 2.2 yr, respectively). This study suggests that a break in humoral immune tolerance is not sufficient to cause pathology and raises intriguing questions about whether there are additional immunologic and environmental modifying factors (e.g., autoantibody post-translational modifications, infections, microbiome perturbations) needed to cause disease.

Systemic Scleroderma

- **Mycophenolate mofetil versus oral cyclophosphamide in scleroderma-related interstitial lung disease (SLS II Study)**. *Lancet Respir Med* 2016;4:708–719.
  - Randomized controlled, double-blind, parallel group trial that randomized patients with scleroderma-related interstitial lung disease to receive mycophenolate mofetil (target dose: 1500 mg twice daily) for 24 months or oral cyclophosphamide (target dose: 2.0 mg/kg per day) for 12 months followed by placebo for 12 months. A post hoc analysis demonstrated significant improvements in lung function (in terms of % FVC) for both groups; however mycophenolate mofetil was better tolerated and demonstrated less toxicity.

Vasculitis

- **Rituximab versus cyclophosphamide for ANCA-associated vasculitis (RAVE Trial)**. *New Engl J Med* 2010;363:221–232.
  - Multicenter, randomized, double-blind, double-dummy, noninferiority trial that studied rituximab vs. cyclophosphamide for patients with ANCA-positive granulomatosis with polyangiitis or microscopic polyangiitis. The primary end point was remission of disease without prednisone at 6 months. The trial demonstrated non-inferiority for rituximab compared with cyclophosphamide.
- **Trial of tocilizumab in giant-cell arteritis**. *New Engl J Med* 2017;377;317–328.
  - Randomized trial that assigned 251 patients with giant cell arteritis to tocilizumab SC weekly, every other week, or placebo, combined with prednisone tapers of various duration. The primary end point was sustained glucocorticoid-free remission at 1 yr. The trial demonstrated tocilizumab (received weekly or every other week) plus a 26-week prednisone taper was superior to either 26-week or 52-week prednisone taper plus placebo.

NOTES

NOTES

General Medicine

INTRODUCTION

This chapter will focus on general outpatient medicine, acknowledging that a whole textbook could be dedicated to this subject alone. We will focus on key symptoms and chief complaints encountered in the outpatient setting, as well as health care maintenance pearls. We have omitted the "Anatomy and Physiology" and "Diagnostics" sections because these concepts are covered in the organ system-based chapters and/or embedded throughout the topics in this chapter.

SYMPTOMS & CHIEF COMPLAINTS

Head and Neck

Sore throat

- **Physical exam:** Inspect the oropharynx (e.g., evaluate for tonsillar inflammation, exudate, soft palate edema, swollen or deviated uvula, oral ulcers); evaluate for lymphadenopathy
- **Differential diagnosis:**
  - **Viral pharyngitis**
    - Epidemiology: More common than bacterial pharyngitis
    - Symptoms: Sore throat. Typically patients with viral pharyngitis are not as sick as patients with bacterial pharyngitis
    - Physical exam: May have tonsillar erythema but usually lack exudate
    - Diagnosis: Rule out bacterial pharyngitis as described below, otherwise it is a clinical diagnosis
    - Treatment: Supportive care, no antibiotics indicated
  - **Strep pharyngitis:** *Group A strep*
    - Symptoms: Fever, odynophagia
    - Physical exam: Tonsillar erythema, edema, and exudate; lymphadenopathy
    - Diagnosis: Centor criteria (1 point each): 1) Fever, 2) Tonsillar exudate, 3) Tender cervical lymphadenopathy, 4) Lack of cough
      - Score 0–2: Low probability for strep pharyngitis, so do <u>not</u> need to send for a rapid strep test
      - Score 3–4: Test with rapid strep antigen test and treat; strep culture is unnecessary per the IDSA guidelines
    - Treatment: Penicillin TID-QID for 10 days
  - **Mononucleosis: EBV**
    - Symptoms: Fever, extreme fatigue
    - Physical exam: Fever, diffuse lymphadenopathy (symmetric; posterior cervical/auricular > anterior), hepatosplenomegaly, pharyngitis, may have palatal petechiae
    - Diagnosis: CBC with differential (lymphocytosis, atypical lymphocytes), +heterophile antibody (although low sensitivity/specificity), serology, peripheral blood smear (large atypical lymphocytes)
    - Treatment: No antibiotics, supportive care
    - Complications: Splenic rupture (refrain from contact sports for at least the first 3 weeks of illness)
  - **Peritonsillar abscess:** Group A strep, *Streptococcus anginosus, S. aureus,* anaerobes
    - Symptoms: Severe, unilateral throat pain; muffled voice; difficulty opening the mouth; drooling
    - Physical exam: Erythema and edema of the affected tonsil and soft palate, trismus
    - Diagnosis: CT/MRI if concerned for deep neck space infection
    - Treatment: Drainage of abscess, IV antibiotics (ampicillin-sulbactam +/– vancomycin)
    - Complications: Airway obstruction, aspiration, extension into the deep neck tissues
  - **GERD**
  - **Post-nasal drip**
  - **Acute HIV**

Sinusitis
- **Physical exam:** Palpate the sinuses (frontal, ethmoid, maxillary); inspect the oropharynx and nasal cavities; perform a cranial nerve exam
- **Differential diagnosis:**
  - **Viral rhinosinusitis**
    - Epidemiology: Most common cause of sinusitis
    - Symptoms: Nasal congestion, sore throat
    - Physical exam: Patients are less sick and lack findings associated with bacterial infection
    - Diagnosis: Clinical diagnosis (no specific labs/imaging required)
    - Treatment: Supportive care, no antibiotics indicated
  - **Acute bacterial rhinosinusitis:** *S. pneumoniae, H. influenzae*
    - Symptoms: Facial pain/pressure/fullness, purulent nasal drainage, nasal congestion, fever
    - Physical exam: Pain with palpation of the facial sinus, nasal turbinate edema, purulent drainage in the nasal cavity/posterior pharynx
    - Diagnosis: Clinical diagnosis (no specific labs/imaging required) based on:
      - Persistent symptoms >10 days, especially if severe/worsening symptoms >3 days; OR
      - Initial improvement followed by worsening of symptoms
    - Treatment: Consider observation for patients who are immunocompetent and have good follow-up; amoxicillin-clavulanate BID (typically not amoxicillin due to increasing resistance of *S. pneumoniae, H. influenzae*) for 5–7 days
    - Complications:
      - Chronic rhinosinusitis: Symptoms that last >12 weeks. Obtain CT scan and refer to ENT.
      - Orbital cellulitis: Pain with extraocular movement of the eyes, diplopia, opthalmoplegia. Urgent management required.
      - Cavernous sinus thrombosis: New headache, focal neurologic findings. Urgent imaging and intervention required.

Rhinitis
- **Physical exam:** Inspect the nasal cavities and oropharynx
- **Differential diagnosis:**
  - **Allergic rhinitis**
    - Symptoms: Watery eyes, rhinorrhea, sneezing, congestion, nasal itching, often with identifiable trigger (e.g., pollen)
    - Physical exam: Nasal mucosa may be normal, pale blue, or with pallor
    - Diagnosis: Clinical diagnosis (no specific labs/imaging required)
    - Treatment:
      - Topical intranasal glucocorticoid (e.g., fluticasone). Must be used daily to be effective. Warn patients about the risk of dry nose which can cause a bloody nose
      - Add a second-generation over-the-counter antihistamine/decongestant if a second line agent is needed
      - Recommend avoidance of identifiable triggers if feasible
      - Add over-the-counter eye drops for allergic conjunctivitis
      - Consider referral to allergy/immunology if no improvement with medical management
  - **Vasomotor rhinitis (aka nonallergic rhinitis)**
    - Symptoms: Nasal congestion, postnasal drainage. Symptoms occur throughout the year without a clear trigger.
    - Physical exam: Nasal mucosa may be normal or boggy
    - Diagnosis: Clinical diagnosis (no specific labs/imaging required)
    - Treatment: Topical intranasal antihistamine, glucocorticoids
  - **Nasal tumors**

Vertigo
- **Physical exam:** Perform a cranial nerve exam and a **HINTS** exam (**H**ead-**I**mpulse, **N**ystagmus, **T**est of **S**kew); perform an otoscopic exam and assess for hearing loss; evaluate the patient's gait; perform the Dix-Hallpike maneuver
- **Differential diagnosis:**
  Peripheral causes
  - **Benign paroxysmal positional vertigo (BPPV)**
    - Symptoms: Dizziness triggered by changing head position, usually intermittent and brief episodes
    - Physical exam: Positive Dix-Hallpike maneuver
    - Diagnosis: Clinical diagnosis (no specific labs/imaging required)
    - Treatment: Epley maneuver

- **Meniere's disease**
  - Symptoms: Ear fullness, tinnitus, unilateral hearing loss. Most patients cycle between periods with active symptoms followed by prolonged remissions.
  - Pathogenesis: Excess fluid buildup in the endolymphatic spaces of the inner ear; the exact mechanism is not entirely clear
  - Physical exam: Nystagmus during the acute attack
  - Diagnosis: Clinical diagnosis (no specific labs/imaging required)
  - Treatment:
    - Avoid substances that cause increased endolymphatic retention (e.g., salt, alcohol, caffeine, nicotine)
    - Consider a trial of a thiazide diuretic
    - Provide symptomatic relief with meclizine or a scopolamine patch (avoid in the elderly given anticholinergic side effects)
  - Complications: Refractory symptoms may require ENT referral to consider surgical interventions
- **Acute vestibular neuritis**
- **Otosclerosis**

Central causes
- **Vestibular migraine**
- **Posterior circulation TIA/stroke** (isolated vertigo from a TIA or stoke is <u>very</u> rare)
- **Medication-induced**

Hearing loss
- **Physical exam:** Otoscopic exam, Weber test (performed by pressing the handle of the tuning fork to the center of the forehead), Rinne test (performed by comparing the sound heard when a tuning fork is placed on the mastoid bone behind the ear to when a tuning fork is held near the ear, in order to compare bone and air conduction)
- **Differential diagnosis:**
  - Conductive hearing loss
    - Symptoms: Decreased perception of sound (especially low frequency), but often can still hear loud noises well
    - Etiologies: Lesion in the external/middle ear
      - <u>External canal</u>: Cerumen impaction, otitis externa, exostoses (bony outgrowths often due to cold water)
      - <u>Tympanic membrane</u>: Perforation secondary to trauma/infection, clot in meatus, tear
      - <u>Middle ear</u>: Effusion (otitis media, allergic rhinitis), otosclerosis (bony immobilization of stapes), neoplasm
    - Physical exam: **CARWA** – **C**onductive hearing loss will have **A**bnormal **R**inne (bone conduction is better than air) and **W**eber with sound lateralizing to **A**ffected side (louder in bad ear)
    - Diagnosis: Clinical diagnosis (no specific labs/imaging required)
    - Treatment: Treat underlying cause, hearing aids, soften and irrigate cerumen, tympanoplasty if needed, stapedectomy for otosclerosis
  - Sensorineural hearing loss
    - Symptoms: Hearing loss; may have more difficulty with high frequency sounds
    - Etiologies: Lesion in the cochlea or CN VIII (auditory branch)
      - <u>Presbycusis</u> (most common): Gradual, symmetric hearing loss (especially at high frequencies) associated with aging, due to degeneration of the sensory cells at the base of the cochlea; most marked at high frequencies with slow progression to lower frequencies
      - <u>Noise-induced</u>: Chronic loud noise damages hair cells in the organ of Corti
      - <u>Inflammatory/infectious</u>: Infection (e.g., viral cochleitis), congenital infections, autoimmune hearing loss
      - <u>CNS</u>: Acoustic neuromas (especially if marked hearing difference between ears), meningitis, multiple sclerosis, syphilis
      - <u>Drug-induced</u>: Aminoglycoside antibiotics, furosemide, ethacrynic acid, cisplatin, quinidine, aspirin (tinnitus)
    - Physical exam: Normal Rinne test (air conduction better than bone); Weber test with sound lateralizing to the unaffected side (louder = good ear)
    - Diagnosis: Clinical diagnosis (no specific labs/imaging required)
    - Treatment: Treat underlying cause, hearing aids, cochlear implants

Ophthalmologic

Vision loss

- **Physical exam:** Perform a fundoscopic exam, pupillary exam, test visual acuity, extraocular motions, and peripheral vision. See anatomy of the eye in Figure 10.1.
- **Differential diagnosis:**
  - **Age-related macular degeneration (ARMD)**
    - Symptoms: Loss of <u>central</u> vision and visual acuity
    - Etiologies:
      - <u>Nonexudative "dry"</u> (more common)
        - Pathophysiology: Poorly understood; potentially primary senescence of the retinal epithelium
        - Symptoms: Gradual loss of unilateral or bilateral vision; often causes difficulty reading or driving
        - Physical exam: Slit-lamp exam with yellow/white deposits (called "drusen") that form under the retinal pigment epithelium
        - Treatment: Smoking cessation, supplementation with zinc/antioxidant vitamins
      - <u>Exudative "wet"</u>
        - Pathophysiology: Choroidal neovascularization, likely due to isoforms of vascular endothelial growth factor (VEGF)
        - Symptoms: Sudden vision loss due to neovascularization which can be rapidly progressive; one of the earliest signs is when straight lines appear wavy (metamorphopsia)
        - Physical exam: Slit-lamp exam with subretinal leakage of serous fluid/blood
        - Treatment: Anti-VEGF intraocular injections (e.g., ranibizumab), supplementation with zinc/antioxidant vitamins
  - **Glaucoma**
    - Symptoms: Loss of <u>peripheral</u> vision, tunnel vision with central sparing; both open-angle and closed-angle ("angle-closure") glaucoma may be primary or secondary (e.g., due to elevated intraocular pressure [IOP] from uveitis, trauma, glucocorticoid therapy, etc.)
    - Subtypes:
      - <u>Open-angle glaucoma</u> (more common)
        - Description: Progressive neuropathy of the optic nerve, due to poorly understood causes, but typically associated with elevated IOP
        - Symptoms: Painless, progressive peripheral vision loss; often initially undetected by patient
        - Physical exam: Fundus exam with evidence of nerve damage ("cupping" = enlargement optic disc)
        - Diagnosis: 1) Evidence of optic disc abnormalities, 2) Adult onset, 3) Open anterior chamber angles, 4) Absence of another known cause for glaucoma (i.e., would result in diagnosis of secondary glaucoma); tonometry with increased IOP can be suggestive but is not always present
        - Treatment:
          - Medical: 1) Increase aqueous outflow (prostaglandin analogues, alpha-agonists), 2) Decrease aqueous production (topical beta-blocker: timolol, alpha-agonist, carbonic anhydrase inhibitor)
          - Interventional: Laser therapy, surgery (trabeculectomy)
      - <u>Closed-angle glaucoma</u>
        - Description: Narrowing or closure of the anterior chamber angle, which normally allows drainage of aqueous humor; thus causing an elevation in IOP and damage to the optic nerve
        - Symptoms: Painful red eye, sudden blurred vision with "halos," associated nausea/vomiting; can be precipitated by dilation with atropine (if a shallow anterior chamber was not recognized)
        - Physical exam: Mid-dilated, minimally reactive pupil; conjunctival redness; corneal edema/cloudiness; shallow anterior chamber
        - Approach: Patients with symptoms and signs of acute closed-angle glaucoma require <u>emergent</u> evaluation by an ophthalmologist, including evaluation of acuity, IOP, slit-lamp examination, and gonioscopy
        - Diagnosis: Gonioscopy to measure the anterior chamber angle is the gold-standard; requires slit lamp with special lens to visualize the angle
        - Treatment: Requires emergent surgical intervention
          - Prior to surgery, attempt to decrease IOP with eye drops (0.5% timolol, 1% apraclonidine, 2% pilocarpine); IV acetazolamide or IV mannitol may be used with specialist assistance
          - Avoid atropine

- **Cataracts**
  - Pathophysiology: The lens of the eye is transparent due to highly organized cytoplasmic proteins called crystallins but cannot shed nonviable cells, which occur with age or due to secondary causes (inflammation, trauma) and become cataracts
  - Symptoms: Slowly progressing loss of visual acuity, blurry vision with glare (e.g., difficulty with night driving due to oncoming headlights). Patients become progressively more near-sighted and may no longer require reading glasses ("myopic shift" or "second sight")
  - Physical exam: Clouding of lens
  - Treatment: Surgery (if cataract interferes with patient functioning)
- **Central retinal vein occlusion (CRVO)**
  - Pathophysiology: Thrombus in the central retinal vein results in venous obstruction, causing retinal capillary nonperfusion and ischemia
  - Symptoms: Subacute painless unilateral vision loss of variable time course (hours to weeks); sometimes preceded by positive visual phenomenon (e.g., scintillations)
  - Physical exam: Optic disc swelling, may also have venous dilation/tortuosity with intraretinal hemorrhage ("blood and thunder" fundus)
  - Treatment: Anti-VEGF intraocular injections, laser surgery

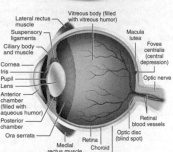

FIGURE 10.1: Anatomy of the eye. The eye has three aspects: the anterior segment, the posterior segment, and the surrounding tissues. The anterior segment includes the conjunctiva, sclera, cornea, iris, ciliary body, and crystalline lens. The posterior segment includes the vitreous humor, retina, choroid, and optic nerve. The eyelids, extraocular muscles, and lacrimal drainage system are other important structures relevant to eye anatomy.

- **Central retinal artery occlusion (CRAO)**
  - Pathophysiology: Occlusion of the central retinal artery (considered a form of stroke), typically due to carotid artery atherosclerosis or cardiogenic embolism, and rarely due to other vascular, hematologic, or inflammatory causes
  - Symptoms: Sudden, painless, unilateral vision loss
  - Physical exam: Pallor of the optic disc, cherry red fovea, boxcar segmentation
  - Treatment: Requires emergent ophthalmology referral for consideration of advanced therapy such as revascularization. Temporizing measures: Instruct the patient to breathe into a paper bag and hold their eye, ocular massage, high-flow O_2, medical therapy for reduction of IOP
- **Retinal detachment**
  - Pathophysiology: Separation of the retina from the underlying retinal pigment epithelium and choroid; vision loss occurs if separation progresses to include the central retina
  - Symptoms: Painless, unilateral vision loss often associated with floaters, black spots, or flashes; symptoms progress at variable pace
  - Physical exam: Elevated retina with folds or tear, abnormal red reflex
  - Treatment: Requires emergent ophthalmology referral and surgical spot welding; if vision is still intact, it is even more emergent to try to save the patient's vision
- **Transient monocular visual loss (aka Amaurosis Fugax)**
  - Etiologies: Carotid pathology, cardioembolic, giant cell arteritis, vasospasm, retinal migraine
  - Symptoms: Sudden transient unilateral vision loss; vision returns when reperfused
  - Physical exam: May have normal exam
  - Diagnosis: Carotid ultrasound, lipids, consider TIA/stroke work-up or evaluation for GCA based on patient risk factors
  - Treatment: Attempt to identify etiology and reduce risk factors

- **Arteritic anterior ischemic optic neuropathy (AAION)**
  - Pathophysiology: Typically, occlusion of the posterior ciliary artery (branch of the ophthalmic artery from the internal carotid, which supplies the optic nerve). Can be associated with giant cell arteritis.
  - Symptoms: Sudden vision loss, jaw claudication, scalp tenderness
  - Physical exam: Pallor and edema of the optic disc
  - Diagnosis: Temporal artery biopsy, elevated ESR/CRP
  - Treatment: High-dose steroids as soon as possible (don't wait for biopsy!)

Acute Red Eye

- **Physical exam:** Fundoscopic exam, pupillary examination, visual acuity, EOM, peripheral vision
- **Differential diagnosis:**
  - **Closed-angle glaucoma:** See previous section
  - **Conjunctivitis**
    - Description: Inflammation of the transparent membrane lining the eyelid and the anterior sclera (i.e., the white part of the eyeball)
    - Etiologies:
      - Viral: Adenovirus
        - Symptoms: Often recent URI, may having itching
        - Physical exam: Watery discharge, may have lymphadenopathy
        - Treatment: Hot compresses, self-limited
      - Bacterial: *S. pneumoniae*, *Pseudomonas*
        - Physical exam: Mucopurulent discharge
        - Treatment: Erythromycin eye drops; if contacts use fluroquinolone for *Pseudomonas* coverage
      - Chlamydial conjunctivitis
        - Symptoms: Often associated with nasal discharge. Assess sexual history and genitourinary symptoms.
        - Etiologies:
          - Trachoma (serotypes A,B,C): Most common cause of blindness worldwide
          - Inclusion (serotypes D-K): Genital hand-eye contact of STD
        - Physical exam: Neovascularization (pannus) of cornea
        - Diagnosis: Giemsa stain
        - Treatment: Oral tetracycline, doxycycline, or erythromycin. Treat sexual partner.
      - Allergic
        - Symptoms: Itching, tearing, nasal congestion, usually bilateral
        - Physical exam: May have eyelid edema
        - Treatment: Remove allergen, topical/systemic antihistamine
      - Irritants
        - Etiologies: Contact lens, chemicals, foreign bodies, dryness
        - Treatment: Irrigation, avoid irritants
  - **Subconjunctival hemorrhage**
    - Description: Bleeding underneath the conjunctiva. May be associated with Valsalva, severe cough, direct trauma. Other risk factors include coagulopathy, anticoagulant use, hypertension.
    - Symptoms: Usually unilateral bleeding underneath the conjunctiva without vision changes
    - Physical exam: Redness in conjunctiva, may be well demarcated
    - Diagnosis: Clinical diagnosis. Check INR if on warfarin.
    - Treatment: Self-limited, may use artificial tears
  - **Hyphema**
    - Description: Pooling or collection of blood inside the anterior chamber of the eye, usually associated with direct trauma or recent eye surgery
    - Symptoms: May have blurred vision/vision loss
    - Physical exam: Layering of blood in anterior chamber of eye
    - Diagnosis: Check intraocular pressure (may be elevated)
    - Treatment: Same day ophthalmology evaluation. Can be medically managed with corticosteroids, beta blockers, or alpha agonists. If failure to improve with medical management, may require surgery.
  - **Keratoconjunctivitis (dry eye)**
    - Description: Inflammation of the cornea and conjunctiva
    - Symptoms: Sensation of "sand in the eyes," bilateral, may have frequent blinking
    - Etiologies: Medications (anticholinergics, antihistamines), autoimmune conditions (Sjögren's syndrome), CN V/VII lesions, allergies

- Diagnosis: Consider testing for anti-Ro and anti-La autoantibodies if risk factors for Sjögren's syndrome
  - Treatment: Treat etiology, symptomatic relief with artificial tears vs gel, avoidance of anticholinergic and antihistamine medications
- **Blepharitis**
  - Description: Inflammation of the eyelids
  - Symptoms: Crusting, burning or itching sensation. Patient may have history of seborrhea or eczema.
  - Physical exam: Inflammation of the eyelids, crusting at the base of the eyelashes
  - Treatment: Lid scrubs (consider non-fragranced baby shampoo), warm compresses, antibiotics if severe (can be associated with *S. aureus* super-infection)
- **Episcleritis**
  - Description: Inflammation of the tissue between the sclera and the conjunctiva
  - Symptoms: Pain, photophobia, may be episodic. Patient may have history of autoimmune conditions (e.g., RA, SLE, psoriatic arthritis).
  - Physical exam: Inflammation of the vessels lining the episclera beneath conjunctiva
  - Treatment: Self-limited
- **Acute anterior uveitis (iritis, iridocyclitis)**
  - Description: Inflammation of the middle layer of the eye (i.e., uvea), which includes the iris and ciliary body. Can be associated with systemic inflammatory conditions (e.g., sarcoidosis, ankylosing spondylitis, IBD, reactive arthritis).
  - Symptoms: Blurred vision, usually unilateral, severe photophobia
  - Physical exam: Inflammation of iris and ciliary body, constricted pupil of affected eye
  - Diagnosis: Consider workup for associated inflammatory conditions depending on risk factors
  - Treatment: Urgent referral to ophthalmology, topical steroids and dilating drops
- **Herpes simplex virus (HSV)**
  - Symptoms: Painful, vision changes (rapidly progressing bilateral necrotizing retinitis can cause blindness)
  - Physical exam: Dendritic ulcer on cornea, peripheral pale lesion
  - Treatment: Trifluoridine eye drops or ganciclovir gel
- **Varicella zoster virus (VZV)**
  - Symptoms: Unilateral painful vesicular rash, eye pain, decreased vision
  - Physical exam: Corneal ulcers, vesicular rash in trigeminal distribution, Hutchinson's sign (lesions on nose)
  - Treatment: Oral acyclovir or valacyclovir (most effective within 72 hours of vesicle outbreak), topical steroids
- **Cytomegalovirus (CMV)**
  - Symptoms: Painless, floaters or flashing lights. Patient may have history of HIV/AIDS or immunosuppresion.
  - Physical exam: Hemorrhages, fluffy granular lesions
  - Treatment: Oral valganciclovir, ensure ART compliance if HIV positive

Musculoskeletal (MSK)
Back pain
- **Physical exam:** Palpate spine for point tenderness, neuro exam (assess strength, reflexes, sensation), straight leg raise test, gait evaluation, consider assessing rectal tone
- **Differential diagnosis:**
  Musculoskeletal:
  - **Lumbar strain/sprain**
    - Symptoms: Diffuse pain, worsens with movement, improves with rest. May have inciting event.
    - Physical exam: May have tenderness to touch over involved muscle/region
  - **Fracture**
    - Symptoms: Sudden onset of pain. May have history of trauma/falls or risk factors for atraumatic fractures (e.g., osteoporosis, osteosclerosis, neoplastic infiltration, osteomyelitis).
    - Physical exam: May have point tenderness, worsened pain with flexion, limited range of motion
  - **Degenerative**
    - Symptoms: Typically chronic pain course
    - Physical exam: May have osteoarthritis in other joints

- **Disc herniation**
  - Symptoms: May worsen with coughing or straining
  - Physical exam: Positive straight leg raise test, worsened pain with flexion
- **Spinal stenosis**
  - Symptoms: Claudication (buttock/leg pain with walking), may have numbness
  - Physical exam: May have decreased pain with leaning forward

Systemic:
- **Malignancy**
  - Symptoms: Constant, dull pain, unrelieved by rest. Pain may be worse at night. May be associated with systemic symptoms including weight loss and generalized fatigue.
  - Etiologies: Metastatic, hematologic, or primary bone tumors
  - Physical exam: May have point tenderness
- **Infection**
  - Symptoms: Back pain sometimes associated systemic symptoms including fever/chills. Patient may have risk factors including IVDU, bacteremia, endocarditis, TB (Pott Disease), or recent instrumentation.
  - Etiologies: Vertebral osteomyelitis, epidural abscess, discitis
- **Inflammatory**
  - Symptoms: Gradual onset back pain that may improve with movement or throughout the day
  - Etiologies: Rheumatoid arthritis, ankylosing spondylitis, psoriatic arthritis, IBD, reactive arthritis

Neurologic:
- **Radicular pain (sciatica)**
  - Symptoms: Pain radiating from back down the posterior leg due to nerve root compression, may have numbness
  - Etiologies: Can be caused by many conditions listed above (disk herniation, spinal stenosis, neoplasm, infection)
  - Physical exam: Positive straight leg raise test, may have sensory or motor deficits
- **Cauda equina syndrome**
  - Symptoms: Bowel/bladder incontinence, urinary retention, lower extremity weakness
  - Physical exam: Loss of anal sphincter tone, saddle anesthesia, weakness
  - Treatment: Emergent surgical evaluation

Other:
- **Congenital:** Spondylosis, kyphoscholiosis, spina bifida occulta, tethered spinal cord
- **Extraspinal:** Pancreatitis, nephrolithiasis, pyelonephritis, prostatisis, psoas abscess, retrocecal appendicitis, fibroids, aortic dissection, postural, psychiatric, referred pain from hip/SI joint

- **Diagnosis:** Consider spinal MRI if any of the following red-flag features are present:
  - Patient history: History of malignancy, intravenous drug use, recent trauma, osteoporosis, prolonged steroid use, immunosuppresion
  - Clinical features: Unexplained weight loss, fever, bowel/bladder incontinence, urinary retention, lower extremity weakness/numbness
  - Physical exam: Neurologic deficits, saddle anesthesia, loss of anal sphincter tone, lower extremity numbness/weakness
- **Treatment:** Generally symptomatic management including non-pharmacologic therapy (patient education, encouraging continued physical activity, physical therapy referral) and pharmacologic therapy (topical agents, APAP/NSAIDs, muscle relaxants, gabapentin for neuropathic) if no red flag symptoms/surgical indications

GENERAL MEDICINE

Gynecologic
Vulvovaginitis
- **Physical exam:** Pelvic exam
- **Differential diagnosis:**
  - Bacterial vaginitis (BV)
    - Etiology: Vaginal inflammation caused by the overgrowth of anaerobic bacteria naturally found in the vagina
    - Symptoms: Malodorous vaginal discharge, may be asymptomatic
    - Physical exam: Fishy odor, grey discharge, no vaginal or vulvar inflammation
    - Diagnosis: Positive whiff test, clue cells on microscopy, pH >4.5
    - Treatment: PO metronidazole
  - Vulvovaginal candidiasis
    - Etiology: Vaginal and vulval symptoms caused by yeast, most often *Candida albicans*
    - Symptoms: Thick "cottage cheese" discharge, pruritus. Can occur in an atrophic/dry form
    - Physical exam: Vulvar inflammation, thick white discharge, may have vaginal dryness
    - Diagnosis: Pseudohyphae/hyphae on microscopy, pH 4–4.5
    - Treatment: PO fluconazole or vaginal clotrimazole
  - Trichomonas
    - Etiology: Sexually transmitted infection caused by the parasite *Trichomonas vaginalis*
    - Symptoms: Frothy yellow/green discharge
    - Physical exam: Petechiae (strawberry patches) in the vagina
    - Diagnosis: Organisms present on microscopy, pH 5–6
    - Treatment: PO metronidazole (for patient AND partner)
- **Additional management:** In addition to condition-specific treatment as above, provide counseling on safe sex practices, offer additional STI testing, discuss contraception options, and screen for intimate partner violence

Urinary Incontinence
- **Physical exam:** Abdominal exam, rectal exam, pelvic exam in females, consider post-void residual
- **Differential diagnosis:**
  - Urge incontinence
    - Symptoms: Sudden urge to urinate such that the patient may not make it to the bathroom, nocturnal bed-wetting. More common in elderly patients.
    - Diagnosis: Urodynamics (incontinence is due to an overactive detrusor muscle)
    - Treatment: Bladder training, anticholinergic (oxybutynin), TCA (imipramine)
  - Stress incontinence
    - Symptoms: Spurts of urine loss during activities that increase intra-abdominal pressure (coughing, laughing, sneezing, exercising). More common in multiparous women.
    - Diagnosis: Positive cough test, weakness of pelvic floor/sphincter leads to loss of bladder support
    - Treatment: Pelvic muscle (Kegel) exercises, pessary placement, surgery (urethropexy)
  - Overflow incontinence
    - Symptoms: Bladder does not empty completely, overdistension may lead to dribbling of urine. The patient may have a history of spinal cord injury or bladder outlet obstruction
    - Diagnosis: Elevated post void residual (PVR) due to obstruction
    - Treatment: Bethanechol, alpha-blockers (tamsulosin), surgical intervention to relieve obstruction
- **Diagnosis:** In addition to the tests above, exclude causes of secondary urinary incontinence:
  - Infection: UA to assess for urinary tract infection
  - Constipation: Rectal exam to assess for stool impaction
  - Functional status: Low mobility may be contributing to physical ability to reach the toilet
  - Mental status: Delirium or dementia may be contributing to cognitive ability to reach the toilet
  - Lifestyle: Assess for alcohol use, uncontrolled diabetes
  - Medications: Diuretics, sedating medications, opioids

GENERAL MEDICINE

Contraception

- **Approach to contraception counseling:** Recommend discussion of contraception with all patients of reproductive age. Counsel patients on the continued use of condoms for protection from STIs, screen for contraindications to certain forms of contraception (e.g., cannot use OCPs if history of DVT/PE), and educate patients about possible side effects. Consider using conversations about the initiation/ continuation of contraception as an opportunity to also offer STI screening and assess for intimate partner violence.
- **Treatment:**
  - **Hormonal birth control**
    - Examples:
      - Combination oral contraceptive pills (OCPs): Progesterone (suppresses LH, thus preventing ovulation) + estrogen (regularizes cycle, prevents breakthrough bleeding), requires daily pill compliance
      - Progestin only ("mini-pill"): Preferred in women who are breast feeding, >40 yr, and those with a history of migraines with aura. Must be very consistent with pill compliance.
      - Transdermal patch: Estrogen + progestin patch. Apply for 3 weeks, remove for 1 week.
      - Vaginal ring: Estrogen + progestin vaginal ring. Patient inserts it and leaves it in place for 3 weeks, then removes it for 1 week.
      - Depot medroxyprogesterone acetate (DMPA): Injectable progesterone that is administered in clinic every 3 months. Safe to use while breast feeding. Long-term risk of osteopenia.
      - Subdermal implant (Implanon): Implanted by a clinician under the skin, effective for up to 3 yr, may cause irregular bleeding
    - Contraindications: Cigarette smoking, history of embolism, heart failure, cerebral vascular disease, migraines with aura, known pregnancy at time of initiation, caution age >35 yr
    - Side effects: VTE, stroke/cardiac event, elevated triglycerides. Decreased risk of ovarian/ endometrial cancer and benign breast disease.
  - **Barrier methods**
    - Examples:
      - Condom: Provides protection from STIs, estimated 5–8% failure rate
      - Diaphragm: Inserted by patient; placed 6 hours before intercourse and should be left in place for 6 hours afterward; may increase risk of UTI
      - Other: Cervical cap, sponge, spermicide
  - **Intrauterine device (IUD)**
    - Mechanism: Inserted by a clinician, prevents fertilization
    - Examples:
      - Mirena (levonorgestrel): Inserted every 5 yr, high rates of amenorrhea
      - Paraguard (copper): Inserted every 10 yr, non-hormonal, preferred if history of breast cancer, may cause heavier menses
    - Side effects: Risk for ectopic pregnancy if patient becomes pregnant with IUD in place
    - Contraindications: Anatomic abnormalities that prevent placement
  - **Emergency contraception**
    - Example:
      - Plan B (levonorgestrel): Effective for up to 120 hours after intercourse to reduce the risk of pregnancy
    - Side effects: Nausea, vomiting
    - Contraindications: Pregnancy, undiagnosed abnormal vaginal bleeding
  - **Sterilization**
    - Examples:
      - Men: Vasectomy (takes 8–10 weeks to be effective, may be reversible)
      - Women: Tubal ligation (effective immediately, non-reversible)

Menopause
- **Diagnosis:**
  - Clinical diagnosis made after 12 consecutive months of amenorrhea. Median age 51 yr.
  - No labs/imaging required for diagnosis
  - If younger age with menopausal symptoms, consider checking a pregnancy test and FSH level
- **Clinical:**
  - Vasomotor symptoms
    - Symptoms: Hot flashes/flushing, night sweats
    - Diagnosis: Consider other etiologies of vasomotor symptoms (e.g., thyroid disorders, medications, alcohol consumption, panic attacks)
    - Treatment: Behavior modification, oral estrogen therapy (aka hormone replacement therapy) can be considered after appropriate patient counseling (typically recommend <5 yr use in total; side effects include increased risk of MI, stroke, DVT/PE, breast cancer)
  - Vaginal symptoms
    - Symptoms: Vaginal dryness/itching, decreased libido, dyspareunia (pain with intercourse)
    - Physical exam: Vaginal atrophy, pallor, dryness
    - Treatment: Vaginal estrogen, lubricants
  - Psychiatric symptoms
    - Symptoms: Mood changes, sleep disturbances, fatigue, difficulty concentrating, anxiety, depression
    - Treatment: Oral estrogen therapy, SSRI

Other Organ Systems
Chronic Noncancer Pain
- **Clinical:**
  - Assess pain: **OPQRST**- **O**nset, **P**rovocation/**P**alliation, **Q**uality, **R**egion/**R**adiation, **S**everity, **T**iming
  - Review past medical history, social history, psychological history (depression, anxiety, stress, ongoing substance abuse can exacerbate chronic pain)
  - Assess functional impairment
- **Physical exam:** Full physical exam, additional maneuvers as appropriate if localized pain (e.g., back or knee)
- **Treatment:** Recommend multi-modal approach:
  - Non-pharmacological: Patient education/reassurance, physical therapy (stretches, exercise), relaxation techniques (meditation, mindfulness practices), sleep hygiene, psychotherapy (cognitive behavioral therapy), acupuncture, massage, heat/cold packs
  - Pharmacological:
    - Topical agents:
      - Good for localized pain, low side effect profile, may be cost-prohibitive for some patients
      - Examples: OTC analgesic balm, lidocaine patches/gel (best evidence in postherpetic neuralgia), diclofenac gel (not systemically absorbed; may be used in ESRD), capsaicin (avoid mucosal surfaces)
    - Acetaminophen:
      - Most patients can take up to 4 grams/day; in liver disease, typically recommend only up to 2 grams/day
    - Non-steroidal anti-inflammatories (NSAIDs):
      - Caution if history of gastritis, AKI/ESRD
      - Examples: Ibuprofen, indomethacin, naproxen
    - Gabapentin/pregabalin:
      - Useful in neuropathic pain
      - Side effects: Sedation, dizziness. Renally cleared (adjust dose if renal impairment).
    - Tricyclic antidepressants (TCAs):
      - Useful in neuropathic pain; okay to use with or without coexisting depression
      - Examples: Nortriptyline, amitriptyline
      - Side effects: Sedation (highest with amitriptyline), anticholinergic side effects
    - Serotonin norepinephrine reuptake inhibitor (SNRIs):
      - Useful in neuropathic pain; okay to use with or without coexisting depression
      - Examples: Venlafaxine, duloxetine
      - Side effects: Nausea, insomnia; avoid duloxetine if hepatic or renal impairment

GENERAL MEDICINE

- Muscle relaxants:
  - May be useful if muscular contractions/spasms (although limited evidence). Typically only pre-scribe a short course
  - Examples: Baclofen, carisoprodol
  - Side effects: Sedation, low muscle tone/weakness, risk of physical dependency and seizures with carisoprodol
- Tramadol:
  - Opioid agonist, lower risk of dependence than opioids
  - Prescribe only short course (maximum 2 weeks)
  - Caution if using other serotonergic agents given the risk of serotonin syndrome
- Opioids:
  - Generally not recommended for chronic non-cancer pain; may be appropriate for acute pain episodes
  - Examples: Oxycodone, hydrocodone, codeine
  - Side effects: Sedation, nausea/vomiting, constipation, tolerance, physical dependence
- **Monitoring:**
  - Recommend frequent visits to monitor progress with pain relief. Use **PEG** scale (**P**ain, **E**njoyment of life, and **G**eneral Activity) during visits.
  - Set realistic expectations and goals
  - Consider early referral to pain specialist for procedural interventions if indicated (e.g., intra-articular injections, nerve blocks)

Edema

- **Definition:** Clinically evident excess of interstitial fluid; recognized as the persistence of an indentation of the skin after pressure (e.g., "pitting edema")
- **Physiology:** Conditions that cause fluid to shift from the intravascular to interstitial space include:
  - Increase in intracapillary hydrostatic pressure
  - Reduction in the oncotic pressure of the plasma
  - Increase in the oncotic pressure in the interstitial space
  - Inadequate lymphatic drainage
  - Damage to the capillary endothelial barrier
- **Etiology:**
  - <u>Generalized/bilateral edema</u>: Heart failure, renal disease, nephrotic syndrome, hypoalbuminemia, hepatic cirrhosis, drug-induced edemia (e.g., amlodipine), nutritional deficiencies, hypothyroidism (e.g., myxedema), hyperthyroidism, venous insufficiency, pregnancy
  - <u>Localized/unilateral edema</u>: Venous obstruction (e.g., deep vein thrombosis), problems with lym-phatic drainage, cellulitis or other unilateral infection
- **Clinical:** Assess onset (acute versus chronic), associated symptoms (dyspnea, pain, skin changes, etc.), relevant PMH (malignancy, clotting disorder, recent immobility, surgery, radiation), current medications
- **Diagnosis:** Based on suspected etiologies above
  - <u>For bilateral edema</u>: Consider TTE to rule out heart failure, LFTs, Cr, albumin, check medication list, TSH
  - <u>For unilateral edema</u>: Consider DVT ultrasound, lymphatic evaluation
- **Treatment:**
  - Treat underlying etiology
  - Often furosemide (Lasix) or another diuretic can be useful to remove edema for certain conditions (e.g., heart failure, cirrhosis), but first determine the etiology of the edema

DISEASES & PATHOPHYSIOLOGY

Hypertension

- Goals Per Joint National Committee 8 (JNC8): See Figure 10.2
  - Patients without diabetes or CKD:
    - Age <60 yr: Goal <140/90 mmHg
    - Age ≥60 yr: Goal <150/90 mmHg
  - Patients with diabetes (no CKD): Goal <140/90 mmHg
  - Patients with CKD (+/− diabetes): Goal <140/90 mmHg (although some nephrologists recommend SBP <130 mmHg, especially if proteinuria)
- Emerging evidence: There is some evidence that targeting a goal SBP <120 mmHg reduces mortality and decreases nonfatal cardiac events, but controversial (SPRINT trial, *New Eng J Med* 2016)
- Etiology:
  - Essential hypertension (estimated 95% of hypertension cases):
    - Risk factors: Older age (M >55 yr, F >65 yr), male gender, black or African American race, obesity, family history, salt intake, alcohol use
  - Secondary hypertension (estimated 5% of hypertension cases):
    - Renal/renovascular: Renal artery stenosis, chronic renal failure, polycystic kidney disease
    - Endocrine: Hyperaldosteronism, Cushing's, pheochromocytoma, hypo/hyperthyroidism, acromegaly
    - Medications/drugs: Oral contraceptive pills, decongestants, estrogen, chronic steroids, TCAs, NSAIDs, cocaine
    - Coarctation of the aorta (differential hypertension in each arm with brachial-femoral pulse delay)
    - Sleep apnea
- Complications:
  - Cardiac: CAD can result in angina/MI; left ventricular hypertrophy, which can lead to CHF
  - Neurologic: Intracerebral hemorrhage or other stroke subtypes: TIAs, ischemic strokes, lacunar stroke; posterior reversible encephalopathy syndrome (PRES)
  - Kidneys: Arteriosclerosis called nephrosclerosis; decreased GFR with eventual renal failure
  - Eyes: AV nicking (discontinuity in retinal vein due to thick artery wall), scotomata, copper wiring, cottonwood, papilledema
- Diagnosis:
  - Two elevated blood pressure measurements at least 1 week apart
    - Accurate blood pressure measurement is dependent upon technique. The patient should be seated, resting (ideally for >5 minutes prior), the arm should be at heart level, and the blood pressure cuff should be the correct size.
  - Physical exam: May be normal, but should evaluate for the following:
    - Eyes: Copper wiring, AV nicks, cottonwood spots
    - Neck: Elevated jugular venous pressure (JVP), carotid bruits
    - Heart: S4 (LVH), S3 (dilated), displaced point of maximal impulse (PMI)
    - Abdominal: Abdominal aortic aneurysm (pulsatile epigastric mass), abdominal bruit, renal bruit
  - At time of initial diagnosis, check the following studies:
    - Urinalysis for occult hematuria, proteinuria
    - Chemistry panel (evalute for renal dysfunction)
    - Lipid profile, hemoglobin A1c
    - Women (age <50 yr): Discuss fertility goals and consider checking a pregnancy test if indicated (important because thiazides diuretics, ACEi/ARBs, and CCBs are contraindicated in pregnancy/ teratogenic)
    - Consider baseline EKG, TTE
    - If severe hypertension, resistant hypertension (hypertension despite three anti-hypertensive agents at adequate doses), or age of onset <30 yr (especially if the patient is not obese and does not have a family history of hypertension) consider further workup for etiologies of secondary hypertension (e.g., consider checking plasma aldosterone to renin ratio, TSH, sleep study)
- Treatment:
  - Lifestyle modifications: Weight loss (most effective), DASH diet (2–4 g salt/day), exercise, smoking and alcohol cessation
  - Anti-hypertensive medications: See Figure 10.2 and medication classes on the next page. There is an increasing preference to counsel patients to take anti-hypertensive medications at night.

GENERAL MEDICINE

- Monitoring:
  - Check blood pressure at every clinic visit and adjust anti-hypertensive medications as needed
  - Consider the use of a home blood pressure kit to compare home BPs to those obtained in clinic and to allow for more frequent BP monitoring
- Hypertensive urgency and emergency: See Cardiology Chapter 1

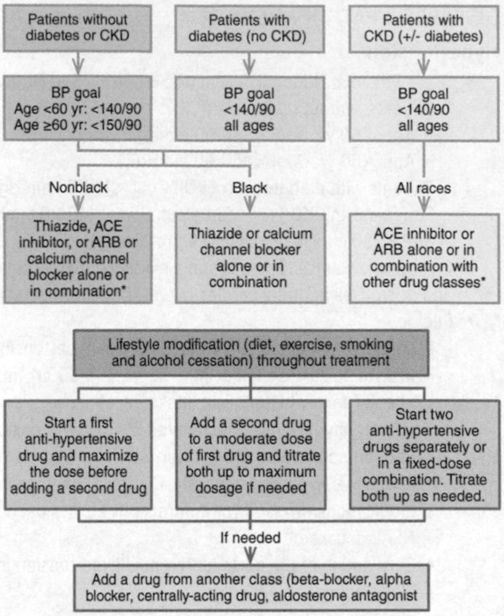

Anti-hypertensive medications:
- **Thiazide diuretics**
  - Examples: Hydrochlorothiazide (12.5 mg/25 mg QD); chlorthalidone (12.5 mg/25 mg QD)
  - Side effects: Hypokalemia (check BMP 3 weeks after initiation), hyperuricemia, hyperglycemia, elevated cholesterol/TG
- **ACE inhibitors (ACEi)**
  - Examples: Lisinopril (QD), enalapril (BID), captopril (TID)
  - Side effects: Hyperkalemia (check BMP three weeks after initiation), increased BUN/CR (ok if increase <35%), cough (5%), angioedema (2%)
  - Contraindication: Teratogenic so avoid in pregnancy and women attempting to get pregnant
- **Angiotensin II receptor blockers (ARB)**
  - Examples: Losartan, valsartan, telmisartan (most potent)
  - Side effects: Decreases uric acid (can be useful in patients who also have gout), cough less common than with ACEi
  - Contraindication: Teratogenic so avoid in pregnancy and women attempting to get pregnant
- **Calcium channel blockers (CCB)**
  - Examples:
    - Dihydropyridine (Lowers BP but not HR): Amlodipine, felodipine, nifedipine
    - Non-dihydropyridine (Lowers BP and HR; useful in patients who also have afib/aflutter): Diltiazem, verapamil
  - Side effects: Edema, gingival hypertrophy
  - Management pearl: Benazepril/amlodipine more effective at decreasing CV events than benazepril (ACCOMPLISH *New Eng J Med* 2008)
- **Beta blockers (BB)**
  - Examples: Atenolol (25–100 mg QD, take at night), metoprolol tartrate (12.5–25 mg BID), metoprolol succinate (25–50 mg QD)
  - Side effects: Bradycardia, bronchospasm (avoid BB in patients with asthma), erectile dysfunction, can increase triglycerides/decrease HDL, may worsen depression
  - Common uses: Generally not used as monotherapy for hypertension. Generally more effective in younger patients. Often used for patients with heart failure. Can be used during pregnancy.
- **Alpha agonists and antagonists**
  - Examples:
    - Central alpha agonist (↓BP and ↓HR): Clonidine (0.1–0.3 mg BID or q7d patch), if patients miss a dose there is a risk of rebound tachycardia
    - Peripheral alpha antagonists: Terazosin (useful in men who also have BPH), doxazosin
- **Vasodilators**
  - Example: Hydralazine (QID)
  - Common uses: Often given to patients who also have heart failure. Can be used during pregnancy.

FIGURE 10.2: Approach to selecting an initial agent in the management of blood pressure using JNC-8 guidelines.

Hyperlipidemia

- Risk factors:
  - Lifestyle: Diet (high saturated fats), inactivity, advanced age, family history, male gender (M>F)
  - Medications that cause/exacerbate hyperlipidemia: Thiazide diuretics (↑LDL, ↑TG, ↑cholesterol), beta-blockers (↑TGs ↓HDL), estrogens (↑TGs), corticosteroids, antiretroviral therapy
  - Other: Endocrine (hypothyroidism, DM, Cushing's), renal (nephrotic, uremia), liver disease
- Types of lipids:
  - **LDL**
    - Calculation: LDL = total cholesterol − HDL − TG/5
    - "Bad" cholesterol − atherogenic
    - Goal <160 mg/dL if no cardiovascular risk factors, <130 mg/dL if some CV risk factors, <100 mg/dL if CVD or DM
  - **HDL**
    - "Good" cholesterol − removes excess cholesterol from arterial walls
    - Goal is high HDL >60 mg/dL (very protective); low HDL <40 mg/dL is an independent risk factor for CAD
  - **Triglycerides (TG)**
    - Higher levels of TGs are associated with an increased risk of ASCVD events; severe TG elevation is associated with an increased risk of pancreatitis
    - Goal <150 mg/dL; considered to be very high if >250 mg/dL
  - **Total cholesterol**
    - Calculation: Total cholesterol = LDL + VLDL (approximately TG/5) + HDL
- Physical exam: Typically no physical exam findings. If severe, may see xanthelasma (yellow plaques on eyelids) and/or xanthoma (on tendons)
- Screening: Recommendations about screening are variable, with some organizations recommending that adults should be screened with a cholesterol lab panel as early as after puberty. For patients with no cardiovascular risk factors, most practitioners start screening men at age 35 yr and women at age 45 yr
- ASCVD risk calculator (aka pooled cohort risk assessment equation):
  - Takes into account age, gender, race, total cholesterol, HDL, SBP, diabetes, smoking
  - Provides a prediction of a patient's 10-yr risk of having a cardiovascular event
  - May overestimate risk especially in older men (extra points assigned for age and gender)
- Guidelines to treat: 2018 ACC/AHA guidelines suggest four groups of patients that warrant treatment:
  - Patients with CAD/CVA/PAD: Prescribe a high-intensity statin
  - Patients with LDL >190 mg/dL: Prescribe a high-intensity statin
  - Patients with DM1 or DM2 + age 40–75 yr + LDL >70 mg/dL: If 10-yr ASCVD risk <7.5%, prescribed a moderate-intensity statin; if 10-yr ASCVD risk >7.5%, prescribe a high-intensity statin
  - Patients age 40–75 yr + LDL cholesterol >70 mg/dL: If 10-yr ASCVD risk >7.5%, prescribe a moderate- or high-intensity statin
- Other factors that may affect treatment decisions: LDL >160 mg/dL + genetic disorder, family history of premature ACS, CRP >2, ABI <0.9, elevated coronary artery calcium score
- Treatment:
  - Lifestyle modifications: Diet, exercise, smoking cessation
  - Statins: HMG-CoA reductase inhibitors, ↓↓LDL
    - High-intensity statin (lowers LDL by 50%): Atorvastatin (Lipitor) 40–80mg QD, rosuvastatin (Crestor) 20–40mg QD
    - Moderate-intensity statin (lowers LDL by 33%): Atorvastatin 10–20 mg QD, rosuvastatin 5–10 mg QD, simvastatin 20–40 mg QD, pravastatin 40–80 mg QD, lovastatin 40 mg QD
    - Timing: Statins should be taken at bedtime since hepatic synthesis of cholesterol is greatest at night
    - Side effects: Rhabdomyolysis/myositis (increased risk in patients with CKD), myalgias; monitor LFTs 12 weeks after initiation
  - Second-line agents:
    - Ezetimibe: Inhibits Niemann-Pick C1-like protein in the GI tract, ↓LDL
      - Used as monotherapy or with a statin
    - Niacin: Inhibits lipolysis, inhibits VLDL formation in the liver, ↓LDL ↑↑HDL ↓TGs
      - Used as monotherapy; no added benefit when used with statin
      - Side effects: Flushing, hepatotoxicity, hyperglycemia, hyperuricemia (don't use in patients with gout)
    - Fibrates (gemfibrozil): ↓LDL ↑HDL ↓↓TGs
      - Used as monotherapy; increased risk of side effects when fibrates are administered with a statin
      - Side effects: GI (mild), gynecomastia, gallstones, weight gain, myopathy
- Monitoring: Repeat lipid panel 4–12 months after initiation of therapy

GENERAL MEDICINE

Osteoporosis

- Bone biology:
  - Osteoblasts promote bone formation and osteoclasts promote bone absorption/breakdown. Bone remodeling is a balance of osteoblast and osteoclast activity
  - Inflammatory diseases cause the upregulation of RANK-ligand, which activates osteoclasts and drives bone loss
- Risk factors:
  - Older age, gender (F>M, accelerated bone loss after menopause due to decreased estrogen), past fractures, family history of osteoporosis, low BMI, smoking, alcohol use, prolonged steroid use
  - Medical conditions: Endocrine disorders (e.g., hyperthyroidism, Cushing's, hypogonadism), GI disorders (e.g., IBD, celiac disease, post gastric bypass), rheumatologic disorders (e.g., rheumatoid arthritis)
- Screening:
  - Screen all women >65 yr; consider screening younger women if risk factors for osteoporosis (fragility fracture, low BMI, high risk medication use)
  - Per USPSTF screening guidelines, there is insufficient evidence to recommend universal screening in men but can consider screening if risk factors for osteoarthritis
- Diagnosis:
  - DEXA: Measures tissue absorption of photons to calculate the bone mineral density (BMD)
  - WHO diagnostic criteria for osteoporosis based on DEXA score:
    - T score >-1.0: Normal bone density
    - T score -1.0 to -2.5: Osteopenia
    - T score <-2.5: Osteoporosis
  - Fracture Risk Assessment Tool (FRAX): Estimates 10-yr probability of fracture if no bone-directed treatment is initiated; incorporates DEXA femoral neck bone mineral density and risk factors
- Treatment:
  - Treatment indicated if osteoporosis or osteopenia AND history of hip or vertebral fracture, 10-yr risk of hip fracture >3% or 10-yr risk of any osteoporosis fracture >20%
  - Universal recommendations:
    - Lifestyle modifications: Exercise, smoking cessation, limiting alcohol intake
    - Calcium supplementation (typically 1200 mg daily)
    - Vitamin D supplementation (typically 800 IU daily)
  - Bisphosphonates:
    - Most common first-line therapy for osteoporosis
    - Mechanism: Inhibits osteoclasts
    - Examples: Alendronate (Fosamax) 5 mg daily or 35 mg weekly orally; ibandronate (Boniva); risedronate (Actonel); zolendronic acid (Reclast, IV formulation)
    - Administration: Most oral bisphosphonates are taken once a week, 30 minutes before eating (need to take on an empty stomach). Consider stopping after 5 yr of treatment.
    - Check calcium and vitamin D before and during treatment and ensure replete
    - Side effects: Heartburn, esophageal irritation, osteonecrosis of the jaw (ensure preventative dental work done prior to starting treatment), atypical sub-trochanteric femur fracture (presents with thigh pain, may be bilateral)
    - Contraindication: Pregnancy, CKD
  - Raloxifene (Evista):
    - Mechanism: Serum estrogen receptor modulator that inhibits bone resorption
    - Clinical use: Only useful in vertebral osteoporosis
    - Side effects: Hot flashes, DVT, leg cramps
    - Contraindications: Pregnancy, prior DVT/PE
  - Calcitonin:
    - Mechanism: Inhibits osteoclasts
    - Administration: Given as a daily intranasal spray
    - Side effects: Risk of anaphylaxis
  - Denosumab (Prolia):
    - Mechanism: Anti-RANK ligand, inhibits osteoclasts
    - Side effects: Hypocalcemia, osteonecrosis of the jaw, atypical sub-trochanteric femur fractures
    - Contraindications: Pregnancy
  - Teriparatide (Forteo):
    - Mechanism: Increases bone remodeling, analog of PTH
    - Administration: Daily injection. Should not be administered for more than 2 yr in duration
    - Side effects: Nausea, leg cramps, dizziness
- Monitoring: Repeat DEXA 2 yr after initiating treatment

KEY TREATMENTS & INTERVENTIONS

Health Care Maintenance and Disease Screening

These health care maintenance and disease screening guidelines summarize recommendations from the U.S. Preventative Services Task Force (USPSTF) guidelines, other guidelines as indicated, and general best practices. Of note, screening tests aim to identify disease in asymptomatic individuals. Recommendations are population-based and may need to be tailored to individual patients based on the clinical context. The decision to stop routine disease screening should be based on shared-decision making with the patient and should take into account the patient's functional status, life expectancy, goals, and preferences.

All patients

- History:
  - Diet/weight, exercise
  - Alcohol, tobacco, substance use
  - Sexual history
  - Depression/anxiety
  - Intimate partner violence
  - Advance care planning: Discuss future health care decisions related to the patient's priorities and values, document code status, identify a surrogate medical decision maker, and complete appropriate documentation (may vary by state: advanced directive, durable power of attorney, physician's orders for life-sustaining treatment [POLST]); Recommended for all adults, and especially important for patients with multiple co-morbidities and/or advanced age
- Screening tests:
  - HIV screening for all patients age 15–65 yr. Offer pre-exposure prophylaxis (PrEP) to persons who are at high risk of HIV acquisition
  - Latent tuberculosis infection (LTBI) screening in persons at increased risk
  - Hepatitis B virus (HBV) screening in persons at increased risk
  - Hepatitis C screening in adults age 18–79 yr
  - Depression screening
- Physical exam: Body mass index (BMI), blood pressure
- Vaccinations: Td(ap) every 10 yr

Women

- 18–39 years:
  - H+P: See list above under "all patients". Also ask about contraception and sexual health.
  - Screening tests:
    - Pap smear (q3 yr if age 21–29 yr; q3 yr or q5 yr if pap/HPV co-testing if age ≥30 yr)
    - If sexually active, gonorrhea/chlamydia screening annually until age 25 yr (and then discretionary). If high risk sexual behavior, offer STD testing more frequently (i.e., q3–6 months)
    - Rubella serology once
  - Vaccinations: Annual flu shot, HBV series, varicella, HPV vaccination if not already completed (recommended for individuals age 9–26 yr, expanded approval up to age 45 yr)
- 40–49 years:
  - H+P: See list above under "all patients"
  - Screening tests:
    - Lipids screening q5 yr starting at age 45 yr, or earlier if risk factors
    - HgA1c q3 yr starting at age 45 yr, or earlier if risk factors
    - USPSTF recommends biennial screening mammogram starting at age 50 yr, but other guidelines recommend starting at age 40 yr so can consider with shared decision-making
    - Pap smear q3 yr or q5 yr if pap/HPV co-testing
  - Vaccinations: Annual flu shot
- 50–64 years:
  - H+P: See list above under "all patients"
  - Screening tests:
    - Lipids q5 yr
    - HgA1c q3 yr
    - Mammogram q2 yr
    - Pap smear q3 yr or q5 yr if pap/HPV co-testing
    - Colon cancer screening (options: FIT q1 yr, flexible sigmoidoscopy q5 yr, colonoscopy q10 yr)
    - Osteoporosis screening if high risk
    - Annual low-dose CT if age 50–80 yr, with >20 pack-yr history and current smoker or quit within the past 15 yr
  - Vaccinations: Annual flu shot, shingles vaccine after age 60 yr

- Age ≥65 years:
  - H+P: See list above under "all patients". Also ask about functional status/falls, safety in current living situation, caregiver support, nutritional status, vision/hearing, memory/cognition, urinary continence, and polypharmacy.
  - Screening tests:
    - Lipids q5 yr
    - HgA1c q3 yr
    - Mammogram q2 yr, insufficient data to support continued mammographic screening in women ≥75 yr
    - Colon cancer screening (options: FIT q1 yr, flexible sigmoidoscopy q5 yr, colonoscopy q10 yr), insufficient data to support continued colon cancer screening in patients ≥75 yr
    - Osteoporosis screening (DEXA)
    - Annual low dose CT if age 50–80 yr, with >20 pack-yr history and current smoker or quit within the past 15 yr
  - Vaccinations: Annual flu shot, pneumococcal vaccine, replace one dose of q10 yr Td booster with Tdap

Men

- 18–39 years:
  - H+P: See list above under "all patients". Also ask about contraception and sexual health
  - Screening tests:
    - Lipid screening q5 yr starting at age 35 yr, or earlier if risk factors
    - Insufficient evidence to assess the benefits/risks of gonorrhea/chlamydia screening in men, but can discuss and offer STD screening
  - Vaccinations: Annual flu shot, HBV series, varicella, HPV vaccination if not already completed (recommended for individuals age 9–26 yr, expanded approval up to age 45 yr)
- 40–49 years:
  - H+P: See list above under "all patients"
  - Screening tests:
    - Lipids q5 yr
    - HgA1c q3 yr starting at age 45 yr, earlier if risk factors
  - Vaccinations: Annual flu shot
- 50–64 years:
  - H+P: See list above under "all patients"
  - Screening tests:
    - Lipids q5 yr
    - HgA1c q3 yr
    - Colon cancer screening (options: FIT q1 yr, flexible sigmoidoscopy q5 yr, colonoscopy q10 yr)
    - Consider discussion about prostate cancer screening with PSA (insufficient evidence per USPSTF, but some societies recommend it so can utilize shared decision making with the patient)
    - Annual low-dose CT if age 50–80 yr, with >20 pack-yr history and current smoker or quit within the past 15 yr
  - Vaccinations: Annual flu shot, shingles vaccine after age 60 yr
- Age ≥65 years:
  - H+P: See list above under "all patients". Also ask about functional status/falls, safety in current living situation, caregiver support, nutritional status, vision/hearing, memory/cognition, urinary continence, and polypharmacy.
  - Screening tests:
    - Lipids q5 yr
    - HgA1c q3 yr
    - Colon cancer screening (options: FIT q1 yr, flexible sigmoidoscopy q5 yr, colonoscopy q10 yr), insufficient data to support continued colon cancer screening in patients ≥75 yr
    - Abdominal aortic aneurysm (AAA) screening in men age 65–75 yr who have ever smoked
    - Consider discussion about prostate cancer screening with PSA in men <75 yr
    - Annual low-dose CT if age 50–80 yr, with >20 pack-yr history and current smoker or quit within the past 15 yr
  - Vaccinations: Annual flu shot, pneumococcal vaccine, replace one dose of q10 yr Td booster with Tdap

Screening recommendations by problem/condition
- Hypertension:
  - Adults ≥18 yr: Screen every 2 yr or annually if pre-HTN
- Hyperlipidemia:
  - Men ≥35 yr, women ≥45 yr, or any patient ≥20 yr with risk factors for HLD (e.g., CAD, diabetes, obesity)
  - If total cholesterol <200 mg/dL and HDL >35 mg/dL, repeat screening in 5 yr
- Diabetes:
  - Screen all patients ≥45 yr; consider earlier screening if risk factors for diabetes (e.g., obesity, family history, history of gestational diabetes, PCOS, HTN, HLD)
  - Testing options: HgA1c, fasting blood glucose, random blood glucose, oral glucose tolerance test
- Abdominal aortic aneurysm (AAA):
  - Perform screening ultrasound for men age 65–75 yr who have ever smoked
- Gonorrhea/chlamydia screening:
  - Women: If sexually active, screen annually until age 25 yr, then discretionary screening after that based on risk factors
  - Men: Insufficient evidence to assess the benefits/risks of gonorrhea/chlamydia screening in men, but can discuss and offer STD screening
- HIV:
  - Screen all adults age 15–65 yr
  - Offer pre-exposure prophylaxis (PrEP) to persons who are at high risk of HIV acquisition
- Hepatitis C:
  - One-time screening for all patients born between 1945 and 1965
- Breast cancer:
  - Breast self-exam: USPSTF recommends *against* self-breast exams (no mortality benefit, more benign breast biopsies)
  - Physical exam: Insufficient evidence for physician breast exam
  - Mammography:
    - Age 40–49 yr: American Cancer Society and others recommend offering mammogram at age 40 yr but USPSTF recommends starting at age 50 yr. Therefore, can consider in women age 40–49 after shared decision-making with the patient.
    - Age 50–74 yr: Screening mammogram q2 yr
    - Age ≥75 yr: Per USPSTF, not recommended (insufficient evidence)
- Cervical cancer:
  - Average risk:
    - Age 21–29 yr: q3 yr pap smear (regardless of whether sexually active, no HPV testing <30 yr)
    - Age 30–65 yr: q3 yr pap smear or q5 yr Pap/HPV co-testing
    - Age >65 yr: Can stop testing if repeated negative tests and not at increased risk (more than one sexual partner in last 5 yr, immunosuppression); also stop if hysterectomy
  - High risk: q1 yr (HIV+, immunocompromised, in-utero DES exposure, CIN 2/3, history of cervical cancer)
- Colorectal cancer:
  - Forms of screening:
    - Fecal occult blood test (FIT) q1 yr (if any one card positive, recommend proceeding to colonoscopy)
    - Flexible sigmoidoscopy q5 yr
    - Colonoscopy q10 yr
  - Average risk: Begin screening at age 50 yr
  - Moderate risk (family history of colorectal cancer or adenomatous polyps in a first degree relative): First colonoscopy age 40 yr or 10 yr younger than the youngest case in family; repeat q3–5 yr
  - Familial adenomatous polyposis: Consider genetic testing at age 10 yr (if positive, consider colectomy) or colonoscopy q1–2 yr starting at puberty
  - Hereditary nonpolyposis colorectal cancer: Consider genetic testing at age 21 yr. If positive, recommend colonoscopy q2 yr until age 40 yr, then annually.
  - Ulcerative colitis: Recommend colonoscopy annually after ≥8 yr of disease
- Prostate cancer:
  - Universal PSA screening is not currently recommended, but can be considered after shared-decision making with the patient
  - No screening if <10 yr predicted survival (50% of men >75 yr)
- Lung cancer:
  - Annual low-dose CT in patients age 50–80 yr, with >20 pack-yr history and currently smoke or have quit within the past 15 yr

- Osteoporosis:
  - All women age >65 yr, or earlier if risk factors. Screen with DEXA scan.
  - Per USPSTF, insufficient evidence to recommend universal screening in men, but can consider if risk factors for osteoporosis
  - Frequency of repeat DEXA scans depends on the presence of low bone mass and risk factors for accelerated bone loss
- Vaccinations:
  - COVID-19: Data forthcoming about recommended vaccination frequency
  - Hepatitis A:
    - Given in two doses 6 months apart
    - Recommended for patients who travel internationally to certain regions and those with certain risk factors (e.g., HCV, chronic liver disease, intravenous drug use)
  - Hepatitis B:
    - Given as a primary series to infants (0, 1, and 6 months)
    - Individuals born outside of the United States may not have been vaccinated as children so consider checking HBV titers
  - HPV:
    - Recommended for men and women ages 9–26 yr
    - Two- or three-dose series depending on the age at initial vaccination
    - Shared decision making for unvaccinated adults age 27–45 yr (consider in high-risk patients)
  - Influenza:
    - Annual flu vaccine recommended. Shot = killed vaccine, nasal spray = live vaccine.
    - Contraindicated: Severe egg allergy
  - Meningococcal:
    - Given as a single dose injection age 11–18 yr
    - Patients at particular risk for meningococcal infection: College students and miliary personnel living in close quarters, asplenic patients, travelers to endemic areas
  - MMR (measles, mumps, rubella):
    - Primary series in children, live vaccine
    - Check prior to pregnancy and administer to patients who are not rubella immune
    - Contraindications: Pregnancy, immunocompromised (ok in HIV if CD4 >200 cells/µl)
  - Pneumococcal: PCV 13 and PPSV 23
    - All adults age ≥65 yr or those age 19–64 yr with certain chronic medical problems (COPD, asthma, cirrhosis, diabetes, history of smoking, high-risk pregnancy, sickle cell disease, asplenia)
    - If a patient is vaccinated at age <65 yr, revaccinate at age 65 yr or 5 yr after the first dose (whichever is longer, for example if vaccinated at age 62 yr revaccinate at age 67 yr)
    - PCV13:
      - Prevents invasive disease *and* pneumonia
      - Ideally administer before PPSV23 if possible
      - If patient received PPSV23 first, wait at least 8 weeks before administering PCV13
    - PPSV23:
      - Prevents invasive disease but not pneumonia
      - Administer 1 yr after PCV13
  - Polio:
    - Primary series in children
    - Not routinely given to unvaccinated adults unless traveling to an endemic area
  - Tetanus/diphtheria:
    - Tdap (tetanus, diphtheria, pertussis) administered as a primary series to infants (1, 2, and 6 months)
    - Td booster q10 yr
    - In adults >65 yr, replace one dose of q10 yr Td booster with Tdap
    - Revaccinate all pregnant women between 27–36 weeks gestation every pregnancy
  - Varicella:
    - Live vaccine given as a primary series in children and adults without a history of chickenpox
    - Two doses; administer the second dose 4–8 weeks after the first dose
    - Contraindications: Pregnancy, immunocompromised patients
  - Zoster:
    - Live vaccine given to adults ≥60 yr
    - Contraindications: Pregnancy, immunocompromised patients
  - Live vaccines:
    - Smallpox, yellow fever, chickenpox, shingles, Sabin's polio, MMR, intranasal influenza, BCG, anthrax

KEY CLINICAL TRIALS & PUBLICATIONS

Hypertension Management

- **SPRINT.** *N Eng J Med* 2015;373(22):2103–2116
  - Multicenter, open-label, randomized controlled trial that randomized patients at high risk for CVD but who did not have a history of diabetes or stroke to an intensive (<120 mmHg) vs. standard (<140 mmHg) SBP target. Intensive BP control (target SBP <120 mmHg) improved CV outcomes and overall survival compared to the standard SBP goal <140 mmHg, with modest increase in the risk of some serious adverse events. Similar benefits were demonstrated in a CKD subgroup analysis (*JASN* 2017:28(9):2561–2563).

Chronic Pain Management

- **Pain Management With Opioids in 2019-2020**. *JAMA* 2019;322(19):1912–1913.
  - This paper offers guidance on the management of patients with chronic pain and currently on opioids: develop and use individualized treatment plans, do not abruptly taper opioid treatment, and consider opioid agonist therapy (e.g., buprenorphine/naloxone) if evidence of opioid use disorder.

Diet and Exercise

- **Association of Step Volume and Intensity With All-Cause Mortality in Older Woman**. *JAMA Intern Med* 2019;179(8):1105–1112.
  - Cohort study of 16,741 women with a mean age of 72 yr, measured steps per day over 7 days. Women who averaged 4,400 steps/day had significantly lower mortality rates during follow up of 4.3 yr (HR 0.75) compared with the less active women (2,700 steps/day). Mortality rates progressively decreased with increasing steps, with a plateau at 7,500 steps/day (HR 0.45).
- **EPIC trial.** *JAMA Intern Med* 2019;179(11):1479–1490.
  - Population-based cohort study of 451,743 individuals from 10 countries in Europe who self-reported intake of soft drinks (diet and regular). Higher all-cause mortality was found among participants who consumed 2 or more glasses/day vs. <1 glass/month (HR 1.17, 95% CI, 1.11–1.22, p < 0.001). Regular and diet soda is associated with mortality, especially CV disease.

Advanced Care Planning

- **Advanced Directives and Outcomes of Surrogate Decision Making Before Death**. *N Engl J Med* 2010;362(13):1211–1218.
  - This study used data from survey proxies in the Health and Retirement Study involving adults ≥60 yr who died between 2000 and 2006 to determine the prevalence of the need for decision making and lost decision-making capacity at the end of life. Many patients needed decision making near the end of life when most lacked the capacity to do so. Patients who had prepared advanced directives received care associated with their preferences, supporting the continued use of advanced directives.

Preventative Health

- **ASPREE**. *N Engl J Med* 2018;379(16):1–10.
  - Multicenter, double-blind, randomized placebo controlled trial that randomized healthy, community-dwelling older adults (age ≥70 yr or ≥65 yr in Hispanic or black patients in the United States) without a history of CVD, cerebrovascular disease, dementia, or any other chronic condition that would likely limit survival to less than 5 yr) to receive either aspirin 100 mg daily or placebo and followed prospectively for all-cause death, dementia, or physical disability. Over almost 5 yr of follow up, rates of disability-free survival were similar between the aspirin and placebo groups (21.5 vs. 21.2 events per 1000 person-years in aspirin and placebo groups, respectively). Aspirin was associated with higher incidence of major hemorrhage (8.6 vs. 6.2 events per 1000 person years respectively).
- **COLONPREV**. *N Engl J Med* 2018;379(16):1–10.
  - Multicenter randomized, controlled noninferiority trial that randomized over 50,000 patients to fecal immunochemical testing (FIT) every 2 yr vs. one-time colonoscopy. In the interim analysis, FIT was non-inferior to baseline colonoscopy in detecting colorectal cancer. 10-yr outcomes will be reported in 2021.

GENERAL MEDICINE

NOTES

Dermatology

ANATOMY AND PHYSIOLOGY

Structure and Function of the Skin

- Function of skin: The skin is a large, complex organ with a variety of important functions: Mechanical barrier, temperature regulation, fluid balance, immune response
- Layers of the skin: The skin has three layers: 1) Epidermis, 2) Dermis, and 3) Hypodermis (adipose tissue, sweat glands, blood vessels, lymphatics)
- Layers of the epidermis: From surface to base – stratum corneum (keratin), stratum lucidum, stratum granulosum, stratum spinosum (desmosomes), and stratum basale

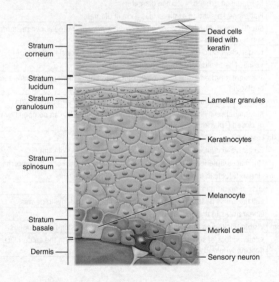

FIGURE 11.1: **Structure of the epidermis.**

DIAGNOSTICS

Physical Exam

- Purpose: The cornerstone of dermatologic diagnosis is the physical exam
- Approach: Identify the skin lesion(s) and try to describe it using specific medical terms (Table 11.1)
  - Be systematic (e.g., head to toe) and try to examine as much of the cutaneous surface as possible
  - Proper lighting is essential
  - It is useful to describe lesions with accurate medical language. A vivid description allows both the internist and the dermatologist to develop an appropriate differential diagnosis.
  - However, when in doubt, simply describe what you see (e.g., multiple raised purple spots on the lower extremities) – this can be translated afterward into medical language

TABLE 11.1 · Dermatologic Terminology to Describe Skin Lesions	
Primary Skin Lesions	
Macule	Flat area of discoloration, <1 cm in diameter and not raised above the surrounding skin
Patch	Flat area of discoloration, >1 cm in diameter (differs from a macule only in size)
Papule	Small, solid lesion, <1 cm in diameter and raised above the surface of the surrounding skin
Nodule	Larger, solid lesion, up to 5 cm in diameter (differs from a papule only in size)
Tumor	Solid, raised growth >5 cm in diameter
Plaque	Flat-topped elevation of the skin, >1 cm in diameter
Vesicle	Small, clear fluid-filled lesion, <1 cm in diameter and raised above the surface of the surrounding skin
Bulla	Larger, clear fluid-filled lesion, >1 cm (differs from a vesicle only in size)
Pustule	Vesicle filled with purulent material
Wheal	Transient, erythematous (e.g., pink-colored and blanchable), and edematous papule or plaque
Telangiectasia	Dilated, superficial blood vessel, not raised above the surrounding skin
Comedone	Keratin debris within the sebaceous gland or hair follicle, can be open ("whitehead") or closed ("blackhead")
Secondary Skin Lesions	
Scale	Excessive accumulation of stratum corneum (e.g., flakes of skin)
Crust	Dried accumulation of body fluids, can be yellow (serous) or red (hemorrhagic)
Excoriation	Linear defects in the epidermis, often caused by scratching
Erosion	Loss of epidermis without loss of dermis
Ulcer	Full thickness destruction of the epidermis into the underlying dermis
Fissure	Linear break in the epidermis, usually along skin lines
Lichenification	Visible thickening of the skin resulting in accentuated skin-fold markings
Atrophy	Acquired loss of substance, may appear as a depression in the epidermis or shiny, delicate wrinkled lesions

APPROACHES AND CHIEF COMPLAINTS

Rash

- Approach to the patient with a rash:
  - General approach: Typically, start with a physical exam before taking an extensive history
  - Where is the rash? (Site of onset? How has it progressed or spread? Is there a specific distribution? Terms: Localized, diffuse, flexural, dermatomal)
  - What does it look like? (Size? Flat or raised? Shape? Color? Terms: Macule, plaque, annular, salmon-colored)
  - Are there any associated symptoms? (Itching or burning? Skin pain? Systemic symptoms?)
  - Recent medications and skin care products? (Ask about prescribed and over-the-counter medications as well as herbal remedies, soaps, and lotions)
  - Allergies?
  - Occupational exposures or recent travel history?
  - Ongoing or recent illnesses?
  - Are there any red flags that warrant urgent dermatologic consultation? (Skin pain? Blistering? Mucous membrane involvement? Extensive body surface area (BSA) involvement? Purpura? Immunocompromise?)
- Steps to describing a rash: It is helpful to have a systematic approach (See Figure 11.2)

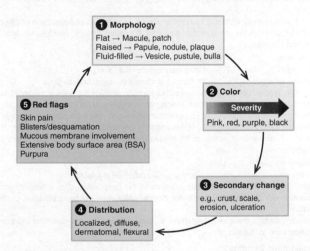

1 Morphology

Flat → Macule, patch
Raised → Papule, nodule, plaque
Fluid-filled → Vesicle, pustule, bulla

2 Color

Severity

Pink, red, purple, black

3 Secondary change

e.g., crust, scale, erosion, ulceration

4 Distribution

Localized, diffuse, dermatomal, flexural

5 Red flags

Skin pain
Blisters/desquamation
Mucous membrane involvement
Extensive body surface area (BSA)
Purpura

FIGURE 11.2: **Five steps to describe a rash.**

DERMATOLOGY

DISEASES AND PATHOPHYSIOLOGY

Eczematous Dermatoses

Dermatitis is red and scaly. The differential is primarily clinical – breakdown the differential by distribution and appearance.

Atopic dermatitis (eczema)

- Pathophysiology: Epidermal barrier dysfunction (e.g., filaggrin mutations), immune dysregulation (skewed Th2 response), and altered skin microbiota; often associated with allergic rhinitis and asthma ("atopic triad")
- Clinical features: Most commonly presents on the face and flexural areas (e.g., popliteal and antecubital fossa)
  - ACUTE: Intensely pruritic erythematous papules and vesicles; may be super-infected with oozing and crusting
  - CHRONIC: Dry, scaly, excoriated papules and plaques; may see lichenification and fissuring
  - Subtypes (descriptive terms of subtypes of atopic dermatitis)
    - <u>Xerotic (asteatotic) eczema</u>: Erythematous lesions with "plate-like" cracked scales, typically on the lower extremities; seen in older adults; associated with dry weather and/or excessive bathing
    - <u>Nummular (discoid) dermatitis</u>: Coin-shaped, pruritic scaly plaques, commonly on the extremities
    - <u>Dyshidrotic eczema</u>: Pinpoint clear vesicles on the lateral sides of the fingers
- Treatment: Emollients (e.g., petroleum jelly, Aquaphor ointment) + topical glucocorticoids. Consider topical calcineurin inhibitors (e.g., tacrolimus) or a less potent steroid for the face, genitals, and skin folds.
- Pearl: History of atopic dermatitis as a child greatly increases the risk of dermatitis in adulthood. Atopic dermatitis increases the risk of contact dermatitis. If a patient's atopic dermatitis worsens, consider co-existing pathologies.

Contact dermatitis

- Pathophysiology: Two types – irritant is more common than allergic
  - <u>Irritant</u>: Direct damage to the skin from harsh chemicals, soaps, or detergents
  - <u>Allergic</u>: Type IV hypersensitivity reaction to a particular antigen (e.g., poison oak/ivy, nickel, iodine, bacitracin); sensitized T-cells trigger an eczematous eruption at the site of contact
- Clinical features: Intensely pruritic erythematous papules and vesicles in the exposed areas
- Treatment: Avoid causative agents; severe eruptions may require topical glucocorticoids or systemic steroids; if dermatitis is severe or life-altering (e.g., job threatening) consider patch testing to determine cause

Stasis dermatitis ("venous eczema")

- Pathophysiology: Innate immune response to fluid collection in tissues
- Clinical features: Pruritic, erythematous lesions on the lower extremities in patients with chronic dependent edema; typically bilateral but may be unilaterally symptomatic; often confused with cellulitis
- Treatment: Reduce the edema (leg elevation, compression stockings) and treat the eczema with emollients and topical steroids

Papulosquamous Dermatoses

Psoriasis

- Pathophysiology: Immune dysregulation (Th1, Th17, excess IFN-gamma) and keratinocyte hyperproliferation
- Clinical features: Thick, well-demarcated salmon-colored plaques with overlying silvery scale; classically on the extensor surfaces (e.g., knees, elbows) but can also be seen on the scalp, palms/feet (palmoplantar psoriasis), nails (pitting, "oil spots") and flexural areas (inverse psoriasis); lesions will bleed if picked (Auspitz sign); 30% of patients have concurrent psoriatic arthritis; associated with metabolic syndrome and greater risk of cardiovascular disease
- Treatment: Depends on disease severity
  - <u>Limited</u>: Topical glucocorticoids, topical vitamin D analogues (calcipotriene, calcitriol), and/or topical retinoids (tazarotene)
  - <u>Moderate/Severe</u>: Phototherapy, methotrexate (+folate), cyclosporine, apremilast, or biologics
    - Anti-TNF: Adalimumab (Humira), etanercept (Enbrel), infliximab (Remicade)
    - Anti-IL-12/23: Ustekinumab (Stelara)
    - Anti-IL-17: Secukinumab (Cosentyx)

Lichen planus
- Pathophysiology: T-cell-mediated
- Clinical features: 4Ps: **P**ruritic, **P**olygonal, **P**urple, **P**apules, most commonly on the ankles, wrists, and membranes; associated with HCV infection
- Treatment: Topical glucocorticoids (mild disease) or systemic steroids, oral retinoids, sulfasalazine, hydroxychloroquine, or phototherapy (severe disease)

Pityriasis rosea
- Pathophysiology: Immune reaction to viral infection or reactivation (e.g., HHV6/7) or less commonly drug-induced pityriasis rosea
- Clinical features: Begins as a red, oval plaque with fine scale ("herald patch"), followed 1–20 days later by numerous similar lesions on the chest and back ("Christmas tree" distribution); typically follows relaxed skin tension lines; does not involve the face, scalp, palms or soles
- Treatment: Time (spontaneously resolves in 6–12 wks) and good skin care (moisturize, gentle soaps); can use topical glucocorticoids (may reduce the itch while waiting for the rash to resolve)
- Pearls: 1) Herald patch is absent in 50% of cases, 2) Consider ruling out syphilis (has a similar appearance)

Seborrheic dermatitis
- Pathophysiology: Associated with *Malassezia furfur*
- Clinical features: Greasy yellow and erythematous scaly patches on the scalp, central face (nose, eyebrows), ears, axillae, chest, and inguinal folds; "cradle cap" in kids, "dandruff" in adults
- Treatment: Selenium sulfide or zinc pyrithione shampoo, ketoconazole cream or shampoo, weak or low-potency topical glucocorticoids if severely inflamed
- Pearl: If severe/refractory seborrheic dermatitis, test for HIV (severity correlates with CD4 count)

Acneiform Eruptions
Acne vulgaris
- Pathophysiology: Inflammation of the hair follicle/sebaceous gland due to increased sebum production (androgen driven), abnormal keratinization, and proliferation of *Cutibacterium acnes* (formerly *P. acnes*)
- Clinical features: Open comedones (blackheads), closed comedones (whiteheads), inflammatory papules and pustules (can progress to nodulocystic lesions and scars) on the face, neck, chest, shoulders, and back
- Treatment:
  - <u>Mild</u>: Topical antimicrobial (benzoyl peroxide, erythromycin, clindamycin) $+/-$ topical retinoid
  - <u>Moderate</u>: Topical combination therapy (antimicrobial $+$ retinoid)
  - <u>Severe</u>: Oral antibiotic (doxycycline, minocycline) or oral isoretinoin (requires birth control if woman of childbearing potential)

Rosacea
- Pathophysiology: Immune dysfunction, *Demodex* mites, and vascular hyperreactivity
- Epidemiology: Common in adults age 30–60 yr with light complexions (Celtic ancestry); much more common in females than males
- Clinical features: Centrofacial erythema (especially the nose and medial cheeks), papules and pustules, flushing, telangiectasias, and phymatous changes (e.g., skin thickening and sebaceous hyperplasia); frequently triggered by stress, alcohol, heat, spicy foods, or sunlight
- Treatment: Avoidance of triggers, topical metronidazole or azelaic acid, oral antibiotics (doxycycline, minocycline), laser therapy

Hidradenitis suppurativa
- Pathophysiology: Inflammatory skin disease of the apocrine glands
- Epidemiology: Begins after puberty, more commonly affects women and prevalence is disproportionately high among African Americans
- Clinical features: Tender inflammatory nodules, abscesses, draining sinuses, and scarring in the intertriginous areas (e.g., axilla, groin, under the breasts, vulva, perineal area)
- Treatment: Weight loss and tobacco cessation, skin decolonization (bleach baths, chlorhexidine), oral antibiotics (tetracyclines, clindamycin, rifampin), TNF-inhibitors (adalimumab, infliximab), surgical excision (although recurrence is common)

DERMATOLOGY

Common Skin Infections

Bacterial

Folliculitis

- Pathophysiology: *Staph aureus* >> *Klebsiella*, *Enterobacter*, and *Pseudomonas* (hot tub exposure). Causes inflammation of the hair follicles
- Clinical features: Perifollicular erythematous papules and pustules on hair-bearing areas
- Treatment: Antimicrobial washes (chlorhexidine), topical antibiotics, or systemic antibiotics if refractory/recurrent

Furuncles/carbuncles

- Pathophysiology: Deeper infections of the hair follicle (i.e., furuncles) may coalesce to form carbuncles
- Treatment: Incision and drainage

Impetigo

- Pathophysiology: Superficial infection of the epidermis, most commonly caused by *Staph aureus* or group A strep
- Clinical features: Characterized by well-demarcated erythema with papules that progress to vesicles or pustules, which break and form a thick, "honey-colored" crust
- Treatment: Topical or oral antibiotics

Cellulitis

- Pathophysiology: Deeper infection involving the dermis, subcutaneous tissue, and superficial lymphatics (termed erysipelas)
- Clinical features: Characterized by an acute, ill-defined red lesion that is tender, warm to the touch, and associated with edema; typically unilateral and can present with systemic symptoms such as fever, tachycardia, and leukocytosis
- Microbiology:
  - Non-purulent cellulitis (~90% *Strep* spp., ~10% *Staph* spp.)
  - Purulent cellulitis/abscess (~75% *Staph aureus* but can be polymicrobial)
- Treatment:
  - Address underlying risk factors (e.g., lymphedema, tinea) and treat with systemic antibiotics
  - Non-purulent cellulitis:
    - Outpatient: Cephalexin ×5 days (alternative = clindamycin). If slow resolution or complicated course consider 7–10 day course
    - Inpatient: IV cefazolin. Add MRSA coverage (e.g., IV vancomycin) if patient is unstable, the cellulitis is over an indwelling medical device, known MRSA colonization, recent prior MRSA infection, significant health care facility exposure (dialysis, long term care), injection drug use, or progression on an antibiotic regimen that does not cover MRSA
  - Purulent cellulitis:
    - Drain abscess, if present, and send for culture
    - Outpatient: TMP/SMX ×7 days (can consider no antibiotics if abscess drained in low risk patient)
    - Inpatient: IV vancomycin
  - Recurrent non-MRSA cellulitis:
    - Address risk factors/try to break cycle (tinea/lymphedema/venous stasis/obesity → impaired drainage, worsening anatomic issues → infection)
  - Animal bite: Wound care + TDAP + prophylactic antibiotics if host risk factors (immunocompromised, e.g., DM, cirrhosis) or bite risk factors (cat bite, severe/deep, high-risk location, e.g., hand, face, joint)
- Pearls:
  - Three general rules for cellulitis:
    - Most cases are unilateral, acute onset, and respond within 72 hours of starting antibiotics. If these features are not present, consider alternative diagnoses and/or a dermatology consult. 30% of cellulitis cases are misdiagnosed. Most common alternative diagnoses: Stasis dermatitis, contact dermatitis, inflammatory tinea
    - Failure of outpatient antibiotics is often due to an unrecognized abscess (need for drainage)
    - Blood cultures are usually unnecessary in the work-up for cellulitis. Exceptions: Severe sepsis, immunocompromised hosts, bites, need for debridement

Necrotizing fasciitis

- Pathophysiology: Infection of the subcutaneous fat and fascia, potentially life threatening (mortality up to 40%) due to rapid spread along fascial planes; may be monomicrobial (commonly *Staph aureus* or *Strep pyogenes*), polymicrobial (aerobic and anaerobic bacteria), or can cause gas gangrene (caused by *Clostridium spp*)
- Clinical features: Early lesions may appear similar to cellulitis but with "pain out of proportion to exam"; rapidly evolves with progressive painful, necrotic lesions and septic shock; may develop hemorrhagic bullae, subcutaneous gas (appreciated on imaging or as crepitus on exam)
- Treatment: Source control (early surgical consultation for debridement) + abx for MRSA, GNRs, and anaerobes (IV vancomycin + pip/tazo +/− clindamycin for toxin production) × 48–72 hrs after source control
- Pearl: Although commonly used, LRINEC score is only ~65% sensitive

Erythrasma

- Pathophysiology: Benign superficial bacterial infection due to *Corynebacterium minutissimum*
- Clinical features: Characterized by mildly pruritic red-brown plaques in the intertriginous areas with a "cigarette paper" appearance
- Treatment: Topical antibiotics

Staphylococcal scalded skin syndrome (SSSS)

- Pathophysiology: Caused by circulating *S. aureus* exotoxin (cleaves desmoglein). Most common in children (age <2 yr), although can occur in adults if renal insufficiency or immunocompromised
- Clinical features: Characterized by diffuse erythema and large flaccid sterile bullae; ALWAYS spares the mucosa
- Treatment: Repletion of fluid/electrolyte losses, skin care with moisture and non-stick dressings, systemic antibiotics if concerned for superinfection; consider adding clindamycin for inhibition of toxin production; consider IVIG in severe cases

Lyme disease

- Pathophysiology: Tick-borne illness due to the spirochete *Borrelia burgdorferi*
- Clinical features: Classically presents with erythema migrans, an erythematous patch with central clearing ("bullseye appearance") that appears 7–14 days after a tick bite
- Treatment: PO doxycycline for primary Lyme disease

Rocky Mountain spotted fever

- Pathophysiology: Tick-borne illness due to *Rickettsia rickettsia*
- Clinical features: Classically presents with a macular eruption involving the palms and soles; associated with systemic symptoms including headache, myalgias, and gastrointestinal symptoms; labs may show leukopenia, thrombocytopenia, and elevated LFTs
- Treatment: PO doxycycline

Syphilis

- Pathophysiology: Infection caused by the spirochete *Treponema pallidum*
- Clinical features:
  - <u>Primary</u>: Red papule that erodes to form a painless ulcer with raised borders ("chancre"), typically on the genitalia; occurs 10–90 days after exposure
  - <u>Secondary</u>: Diffuse "ham-colored" macules on the trunk and extremities, frequently involving the palms and soles; occurs 2–10 weeks after developing the chancre
- Treatment: See Infectious Diseases Chapter 10

Viral

Herpes simplex virus (HSV)

- Pathophysiology: HSV-1 infection is typically above the waist (oral, facial). HSV-2 infection is typically below the waist (genital); can be primary or recurrent. Typically, first infection with HSV-1 is during childhood (0–5 yr), whereas HSV-2 infection may occur with onset of sexual activity.
- Clinical features: Presents as painful clear vesicles on an erythematous base. May be asymptomatic (subclinical) or have fever, malaise, local lymphadenopathy (primary >> recurrence). Widespread infection can occur in immunocompromised patients (e.g., patients with HIV). Can infect established dermatoses (e.g., eczema herpeticum) or involve cranial nerves (Maurice syndrome).
- Treatment: Acyclovir, valacyclovir

Varicella zoster virus (VZV)
- Pathophysiology: Primary varicella ("chickenpox") → herpes zoster ("shingles")
- Clinical features: Herpes zoster presents as localized burning, tingling, or stinging followed by a dermatomal eruption of vesicles and pustules on an erythematous base; considered disseminated if there are vesicles outside the primary dermatome or if involving the CNS (meningitis, encephalitis), liver (hepatitis), or lungs (pneumonia). Ophthalmology consult required if involvement occurs near the eye
- Treatment: Acyclovir, valacyclovir, gabapentin and TCAs for post-herpetic neuralgia

Warts
- Pathophysiology: Common warts (*Verruca vulgaris*) and anogenital warts (*Condyloma acuminata*) caused by HPV
- Clinical features: Presents as skin-colored papules with thrombosed capillaries
- Treatment: Salicylic acid, cryotherapy

Molluscum contagiosum
- Pathophysiology: Infection caused by a poxvirus; occurs in children, sexually transmitted in adults; can be severe in HIV/AIDS
- Clinical features: Presents as pink-white smooth papules with an umbilicated center
- Treatment: Typically self-resolves but can use cryotherapy, curettage

Fungal
Tinea
- Pathophysiology: Superficial fungal infection classified by body site involved (pedis = feet, manuum = hands, cruris = groin, capitis = scalp, corporis = body)
- Clinical features: Characterized by annular (ring-like) scaly patches with well-demarcated edges and central clearing; may be pruritic
- Diagnosis: +KOH stain
- Treatment: Topical azoles or terbinafine
- Pearl: Use terbinafine (or another allylamine) as first line for tinea pedis, cruris, and corporis. Allylamines are fungicidal whereas topical azoles are fungistatic.

Pityriasis (tinea) versicolor
- Pathophysiology: Caused by *Malassezia furfur*
- Clinical features: Presents as non-pruritic oval/round hypo- or hyper-pigmented lesions on the trunk and upper extremities
- Diagnosis: KOH prep with "spaghetti and meatball" appearance
- Treatment: Ketoconazole shampoo or selenium sulfide

Candidiasis/intertrigo
- Pathophysiology: Superficial fungal infection due to *Candida* spp.
- Clinical features: Presents as bright red (often macerated) patches with satellite pustules in areas of moist occluded skin (intertriginous areas, oropharynx, genitals)
- Treatment: Topical azoles, nystatin, drying/absorbent powders or zinc oxide paste. If widespread, can consider oral fluconazole

Ectoparasites
Scabies
- Pathophysiology: Highly contagious infestation caused by the mite *Sarcoptes scabiei hominis*
- Clinical features: Characterized by intensely pruritic erythematous papules, excoriations and linear burrows in the interdigital spaces, wrists, ankles, breasts, periumbilical area, and genitals
- Treatment: Permethrin 5% cream, decontamination of clothes and bedding

Lice
- Pathophysiology: Infestation caused by the louse *Peduculus humanus*; can affect the head, body, or pubic area
- Clinical features: Presents with excoriations and crusted papules on the neck, trunk, proximal arms, or groin; may find live lice on the scalp or eggs (nits) in the hair
- Treatment: Permethrin 1% cream, decontamination of clothes and bedding

Bedbugs
- Pathophysiology: Infestation caused by the insect *Cimex lectularis*
- Clinical features: Presents with linearly arranged pruritic papules ("breakfast, lunch, and dinner")
- Treatment: Professional extermination

Cutaneous Drug Reactions

Morbilliform drug eruption

- Pathophysiology: Most common type of cutaneous drug reaction (~75 to 90% of cases); common culprits include antibiotics, antiepileptics, NSAIDs, and calcium channel blockers
- Clinical features: Presents with erythematous macules and papules coalescing into patches on the trunk, back, and extremities ("morbilliform" = measles-like)
- Treatment: Discontinue unnecessary medications, treat symptoms with oral antihistamines +/− topical steroids, may attempt to "treat through" if mild and no substitute medication is available

Erythema multiforme

- Pathophysiology: Immune-mediated eruption that can mimic SJS/TEN; typically caused by infection (~90% of cases) but can also be due to a drug reaction; commonly associated infections such as HSV, Mycoplasma
- Clinical features: Characterized by "true target" lesions with three distinct zones on the extremities including the palms and soles; may have mucocutaneous involvement
- Treatment: Discontinue unnecessary medications, treat infection if applicable, treat symptoms with oral antihistamines +/− topical steroids

Severe Cutaneous Drug Reactions

Can be life threatening due to profound insensible losses and resultant fluid and electrolyte shifts.

Stevens-Johnson syndrome (SJS) / Toxic epidermal necrolysis (TEN)

- Pathophysiology: Life-threatening drug reaction with mucocutaneous involvement; common medication triggers include TMP-SMX, PCN, lamotrigine, carbamazepine, and allopurinol
- Clinical features: Presents with painful "targetoid" lesions on the face, trunk, and extremities; can progress to dusky blisters with widespread skin sloughing (+Nikolsky sign); majority of patients have mucosal involvement (ocular, oral, genital). SJS <10% body surface area (BSA), SJS/TEN overlap 10–30% BSA, TEN >30% BSA.
- Treatment: Discontinue suspected agents, early dermatology consultation (associated with improved outcomes), supportive care in ICU or burn unit if needed

Drug-induced hypersensitivity syndrome (DIHS)

- Pathophysiology: Potentially life-threatening drug reaction (mortality 10%) associated with antiepileptic drugs (carbamazepine, lamotrigine, phenytoin), TMP-SMX, NSAIDs, minocycline, allopurinol, and abacavir
- Clinical features: Presents most commonly with a morbilliform drug eruption with facial swelling (nasolabial folds); eosinophilia is NOT a requirement for diagnosis (although present in 90% of cases); may have fever, lymphadenopathy, and evidence of organ involvement (liver, kidney, heart, lungs)
- Treatment: Discontinue suspected agents, prolonged systemic steroids

Acute generalized exanthematous pustulosis (AGEP)

- Clinical features: Rapidly progressive morbilliform drug eruption with innumerable pinpoint sterile pustules; common drug triggers include penicillins, macrolides, CCBs, and radiocontrast dye
- Treatment: Discontinue unnecessary medications, treat symptoms with oral antihistamines +/− topical steroids

Autoimmune Bullous Diseases

Bullous pemphigoid (BP)

- Pathophysiology: Chronic autoimmune blistering disease most commonly seen in the elderly due to autoantibodies targeting hemidesmosomes on the basement membrane, resulting in sub-epidermal blistering ("bullow").
- Clinical features: Pruritic plaques and urticarial lesions with tense, intact blisters on the thighs and flexural areas
- Histology: Direct immunofluorescence (DIF) shows linear IgG deposition at the basement membrane zone
- Treatment: Topical high-potency glucocorticoids, oral steroids, methotrexate, mycophenolate mofetil

Pemphigus vulgaris

- Pathophysiology: Rare autoimmune blistering disease with mucocutaneous involvement due to autoantibodies targeting desmoglein proteins in the epidermis, resulting in suprabasal (interepidermal) blistering.
- Clinical features: Flaccid blisters that easily rupture (+Nikolsky sign) leaving painful, bright red erosions; most patients have oral involvement but can also see esophageal, urethral, vulvovaginal, and penile lesions
- Histology: DIF shows intracellular IgG deposition; may also see "tombstones" of basal cells attached to the basement membrane
- Treatment: Systemic steroids, azathioprine, or mycophenolate, plasmapheresis, cyclophosphamide, or rituximab for severe disease

DERMATOLOGY

Dermatitis herpetiformis

- Pathophysiology: Autoimmune blistering disease due to IgA autoantibodies targeting epidermal tissue transglutaminase; >90% of patients have gluten insensitivity
- Clinical features: Presents with severe pruritus and excoriated papulovesicles on the extensor surfaces (elbows, knees)
- Treatment: Gluten avoidance, dapsone

Inflammatory and Autoimmune Conditions

Pyoderma gangrenosum (PG)

- Pathophysiology: Neutrophilic dermatosis; often associated with underlying systemic disease (IBD, RA, malignancy)
- Clinical features: Classically presents as a rapidly expanding ulcer with a purulent base and violaceous overhanging borders; often occurs at sites of prior trauma (+pathergy)
- Treatment: Search for underlying disease, treat with topical/intralesional steroids, oral steroids, oral antineutrophilic agents (dapsone), and wound care

Sweet syndrome

- Pathophysiology: Acute febrile neutrophilic dermatosis; often occurs after an upper respiratory or gastrointestinal infection but can be associated with malignancy (MDS, AML, solid tumor) or GM-CSF
- Clinical features: Presents with high fevers, peripheral neutrophilia, and painful, edematous "juicy" red-violaceous papules on the face, neck, and extremities
- Treatment: Systemic glucocorticoids (should see rapid improvement)

Erythema nodosum (EN)

- Pathophysiology: Panniculitis; can occur due to an underlying condition (*Strep* spp. infection, oral contraceptive pills, IBD, malignancy, sarcoidosis, pregnancy) but etiology is unknown in ~50% cases
- Clinical features: Presents as an ill-defined, red subcutaneous nodule, often on the lower extremity
- Treatment: Search for underlying condition, treat symptoms with leg elevation and NSAIDs

Dermatomyositis

- Pathophysiology: Autoimmune disease with characteristic skin findings, +/− muscle involvement, and systemic symptoms; skin-limited disease (amyopathic dermatomyositis) in up to 30% of patients
- Clinical features: Presents with violaceous lesions around the eyes (heliotrope sign), on the anterior chest and back (shawl sign), over the finger and hand joints (Gottron's papules), and lateral hips (holster sign)
- Treatment: Age-appropriate cancer screening, chest imaging to evaluate for ILD, sun protection, topical glucocorticoids, systemic steroids if extensive disease

Cutaneous lupus

- Subtypes:
  - Acute cutaneous lupus: Classic sun-exacerbated malar erythema (butterfly rash); spares the nasolabial folds; associated with active systemic disease
  - Sub-acute cutaneous lupus: Photo-distributed erythematous plaques on the trunk, back, and extremities; can be annular or look like psoriasis; may be drug-induced (hydrochlorothiazide, PPIs, terbinafine)
  - Chronic cutaneous lupus: Most common; well-demarcated erythematous macules and papules on the face, scalp, and extremities that can develop into indurated discoid plaques
- Treatment: Rheumatology involvement if systemic disease, treat skin symptoms with sun protection, topical/intralesional glucocorticoids, hydroxychloroquine, methotrexate

Vasculitis and Vasculopathy

- Leukocytoclastic vasculitis (LCV): Histopathologic term that describes nuclear debris from an inflammatory infiltrate; often used interchangeably with small vessel or cutaneous vasculitis

Cutaneous small vessel vasculitis (CSVV)

- Pathophysiology: Skin-isolated small vessel vasculitis without systemic vasculitis or glomerulonephritis; typically with LCV histology; most often idiopathic (~50%) but can be caused by infection (HBV, HCV, bacteremia), autoimmune disease, or drug-induced (penicillins, cephalosporins, sulfa drugs, diuretics)
- Clinical features: Presents with palpable purpura (non-blanching purple papules) in dependent areas (lower extremities, buttocks, posterior thigh)
- Treatment: Eliminate potential triggers, leg elevation, compression stockings, topical steroids

Cholesterol emboli
- Pathophysiology: Vasculopathy due to arterial embolization of cholesterol crystals
- Clinical features: Presents with retiform ("net-like") purpura or livedo reticularis in the distal lower extremities; classically occurs after endovascular procedures or thrombolysis
- Treatment: Supportive care

Cryoglobulinemia
- Pathophysiology: Small- and medium-vessel clot formation (vasculopathy) and inflammation (vasculitis) due to precipitation of intravascular proteins (cryoglobulins); associated with HCV, autoimmune diseases, and plasma cell dyscrasias (MGUS, multiple myeloma, Waldenstrom macroglobulinemia)
- Clinical features: Presents with stellate ("star-like"), reticular, or palpable purpura which may progress to ulcers, ischemia, or necrosis. Typically occurs on the lower legs, feet, digits, and ears due to exposure to colder temperatures
- Treatment: Treat underlying disease

Calciphylaxis
- Pathophysiology: Progressive vascular calcification most commonly due to ESRD (uremic calciphylaxis), although also can be seen in hyperparathyroidism, malignancy, and with warfarin use
- Clinical features: Exquisitely painful purpuric lesions with associated ischemia, necrosis, and bullae
- Treatment: Pain management, wound care, remove potential triggers, sodium thiosulfate, dialysis if appropriate

Common Skin Cancers

Benign skin conditions
- Seborrheic keratosis (SK): Benign pigmented neoplasm; common after age 50 yr; presents as tan-brown "stuck on" papules or plaques. Sudden appearance of multiple SK's is associated with underlying malignancy (Leser-Trelat sign). Treatment: Cryotherapy or shave removal if symptomatic.
- Melanocytic nevi ("mole"): Benign neoplasm composed of melanocytes; can occur anywhere on the body and can mimic melanoma. Treatment: Biopsy to rule out melanoma if concerning appearance.
- Acrochordon ("skin tag"): Skin-colored pedunculated papules on the neck and skin folds; associated with obesity and insulin resistance. Treatment: Cryotherapy or snip excision.
- Cherry angioma: Benign vascular lesion that presents as a red-violaceous papule
- Dermatofibroma: Benign fibrohistiocytic lesion; presents as a tan-brown papule that "dimples" with pressure; often on the lower extremities; F>M

Basal cell carcinoma (BCC)
- Epidemiology: Most common skin cancer; due to UV light exposure; rarely metastasizes but can cause significant local tissue destruction
- Clinical features: Presents as a pearly nodule with arborizing telangiectasias and ulceration (nodular type, most common), a pink-red patch (spreading type), or shiny black-blue papules (pigmented type)
- Diagnosis: Confirm histologically with biopsy
- Treatment: Surgical excision (standard versus Mohs), electrodessication and curettage, or topical chemotherapy

Actinic keratosis (AK)
- Definition: Precancerous lesion of the epidermis (<5% progress to squamous cell skin cancer)
- Clinical features: Presents as pink, scaly, "sandpaper-like" papules and plaques in sun exposed areas
- Treatment: Cryotherapy, topical 5-FU, imiquimod

Squamous cell carcinoma (SCC)
- Epidemiology: Second most common skin cancer; risk factors include UV light exposure, radiation, chemicals (coal, soot, arsenic), HPV, and immunosuppression (e.g., solid organ transplantation).
- Clinical features: Presents as a pink, scaly papules, plaques, and nodules that ulcerate, bleed, and become crusty; may arise from a chronic wound/scar (Marjolin ulcer)
- Diagnosis: Confirm histologically with biopsy
- Treatment: Surgical excision (standard versus Mohs) is first line, radiation if surgery is contraindicated, systemic chemotherapy if metastasis

DERMATOLOGY

Malignant melanoma
- Epidemiology: Most deadly skin cancer; histologically aggressive and has a high risk of metastasis; lifetime risk is 1 in 50 individuals
- Clinical features: **ABCDE** – **A**symmetry, **B**order irregularities, **C**olor variation, **D**iameter >6 mm, **E**volution over time
- Subtypes include:
  - Superficial spreading (~70% of melanomas): Presents as variably pigmented macules with irregular borders; commonly located on the back (men) or posterior legs (women)
  - Nodular (15–30% of melanomas): Presents as darkly pigmented "berry-like" papules or nodules
  - Lentigo maligna (10–15% of melanomas): Presents as atypical pigmented macules, typically in chronically sun-damaged areas in older adults
  - Acral lentiginous (<5% of all melanomas): Most common melanoma among dark-skinned individuals; presents as dark brown macules or patches on the palmar, plantar, and subungual surfaces (e.g., beneath the nail plate)
  - Uveal melanoma: Melanoma of the eye involving the iris, ciliary body, or choroid (collectively referred to as the uvea)
  - Mucosal melanoma: Rare type of melanoma that occurs on mucosal surfaces (e.g., GI tract, GU tract, respiratory tract)
- Staging: Via TNM system. Based on tumor depth, lymph node involvement, and presence of metastatic spread
- Prognosis: Poor prognostic factors include: male gender, older age, increased tumor thickness (Breslow depth), ulceration, increased tumor mitotic rate, and tumor location on head/neck
- Treatment:
  - Stage I–II: Wide local excision, consider sentinel lymph node biopsy if stage IB or higher (e.g., tumor thickness ≥1 mm)
  - Stage III: Wide local excision + lymph node dissection + adjuvant systemic therapy
  - Stage IV: Systemic immunotherapy (nivolumab, pembrolizumab) or targeted therapy (e.g., BRAF/MEK inhibitors if BRAF V600 mutant)

Hair and Nail Disorders
- Hirsutism: Excess hair growth in androgen-dependent areas (upper lip, lateral cheeks, chin, chest, lower abdomen, groin, and buttocks); most commonly caused by polycystic ovary syndrome (~60% of cases) but can also be due to other forms of androgen excess (e.g., adrenal hyperplasia, androgen-secreting tumors). Treatment: OCPs, antiandrogens (spironolactone, finasteride), hair removal
- Alopecia: Localized or generalized hair loss; categorized as nonscarring (alopecia areata, traumatic alopecia, androgenic alopecia) or scarring (discoid lupus, lichen planopilaris)
- Onychomycosis: Dermatophyte infection of the nail; presents as nail plate discoloration (yellow, white, or brown) with thickening and subungual debris. Treatment: Oral therapy with terbinafine or itraconazole, topical antifungals have limited efficacy
- Paronychia: Infection of the nail fold; most commonly caused by *Staph aureus*. Treatment: Warm compresses, incision and drainage, oral antibiotics if severe

Disorders of the Mucous Membranes
- Aphthous ulcers ("canker sores"): Painful, shallow oral ulcers with a gray base and a red surrounding halo; if recurrent or severe may suggest underlying disease such as Behçet's syndrome, Crohn's disease, or HIV. Treatment: Self-resolves
- Oral candidiasis: Painful white Non-adherent plaques; risk factors include immunosuppression, DM, and glucocorticoids. Treatment: Azole troches or nystatin swish and swallow
- Leukoplakia: Adherent white patches in the oral mucosa; pre-malignant lesion. Requires biopsy to rule out dysplasia
- Erythroplakia: Red mucosal patches; high risk of malignant transformation. Requires biopsy to rule out dysplasia
- Black hairy tongue: Benign condition due to elongation and defective desquamation of filiform papillae. Treatment: Oral care/hygiene
- Geographic tongue: Benign condition; presents with migratory smooth red surfaces and white patches on the tongue; may be sporadic, familial, or associated with psoriasis
- Lichen planus: Erythematous patches with overlying white lacelike pattern (Wickham striae); may be isolated to oral mucosa or can be associated with skin or vulvovaginal lesions. Treatment: Topical glucocorticoids and systemic steroid-sparing agents
- Lichen sclerosus: White atrophic patches involving the vaginal introitus and perianal area ("figure 8" morphology); typically affects women age 50 to 60 yr. Treatment: Topical glucocorticoids

DERMATOLOGY

Miscellaneous

- Milaria ("heat rash"): Numerous non-follicular papules or pustules; caused by occlusion of the sweat ducts. Treatment: Removal of occluding agents
- Transient acantholytic dermatosis (Grover disease): Discrete pruritic papulovesicles on the trunk and back; especially common in older Caucasian men. Treatment: Moisturizers and topical glucocorticoids
- Vitiligo: Autoimmune condition resulting in the absence or loss of function of melanocytes; presents as well-demarcated depigmented macules and patches; associated with type 1 diabetes and autoimmune thyroid disease. Treatment: Topical glucocorticoids, phototherapy
- Venous stasis ulcer: Most common cause of leg ulceration (~70% of cases); presents as irregularly shaped shallow ulcers on the lower extremities; often occurs with other findings to suggest chronic venous stasis, including edema, eczematous change, hyperpigmentation, and varicosities. Treatment: Leg elevation, compression therapy, wound care
- Arterial insufficiency ulcer: Less common cause of leg ulceration (~25% of cases); presents as painful, sharply demarcated ulcers with a "punched out" appearance. Diagnosis: Ankle-brachial index. Treatment: Wound care and surgical revascularization

KEY MEDICATIONS AND INTERVENTIONS

TABLE 11.2 · Topical Steroid Ointments, Creams, and Lotions by Strength	
Strength	**Common examples: Medication, strength, (formulation)**
Group 1: Super-high potency	betamethasone dipropionate 0.05% (O)
	clobetasol propionate 0.05% (O, C, L)
Group 2: High potency	betamethasone dipropionate 0.05% (C)
	desoximetasone 0.25% (C)
	fluocinonide 0.05% (O, C)
Group 3: High potency	betamethasone valerate 0.1% (O)
	mometasone furoate 0.1% (O)
	triamcinolone acetonide 0.5% (O, C)
Group 4: Medium potency	hydrocortisone valerate 0.2% (O)
	mometasone furoate 0.1% (C, L)
	triamcinolone acetonide 0.1% (O, C)
Group 5: Lower-mid potency	desonide 0.05% (O)
	hydrocortisone valerate 0.2% (C)
	triamcinolone acetonide 0.1% (L)
Group 6: Low potency	desonide 0.05% (C, L)
	triamcinolone acetonide 0.25% (C, L)
Group 7: Least potent	hydrocortisone 1–2% (C, L)

Formulation of topical steroid: Ointment (O), Cream (C), Lotion (L)

- Treatment pearls:
  - Steroid strength typically: Ointment > Cream > Lotion
  - Steroid comfort for most patients (less occlusive): Lotion > Cream > Ointment
  - The best topical medication is the one that the patient will use. As most medications come in different vehicles (e.g., cream, ointment, lotion, shampoo), ask your patient what he/she prefers.
  - Typically, a solitary lesion should respond to correct treatment within 2 weeks. If a lesion does not resolve completely with treatment by 4 weeks, re-evaluate the diagnosis and consider malignancy.

KEY CLINICAL TRIALS AND PUBLICATIONS

Inpatient Dermatology

- **Prevalence of cutaneous findings in hospitalized medical patients.** *J Am Acad Dermatol* 1995;33(2 Pt 1):207–211.
  - Observational study in which patients admitted to medical services were examined by a dermatologist within 48 hours to determine if cutaneous findings had been overlooked. Of examined patients (n = 231), 31 patients (13.4%) had cutaneous signs related to the reason for hospitalization or associated with a systemic disorder. For 14 patients, the primary team had not recognized these skin findings.
- **Association of dermatology consultation with accuracy of cutaneous disorder diagnoses in hospitalized patients.** *JAMA Dermatol* 2016;152(4):477–480.
  - Observational study in which primary teams' vs. dermatology teams' final diagnoses were compared at multiple academic centers. Dermatology consultation changed the final diagnosis in 71% of consultation requests. Cellulitis, leg ulceration, and viral infections were the three most commonly undiagnosed and misdiagnosed conditions by the referring team. The authors conclude that dermatology consultation is associated with improved diagnostic accuracy of cutaneous disorders in hospitalized patients and facilitates early appropriate intervention.
- **Association of dermatology consultations with patient care outcomes in hospitalized patients with inflammatory skin diseases.** *JAMA Dermatol* 2017;153(6):523–528.
  - Retrospective, single-center study that examined the impact of dermatology consultation on readmission within 1 year and length of stay for patients with inflammatory skin conditions. Findings demonstrated that dermatology consultations were associated with reduction in readmission within 1 year and reduction in length of stay by 2.6 days (95% CI 1.75–3.5 days).
- **Outcomes of early dermatology consultation for inpatients diagnosed with cellulitis.** *JAMA Dermatol* 2018;154(5):537–543.
  - Prospective cohort study that enrolled 116 patients with presumed cellulitis in the emergency department, in the emergency department observation unit, or within 24 hours of inpatient admission to receive a dermatology consult. For patients with presumed cellulitis, early consultation by dermatologists improved health-related outcomes through the reduction of inappropriate antibiotic use and hospitalization.

Cellulitis and Cellulitis Mimickers

- **Effect of dermatology consultation on outcomes for patients with presumed cellulitis.** *JAMA Dermatol* 2018;154(5):529–536.
  - Randomized clinical trial of 175 hospitalized adults where patients were randomized to intervention (dermatology consult) vs. control (no dermatology consult, standard of care). The length of intravenous antibiotic use was significantly shorter, and the 2-week improvement rate was significantly higher in patients in the intervention group (dermatology consult), suggesting that inpatient dermatology consult may enhance patient outcomes by improving diagnostic accuracy and facilitating antibiotic stewardship in hospitalized patients with suspected cellulitis.

DERMATOLOGY

NOTES

Neurology

12

ANATOMY & PHYSIOLOGY

In neurology, we talk about "localizing" a lesion.
- Step 1: Where is the lesion that is responsible for a patient's signs and symptoms?
- Step 2: Based on the location, what are the possible etiologies of the signs and symptoms?

These steps require a clear understanding of the anatomy and pathophysiology of the central and peripheral nervous systems and blood supplies. A helpful tip is to learn to map signs and symptoms to a location (e.g., vertigo, diplopia, and nystagmus = brainstem).

Central Nervous System (CNS)
Tracts of the CNS

The CNS includes the brain and spinal cord. It is composed of gray matter (cell bodies) and white matter (axons). The brain and spinal cord are somatotopically organized. Signals travel on "tracts" – i.e., descending motor tracts and ascending sensory tracts. Here is a summary of the main tracts.

Motor tracts
- Pyramidal: Corticospinal and corticobulbar tracts (Figure 12.1A)
  - **Corticospinal tracts:**
    - Anatomy: Neurons in the primary motor cortex (precentral gyrus), pre-motor and supplemental motor cortex $\rightarrow$ axons descend through the posterior limb of the internal capsule $\rightarrow$ enter the brainstem (cerebral peduncle in the midbrain) $\rightarrow$ basis pontis $\rightarrow$ medullary pyramids $\rightarrow$ tract divides into two tracts at the cervicomedullary junction: the contralateral lateral spinal tract and ipsilateral anterior spinal tract $\rightarrow$ descend and synapse onto the lower motor neuron (LMN).
    - Function: Voluntary control of movement from the neck to the feet
  - **Corticobulbar tracts:**
    - Anatomy: Same pathway origins, synapse onto the brainstem motor nuclei
    - Function: Voluntary control of face, head and neck movement
- Extra-pyramidal: Ventromedial bulbospinal and ventrolateral bulbospinal

Sensory Tracts
- Anterolateral: **Anterior and lateral spinothalamic tracts** (Figure 12.1B)
  - Anatomy: Smaller afferent fibers of the peripheral nerves enter the dorsal horn of the spinal cord $\rightarrow$ cross and ascend in the opposite anterior and lateral columns $\rightarrow$ enter the brainstem $\rightarrow$ thalamus (VPL nucleus $\rightarrow$ postcentral gyrus of the parietal cortex)
  - Function: Nociception (pain), temperature sensibility, touch
- Posterior column-medial lemniscal pathway:
  - Anatomy: Larger afferent fibers of the peripheral nerves enter the spinal cord $\rightarrow$ ascend in the ipsilateral posterior column $\rightarrow$ first synapse in the gracile or cuneate nucleus in the lower medulla $\rightarrow$ cross and ascend in the medial lemniscus (located in the medial medulla and tegmentum of the pons and midbrain) $\rightarrow$ synapse in the thalamus (VPL nucleus) $\rightarrow$ parietal cortex
  - Function: Tactile, position sense, and kinesthesia

* Note: Other fibers carrying sensory information about pain, touch, vibration, and proprioception ascend in a diffuse pattern; therefore, a lesion in the posterior column may not result in sensory deficit.

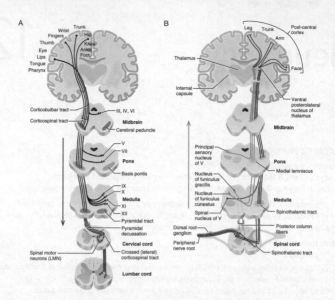

FIGURE 12.1: A) **The main descending motor pathways.** Shown is the brain and spinal cord with a depiction of the corticospinal (maroon) and corticobulbar (red) tracts. These tracts carry motor signals from the brain to the periphery (descending). B) **The main ascending somatosensory pathways.** Shown is the brain and spinal cord with a depiction of the spinothalamic tract (dark blue; pain, thermal sense) and the posterior column-medial lemniscus pathway (light blue; proprioception, vibration). These tracts carry sensory signals form the periphery to the brain (ascending).

Brain

Cerebral cortex
- Functions: Higher processing
- Clinical effects of a lesion: <u>Contralateral</u> motor, sensory, visual symptoms
- Regions: See Figure 12.2
  - **Frontal:**
    - Function: Motor, social judgment, executive function, voluntary horizontal gaze initiation
    - Vascular supply: ACA (legs), MCA (face/arms > legs)
    - Lesion: Disinhibition, apathy, personality/behavioral change; contralateral motor weakness
  - **Parietal:**
    - Function: Sensory, visuospatial, attention, vision
    - Vascular supply: ACA, MCA
    - Lesion: Contralateral visual, tactile, and auditory neglect
  - Temporal:
    - Function: Hearing, emotion, memory
    - Vascular supply: MCA, PCA
    - Lesion: Problems with speech and language, memory loss
  - Occipital:
    - Function: Vision
    - Vascular supply: PCA (macula supplied by the MCA)
    - Lesion: Contralateral hemifield vision loss

Cerebellum
- Function: Detects "motor error" and helps correct it. Vermis = trunk. Hemisphere (lateral) = limbs
- Lesion: Vertigo, nystagmus, nausea/vomiting, (usually) <u>ipsilateral</u> ataxia

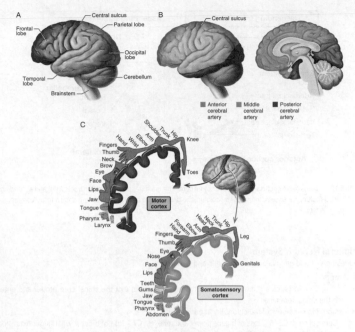

FIGURE 12.2: The cerebrum. A) Regions of the cerebrum. B) Vascular supply to the cerebrum. C) The cortical homunculus, which is a distorted representation of the human body based on the neurologic "map" of the areas of the human brain dedicated to processing motor (red) and sensory (blue) functions for different parts of the body.

Brainstem
- Description: Includes midbrain, pons, and medulla
- Function: Cranial nerves, motor and sensory tracts
- Lesion: Diplopia, facial weakness, facial sensory loss, dysphagia, dysarthria; contralateral weakness and numbness in the body; "crossed" weakness (with UMN signs) and sensory abnormalities of the head and limbs (e.g., weakness in the right face and the left arm and leg)

Thalamus
- Function: Sensory and motor relay station; emotion
- Lesion: Contralateral symptoms, based on nuclei affected

Basal ganglia
- Function: Initiation of purposeful movement; suppresion of unwanted movement. Dopamine = movement
- Lesion: Difficulties with speech, posture, movement on the contralateral side. Forms a circuit with the cortex on the SAME side

Hypothalamus
- Function: **TAN HATS to Bed** (**T**hirst/water balance, **A**denohypophysis control, **N**eurohypophysis and **H**ormones, **H**unger, **A**utonomic regulation, **T**emperature regulation, **S**exual urges, **C**ircadian rhythm)
- Lesion: Depends on the nuclei affected

Limbic system
- Description: Includes hippocampus (first affected by anoxic damage), amygdala, cingulate gyrus, fornix, mammillary bodies, septal nucleus
- Function: Emotions, behavior, eating, memory
- Lesion: Change in the ability to perceive hunger/satiety, emotional changes, amnesia, seizures

Spinal cord
- Description: Includes the white matter tracts which contain the ascending sensory pathways, descending motor pathways, and nerve cell bodies (Figure 12.3)
- Lesion: Presence of a horizontal level below which sensory, motor, and autonomic function is impaired

NEUROLOGY

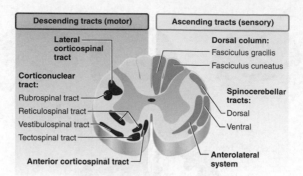

FIGURE 12.3: Transverse section through the spinal cord. The main descending motor tracts (red) and ascending sensory tracts (blue) are shown. In the dorsal column, the gracilus and cuneatus tracts are shown (gracilus = legs, cuneatus = arms).

Peripheral Nervous System

Includes nerves and ganglia outside the brain and spinal cord.

Spinal roots

- Description: Includes the motor and sensory nerve roots that exit the spinal cord proper and enter into the spinal foramina
- Lesion: Main features of radiculopathy at each level:
  - <u>Cervical cord:</u> C5–6 – loss of biceps power and reflexes; C7 – loss of triceps, wrist/finger extension power; C8 – impaired wrist/finger flexion
  - <u>Thoracic cord:</u> Localize using site of back pain and sensory level; T4 – nipples, T10 – umbilicus; lesion causes paralysis with leg weakness, disturbances of bowel/bladder function
  - <u>Lumbar cord:</u> L2–4 – paralysis of flexion/adduction of thigh, leg extension at knee, absent patellar reflex; L5–S1 – paralysis of extension of thigh, leg flexion at knee, movements of ankle/foot, absent ankle jerk (S1)
  - <u>Sacral cord/conus medullaris:</u> S3–5 – bilateral saddle anesthesia, urinary retention/lax anal tone; S2–4 – absent bulbocavernosus reflex; S4–5 – absent anal reflex
  - <u>Cauda equina:</u> Low back and radicular pain, asymmetric leg weakness and sensory loss, variable areflexia of the lower extremities

Peripheral nerves

- Lesion: Mid or distal limb pain, weakness (with LMN signs) or sensory abnormalities following the nerve distribution, "stocking or glove" distribution, loss of reflexes

Neuromuscular junction

- Lesion: Proximal weakness, diplopia, possible bulbar weakness (dysarthria, dysphagia, facial weakness) that may get worse with use (aka fatiguability); sensation is spared

Muscle

- Lesion: Bilateral proximal or distal weakness (typically proximal weakness is more than distal weakness); sensation is spared

Cranial nerves

- Description: See Table 12.1
- Cranial nerve reflexes: Automatic response to a stimulus that does not require conscious thought
  - Pupillary light reflex (direct and consensual pupil constriction to light): II → III
  - Corneal reflex (touch cornea → blink): V → VII
  - Jaw jerk (tap chin with reflex hammer → jaw protrudes forward): V3 (sensory) → V3 (motor, masseter)
  - Vestibulo-ocular reflex (turn head laterally, eyes remain fixated on target): VIII → III, VI
  - Gag reflex (touch posterior pharynx → gag): IX → X
  - Cough reflex (advanced suction tube through endotracheal tube and suction deep in trachea → cough): X (sensory) → X (motor)

TABLE 12.1 · Cranial Nerves and their Functions		
Cranial Nerve (number, name)	**Primary Function**	**Dysfunction**
1. Olfactory	**Special sensory:** Smell (only CN without thalamic relay to cortex)	Anosmia
2. Optic	**Special sensory:** Vision	Vision loss
3. Oculomotor	**Somatic motor:** Eye movement (SR, IR, MR, IO), accommodation, eyelid opening (levator palpebrae) **Visceral motor (parasympathetic):** Pupillary constriction (parasympathetic: Edinger-Westphal nucleus)	Eye down and out Dilated pupil No accommodation
4. Trochlear	**Somatic motor:** Eye movement (SO) – depression and intorsion	Extorted eye that is hypertropic
5. Trigeminal Ophthalmic (V1) Maxillary (V2) Mandibular (V3)	**Somatic sensory:** V1: Sensation to upper face, nasal cavity, frontal, sphenoid, ethmoid sinus V2: Sensation to middle face and maxillary sinus V3: Sensation to lower portion of the face: jaw, anterior 2/3 of tongue, oral floor **Somatic motor:** V3 innervates muscles of mastication	Loss of facial sensation V3: Lose sensation to tip of tongue, difficulty chewing Jaw deviation <u>towards</u> lesion
6. Abducens	**Somatic motor:** Eye movement (LR)	Impaired abduction
7. Facial	**Somatic motor:** Facial movement, eyelid closure, stapedius in ear **Somatic sensory:** Outer ear **Visceral motor (parasympathetic):** Lacrimation and salivation (submandibular, sublingual) **Special sensory:** Taste to anterior 2/3 of tongue and palate	Facial palsy Central (upper 1/3 face spared) vs. peripheral (upper and lower face affected) Loss of taste to anterior 2/3 of tongue
8. Vestibulocochlear	**Special sensory:** Hearing from cochlea; balance from semicircular canals	Hearing loss, vertigo and loss of balance
9. Glossopharyngeal	**Somatic motor:** Innervates stylopharyngeus (elevates pharynx, larynx); swallowing **Somatic sensory:** Pharyngeal region above epiglottis – "gag" reflex **Visceral motor (parasympathetic):** Salivation (parotid gland) **Visceral sensory:** Baro/chemoregulation from the carotid body and sinus **Special sensory:** Taste to posterior 1/3 of tongue	Impaired palate elevation Loss of taste in posterior 1/3 of the tongue/pharynx
10. Vagus	**Somatic motor:** Pharyngeal movement except stylopharyngeus- swallowing, palate elevation, midline uvula, recurrent laryngeal nerve to laryngeal muscles **Somatic sensory:** Below epiglottis **Visceral motor (parasympathetic):** Innervates smooth muscles/gland in the respiratory and GI tracts **Visceral sensory:** Baro/chemoreception from the aortic arch **Special sensory:** Taste at the epiglottis	Impaired cough reflex, swallow. Uvula deviates <u>away</u> from the lesion
11. Accessory spinal	**Somatic motor:** Innervates sternocleidomastoid and trapezius muscles: Turn head and shoulder	Can't turn head to contralateral (SCM); <u>ipsilateral</u> shoulder droop
12. Hypoglossal	**Somatic motor:** Tongue movement (all except palatoglossus – CNX)	Tongue deviates <u>towards</u> the lesion

DIAGNOSTICS

The Neurologic Exam

Mental status
- Orientation: Person, place, time, situation
- Language: Fluency, repetition, naming (high and low frequency items), comprehension (axial ["close eyes, stick out tongue"] and appendicular ["show two fingers, give thumbs up"] commands, complex commands ["take your right thumb, touch your left ear, and stick out your tongue"])
- Attention: Ask patient to spell "WORLD" forward, then backward. Alternatively: Recite months of the year or days of the week backward.
- Memory: Working (digit span forward (normal >5–7 digits), backward) and delayed (remember three words ×5 minutes)

Cranial nerves
- I – Olfactory nerve: Not frequently tested
- II – Optic nerve/III parasympathetic fibers: Visual fields/pupillary constriction (afferent – optic nerve, efferent parasympathetic fibers)
- III, IV, VI – Oculomotor, trochlear, and abducens nerves: Extraocular muscle movements
- V – Trigeminal nerves: Facial sensation, motor for muscles of mastication
- VII – Facial nerve: Facial movement, eyelid closure, lacrimation and salivation, taste in the anterior 2/3 of the tongue
- VIII – Vestibulocochlear nerve: Hearing from the cochlear nerve, balance from the vestibular nerve
- IX, X – Glossopharyngeal and vagus nerve: Palate elevation, gag, cough

Motor
- Bulk and tone: Increased = spasticity, rigidity, or paratonia; decreased = flaccidity
- Screening motor exam: Pronator drift (sign of upper motor neuron weakness; evaluate for finger flexion and/or pronation with arms outstretched and eyes closed), finger taps and toe taps (evaluate for large, symmetric, rapid movements)
- Confrontational strength testing:
  - Power: Score motor strength in each muscle group from 0 to 5:
    - 0: No contraction
    - 1: Trace movement
    - 2: Full range of motion when gravity is eliminated
    - 3: Full range of motion against gravity
    - 4: Movement against gravity with resistance, but still less than full strength
    - 5: Full/normal strength
  - Preferential muscle groups to test:
    - Upper extremity: Shoulder abduction (deltoids), flexion and extension at elbow (biceps, triceps, resp), wrist extension, finger extension and abduction
    - Lower extremity: Hip flexion (iliopsoas), knee flexion and extension (hamstrings, quads), ankle dorsiflexion (tibialis anterior)

Sensory
- Screening exam: Assess ability to sense light touch
- Small fiber: Pain (safety pin) and temperature (alcohol swab, cold tuning fork)
- Large fiber: Vibration (tuning fork) and proprioception (joint position sense)

Reflexes
- Upper extremity reflexes: Biceps (C5–6), triceps (C7–8)
- Lower extremity reflexes: Patellae (L3–4), Achilles tendon (S1–S2)
- Plantar response: Apply noxious stimulus starting at the lateral aspect of the sole of the foot, moving medially across the ball of the foot. Normal response is flexor (toes down); abnormal response is extensor (large toe goes up and remaining toes fan out = Babinski sign)

Coordination
- Appendicular (limb) ataxia: Finger-nose-finger, heel-knee-shin
- Truncal ataxia: Sitting upright unsupported, gait ataxia

Gait
- Description of gait: Stance (normal, wide, or narrow-based), stride length, foot clearance (shuffling; foot drop → steppage gait), arm swing (decreased in parkinsonism)
- Romberg test: Balance requires visual, vestibular (inner ear), and proprioceptive (positional sense) systems. Romberg testing eliminates vision and tests the remaining two; this is NOT a test of cerebellar function!

Imaging

Non-contrast head computed tomography (NCHCT)
- Description: CT scanning is particularly useful for evaluation of bony defects, metallic objects, calcifications, hemorrhage, and hydrocephalus
- Common indications: Acute stroke (to exclude hemorrhage), tumor, hydrocephalus, trauma, subarachnoid hemorrhage, bony or sinus disease
- Pitfalls: Insensitive for early ischemic stroke changes and posterior fossa and spinal cord lesions, among others

Magnetic resonance imaging (MRI)
- Description: MRI does not involve ionizing radiation and provides superior soft tissue sensitivity
- Common indications: Stroke, tumor, parenchymal pathology (ischemia, demyelinating, lesions, edema, infection, etc.) of the brain or spinal cord
- Sequences:
  - T1: Gray matter is gray, white matter is white, CSF is black
  - T2: Gray matter is white, white matter is gray, CSF is white
  - T2/FLAIR: Same as T2 except CSF is black
    - Pearl: T1 is usually helpful for anatomy only. On T2, because CSF is white (water), then edema is also white, which means pathology appears bright and is typically easier to see. T2/FLAIR subtracts the bright CSF signal to make pathology even easier to appreciate

Lumbar Puncture

- Common indications: Concern for CNS infection, autoimmune or inflammatory condition, or malignancy; also can be used to diagnose subarachnoid hemorrhage, intracranial pressure abnormalities, or to reduce CSF pressure therapeutically
- Obtain NCHCT prior to LP if: Patient >60 yr, immunocompromised state, history of CNS disease (e.g., mass lesion, stroke, focal infection), seizure within one week of presentation, focal neurologic deficit
- CSF studies:
  - Always send: Cell count with differential, protein, glucose (check serum glucose simultaneously)
  - Additional CSF testing to consider based on clinical suspicion:
    - Autoimmune or inflammatory: Oligoclonal bands, IgG index, targeted autoantibody tests
    - Infection: Bacterial gram stain and culture, targeted infectious studies (PCR, serology, AFB, fungal, or viral culture)
    - Malignancy: Cytology and flow cytometry
- Contraindications:
  - Local infection over the site of puncture
  - Coagulopathy: Platelet goal >50K/μL, INR < 1.7
  - If known intracranial or spinal cord mass lesion, always obtain imaging first. Mass lesions are not always a contraindication for LP, but imaging should be reviewed prior to attempted LP

Electroencephalogram (EEG)

- Definition: Test used to evaluate the electrical activity in the brain, particularly for seizure or "interictal" (between seizures) epileptiform discharges
- Indications:
  - Evaluation of suspected epilepsy and classification of seizure disorders
  - Management of status epilepticus
  - Evaluation of altered mental status

Electromyography (EMG) and Nerve Conduction Studies

- Definitions:
  - EMG: Clinical study of electrical activity of muscle fibers
  - Nerve conduction study: Clinical study of electrical activity from nerve roots, plexus, peripheral nerves +/– neuromuscular junction
- Indications:
  - Localization of lower motor neuron disorders, including anterior horn, nerve root, plexus, peripheral nerve, neuromuscular junction, or muscle
  - Classification of peripheral nerve disorders as axonal or demyelinating
  - Prognostication of clinical course

NEUROLOGY

Altered Mental Status

There are many approaches to altered mental status (AMS). Here is one of them:

- Step 1: First assess for acute/emergent situations
  - Is the patient protecting their airway? If not, intubate.
  - Does the patient have signs of elevated intracranial pressure (ICP) such as acute loss of brainstem reflexes, particularly with fixed and dilated pupils? If so, perform NCHCT and consult neurosurgery stat. Consider the need for intubation, mannitol, hypertonic saline.
  - Concern for opioid overdose? Administer naloxone.
  - Check a fingerstick glucose? If <70 mg/dL, administer D50 and thiamine.
- Step 2: Consider the differential diagnosis using the mnemonic **"MISTO"**:
  - **M**etabolic:
    - Electrolyte abnormalities: Check sodium, calcium
    - Endocrine abnormalities: Check TSH, glucose (hypoglycemia or hyperglycemia [consider DKA/HHS])
    - Organ dysfunction: Kidney, liver, heart (ACS), lung (low oxygen, high CO_2)
    - Vitamin deficiencies: B1 (thiamine), B12
    - Other: Urinary retention, constipation
  - **I**nfection:
    - CNS infection: Meningitis, encephalitis, abscess
    - Non-CNS infection: UTI, pneumonia, bacteremia
  - **S**tructural/seizure:
    - Structural: Stroke, hemorrhage, tumor
    - Seizure
  - **T**oxin:
    - Medications
      - Perform a complete medication reconciliation; polypharmacy is a common cause of AMS in elderly patients
      - Consider drug overdose, drug withdrawal, associated syndromes (e.g., serotonin syndrome)
    - Alcohol/substances
      - Check serum alcohol level and serum osms
      - Check urine toxicology screen
  - **O**xygenation:
    - Low O_2
    - High CO_2
- Step 3: Based on this differential, perform diagnostic tests to further evaluate. Diagnostics to consider:
  - Labs: CBC, BMP, LFTs, TSH, serum alcohol level, serum osms, ABG/VBG, ammonia, Utox
  - Imaging: Choose based on differential diagnosis – NCHCT, contrast-enhanced head CT, MRI brain

Weakness

- Step 1: Delineate neurologic versus non-neurologic causes of weakness and take a detailed history
  - Non-neurologic causes of weakness:
    - Generalized weakness/deconditioning from prolonged bedrest or systemic illness
    - Asthenia (motor impairment due to pain or joint dysfunction)
    - Functional/psychogenic weakness – diagnosis of exclusion!
  - History of present illness:
    - Be specific! Describe the weakness; are there specific tasks the patient has difficulty performing? Are they limited by fatigue, shortness of breath, joint pain, etc.?
    - Tempo: Hyperacute, acute, subacute, chronic, episodic, fatigable?
    - Distribution: Generalized, proximal vs. distal, unilateral vs bilateral, symmetric vs. asymmetric?
    - Progression over time: Have symptoms remained localized? Or have they spread over time?
    - Sensory involvement: Numbness, paresthesia, allodynia
    - Autonomic symptoms: Orthostasis, palpitations, bowel/bladder dysfunction, pupil abnormalities
    - Associated symptoms: Recent fever, URI, gastroenteritis, or vaccinations (rarely trigger Guillain-Barré), neck/back pain, spine trauma, tenderness, breathing difficulties
  - Review other history/comorbidities:
    - Medications: Perform a complete medication reconciliation. In particular, ask about medications which may contribute to weakness (e.g., statins, colchicine)
    - Past medical history: Certain medical conditions can contribute to weakness (e.g., DM, thyroid disease, HIV, syphilis, B12 deficiency)
    - Social history: Ask about alcohol use, recreational drug use
    - Family history: Ask about family history of neuromuscular disorders, such as myopathy, ALS, multiple sclerosis
- Step 2: Localize the lesion. See Table 12.2 and the following information about CNS and PNS causes of weakness

TABLE 12.2 · Upper Motor Neuron (UMN) vs. Lower Motor Neuron (LMN) Clinical Findings		
Characteristic	**Upper Motor Neuron (UMN) Pattern**	**Lower Motor Neuron (LMN) Pattern**
Pattern of weakness	Distal > proximal, extensors in UE, flexors in LE	Varies by muscle innervated
Bulk	Less prominent atrophy	More prominent atrophy, fasciculations
Reflexes	Hyperreflexia, clonus, Babinski sign	Hyporeflexia or normal*
Tone	Spastic or normal**	Flaccid or normal

*Muscle and neuromuscular junction diseases typically have intact reflexes
**Hyperacute brain and spinal cord pathology can result in flaccid weakness

CNS causes of weakness
- Brain: Suspect if UMN signs (hyperreflexia, spasticity, distal>proximal weakness in pyramidal distribution, +Babinski sign), cortical signs (language deficits, neglect, visual field cut), etc.
- Spinal Cord: Suspect if UMN signs that are symmetric or asymmetric without facial involvement

PNS causes of weakness
- Motor neuron (anterior horn cell): LMN signs (+/– UMN signs if ALS), patchy weakness, no sensory involvement
- Peripheral nerve: LMN signs (hypo- or areflexia, decreased tone, atrophy, fasciculations), symmetric or asymmetric, axonal neuropathy typically length-dependent, demyelinating neuropathy patchy
- Neuromuscular junction: LMN, usually symmetric, proximal muscle weakness, check for bulbar signs/ symptoms ("D" symptoms – dysphagia, diplopia, dysarthria); extraocular movement restriction, ptosis, and shortness of breath (especially orthopnea and with bending over)
- Muscle (myopathy): LMN, often symmetric, tends to be proximal (axial muscles, deltoids, hip flexors) > distal (decreased grip strength, weakness of wrist flexion/extension)

Headache
Approach to Headaches
- History:
  - Is this an old or new headache? If old, how do the current headaches differ?
  - What's the headache phenotype?
    - **PQRST:**
      - **P**rovocation – associated with stress, foods, posture, menstruation, lack of sleep?
      - **P**alliation – which medications have been tried, how often, treatment response?
      - **Q**uality
      - **Q**uantity
      - **R**egion – unilateral or bilateral?
      - **R**adiation – from neck or jaw? (may suggest cervicogenic headache or TMJ-associated headache)
      - **S**ymptoms – nausea/vomiting, photo/phonophobia, lacrimation/rhinorrhea, aura?
      - **T**iming – frequency (including # of h/a per month), duration, onset (gradual or thunderclap), worse in morning (suggests increased ICP)?
  - Are there features suggestive of a primary headache disorder?
    - Associated features: Photo/phono/osmophobia, N/V, restlessness/agitation (TACs), allodynia?
    - Aura: Visual scotoma, scintillations, wavy lines in vision, photopsia, paresthesias?
    - Autonomic features (unilateral): Eye tearing, periorbital discoloration, ptosis or eyelid edema, conjunctival injection, nasal congestion/discharge, forehead/face sweating/flushing?
    - Triggers: Menses, alcohol, bright lights, loud sounds, weather changes, dehydration, skipped meals, stress, poor sleep?
    - Are there any headache red flags? **SNOOP**
      - **S**ystemic symptoms
      - **N**eurologic signs/symptoms
      - **O**lder age of onset (>50 yr)
      - **O**nset (sudden "thunderclap" headache)
      - **P**apilledema, **P**ositional (worse when supine → intracranial hypertension; worse when upright → intracranial hypotension), **P**recipitated by Valsalva, **P**regnant or **P**ost-partum, **P**attern change)

NEUROLOGY

- Physical exam:
  - Blood pressure and heart rate, palpate neck/shoulder for trigger points, evaluate spine and paraspinal musclces, palpate temporal arteries, ascultate for bruits, neurologic exam (including fundoscopic exam)
- Imaging:
  - Indications for imaging include focal neurologic deficients, onset with exertion, new onset >50 yr, recent change in headache pattern, positional headache
  - MRI preferred but start with NCHCT in the acute setting
- Labs:
  - Consider checking ESR/CRP in patients >50 yr given risk of giant cell arteritis

Primary Headache Disorders

Migraine headache

- Symptoms:
  - **POUND: P**ulsatile quality, **O**ne day duration, **U**nilateral, **N**ausea/vomiting, **D**ebilitating
  - Increased stroke risk if migraines are associated with aura, so avoid oral contraceptive pills in these patients
- Treatment:
  - Acute migraine treatment:
    - Mild to moderate attacks: NSAIDs (i.e., ibuprofen 400 mg, naproxen 500/550 mg, level A), acetaminophen (1000 mg, level A), combination analgesics (i.e., acetaminophen-aspirin-caffeine, level A); if severe nausea/vomiting, also prescribe an oral or rectal antiemetic
    - Moderate to severe attacks: Triptans (especially combination of sumatriptan and naproxen, level A; can be given subcutaneously or intranasally if severe vomiting), nonoral antiemetics
    - Emergency settings: Sumatriptan 6 mg subcutaneously, antiemetics/dopamine receptor blockers (metoclopramide 10 mg IV, prochlorperazine 10 mg IV/IM, chlorpromazine 0.1 mg/kg IV [total 25 mg IV], level B), dihydroergotamine 1 mg IV, with metoclopramide, ketorolac 30 mg IV or 60 mg IM (level C)
  - Prophylactic migraine treatment:
    - Indication: Frequent, prolonged, or debilitating migraines with contraindication to or failure of acute therapies above
    - Medications: Propranolol, valproic acid, topiramate
    - Efficacy: Effectiveness only apparent after taking medication for 1–3 months
    - Refer to a neurologist: Pregnancy, known structural brain anomalies, chronic daily headaches >15× per month, failure of multiple medications, consideration of calcitonin gene-related peptide (CGRP) receptor antagonists, or hospitalizations

Tension headache

- Symptoms: Described as "boring," "tightening," or "vice-like"; non-pulsatile, bilateral, featureless headache
- Treatment: Acetaminophen, NSAIDs, aspirin. Amitriptyline can be helpful for prevention

Trigeminal autonomic cephalgias (TACs)

- Definitions:
  - Trigeminal autonomic cephalgias (TACs): Headache disorders characterized by trigeminal and cranial autonomic activation with unilateral pain and autonomic features.
  - Cluster headaches: Most common subtype of TAC (90%); onset typically 20–40 yr; M:F = 3:1. Clinically, patient reports a knife-like pain (often behind the eye) that is maximal at onset or achieves maximal intensity within minutes. Associated with autonomic features and restlessness. Headaches often cluster in periods of 2–12 weeks, followed by long periods of remission.
- Treatment:
  - Acute: Sumatriptan 4–6 mg subcutaneously or 22 mg inhaled (max 2 doses/24 hr), high-flow oxygen >7 liters per minute face mask
  - Prophylaxis: Verapamil 80 mg TID (starting dose)

Secondary Headache Disorders

Medication overuse headache ("rebound headache")

- Drugs that cause rebound headaches: Abortive medications taken ≥2 times per week, such as acetaminophen-butalbital-caffeine, APAP, NSAIDs, caffeine, ergotamine, opioids, triptans
- Treatment: Taper off medication; reduce 10% every 1–2 wks, can treat with naproxen 500 mg BID to bridge

Post-traumatic headache

- Vascular etiologies:
  - Arteriovenous malformation (AVM), subarachnoid hemorrhage (SAH), dissection
  - Giant cell arteritis
  - Reversible cerebral vasoconstriction syndrome (RCVS)
  - Posterior reversible encephalopathy syndrome (PRES, associated with malignant hypertension, pre-eclampsia, certain medications)
  - Pituitary apoplexy
  - Cerebral venous sinus thrombosis
- Intracranial hypotension/low CSF volume:
  - Symptoms: Positional headaches
  - Etiologies: Post-LP, postural orthostatic tachycardia syndrome (POTS), spontaneous
  - Treatment: Epidural blood patch if CSF leak
- Intracranial hypertension:
  - Etiology: Idiopathic intracranial hypertension (pseudotumor cerebri) vs. secondary
  - Risk factors: Obesity, vitamin A excess, tretinoin use
  - Diagnosis: Test visual fields and acuity, evaluate optic discs for papilledema
  - Treatment: Acetazolamide or topiramate, VP shunt, optic nerve fenestration if vision loss

Dizziness and Vertigo

- Definitions:
  - <u>Vertigo</u>: "Room spinning," falling, rocking, or a sense of being pushed or pulled
  - <u>Disequilibrium</u>: Loss of balance that results from visual disturbance, sensory ataxia, cerebellar ataxia, or extrapyramidal syndrome (e.g., Parkinsonism)
  - <u>Presyncope</u>: Feeling of impending loss of consciousness, faintness, lightheadedness, often with tunnel vision, diaphoresis, and palpitations
- Etiologies of vertigo: Can have a central or peripheral cause. See Table 12.3.
- Exam:
  - Focal neurologic deficits are concerning for a central vestibular lesion (gaze or saccade impairment, past-pointing, cranial nerve deficit, dysmetria, ataxia, or face/limb weakness/numbness)
  - **HINTS** exam: Screening test that can help differentiate central vs. peripheral causes of vertigo
    - **H**ead **I**mpulse test: In the setting of unilateral vestibular dysfunction, a rapid rotation of the head horizontally 10–20° toward the lesioned side (with the patient continuing to stare at a fixed point straight ahead) will result in a corrective catch-up saccade, indicative of a peripheral lesion
    - **N**ystagmus:
      - <u>Features of peripheral-etiology nystagmus</u>: Unidirectional torsional or horizontal nystagmus, fatigues over time, goes away with fixation after a 5–10 second latency
      - <u>Features of central-etiology nystagmus</u>: Vertical or direction-changing nystagmus
    - **T**est of **S**kew: Ask the patient to fixate on a central target (e.g., examiner's nose). Alternate occluding each eye with your hand. Observe for a vertical corrective saccade (= abnormal test of skew), which suggests brainstem involvement
  - <u>Dix-Hallpike maneuver</u>: To evaluate for BPPV, with the patient in the seated position, turn the head 45° to one side; then lie the patient supine with their head hanging 30° below the horizontal. A positive test = brief latency, and then vertigo with rotary upbeating nystagmus lasting <30 seconds which fatigues with repeated testing. Low positive predictive value. Purely vertical nystagmus, absence of latency, or lack of fatigability raise concern for a central cause
- Imaging: MRI brain is REQUIRED if there is suspicion for a central cause of vertigo (e.g., abnormal exam, focal neurologic deficits, and/or vascular risk factors)

NEUROLOGY

TABLE 12.3 · Etiologies of Vertigo

Disease	Pathophysiology	Duration	Notable Clinical Features	Symptoms	Treatment
Peripheral					
Benign paroxysmal positional vertigo (BPPV)	Otolith displaced from utricle into the semicircular canal	30 to 90 seconds	Can recur over years; most common cause of peripheral vertigo. + Dix Hallpike maneuver	Vertigo often triggered by changing position (rolling in bed, looking up/bending over)	Epley maneuver (bedside maneuver that aims to use gravity to move the displaced otolith back into the utricle)
Vestibular neuritis/ labyrinthitis	Post-viral inflammation of the vestibular nerve or entire labyrinthine apparatus	Days	Most severe in the first 24 to 72 hr	Aural fullness, tinnitus, severe nausea/ vomiting Neuronitis = no hearing loss Labyrinthitis = hearing loss	Short course of steroids and/or anti-histamines, benzodiazepines if severe, vestibular rehabilitation
Meniere's disease	Abnormal endolymph flow	Hours	Triad of hearing loss, tinnitus, vertigo is classic; but they do not necessarily occur together	Low-frequency hearing loss, tinnitus	Salt restriction, vestibular rehabilitation, diuretics
Drug toxicity	Oto- or vestibulo-toxic medications	Variable	Insidious onset	Vertigo; additional features vary with offending agent	Withdraw offending agent
Central					
TIA/stroke	Ischemia or hemorrhage in the brain stem or cerebellum	Variable, usually continuous	Acute onset, usually maximal at onset	Weakness, numbness, dysarthria, dysphagia, diplopia, ataxia	Secondary stroke prevention, antiemetics/benzodiazepines in the acute setting
Vestibular migraine	Same as migraine	Hours-days	Vertigo can precede headache	Headache, photo/phono/osmophobia, motion sickness; can be provoked by dehy-dration, alcohol, inadequate sleep	Acute migraine treatment, benzodiazepines if severe
Drug toxicity	Cerebellar toxicity	Variable	Insidious onset if chronic exposure, acute if suddenly supratherapeutic	Ataxia, nausea, vomiting	Withdraw offending agent

Seizures

- History (to distinguish from syncope):
  - Tongue biting or incontinence, unexplained injuries, or lack of recollection of the event? Did the entire body jerk or twitch? Did the eyes or head turn to one side? Was there a noise (ictal cry)? Prolonged confusion afterwards? Any history of seizures?
  - History of febrile seizures, CNS infections, tumors, stroke, and/or head trauma? (all increase the likelihood of seizures)
- Classification: Generalized vs. focal onset
  - <u>Generalized onset</u>: Tonic, clonic, tonic-clonic, myoclonic, atonic, absence
  - <u>Focal onset</u>: $+/-$ impairment in consciousness/awareness, $+/-$ motor components, subjective phenomena, evolving to bilateral convulsive seizure (previously secondarily generalized)
- Etiologies:
  - <u>Provoked seizure</u>: Systemic process leading to seizures
    - Metabolic ($\uparrow/\downarrow$ Na^+, $\uparrow/\downarrow$ glucose, $\downarrow$ Mg^{2+}, $\downarrow$ Ca^{2+}, $\uparrow$ NH_3^-, thyroid disorders, renal dysfunction, hyperthermia)
    - Cerebrovascular: Hypertensive encephalopathy
    - Systemic infection
    - Toxic: Alcohol withdrawal, barbiturate or benzodiazepine withdrawal, sympathomimetics, PCP
    - Medications: Tramadol, imipenem, theophylline, bupropion, clozapine, among others
  - <u>Symptomatic seizure</u>: Localized process in the brain that causes seizures
    - Acute symptomatic:
      - Cerebrovascular: Ischemic stroke, intracranial hemorrhage, hypoxic-ischemic injury, vasculitis, posterior reversible encephalopathy syndrome (PRES)
      - Infection: Meningitis/encephalitis, abscess, neurocysticercosis, fungal infections, TB
      - Autoimmune/paraneoplastic: NMDA receptor encephalitis, SLE, Hashimoto's
      - Structural: Tumor, metastases
    - Remote symptomatic: Prior stroke, traumatic brain injury (TBI), meningitis/encephalitis
  - <u>Epilepsy syndrome</u>: Idiopathic or genetic epilepsy. See epilepsy section later in this chapter
- Diagnosis:
  - CBC, CMP, LFTs, ammonia, Utox, alcohol level, UA, CXR
  - Perform a lumbar puncture if suspicion for meningitis
  - If the patient is on antiepileptic medications, check antiepileptic levels (e.g., phenytoin, valproate, carbamazepine, phenobarbital)
  - Imaging: In the acute setting, NCHCT ($+/-$ CTA if concerned for stroke, AVM or vasculitis, CTV if concerned for venous sinus thrombosis); in the outpatient setting, MRI brain is preferred
- Treatment:
  - Medication choice is based on multiple variables. Narrow choices by seizure type (focal vs general), as well as consideration of drug effectiveness, tolerability, cost, and drug interactions. See treatment section at the end of this chapter.

DISEASES & PATHOPHYSIOLOGY

Neurologic Emergencies

Transient Ischemic Attack and Acute Ischemic Stroke

Transient ischemic attack (TIA)

- Definition: Transient neurologic deficit that lasts <24 hr with a normal brain MRI
- Management: **ABCD²** score (**A**ge, **B**P, **C**linical presentation, **D**uration, **D**M2) helps risk stratify patients. If score >3, consider hospitalization. Workup same as for stroke (see below).

Acute ischemic stroke

- Etiology:
  - <u>Thrombotic</u>: Rupture of atherosclerotic plaque
  - <u>Embolic</u>: Cardioembolic event due to atrial fibrillation, cardiac thrombus, aortic atheroma, or paradoxical emboli from an intracardiac shunt
  - <u>Lacunar</u>: Due to lipohyalinosis of small vessels which occurs in the setting of hypertension and/or diabetes
  - <u>Arterial dissection</u>: Arterial wall compromise leading to thrombus formation. Common cause of stroke in young people in the setting of trauma, neck manipulation (e.g., during a chiropractor visit), connective tissue disease
- Symptoms: See Table 12.4. Symptoms depend on the vascular territory involved and thus which anatomic areas are affected.
- Diagnosis:
  - If concern for a stroke, call a `code stroke`. If a code stroke is activated, simultaneously:
    - Perform a complete neurologic exam and document any new neurologic deficits
    - Establish the "time last seen normal" (i.e., time when the patient was last seen by another person at their neurologic baseline; not the same as when the patient was found to be symptomatic)
    - Check vital signs and point of care glucose
    - Order CT stroke protocol
    - Review medication list. If the patient is confused, in particular check for administration of any delirium-inducing medications. Determine whether the patient is on any anticoagulants as an inpatient or outpatient
    - Establish whether the patient has a history of stroke (and subsequent deficits) or seizure
    - Determine if the patient underwent any recent invasive procedures/surgeries
  - Imaging:
    - CT stroke protocol (CT brain w/o contrast, CT angiogram head/neck, CT perfusion) to rule out hemorrhage, evaluate for early signs of ischemia, and diagnose large vessel occlusion
    - MRI brain w/o contrast: Ischemia is bright on DWI and dark on ADC sequences
- Treatment:
  - Tissue plasminogen activator (tPA): If no contraindications for administration and last seen normal time <4.5 hours prior
  - Consider thromectomy if large vessel occlusion
- Work-up: Telemetry/cardiac event monitor, TTE (with bubble if age < 60 yr), carotid ultrasound (for anterior circulation strokes if no CTA neck), fasting lipid panel, HgA1c
- Secondary prevention:
  - Lifestyle changes (exercise, diet)
  - Management of risk factors (e.g., hypertension, hyperlipidemia, diabetes, smoking cessation)
  - Antiaggregant/anticoagulation:
    - Aspirin
    - If stroke while on aspirin, consider switching to clopidogrel
    - If acute stroke with minor deficits, consider aspirin + clopidogrel (clopidogrel for 21 days per the POINT trial *N Eng J Med* 2018 or clopidogrel for 3 months per the SAMPRISS *N Eng J Med* 2015)
    - If atrial fibrillation/valvular disease, recommend anticoagulation

TABLE 12.4 • Vascular Territories and Corresponding Symptoms/Deficits If Injury	
Vascular Territory	**Symptoms/Deficits If Injury**
Anterior cerebral artery (ACA)	Motor/sensory legs
Middle cerebral artery (MCA)	Motor/sensory face/arm > leg, aphasia (L frontal or temporal), neglect (R parietal), visual field cut (optic radiations), and/or gaze preference (frontal eye fields)
Posterior cerebral artery (PCA)	Visual field cut (occipital lobes)
Internal capsule	Pure motor syndrome, face = arm = leg weakness
Thalamus	Pure sensory syndrome
Brain stem/cerebellum	Dysarthria, dysphagia, diplopia, weakness, numbness, ataxia, vertigo

Intracranial Hemorrhage

Epidural hematoma
- Etiology: Rupture middle meningeal artery due to head trauma. Can have periods of unresponsiveness with interval lucidity; CSF is often yellow because bilirubin is present (xanthochromia)
- NCHCT: Convex, lens-shaped hematoma that respects suture lines
- Treatment: Reverse coagulopathy, consult neurosurgery, craniotomy may be indicated

Subdural hematoma (SDH)

Acute subdural
- Etiology: Head trauma resulting in injury to small bridging veins
- NCHCT: Crescent shaped hematoma that crosses suture lines
- Treatment: Reverse coagulopathy, consult neurosurgery, craniotomy may be indicated

Chronic subdural
- Etiology: Typically occurs in elderly patients or patients on anticoagulation who have mild head trauma
- NCHCT: Crescent-shaped hematoma
- Treatment: Reverse coagulopathy, consult neurosurgery, can sometimes observe or may need craniotomy

Subarachnoid hemorrhage (SAH)
- Etiology: Ruptured aneurysm or due to an AV malformation (e.g., in the setting of Marfan's syndrome, ADPKD), trauma, arterial dissection
- Symptoms: "Worst headache of my life," meningismus, focal neurologic deficits, encephalopathy, seizure
- Diagnosis: NCHCT, LP needed to definitely rule out if head imaging is negative
- Treatment: Reverse coagulopathy, consult neurosurgery, maintain SBP goal <140 mmHg, nimodipine, clip or coil aneurysm
- Complications: Rebleed (highest risk during the first 24 hr), vasospasm (highest risk 3–14 days after SAH), hydrocephalus, seizures, hyponatremia (SIADH)

Intracerebral hemorrhage (ICH)
- Etiology: Intraparenchymal bleed, which is most often due to hypertension
- Symptoms: Focal neurologic symptoms and then signs of ↑ICP (somnolence, vomiting, headache, bradycardia, hypertension, coma)
- Diagnosis: CT angiogram, repeat NCHCT at 6 hours
- Treatment: Reverse coagulopathy, consult neurosurgery, maintain SBP < 160 mmHg

Other Neurologic Emergencies

Elevated intracranial pressure (ICP)
- Definition: Elevation of the pressure in the cranium. ICP is normally 7–15 mmHg; at 20–25 mmHg, treatment to reduce ICP may be needed
- Etiologies: Tumor, infection, trauma, venous sinus thrombosis, surgical complication
- Symptoms: Headache, nausea/vomiting, hypertension, blurry vision, seizures, papilledema, encephalopathy
- Treatment:
  - Consult neurosurgery to help guide medical management and to determine if a surgical intervention is needed
  - Elevate head of bed 30°, keep head midline, provide sedation (reduced demand)
  - Hyperventilate (CO_2 washout causes cerebral vasoconstriction, which can be a temporizing measure)
  - Mannitol or hypertonic saline (osmotic diuresis)
  - Surgical intervention

Status epilepticus
- Definition: A single seizure lasting more than 2–3 minutes or ≥2 seizures back-to-back without the patient returning to their baseline mental status in between them
- Risk factors:
  - Acute: Ischemic or hemorrhagic stroke, traumatic brain injury, sympathomimetic intoxication, alcohol withdrawal, CNS infection, metabolic disturbance, paraneoplastic or autoimmune CNS disease
  - Chronic: Non-adherence to antiepileptic drugs, prior stroke, prior traumatic brain injury
- Diagnosis: Head imaging, labs (see seizure section), EEG
- Differential diagnosis: Other conditions that may present similarly include hypoglycemia, movement disorders, meningitis, delirium, psychogenic nonepileptic seizures (PNES)
- Treatment: Progress through each treatment tier below until the clinical seizures stop
  - 1st tier: Benzodiazepines (lorazepam 0.1 mg/kg [2–4 mg, max 8 mg in two doses], diazepam or midazolam)
  - 2nd tier: Fosphenytoin (20 mg PE/kg IV), valproic acid (40 mg/kg IV), OR levetiracetam (30–60 mg/kg IV)
  - 3rd tier: Propofol bolus and gtt, midazolam bolus and gtt, pentobarbital. Patients will need to be intubated and undergoing EEG monitoring by this stage.

Neuromuscular Disorders
Motor Neuron Diseases
Amyotrophic lateral sclerosis (ALS)
- Pathophysiology: Degeneration of upper and lower motor neurons leading to a combination of hyperreflexia/spasticity and atrophy/fasciculations
- Diagnosis: EMG; rule out mimics with MRI brain/C-spine, B12/MMA, TSH, PTH, Lyme ab, heavy metals
- Treatment: Riluzole (survival benefit of 2–3 months)

Peripheral Neuropathies
Exam is notable for LMN signs (hypo- or areflexia, decreased tone, atrophy, fasciculations); may be symmetric or asymmetric. Axonal neuropathy is typically length-dependent, demyelinating neuropathy is patchy.

Mononeuropathy
- Etiology: Usually due to nerve compression (e.g., carpal tunnel, cubital fossa). Progressive sequential mononeuropathy suggests mononeuritis multiplex and requires an urgent work-up

Polyneuropathy
- Etiology: Approximately 1/3 due to complications of diabetes, 1/3 due to complications of chronic alcohol use, and 1/3 due to other causes including:
  - Immune mediated (Guillain-Barré, chronic inflammatory demyelinating polyneuropathy [CIDP])
  - Metabolic (thyroid disease, uremia, vitamin B12 deficiency, paraproteinemia)
  - Rheumatologic (SLE, vasculitis)
  - Malignancy/monoclonal gammopathy (paraneoplastic, leukemia, MGUS, amyloid)
  - Infection (HIV, syphilis, lyme, leprosy)
  - Toxin/medications (heavy metals, amiodarone, chemotherapy)
  - Inherited (Charcot-Marie Tooth disease)

Neuromuscular Junction Disorders
Exam is notable for LMN signs which are usually symmetric; may have proximal muscle weakness; check for bulbar signs/symptoms (**"D"** symptoms – **D**ysphagia, **D**iplopia, **D**ysarthria); may have extraocular movement restriction, ptosis and shortness of breath (especially orthopnea). No fasciculations or atrophy because there is no denervation.

Myasthenia gravis
- Pathophysiology: Autoantibodies against the Ach receptor on the post-synaptic membrane
- Symptoms: Weakness after extended muscle use (e.g., worse with use, improves with rest). Can involve ocular muscles (causing ptosis, diplopia) or bulbar muscles (causing dysarthria, dysphagia). Respiratory weakness = myasthenic crisis = emergency!
- Physical exam: Fatigable weakness (e.g., more pronounced ptosis with sustained upgaze, more weakness with repeated maneuvers), proximal muscle weakness. Monitor for respiratory compromise with MIF/MEP.
- Diagnosis: Acetylcholine receptor antibody panel, CK (normal), EMG with repetitive stimulation, CT chest to rule out thymoma
- Treatment: Pyridostigmine, immunosuppression. If concern for myasthenic crisis, perform plasmapheresis or administer IVIG. If a thymoma is present, remove the thymus.

Lambert-Eaton myasthenic syndrome (LEMS)
- Pathophysiology: Small cell lung cancer cells can produce antibodies against the pre-synaptic Ca^{2+} channels, which decreases ACh release.
- Symptoms: Proximal muscle weakness that improves with use
- Physical exam: Proximal muscle weakness, areflexia
- Diagnosis: Voltage-gated calcium channel antibodies. EMG with repetitive stimulation. Evaluate for malignancy.
- Treatment: Remove malignancy, immunosuppression

Botulism
- Etiology: Rare illness caused by toxins produced by *Clostridium botulinum* bacteria; can be spread by food (e.g., home-canned foods) or infect a wound (e.g., occurs with IV drug use)
- Symptoms: Bulbar symptoms (diplopia, dysarthria, dysphagia), blurry vision followed by descending weakness, urinary retention/constipation
- Physical exam: Ophthalmoplegia with fixed/dilated pupils (vs. normal pupils in myasthenia gravis), facial weakness no sensory involvement
- Diagnosis: EMG with repetitive stimulation. Stool and serum botulinum toxin testing
- Treatment: Medical emergency; intubate if needed; administer antitoxin (local Department of Public Health often maintains supply)

Myopathies

- **Definition:** Myopathy refers to any disease that affects the muscle tissue, which can occur due to inherited or acquired causes
- **Physical exam:**
  - LMN signs, often symmetric. Typically proximal weakness with relatively preserved reflexes
  - Typically no fasiculations because no denervation
  - May have atrophy, but typically less prominent than atrophy associated with motor neuropathy
- **Diagnosis:**
  - Primarily a clinical diagnosis
  - Serum creatine kinase (CK) is typically elevated
  - Additional work-up may include: EMG (may or may not be abnormal), muscle biopsy, and/or genetic testing
- **Etiologies:**
  - Toxin induced: Chronic alcohol use
  - Endocrinopathies: Hyper- or hypothyroidism, Cushing's disease
  - Autoimmune/inflammatory: Dermatomyositis (DM), polymyositis (PM), and inclusion body myositis (IBM). See Table 12.5.
  - Genetic: Muscular dystrophies, mitochondrial myopathies, congenital myopathies
  - Infections: Myositis (especially with viral infections)
  - Medications: Statins
  - Rhabdomyolysis
- **Treatment:** Correct the underlying disorder if present. See Table 12.5 for treatment of autoimmune/inflammatory conditions.

TABLE 12.5 · Dermatomyositis, Polymyositis, and Inclusion Body Myositis			
	Dermatomyositis (DM)	**Polymyositis (PM)**	**Inclusion Body Myositis (IBM)**
Etiology	Humorally mediated inflammation of blood vessels that supply the muscle	CD8+ T cell-mediated invasion of the muscle	CD8+ T cell-mediated invasion of the muscle
Symptoms	• Symmetric proximal muscle weakness • Heliotrope rash on the eyelids • Gottron's papules on the finger extensors • Shawl sign (rash over shoulders and arms)	• Symmetric proximal muscle weakness	• Asymmetric finger flexor and proximal leg muscle weakness, especially the quadriceps • CK may be normal or mildly elevated (<10x ULN) • Typically age > 50 yr
Diagnosis	• High association with malignancy: consider cancer screening • Obtain CT chest to assess for ILD • Labs: ESR, CRP, ANA, myositis associated and specific antibodies (e.g., anti-Ro and Jo)	• Similar to dermatomyositis, but less likely to be associated with malignancy	• Similar to dermatomyositis, but less likely to be associated with malignancy
Treatment	Steroids, followed by steroid-sparing agents	Steroids, followed by steroid-sparing agents	No effective treatments

Movement Disorders
Hypokinetic Movement Disorders
Parkinsonism

- Symptoms: Syndrome of bradykinesia (#1), rigidity, tremor, postural instability
- Physical exam: Slowed responses (bradyphrenia), decreased blink rate, hypomimia ("masked facies"), slowed finger and toe taps, pill-rolling tremor (resting > postural), rigidity (cogwheel rigidity = rigidity with superimposed tremor), stooped posture, shuffling gait, en bloc turning, reduced arm swing

Idiopathic Parkinson's disease

- Pathophysiology: Gradual loss of dopamine-producing neurons in the substantia nigra due to both genetic and environmental factors
- Symptoms: Asymmetric resting tremor, bradykinesia, postural instability with falls, anosmia (lack of smell, often precedes motor symptoms), REM sleep behavior disorder, constipation, orthostatic hypotension, urinary retention, nocturia
- Treatment:
  - <u>Carbidopa-levodopa</u>: Start 0.5–1 tablet TID. Side effects: Worsened orthostatic hypotension, nausea, visual hallucinations. Comes in extended release formulation (good for motor fluctuations)
  - <u>Entacapone</u>: COMT inhibitor, prolongs effectiveness of carbidopa-levodopa
  - <u>MAO-B inhibitors</u>: Selegiline, rasagiline. Side effects: Hallucinations, orthostasis, insomnia
  - Dopamine agonists: Pramipexole, ropinirole, rotigitine. Side effects: Hallucinations, impulse control disorder

Parkinson-plus syndromes (atypical parkinsonism)

- Lewy body dementia (LBD): Parkinsonism + fluctuating mental status + visual hallucinations
- Progressive supranuclear palsy (PSP): Early falls + vertical gaze limitation
- Multiple aystem atrophy (MSA): Parkinsonism + prominent, early autonomic dysfunction
- Corticobasal syndrome (CBS): Asymmetric rigidity/dystonia + cortical signs

Hyperkinetic Movement Disorders
Tremor

- Essential tremor: Postural and action tremor that usually starts in the hands/arms and spreads to the head, voice, and legs; often improves with alcohol intake. Treatment: Propranolol or primidone
- Dystonic: Concomitant contraction of agonist and antagonist muscles causing abnormal postures; can be associated with tremor
- Parkinsonian: Resting > postural tremor
- Cerebellar: Appendicular ataxia when cerebellar hemispheres are involved; intention tremor (higher amplitude tremor when getting closer to target)
- Physiologic: Low amplitude not visible under normal conditions, more obvious with drugs/caffeine

Other hyperkinesias

- Chorea: Involuntary continual, irregular "dance-like" movements. Etiologies include genetic diseases (e.g., Wilson's disease, Huntington's), drug-induced (especially neuroleptics, cocaine), metabolic (e.g., HHS, hyperthyroidism), infectious (e.g., HIV, viral encephalitis), autoimmune (e.g., Sydenham chorea), nutritional (e.g., thiamine deficiency)
- Restless leg syndrome (RLS): Typically nocturnal discomfort in the legs that is partially or totally relieved by movement. Screen for iron deficiency, uremia, anemia, and neuropathies and treat the underlying condition if present. Treatment: Dopamine agonists (e.g., pramipexole, ropinirole, rotigotine patch)
- Tics: Irresistible, repetitive, purposeless, temporarily suppressible movements with urge to complete and relief after completing the movements

Cognitive Impairment

Alzheimer's disease

- Epidemiology: Most common form of dementia. Typically symptoms appear after age 60 yr. Increasing prevalence with increasing age.
- Pathophysiology: Loss of neurons and synapses in the cerebral cortex (particularly in the temporal/parietal lobes); thought to be due to misfolding of amyloid beta protein, although poorly understood
- Symptoms: Memory loss (particularly short term memory), decreased attention, visuospatial dysfunction, disorientation
- Treatment:
  - Mild/moderate: Cholinesterase inhibitor – donepezil, galantamine, rivastigmine
  - Severe: NMDA antagonist – memantine

Other etiologies of dementia

- Vascular dementia: Second most common cause of dementia; often multiple infarcts cause a stepwise decline. Treatment: Aspirin; control vascular risk factors
- Atypical parkinsonian syndromes: See movement disorders section above
- Normal pressure hydrocephalus (NPH): Idiopathic or due to hydrocephalus out of proportion to brain parenchymal atrophy with normal opening pressure. Typically, gait instability occurs first (magnetic gait due to apraxia), followed by urge incontinence, cognitive impairment (executive dysfunction, apathy). Diagnosis: Large volume LP with pre- and post-MOCA and motor testing. Treatment: VP shunt
- Creutzfeldt-Jakob disease (CJD): Median onset 60 yr. Rapidly progressive ataxia/dementia that is uniformly fatal (70% die within 1 yr). Diagnosis: LP – 14-3-3 protein, RT-Quic; EEG = periodic sharp waves. No effective treatments
- Pseudodementia: Depression can cause memory loss. Patients may be apathetic with formal testing and thus may perform poorly and out of proportion to their actual deficits

Neuroimmunology

Multiple sclerosis (MS)

- Diagnostic criteria:
  - Relapsing-remitting MS: An attack, relapse, or exacerbation of symptoms typical of acute inflammatory demyelinating event with duration of at least 24 hours in the absence of fever or infection and clinical and/or radiographic evidence of dissemination in space and time
  - Primary-progressive MS: Progressive accumulation of disability from onset without clear relapses
  - Secondary-progressive MS: Progressive accumulation of disability after an initial relapsing course
- Symptoms: Optic neuritis (painful vision loss or blurring, color desaturation), internuclear ophthalmoplegia, transverse myelitis
- Diagnosis: MRI brain (+/– MRI cervical/thoracic spine depending on symptoms) w/wo contrast, LP with basic studies, IgG index, and oligoclonal bands. Rule out other etiologies with labs including HIV antibody, RPR, TSH, B12 with MMA + homocysteine, ESR, CRP, ANA, Sjogren's antibodies, ACE
- Treatment:
  - Acute: Optic neuritis- PO and IV steroids are equally efficacious. Severe symptoms such as bilateral optic neuritis or transverse myelitis with paraparesis/quadriparesis may require IV steroids or plasma exchange
  - Chronic: Numerous disease modifying therapies, prescribed by a neurologist
  - If known MS: Rule out pseudoflare (infection, metabolic disturbance, etc.), which worsens previous MS symptoms in the absence of a new or enhancing lesion on imaging

Neuromyelitis optica (NMO)

- Symptoms: Optic neuritis (often bilateral), acute myelitis, area postrema syndrome (hiccups, nausea, vomiting), acute brainstem syndrome, narcolepsy, symptomatic cerebral syndrome
- Diagnosis: Serum aquaporin 4 IgG

Acute disseminated encephalomyelitis (ADEM)

- Description: Acute demyelination within the white matter of the brain and spinal cord following a viral infection or vaccination
- Symptoms: Often affects children/young adults; causes encephalopathy, weakness
- Treatment: Steroids, plasmapheresis

Progressive multifocal leukoencephalopathy (PML)

- Description: Progressive damage of the white matter of the brain caused by the JC virus in immunosuppressed patients
- Symptoms: Weakness, visual changes, speech changes, personality changes
- Treatment: No cure. Treatment aimed at reversing the immune deficiency to slow or halt disease progression
- Prognosis: Poor prognosis, 30–50% fatality

Myelopathy and Radiculopathy
- Description: Neurologic deficit related to the spinal cord
- Physical exam:
  - Myelopathy: Pyramidal weakness in the arms/legs, bowel or bladder dysfunction, numbness including saddle anesthesia, hyperreflexia below the level of the lesion (may be hyporeflexive at the level of the lesion or if hyperacute), spasticity, +Babinski sign
  - Radiculopathy: Sensory and motor symptoms referable to an individual nerve root
- Key clinical syndromes:
  - Conus medullaris syndrome: Diseases affecting spinal cord levels S2–S5 resulting in back pain, bowel/bladder dysfunction, bilateral sensory loss, and spastic or flaccid weakness.
  - Cauda equina syndrome: Diseases affecting the lumbosacral nerve roots resulting in leg weakness, saddle anesthesia, urinary retention/incontinence, fecal incontinence, impotence, reduced patellar and ankle reflexes
- Etiologies:
  - Compressive: Spondylotic (degenerative/arthritic), tumor, infection (abscess), trauma/hemorrhage
  - Non-compressive:
    - Non-inflammatory (CSF with normal WBC, normal IgG index, no oligoclonal bands)
      - Vascular: Cord ischemia (e.g., during aortic surgery), dural arteriovenous fistula (slowly progressive myelopathy, common in older men), arteriovenous malformation (often presents with subarachnoid hemorrhage, common in patients 20–30 yr)
      - Infectious: HIV vacuolar myelopathy
      - Toxic/metabolic: B12 deficiency (can be due to pernicious anemia, gastrectomy, Crohn's, malnutrition, medication effect), nitrous oxide toxicity (functional B12 deficiency), vitamin E deficiency, copper deficiency (can be due to zinc excess [denture cream!])
      - Inherited: Friedreich ataxia, adrenoleukodystrophy
      - Structural: Syringomyelia (post-traumatic or associated with Chiari malformation; areflexia at level of lesion, "cape-like" distribution of sensory loss to pain and temperature)
    - Inflammatory (CSF with abnormal WBC or abnormal IgG index/oligoclonal bands)
      - Autoimmune: Multiple sclerosis, neuromyelitis optica (NMO), SLE, Sjogren's, sarcoid, ADEM
      - Infectious: HSV, CMV, VZV, HIV, HTLV-1, enterovirus, fungal infections, tuberculosis, Lyme, syphilis (tabes dorsalis, affects dorsal columns)
      - Neoplastic: Lymphoma, paraneoplastic, solid tumor malignancies (may also have bland CSF)

Neuro-oncology
Metastatic brain tumors
- Radiographic findings: Multifocal lesions at the gray-white junction, ring enhancement with contrast
- Common malignancies that metastasize to the brain: Lung cancer, breast cancer, melanoma, GI malignancies, GU malignancies

Primary CNS tumors
- See Hematology/Oncology Chapter 7

Paraneoplastic neurologic syndromes
- Clinical presentation: Consider paraneoplastic (or autoimmune) encephalitis in patients with subacute onset neurologic symptoms including limbic encephalitis (memory loss, behavior changes, seizures), movement disorders, myelopathy, and/or neuropathy. Higher risk if the patient has a known history of malignancy. Typically, CSF is acellular (though often have abnormal IgG index and oligoclonal bands). MRI brain/spine may show abnormal findings in the limbic system, brainstem, or spinal cord.
- Diagnosis: MRI, lumbar puncture with IgG index and oligoclonal bands, serum and CSF autoimmune encephalitis panel, CT chest/abdomen/pelvis, testicular/vaginal ultrasound and/or PET if unknown primary site of malignancy
- Treatment: Treat underlying malignancy, may require immunosuppression

KEY MEDICATIONS & INTERVENTIONS

TABLE 12.6 · Key Medications Used in Neurology				
Class	**Medication**	**Mechanism of Action**	**Uses**	**Adverse Reactions**
Thrombolytic	alteplase (tPA)	Binds to fibrin in the thrombus and converts entrapped plasminogen to plasmin	Acute ischemic stroke with last seen normal within 4.5 hours	Hemorrhage (intracranial and otherwise)
Antiplatelet	aspirin	Irreversible inhibition of COX-1 and -2 enzymes → inhibited formation of prostaglandin derivative (thromboxane A2) → inhibition of platelet aggregation	Stroke, TIA	Bleeding, GI ulcer, gastritis, hepatitis, allergic reaction, tinnitus, hearing loss
	clopidogrel (Plavix)	Irreversible inhibition of P2Y12 component of ADP receptors on platelet surface → prevents activation of GPIIb/IIIa receptor complex → reduced platelet aggregation	Stroke, TIA	Hemorrhage
Antilipidemic	atorvastatin	Inhibition of HMG-CoA reductase enzyme → increased expression of LDL receptors → stimulation of LDL catabolism; additionally, reduces inflammation at the plaque site and improves endothelial function	Stroke, TIA	Increased transaminases, myalgia, myopathy
Anticonvulsants	phenytoin (Dilantin)	Na^+ channel blocker → neuronal membrane stabilization	Seizures, trigeminal neuralgia	Dizziness, ataxia, cardiac arrhythmia, sedation, slurred speech, rash, gingival hyperplasia; teratogenic
	valproic Acid (Depakote)	Enhances action of GABA on neurons, blocks voltage-dependent Na^+ channels	Seizures, migraine prophylaxis	Thrombocytopenia, increased transaminases, tremor, rash, hirsutism, weight gain; teratogenic
	levetiracetam (Keppra)	Modulation of synaptic neurotransmitter release through binding to the synaptic vesicle protein SV2A	Seizures	Aggression, agitation, anxiety, irritability, headache, sedation
	carbamazepine (Tegretol)	Na^+ channel blocker	Seizure, neuropathic pain (including trigeminal neuralgia)	Rash (including SJS/TEN), dizziness, ataxia, sedation
Anti-parkinson agent	carbidopa-levodopa	Levodopa converted to dopamine; carbidopa inhibits peripheral conversion and increases available levodopa at the blood-brain barrier	Parkinsonism	Orthostatic hypotension, dizziness, nausea, depression, dyskinesia, hallucinations, insomnia

(Continued)

TABLE 12.6 · Key Medications Used in Neurology (*Continued*)				
Class	**Medication**	**Mechanism of Action**	**Uses**	**Adverse Reactions**
Acetylcholine-sterase inhibitor	donepezil	Reversible and non-competitive inhibition of centrally active acetylcholinesterase → increased concentrations of acetylcholine available for synaptic transmission in the CNS	Alzheimer disease, Parkinson-related dementia, Lewy body dementia, vascular dementia	Diarrhea, insomnia, anorexia, abnormal dreams
Antidepressants	amitriptyline	Increases synaptic concentration of serotonin/norepinephrine in the CNS by inhibiting reuptake by the presynaptic neuron	Migraine, neuro-pathic pain	Orthostatic hypotension, sedation, dizziness, confusion, cardiac conduction disturbance
	venlafaxine	Inhibitor of serotonin and norepinephrine reuptake	Migraine, neuro-pathic pain	Anorexia, sexual dysfunction, tremor
Antihypertensive	propranolol	Non-selective beta-adrenergic blocker	Migraine, essential tremor	Bradycardia, orthostatic hypertension, depression, bronchospasm; can mask symptoms of hypoglycemia in insulin-dependent diabetics
Serotonin receptor antagonist	sumatriptan	Serotonin receptor agonist on intracranial blood vessels → vasoconstriction	Migraine, cluster headache	Paresthesia, dizziness, flushing, chest discomfort; contraindicated in patients with CAD/CVD/PVD, cardiac conduction disorders
Vitamins	thiamine	Essential enzyme in carbohydrate metabolism, combines with ATP to form thiamine pyrophosphate	Thiamine deficiency, alcohol withdrawal syndrome, Wernicke encephalopathy	Flushing, hypersensitivity reaction (IV)
	cyanocobalamin	Coenzyme for numerous metabolic functions	Vitamin B12 deficiency	Headache (IM)
Neuromuscular blocking agent	botox	Prevents Ca^{2+}-dependent release of acetylcholine	Migraine, spasticity due to stroke, multiple sclerosis, dystonia	Weakness, ptosis, strabismus, URI

KEY CLINICAL TRIALS & PUBLICATIONS

Stroke

- **Tissue Plasminogen Activator for Acute Ischemic Stroke (NINDS Trial).** *N Eng J Med* 1995;333: 1581–1588.
  - Double-blinded, randomized controlled trial that randomized 624 patients to receive tissue plasminogen activator (tPA) vs. placebo within 3 hours of an ischemic stroke. This trial was the first to establish the efficacy of thrombolysis within 3 hours of an ischemic stroke, demonstrating improvements in functional outcomes at 3 months. There was a tenfold increase in symptomatic intracranial hemorrhage (ICH) with tPA administration, but no significant difference in mortality.
- **European Cooperative Acute Stroke Study: Thrombolysis with Alteplase 3 to 4.5 Hours After Acute Ischemic Stroke (ECASS III).** *N Eng J Med* 2008;359:1317–1329.
  - Multicenter, double-blinded, randomized placebo-controlled trial that randomized 821 patients to receive tPA or placebo within 4.5 hours of the onset of ischemic stroke symptoms. Treatment with tPA at 3–4.5 hours from stroke onset was associated with more favorable outcomes and more symptomatic ICH compared to placebo, extending the window of tPA administration to 4.5 hours.
- **Multicenter Randomized Clinical Trial of Endovascular Treatment for Acute Ischemic Stroke in the Netherlands (MR CLEAN).** *N Eng J Med* 2008;372:11–20.
  - Multicenter open-label randomized controlled trial that randomized 500 patients with acute ischemic stroke and imaging proven proximal anterior intracranial circulation large vessel occlusion to receive usual care or usual care plus intra-arterial therapy within 6 hours. In patients with large proximal anterior circulation strokes, usual care plus endovascular therapy was both safe and superior to usual care at 90 days.
- **Beneficial Effect of Carotid Endarterectomy In Symptomatic Patients with High-Grade Stenosis (NASCET).** *N Eng J Med* 1991;325(7):445–453.
  - Multicenter parallel group randomized controlled trial that randomized over 2000 patients with symptomatic cervical ICA stenosis to undergo carotid endarterectomy (CEA) versus medical therapy. CEA reduced the 5 yr risk of death or stroke by 29% in patients with 50–69% stenosis. Patients with $\geq$70% stenosis received such a dramatic benefit that this study arm was closed prematurely and all patients with severe stenosis were referred for CEA.
- **Randomized Placebo-Controlled Trial of Early Aspirin Use in 20,000 Patients with Acute Ischemic Stroke (CAST).** *Lancet* 1997;349(9066):1641–1649.
  - Multicenter randomized placebo controlled trial that randomized patients with suspected acute ischemic stroke to receive aspirin 160 mg daily within 48 hours and continue for 4 weeks vs. placebo. Patients randomized to the aspirin arm had a small (1%) but statistically significant reduction in death and recurrent ischemic stroke compared to the placebo group.
- **High-dose Atorvastatin After Stroke or Transient Ischemic Attack (SPARCL).** *N Eng J Med* 2006;355:549–559.
  - Multicenter double blind placebo-controlled trial that randomized patients with a history of stroke/TIA in the preceding 1–6 months to receive atorvastatin 80 mg daily or placebo. Atorvastatin reduced the composite primary endpoint of fatal or non-fatal stroke by 16%, and also reduced the secondary endpoint of fatal stroke by 43% at 5 yr compared to placebo.
- **Apixaban Versus Warfarin in Patients with Atrial Fibrillation (ARISTOTLE).** *N Eng J Med* 2011;365:981–992.
  - Multicenter double blind comparative clinical trial that randomized 18,201 patients with nonvalvular atrial fibrillation and $\geq$1 stroke risk factor(s) to apixaban 5 mg BID or warfarin (INR 2–3). Apixaban was superior to warfarin for the prevention of stroke and systemic embolism and was associated with less ICH, major bleeding, and death.
- **Thrombectomy 6–24 hours After Stroke with a Mismatch Between Deficit and Infarct (DAWN).** *N Eng J Med* 2018;378(1):11–21.
  - Multicenter randomized controlled trial that enrolled patients who had evidence of an occluded intracranial internal carotid artery (ICA) or proximal middle cerebral artery (MCA) and an infarct to clinical severity mismatch assessed by MR or CT who presented within 6–24 hours from the time when they were last seen well to receive standard of care vs. standard of care + thrombectomy. Patients treated with thrombectomy + standard of care had a higher rate of functional independence at 90 days.
- **Thrombectomy for Stroke At 6 to 16 Hours with Selection by Perfusion imaging (DEFUSE 3).** *N Eng J Med* 2018;378:708–718.
  - Multicenter randomized open-label clinical trial that randomized patients with anterior circulation large vessel occlusion, favorable perfusion imaging, and last known well of 6–16 hours to receive standard medical therapy alone or standard medical therapy + endovascular treatment (thrombectomy). Endovascular thrombectomy was superior to standard medical therapy alone with better functional outcome at 90 days.

NEUROLOGY

- **Stenting versus Aggressive Medical Therapy for Intracranial Arterial Stenosis (SAMMPRIS).** *N Eng J Med* 2015;365:993–1003.
  - Randomized multicenter clinical trial which demonstrated that dual antiplatelet therapy (aspirin and clopidogrel) for 90 days was superior to stenting in symptomatic intracranial stenosis (70–99% stenosis) for prevention of stroke and death in perioperative period and long-term.
- **Clopidogrel and Aspirin in Acute Ischemic Stroke and High-Risk TIA (POINT).** *N Eng J Med* 2018;379(3):215–225.
  - International randomized controlled trial which randomized 4881 patients with minor stroke or high-risk TIA to clopidogrel and aspirin (dual antiplatelet therapy, DAPT), vs aspirin and placebo within 12 hours of symptom onset. Treatment with a loading dose of clopidogrel along with aspirin for 90 days was superior to aspirin alone for composite risk of MI, stroke, or death from vascular case at 90 days with significant increase in major hemorrhage. The greatest risk reduction was in the first 7 days with increasing hemorrhage risk over time. Subgroup analysis determined that the highest benefit was conferred in the first 21 days.

Epilepsy

- **Veterans Affairs Status Epilepticus Cooperative Study Group: A comparison of four treatments for generalized convulsive status.** *N Eng J Med* 1998;339(12):792–798.
  - Multicenter, double-blind, randomized controlled clinical trial that assessed the use of four different IV antiepileptic regimens for the initial treatment of generalized convulsive status epilepticus. In this study, IV lorazepam was more effective than phenytoin.
- **Randomized Trial of Three Anticonvulsant Medications for Status Epilepticus (ESETT).** *N Eng J Med* 2019;381:2103–2113.
  - Multicenter, blinded randomized controlled trial that randomized patients with status epilepticus refractory to benzodiazepines to second-line anticonvulsive agents: levetiracetam, fosphenytoin, or valproate. All were equally efficacious with a seizure cessation rate of approximately 50%, with similar incidences of adverse events.

Multiple Sclerosis

- **Oral versus Intravenous Steroids for Treatment of Relapses in Multiple Sclerosis [Cochrane Review].** *Cochrane Database of Systematic Reviews* 2012;(3):CD006921.
  - Meta-analysis of 167 randomized or quasi-randomized trials comparing oral and intravenous steroids for acute multiple sclerosis relapses. The trials reviewed support the hypothesis that oral steroids are equally efficacious to IV steroids in treating MS exacerbations.
- **A Randomized, Controlled Trial of Corticosteroids in the Treatment of Acute Optic Neuritis.** *N Eng J Med* 1992;326:581–588.
  - Multicenter randomized placebo-controlled trial that randomized patients with acute optic neuritis to receive high-dose IV methylprednisolone followed by oral prednisone vs. placebo. High-dose IV methylprednisolone followed by oral prednisone accelerated visual recovery but did not improve 6-month or 1-yr visual outcomes compared to placebo.

Neurocritical Care

- **Mild Therapeutic Hypothermia to Improve the Neurologic Outcome After Cardiac Arrest (HACA).** *N Eng J Med* 2002;346(8):549–556.
  - Multicenter unblinded randomized controlled trial that randomized patients with return of systemic circulation (ROSC) after cardiac arrest due to ventricular fibrillation or pulseless ventricular tachycardia to normothermia vs. 12–24°C of cooling to 32–34°C. Patients who underwent therapeutic hypothermia (32–34°C) had improved neurologic outcomes and reduced mortality at 6 months.

Neuromuscular

- **Intravenous immunoglobulin for Guillain-Barré syndrome. [Cochrane Review].** *Cochrane Database of Systematic Reviews* 2014;(9):CD002063.
  - Meta-analysis of 12 randomized or quasi-randomized trials comparing IVIG vs. no treatment, placebo treatment, or plasma exchange in children and adults with Guillain-Barré syndrome (GBS) of all degrees of severity. Treatment with either IVIG or plasma exchange was equally efficacious.

Migraine

- **A Controlled Trial of Erenumab for Episodic Migraine.** *N Eng J Med* 2017;377:2123–2132.
  - Multicenter, randomized, placebo-controlled trial that randomized patients with episodic migraine to received erenumab, a calcitonin gene-related peptide (CGRP) receptor antagonist vs. placebo. Patients who received erenumab administered subcutaneously monthly had significantly reduced migraine frequency, severity, and use of migraine-specific medications over a 6-month period.

NOTES

NOTES

Psychiatry

ANATOMY & PHYSIOLOGY

Mechanisms of Psychiatric Disease

- Mechanisms of psychiatric disease remain partially understood
- Complementary mechanistic hypotheses exist for many disorders (e.g., dysfunction in the stress axis, altered glutamatergic neurotransmission, reduced GABAergic transmission, abnormal circadian rhythms, thyroxine abnormalities, etc.) and these data inform current psychopharmacotherapy (Table 13.1)
- Advanced imaging techniques offer increasingly refined descriptions of neurobiological mechanisms and can help uncover novel targets for advanced therapies such as deep brain stimulation or operative interventions (Figure 13.1)
- Researchers have begun to use behavioral domains to characterize psychiatric disease (e.g., reframing obsessive compulsive disorder [OCD] as dysfunction of performance monitoring, response inhibition, goal selection, and reward learning), which may help refine therapeutic management in the future

DIAGNOSTICS

Mental Status Exam

- Appearance: Apparent age, weight, clothing, personal hygiene, odor, skin markings, etc. (Goal: Document a description with enough salient details that another provider could identify the patient on sight.)
- Behavior: Movements (i.e., resting comfortably vs. fidgeting, tics, stereotyped movements), facial expression, eye contact, attitude (i.e., cooperative vs. hostile)
- Speech: Rate, rhythm, volume, tone, articulation, quantity (i.e., hyper-verbal or pressured vs. paucity of speech/content)
- Mood: "How would you describe your mood right now?" Document the patient's own words. (Goal: Capture the subjective state of the patient at the time of the interview.)
- Affect: Assessment of how the patient's mood appears to the examiner – quality (flat, blunted, constricted, full, intense), motility (sluggish, supple, labile), appropriate/not appropriate
- Thought process: Progression and form of thought. Normal thought process is linear and goal-oriented. Abnormal thought processes include disorganized, tangential, circumstantial, loosened associations, flight of ideas, neologisms (i.e., made up words), word salad, clanging (e.g., "bed, red, fed, led")
- Thought content: Suicidal ideation (SI), homicidal ideation (HI), paranoia, poverty of thought (the absence of content (such as a one-word response to a complex question, reduced spontaneity of speech/thought, or the use of vague/stereotyped phrases), delusions, phobias, obsessions, compulsions
- Perception: Hallucination (i.e., sensory experience not based in reality; can be auditory, visual, or tactile), illusions (i.e., inaccurate perception of real sensory stimuli, such as a shadow misperceived as a cat)
- Sensorium: Alertness, orientation, memory (3 words), calculations, fund of knowledge (e.g., presidents), attention (e.g., spelling "WORLD" backward), abstract thinking (e.g., what does it mean to say, "The grass is always greener?")
- Insight: Intact, fair, or impaired. The patient's understanding of their illness and or current mental state, as well as the impact on their well-being.
- Judgment: Intact, fair, or impaired. The patient's ability to make rational decisions (i.e., weigh evidence, assess pros and cons, anticipate consequences, etc.).

TABLE 13.1 · Selected Psychiatric Diseases and Classically Associated Neurotransmitter Changes	
Disease	**Neurotransmitter pattern**
Anxiety	• Decreased GABA, serotonin • Increased norepinephrine
Depression	• Decreased dopamine, norepinephrine, serotonin
Schizophrenia	• Increased dopamine (for positive symptoms)

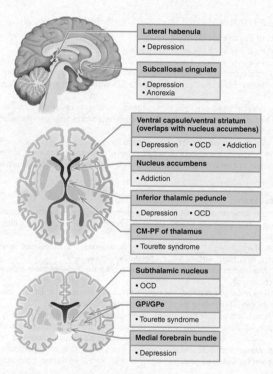

FIGURE 13.1: Deep brain stimulation targets by psychiatric disease. Deep brain stimulation targets are selected based on historical ablation targets as well as emerging understandings of which neuroanatomical structures and tracts are involved in the pathophysiology of specific psychiatric diseases. Abbreviations: CM-PF, centromedian nucleus; GPi, globus pallidus internus; GPe, globus pallidus externus; OCD, obsessive-compulsive disorder

APPROACHES & CHIEF COMPLAINTS

Depressed Mood/Suicidal Ideation

- Definitions:
  - Suicidal ideation (SI)
    - Active SI: Thoughts about acting to kill oneself with intent and/or plan (e.g., considering whether to shoot oneself with an owned gun, etc.)
    - Passive SI: Thoughts about dying without intent and/or plan; an expression of despair/not wanting to be in a current mood, state, or situation (e.g., thoughts of "being better off dead," thoughts of being hit by a car, etc.)
    - Conditional SI: Thoughts of suicide that are dependent on specific conditions, such as satisfying a need, obtaining secondary gain, or remaining in the sick role (e.g., "If you don't prescribe pain medications, I'm going to kill myself")
  - Suicide attempt: Self-injury made in an attempt to kill oneself that does not result in fatality
  - Suicidal gesture: Self-injury made in an attempt to lead others to think that one wants to kill oneself even though there is no intention of dying; clinical feature of borderline personality disorder (e.g., holding a knife to one's neck, putting a rope around one's neck)
- Risk factors for suicide: Prior attempts, psychiatric disease (>90% of patient who attempt), hopelessness, married, member of sexual minority, certain occupations, veterans, chronic pain, traumatic brain injury, access to firearms
- Differential diagnosis for depressed mood:
  - Psychiatric disease:
    - Major depressive disorder
    - Bipolar disorder
    - Anxiety disorders
    - Personality disorders (e.g., borderline personality disorder)
    - Post-traumatic stress disorder (PTSD)
    - Psychotic disorders (e.g., schizophrenia)
    - Substance use disorders
  - Other causes:
    - Depression due to another medical condition
      - Cardiac disease
      - Malignancy (especially oropharyngeal and pancreatic)
      - Neurologic disease (including stroke, movement disorders)
      - Diabetes
      - Hypothyroidism
      - Chronic infection (including HIV, HCV)
    - Depression due to medication effect
    - Traumatic brain injury
    - Chronic pain
    - Malingering
- Approach:
  - Safety assessment:
    - Assess the suicidal ideation (i.e., passive vs. active; assess for plan, intent, means, lethality of means, rehearsal [i.e., elements of the plan being practiced, making preparations for one's death])
    - Assess protective factors (e.g., children or pets who rely on the person, loved ones who would be affected by their death, willingness to engage in safety planning/contingency planning for worsening symptoms, having hopes for the future ["future-oriented"], etc.)
    - Assess for risk factors (see list of risk factors above), especially for prior suicide attempts
  - Assess for triggers/stressors
- Work-up: CBC, BMP, LFTs, TSH (assess baseline organ function in anticipation of pharmacotherapy; rule out fatigue due to medical comorbidities, e.g., anemia or hypothyroidism mimicking depression). Consider additional testing based on exam/review of symptoms.

- Management:
  - Medical stabilization (if patient has attempted suicide and attempt was non-fatal) with involvement of psychiatry to make appropriate holding plan
  - Determine appropriate level of care (e.g., inpatient, day program, intensive outpatient therapy, outpatient): Inpatient hospitalization always indicated for recent attempt or high imminent risk (e.g., patients with plan/intent, poor social support, inability to discuss safety planning)
  - Create a safety plan
    - Know warning signs and precipitants
    - Secure/remove lethal agents
    - Utilize individual coping strategies, such as reflecting on reasons to live, distraction activities, relaxation, and exercise
    - Utilize interpersonal coping, such as friends or family who lift mood
    - Create a list of professionals who can help and how to contact them
  - Initiate pharmacotherapy: See Table 13.3

Psychosis (e.g., Delusions and/or Hallucinations)

- Definitions:
  - Delusions: False, fixed beliefs that persist in the face of challenging/contrary evidence and which are not typical of a patient's culture or religion; subtypes include erotomanic, grandiose, jealous, persecutory, somatic, mixed, and unspecified
  - Hallucinations: Perceptions of sensory experiences in the absence of external stimuli
- Differential diagnosis:
  - Primary psychotic disorder
  - Substance use disorder
  - Mood disorder with psychotic symptoms
  - Delirium
  - Dementia (especially Lewy body dementia)
  - Psychosis due to another medical condition
    - Endocrine (hyperparathyroidism, hyperthyroidism)
    - Metabolic (hepatic encephalopathy, uremic encephalopathy, vitamin B12 deficiency, Wilson's disease, acute intermittent porphyria)
    - Infectious (HIV, neurosyphilis, herpes simplex encephalitis, Lyme's disease)
    - Inflammatory or demyelinating disorders (anti-NDMA encephalitis, systemic lupus erythematosus, multiple sclerosis)
    - Neurodegenerative disease (particularly Lewy body dementia; also Alzheimer's disease, Parkinson's disease, Huntington's disease)
    - Other neurological disorders (epilepsy, intracranial tumor, prion disease)
- Approach by hallucination subtype:
  - Auditory: More commonly a feature of primary psychiatric illness, but other causes also occur
  - Visual: More commonly a feature of substance use or medical illness, but other causes also occur, including primary psychiatric disease
  - Tactile: Most common in setting of substance use (e.g., alcohol withdrawal; stimulant intoxication), although delusional parasitosis (the belief that one is infested with a pathogen) is on the differential diagnosis as well
  - Olfactory: Most commonly an aura of temporal lobe epilepsy or in the setting of an intracranial mass
  - Gustatory: Very rare; occurs occasionally in epilepsy
  - Hypnagogic: Occurs while going to sleep; not typically pathologic
  - Hypnopompic: Occurs while waking from sleep; not typically pathologic
- Work-up: Basic labs, UA, urinary toxicology; consider other testing, such as head imaging, based on clinical features and context
- Management:
  - Acute therapy
    - Treat underlying cause if identified
    - If risk of harm, consider rapid sedation with benzodiazepine, antipsychotics (PO or IM)
  - Maintenance therapy for primary psychotic disorder: See Table 13.4

DISEASES & PATHOPHYSIOLOGY

Psychotic Disorders

Schizophrenia

- Etiology: Likely multiple diseases with similar signs/symptoms (*Neuropsychopharmacol* 2009;34(9): 2081).
- Pathophysiology: Dopamine hypothesis of schizophrenia suggests that excess dopamine in mesolimbic tract causes positive psychotics symptoms, although other neurotransmitters are likely involved; antipsychotics used for treatment block dopamine, consistent with the dopamine hypothesis
- Epidemiology: ~1% population. M:F = 1.4:1. Onset in men 18–25 yr, women 25–35 yr. Better prognosis if late onset, positive symptom predominant, and good social support.
- Symptoms: Divided into positive and negative symptoms; negative are more difficult to treat
  - (+) Hallucinations, disorganized speech
  - (−) Blunted affect, apathy, isolation, cognitive impairment
- Phases: 1) Prodromal (irritable, isolation); 2) Psychotic; 3) Residual (persists between psychotic episodes: Flat affect, isolation) (Figure 13.2)
- Diagnosis: ≥6 months with two or more of 1) Delusions; 2) Hallucinations; 3) Disorganized speech; 4) Disorganized or catatonic behaviors; 5) Negative symptoms (flat affect). Significantly affects function. Imaging not required for diagnosis, but MRI brain may show enlargement of the cerebral ventricles.
- Subtypes: 1) Paranoid; 2) Disorganized; 3) Catatonic; 4) Residual (mostly negative symptoms); 5) Undifferentiated
- Treatment:
  - **Typical antipsychotics**: Haloperidol, chlorpromazine, thioridazine; use depot/decanoate versions of drugs if poor compliance. Several clinically important clinical syndromes can result as side effects:
    - Acute dystonia: Involuntary contraction of major muscle groups. Treatment: Benztropine, diphenhydramine
    - Akathisia: Motor restlessness. Treatment: Propranolol
    - Parkinsonian: Mask-like facies, resting tremor, cogwheel rigidity, shuffling gait; Treatment: Benztropine, amantadine
    - Tardive dyskinesia: After chronic use; sucking/smacking lips, facial grimacing, choriform movements. Treatment: Stop medication
    - Neuroleptic malignant syndrome (NMS): Tetrad of fever, rigidity, mental status changes, and autonomic instability. Treatment: Stop medication and admit to ICU
  - **Atypical antipsychotics**: Olanzapine, quetiapine, risperidone, aripiprazole, clozapine, ziprasidone. Side effects: Metabolic syndrome especially olanzapine and clozapine. Only use clozapine if patient has failed other options, due to risk of agranulocytosis.

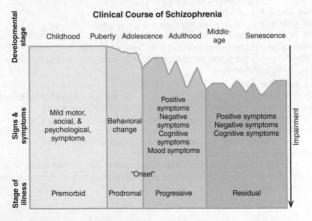

FIGURE 13.2: Clinical course of schizophrenia. Schizophrenia progresses through premorbid, prodromal, progressive, and residual stages. Typical period of onset, symptoms, and signs differ for each stage.

Other psychotic disorders

- Schizophreniform: Same as schizophrenia but only <u>1–6 months</u> (Think "forming")
- Brief psychotic disorder: <u><1 month</u>. Rare, often in response to trauma or stress.
- Schizoaffective: Schizophrenia + mood disorder (depression or mania). Mostly mood symptoms, but must be psychosis in the absence of mood symptoms 2+ wks (i.e, if psychotic features <u>only</u> occur during mood symptoms, then appropriate diagnosis is MDD or bipolar disorder with psychotic features).
- Delusional disorder: Non-bizarre fixed delusion for 1+ month (e.g., thinks food is poisoned) but does NOT interfere with daily function.
- Shared psychotic disorder: Folie a duex ("madness for two"). Same symptoms as loved one. Treatment: Separation.
- Secondary to medical condition: 1) CNS disease; 2) Endocrinopathy; 3) Nutritional deficiency (B12, folate, niacin); 4) Other: SLE, porphyria
- Secondary to medications or substance abuse: Steroids, antiparkinsonians, anticonvulsants, antihistamines, anticholinergics

Mood Disorders

Major depressive disorder (MDD)

- Etiology: Multiple synergistic biopsychosocial risk factors at play. Abnormal functioning of many neurotransmitters (serotonin, norepinephrine, dopamine, GABA, and glutamate) and complex intracellular cascades involved in both pathogenesis and response to antidepressant medications.
- Epidemiology: Lifetime prevalence 20.6% (*JAMA Psychiatry* 2018;75(4):339), F:M = 2:1.
- Diagnosis: Patient experiences a depressive episode, which requires 5+ depressive symptoms for >2 weeks (with at least one symptom being either depressed mood or anhedonia); no history of hypomanic/manic episodes
- Depressive symptoms: **SIG E CAPS** – **S**leep (↑ or ↓, multiple or early awakenings), **I**nterest (↓), **G**uilt, **E**nergy (↓), **C**oncentration (↓), **A**ppetite (↑ or ↓) **P**sychomotor slowing, **S**uicidal
- Subtypes:
  - <u>Melancholic</u>: Anhedonia, motor agitation/retardation, cognitive impairment, interrupted sleep, loss of appetite, diurnal variation-mood/energy worse in the AM, affect does not respond to positive events
  - <u>Atypical</u>: Hypersomnia, hyperphagia, leaden paralysis, longstanding history of rejection sensitivity, reactivity to pleasurable stimuli (i.e., feels better when positive events occur)
  - <u>Catatonic</u>: Immobility, mutism, decreased alertness, resistance to all instructions/attempts to be moved, waxy flexibility, staring, purposeless motor activity, echolalia (senseless verbal mirroring), echopraxia (senseless physical mirroring)
  - <u>Psychotic</u> ("with psychotic features"): Accompanied by delusions and/or hallucinations concurrent with mood symptoms
- Treatment: Screen with **PHQ9** – goal is to get PHQ9 score <5
  - 5–9: Mild → Reassurance
  - 10–14: Moderate → Watchful waiting, supportive counseling
  - 15–19: Moderately severe → Antidepressant (See Table 13.3) +/− psychotherapy (SSRI takes 4–8 wks to achieve maximal effect; for first episode, continue for at least 6–12 months)
  - 20+: Severe → Antidepressant, psychotherapy, hospitalize if SI/HI; consider electroconvulsive therapy (ECT) if refractory

Other depressive disorders

- Persistent depressive disorder (dysthymia): ≥2 yr with depressed mood and at least two other symptoms, never symptom-free for >2 months. No history of mania/hypomania.
- Acute grief: Typically occurs following a death although other loss or anticipatory loss can precipitate; symptoms can include yearning for the deceased, loneliness, crying, disrupted sleep, social withdrawal, disbelief/shock, impaired attention/concentration/memory. Usually improvement seen within 6 months; if longer, consider complicated grief.
- Complicated grief: 6 months or more (though longer duration, up to 12 months, may be appropriate in some cultures) with symptoms of grief that cause significant distress or psychosocial impairment. Treatment: Therapy, SSRI.

Bipolar I disorder
- Etiology: Strong genetic component, 5–10% risk with first-degree relative
- Epidemiology: 2–3% of world population affected by bipolar spectrum disorders; average age of onset 21 yr
- Diagnosis: Patient experiences a manic episode, which requires 3+ manic symptoms that require hospitalization or persist for >1 week (with at least one symptom being euphoric mood or agitation)
- Manic symptoms: **DIG FAST** – **D**istractibility, **I**mpulsivity, **G**randiosity, **F**light of ideas, **A**ctivity/agitation, **S**leeplessness (i.e., goes days without need to sleep), **T**alkativeness (i.e., pressured speech); psychotic symptoms may or may not be present
- Treatment: See Tables 13.4 and 13.5
  - Acute: Hospitalize. Anticonvulsant (e.g., valproic acid) + atypical antipsychotic (e.g., olanzapine).
  - Long term: Lithium is typically first line. If the patient has CKD or develops renal failure, lithium is contraindicated and use valproic acid instead. If only 1 manic episode, can attempt to taper after 1 yr; if 2 manic episodes, typically requires years of treatment; if 3+ manic episodes, typically requires lifelong treatment.

Other disorders with mania
- Bipolar II disorder: 1+ hypomanic episode (DIGFAST symptoms for >4 days but <1 week without any psychotic symptoms) AND 1+ episode major depression
- Cyclothymic disorder: ≥2 yr of alternating hypomanic + depressive symptoms that DO NOT meet criteria for major depression, mania, or hypomania AND never symptom free 2+ months

Personality Disorders
Definitions:
- Personality: Patterns of relating to and perceiving the world and oneself that persist across multiple contexts
- Personality disorder: The presence of traits that are maladaptive and inflexible across enough contexts to cause distress and impaired functioning within an individual's environment/culture

Cluster A ("weird")
- Paranoid: Distrust, suspiciousness of others (often directed towards a spouse)
- Schizoi**D**: **D**istant, socially withdrawn, has few friends and prefers to be alone ("happy loner")
- Schizo**T**ypal: Socially withdrawal and eccentric behavior, magical **T**hinking; 10–20% children with schizotypal personality disorder ultimately develop schizophrenia

Cluster B ("wild")
- Antisocial: Violates rights of others without remorse; often history of malingering, arrests/incarcerations, and substance use disorder. Must be ≥18 yr (in children, this behavior is instead called conduct disorder). Treatment: Cognitive behavioral therapy (CBT), although two trials have not demonstrated benefit (*Psychol Med* 2009;39(4):569; *Br J Psychiatry* 2007;190:307). Other modalities not studied.
- Borderline: Unstable mood, labile intense relationships, poorly defined sense of self, chronic feelings of emptiness, intense fear of abandonment/rejection, black/white thinking, suicidal gestures common. Treatment: dialectical behavior therapy (DBT).
- Histrionic: Attention-seeking, provocative, exaggerated, regression to childlike behavior
- Narcissistic: Grandiose, limited empathy, often conveys a sense of superiority but the individual actually has fragile self-esteem. Desires recognition/admiration.

Cluster C ("worried")
- Avoidant: Shy and fear of rejection but would prefer to have friends (in contrast to schizoid); very isolated
- Dependent: Need for others to make decisions and/or care for them. Fear rejection/abandonment.
- Obsessive-compulsive personality: Perfectionism, inflexibility, orderliness, ego-syntonic (i.e., behavior does not threaten the ego; patient does not experience behavior as an external force/impulse, in contrast with obsessive-compulsive disorder)

Anxiety Disorders
- Panic disorder: Recurrent <u>unexpected</u> panic attacks, resulting in a fear of future panic attacks and avoidance of potential panic triggers. Symptoms: Chest pain/tightness, tachycardia, palpitations, which frequently requires ruling out an acute coronary syndrome first. Proposed etiology: Overactive amygdala-hypothalamus circuits. Treatment: Acute: benzodiazepines (lorazepam, clonazepam), but ideally discontinue as soon as possible. If history of substance abuse, consider gabapentin or hydroxyzine. Chronic: 1st-line SSRIs (e.g., escitalopram, sertraline).

- Specific phobia: Fear of specific trigger (animal, heights, flying). Treatment: CBT with exposures; benzodiazepines if exposures cannot be tolerated.
- Agoraphobia: Fear and/or avoidance of situations that are difficult to leave/escape in the event of panic or other embarrassing symptoms. Situations commonly include crowds, shopping areas, public transport, being outside of the home in general. Treatment: CBT and/or SSRIs.
- Social anxiety disorder: Excessive fear of social situations, embarrassment/humiliation. Treatment: SSRI (escitalopram, sertraline), CBT. If for public speaking only, can consider using propranolol 30 min before the event.
- Generalized anxiety disorder: 6+ months with worries/anxiety across multiple domains. Associated with impaired sleep, poor concentration, easy fatigability, irritability, muscle tension, restlessness. Treatment: CBT, SSRI, buspirone.
- Obsessive compulsive disorder (OCD): Obsessions and compulsions that are time consuming, distressing, and/or impair function. Obsession: Recurrent intrusive thought. Compulsion: Conscious repetitive behavior to relieve anxiety. Ego-dystonic (i.e., bothers patient, in contrast to obsessive-compulsive personality disorder). Proposed etiology: Serotonin, glutamate, and dopamine involved. Treatment: SSRI, TCA (e.g., clomipramine). Exposure and response prevention therapy (ERP).
- Body dysmorphic disorder: Preoccupation with body parts that the patient thinks are flawed; very distressing. Surgical correction does not satisfy.
- Trichotillomania: Recurrent pulling out of hair causing distress and/or impairing daily function. May present with bald spots, most commonly scalp, eyebrows, and/or eyelashes. Treatment: CBT, habit-reversal therapy.
- Acute stress disorder: Reaction within 3 days to 1 month of trauma including re-experiencing, negative mood, dissociation, avoidance, and hyper-vigilance. Treatment: Trauma focused cognitive therapy; short-term benzodiazepine if severe.
- Post-traumatic stress disorder (PTSD): Reaction lasting 1+ month. Response to trauma (experienced, threatened, or witnessed) including re-experiences, avoidance, cognitive/emotional disturbances, hyper-arousal, dissociative symptoms. Imaging not required for diagnosis, but MRI brain may show decreased hippocampal volume. Treatment: Trauma-focused CBT ("TF-CBT"), SSRIs (e.g., sertraline, fluoxetine).
- Adjustment disorder: Low mood and/or anxiety within 3 months of a stressor AND does not meet criteria for another disorder (i.e., MDD or generalized anxiety disorder [GAD]) but still causes significant impairment. Treatment: Supportive psychotherapy, cognitive or psychodynamic psychotherapy.

Dissociative Disorders

- Dissociative amnesia: Episodes of inability to remember salient details about one's self. Retrograde amnesia most common
- Dissociative fugue: Sudden, unexpected, and purposeful travel with inability to recall one's identity or past (think "fugitive" with new identity). Unaware of amnesia and does not recall the period of fugue. Low anxiety despite confusion. Associated with trauma, war exposure.
- Depersonalization: Sense of disconnection from one's self/body/actions. Often vague/difficult for one to describe.
- Derealization: Sense of disconnection from reality/one's surroundings. Feeling of "unreality." Often vague/difficult for one to describe.

Impulse Control Disorders

- Intermittent explosive disorder: Recurrent aggressive outbursts, out of proportion with stressor, then remorse (unlike antisocial personality). Treatment: CBT, pharmacotherapy (anticonvulsants, antidepressants, anti-psychotics, beta-blockers, anxiolytics).
- Kleptomania: Uncontrollable urge to steal objects not needed for money or use. Pleasure/relief when stealing, but shame/guilt afterward. Treatment: CBT or insight-oriented psychotherapy, pharmacotherapy (anti depressants, anticonvulsants, or anxiolytics).
- Pyromania: Multiple episodes of deliberate fire setting; often tension/arousal before, then pleasure/relief afterward. Fascination with fires. Better prognosis in children. Treatment: CBT, pharmacotherapy (anti-depressants, anticonvulsants).

Somatic Symptom and Related Disorders

- Somatic symptom disorder: Somatic symptoms with excessive thoughts, anxieties, or behaviors causing significant disruption to social, occupational, and/or other areas of functioning lasting >6 months. Treatment: Regularly-scheduled visits with providers (i.e., not PRN when symptoms and/ or related anxiety spikes), CBT, limited evidence for SSRIs but should be considered in patients with comorbid psychiatric illnesses.

- Conversion disorder (functional neurological symptom disorder): 1+ "real" (i.e., not intentionally feigned) neurologic symptom (e.g., blindness, deafness, mutism, paralysis) not otherwise explained by a medical disorder (think "converts" a psychiatric disorder into a neurologic disorder). Typically patient is calm/unconcerned about symptom(s) ("la belle indifference"). Diagnosis of exclusion. Treatment: Patient education, CBT, physical therapy (i.e., for motor deficits); antidepressants may be helpful.
- Illness anxiety disorder: Preoccupation and anxiety of having an undiagnosed serious disease to the point where the concern interferes with functioning. May have mild or no symptoms. Treatment: Goal is to improve tolerance/ability to cope with anxieties. Regularly scheduled visits with providers (i.e., not PRN when anxieties spike), reassurance, CBT, SSRIs may be helpful.
- Factitious disorder: Consciously feigning/producing symptoms in the absence of external reward to assume the role of the sick patient (i.e., primary gain is assuming the sick role without external reward). Treatment: 1) Use only objective signs/data to decide on diagnostics/procedures (i.e., do NOT rely on subjective reporting); 2) Communicate frequently with the patient as a "united front" with all members of the care team to prevent splitting; 3) Supportive confrontation once rapport is established (or, if admitted inpatient, pursue a therapeutic discharge).
  - Munchhausen syndrome: Repeated episodes of simulated/feigned illness, peregrination (i.e., visiting multiple medical settings), and pseudologia fantastica (i.e., patient provides detailed, colorful/ fantastical stories associated with feigned illness)
  - Factitious disorder imposed on another ("Munchhausen syndrome by proxy"): Typically the caregiver is causing harm to another and/or giving false report of symptoms to providers; victims are typically <4 yr, but adults can also be victimized
- Malingering: Consciously feigning/producing symptoms for external reward (e.g., to avoid jail, to gain disability, to acquire pain medications). Symptoms stop when reward is obtained.

Eating Disorders

Anorexia nervosa

- Definition: Intense fear of gaining weight leading to low body weight (<85% ideal, BMI <18.5)
- Subtypes: Restricting (little intake, no purging); binging and purging (binge eating then self-induced vomiting, laxatives, or excessive exercise)
- Clinical features: Preoccupation with avoiding weight gain; may result in amenorrhea, cold intolerance, hypotension, bradycardia, decreased bone density
- Treatment: Goal = improve nutritional status. 1) Psychotherapy (e.g., family-based, CBT, interpersonal psychotherapy [IPT]); 2) Nutritional rehab with careful weight gain schedule; 3) Off-label pharmacotherapy (no approved medications; in clinical practice, SSRIs are often used to target mood symptoms and olanzapine may be used to target weight gain and rigid/obsessional thinking around weight).
- Common criteria for inpatient admission: Abnormal vitals/electrolytes/EKG, BMI <14, precipitous weight loss

Bulimia nervosa

- Definition: Binge eating *plus* reactive behavior to prevent weight gain, i.e., purging (vomiting, laxatives, diuretics) or non-purging (excessive exercise, fasting) behavior; normal body weight (BMI 18.5–30) but excess worry about body appearance
- Clinical features: Preoccupation with body appearance, parotid gland enlargement (dialadenosis), dental caries, "Russell's sign" (calluses on knuckles due to purging), peripheral edema
- Treatment: 1) Psychotherapy (CBT, IPT, DBT, nutrition education); 2) Fluoxetine (only approved medication for bulimia nervosa, though other SSRIs are used 2nd line in clinical practice). Note: Bupropion contraindicated due to increased risk of symptoms.

Binge eating disorder

- Definition: Binging (eating more than normal sometimes without feeling hungry, feeling out of control, followed by feelings of disgust or guilt) at least 1 time per week for 3 months but without regular use of compensatory behaviors afterward. Associated with obesity but can be overweight or normal weight.
- Treatment: 1) Psychotherapy (e.g., CBT, IPT, DBT, nutrition education); 2) Off-label pharmacotherapy (no approved medications; in clinical practice, SSRIs are often used to target comorbid mood symptoms and antiepileptics are often used to target reduction of binging episodes)

Sleep Disorders

Dyssomnias

<u>Definition</u>: Disturbance in the amount, quality, or timing of sleep

- Insomnia:
  - Subtypes: Acute/short-term (symptoms for <1 month; often related to a stressor or jet lag); chronic/long-term (symptoms for >1 month)
  - Treatment:
    - Cognitive Behavioral Therapy for Insomnia ("CBT-I"). First line, gold standard treatment of <u>chronic</u> insomnia (*J Clin Sleep Med* 2017;13(2):307. *Ann Intern Med* 2016;165(2):125).
    - Benzodiazepines. Can be used effectively, but generally try other medications first. Side effects include daytime sedation, drowsiness, dizziness, lightheadedness, cognitive impairment, motor incoordination, tolerance, dependence, rebound insomnia with discontinuation; increased risk of adverse events in older patients
    - Non-benzodiazepines (e.g., **Z**olpidem, es**Z**opiclone, **Z**aleplon). Side effects similar to benzodiazepines; can also cause complex sleep related behaviors (e.g., sleepwalking, sleep driving); increased risk of adverse events in older patients
    - Antidepressants (e.g., mirtazapine, trazodone, amitriptyline, doxepin).
- Obstructive sleep apnea (OSA): Apnea during sleep that last 20–30 seconds; may cause hypoxia that arouses the patient from sleep, snoring, daytime sleepiness, decreased libido, morning headaches, polycythemia, secondary hypertension. Etiologies include obesity, structural causes (e.g., enlarged tonsils, nasal polyps), alcohol use. Diagnosis: Polysomnography (overnight sleep study). Treatment: Mild/moderate (<20 apneic spells) – weight loss, avoid alcohol. Severe (>20) – CPAP
- Narcolepsy: REM sleep right away. Causes excessive daytime sleepiness, involuntary sleep attacks, cataplexy (loss of muscle tone with emotional stimuli), sleep paralysis (can't move when wake up), hypnagogic hallucinations (visual/auditory hallucinations: "dreams while awake"). Treatment: 1) Pharmacotherapy for sleepiness (e.g., modafinil, methylphenidate [Ritalin]); 2) Pharmacotherapy for cataplexy (e.g., sodium oxybate); 3) Planned naps.
- Idiopathic hypersomnia: Excessive daytime sleepiness as well as prolonged nocturnal sleep; rule out medical disorders first
- Kleine-Levin syndrome: Extremely rare. Recurrent hypersomnia, hyperphagia, hypersexuality, aggression.

Parasomnias

<u>Definition</u>: Unwanted events or experiences that occur during sleep

- Sleepwalking: Slow-wave sleep, eyes open/glassy. Don't remember.
- Sleep terrors: **N**on-REM, **N**o memory. Episodes of sudden arousal with screaming. Don't remember, return to sleep. Treatment: Reassurance.
- Nightmare disorder: **R**EM, **R**emember. Recurrent frightening dreams; end when awake with vivid recall. Treatment: Imagery rehearsal therapy.
- REM sleep behavior disorder: Sleep talking, yelling, limb jerking, dream enactment. Treatment: Ensure safety of sleeping environment; consider melatonin, clonazepam.

Substance Use Disorders

- Overview: Named by type of substance involved in problematic use (i.e., alcohol use disorder, cocaine use disorder, etc.); however, clinical criteria for diagnosis of each disorder is the same
- Diagnosis: 2+ symptoms within 1 yr (severity assigned based on number of symptoms: Mild 2–3, moderate 4–5, severe 6+):
  - Using larger amounts or for longer periods of time than intended
  - Desire/attempts to reduce or abstain from use
  - Large amount of time spent on obtaining, using, and/or recovering from use
  - Strong cravings
  - Use that impairs ability to fulfill responsibilities
  - Persistent use despite problems caused by or worsened by use
  - Stops or reduces daily activities due to use (e.g., social, occupation or recreational)
  - Use in dangerous situations or settings
  - Persistent use despite awareness of physical or psychiatric problems that are caused or worsened by use
  - Tolerance
  - Withdrawal
- Clinical presentation: See Table 13.2

TABLE 13.2 • Recreational Substances: Intoxication, Withdrawal, and Treatment

Substance	Intoxication	Withdrawal	Treatment
Alcohol	• Slurred speech • ↓Coordination • Horizontal nystagmus • ↓Attention/memory • stupor/coma	• ↑Autonomic (HR, BP, RR, Temp) • Anxiety • Insomnia • Nausea/vomiting • Tremor • Agitation	**Withdrawal** • Symptom-triggered benzodiazepines (i.e., CIWA Protocol) • High-dose thiamine (vitamin B1) + volume/electrolyte repletion if Wernicke's on differential diagnosis **Use Disorder** • Use motivational interviewing to determine patient's goals • Pharm: 1st-line, naltrexone or acamprosate; monthly IM naltrexone if compliance concerns. 2nd-line, disulfiram • Psycho-social: CBT, couple's/family therapy, contingency management (incentives provided contingent on treatment/abstinence), mutual support groups (e.g., Alcoholics Anonymous)
Cannabis	• Conjunctival injection • ↑Appetite • Dry mouth • ↑HR	• Insomnia • Vivid dreams • Dysphoria • ↓Appetite • Anxiety • Irritability • Flu-like symptoms • Restlessness	**Intoxication** • Calming environment (quiet, dim lighting), reassurance, can consider benzodiazepine for anxiety **Withdrawal** • Gabapentin, dronabinol **Use Disorder** • Use motivational interviewing to determine patient's goals • Pharm: No FDA approved treatments, N-acetylcysteine (NAC) used in clinical practice but limited evidence • Psycho-social: CBT, mutual support groups
Tobacco		• Anxiety • Depression • Irritability • Restlessness • ↓Concentration • Headache • Insomnia • ↑Appetite/weight gain	**Use Disorder** • Use motivational interviewing to determine patient's goals • Pharm: Nicotine replacement therapy (NRT) with long-acting agent (i.e., patch) and short-acting agent (i.e., gum), varenicline (partial nicotine agonist), or bupropion.

(Continued)

TABLE 13.2 · Recreational Substances: Intoxication, Withdrawal, and Treatment *(Continued)*

Substance	Intoxication	Withdrawal	Treatment
Cocaine	• ↑Energy • ↑Confidence • Anxiety/panic • Agitation • Tremors • Insomnia • ↑HR, BP • Diaphoresis • Mydriasis	• Dysphoria +/− SI • Anhedonia • Vivid dreams • Insomnia or hypersomnia • ↑Appetite • Psychomotor agitation or retardation	**Intoxication** • Anxiety/Panic/Agitation → benzodiazepines • Psychosis → 1st/2nd generation antipsychotic • *Avoid β-blockers for HTN management (risk of unopposed α-agonism) **Withdrawal** • Suicide risk assessment, hospitalization if needed • Supportive treatment **Use Disorder** • Use motivational interviewing to determine patient's goals • Pharm: No FDA approved treatments • Psycho-social: CBT, contingency management, mutual support groups
Methamphet-amine	• Euphoria • ↑Sexuality • ↓Sleep • Distractibility • Agitation/Anxiety • Psychosis • Violent behavior • SI/HI • ↑Autonomic (HR, BP, RR, Temp, diaphoresis) • Mydriasis • Myoclonus • Tremors • ↑Seizure risk	• Dysphoria • Anhedonia • Insomnia • ↓Concentration • Irritability • ↑Appetite *Duration: 1–4 wks, if chronic long-term user can last for months	**Intoxication** • Anxiety/panic/agitation → benzodiazepines (PO, IM, or IV) • Psychosis → 1st/2nd-generation antipsychotic (PO, IM, or IV) • **"5-2-50"** = IM 5 mg haloperidol, 2 mg lorazepam, 50 mg diphenhydramine for severe acute agitation (i.e., acute risk of harm to self or others); aka "HAC" where 1 mg of Cogentin (benztropine) is substituted for diphenhydramine **Withdrawal** • Supportive treatment **Use Disorder** • Use motivational interviewing to determine patient's goals • Pharm: No FDA approved treatments, some evidence for mirtazapine • Psycho-social: CBT, contingency management, mutual support groups

(Continued)

TABLE 13.2 • Recreational Substances: Intoxication, Withdrawal, and Treatment (*Continued*)

Substance	Intoxication	Withdrawal	Treatment

Opioids	• Pupillary constriction
	• Drowsiness
	• Coma
	• Slurred speech
	• Impairment of attention/memory
		• Dysphoria
		• Irritability
		• Nausea/vomiting
		• Diarrhea
		• Fever
		• Muscle aches
		• Rhinorrhea/lacrimation
		• Piloerection (goosebumps)
		• Diaphoresis
		• Insomnia
		• Yawning
		*Can be assessed with COWS (Clinical Opioid Withdrawal Scale)
		Overdose signs
		= CPR+3HYPOs
		• Coma
		• Pinpoint pupils
		• Respiratory depression
		• Hypotension
		• Hypothermia
		• Hyporeflexia
			Intoxication
			Life-threatening overdose → initiate CPR + IV naloxone (IM, SubQ, or intranasal if no IV access)
			• If no initial response continue CPR
			• Should see resolution of symptoms within 2–3 minutes
			• May need repeat dose if no response after 2–3 minutes
			Goal = adequate ventilation
			• If RR ≥ 12 & O_2 sat ≥ 90% RA → observe w/ freq rechecks
			• If O_2 sat <90% RA but breathing spontaneously → supplemental O_2 + naloxone
			• If apneic → ventilate using bag-valve mask + supplemental O_2 + naloxone
			• If no response after 5–10 mg naloxone → intubate + reconsider diagnosis
			Withdrawal
			• Management with opioids OR non-opioids
			  - Opioids: Methadone 10–20 mg IM, buprenorphine 4–8 mg SL
			  - Non-opioids: Clonidine 0.1–0.3 mg q1h not to exceed 1.2 mg per 24 hrs
			• Supportive management of other symptoms
			  - Nausea/vomiting → promethazine, ondansetron
			  - Diarrhea → loperamide
			  - Anxiety → diazepam
			  - Insomnia → mirtazapine
			Use Disorder
			• Use motivational interviewing to determine patient's goals
			• Pharm: Medication assisted treatment (MAT); methadone or buprenorphine
			• Harm reduction by prescribing rescue naloxone
			• Psychosocial: CBT, contingency management mutual support groups, random drug screening, patient and patient family education

KEY MEDICATIONS & INTERVENTIONS

TABLE 13.3 · Antidepressant Medications

Class	Drug: Generic (Trade Name)	Mechanism of Action	Use	Side Effects
Selective serotonin reuptake inhibitor (SSRI)	fluoxetine (Prozac) sertraline (Zoloft) escitalopram (Lexapro)	Serotonin-specific reuptake inhibitor	Depression, OCD, panic, anxiety, PTSD	• Nausea, diarrhea, sexual dysfunction, GI bleeds (platelet inhibition), hyponatremia (especially in the elderly), possible initial increase in anxiety • Withdrawal symptoms when stop (especially fluoxetine, which has a long half life) • Fluoxetine/sertraline: CYP450 inhibitors
Serotonin-norepi-nephrine reuptake inhibitor (SNRI)	venlafaxine (Effexor) duloxetine (Cymbalta) desvenlafaxine (Pristiq)	Serotonin + norepineph-rine reuptake inhibitor	Depression, anxiety. Venlafaxine also used for fibromyalgia and chronic pain	• Nausea, sexual dysfunction, hypertension at higher doses • Desvenlafaxine = active metabolite of venlafaxine
Tricyclic antidepres-sant (TCA)	amitriptyline (Elavil) clomipramine (Anafranil) nortriptyline (Pamelor) imipramine (Tofranil) doxepin (Sinequan)	Serotonin + norepineph-rine reuptake inhibitor	Depression Amitriptyline and nortriptyline also used for chronic pain; imipramine also used for enuresis and panic disorder; clomipramine also used for OCD (1st line)	• Anticholinergic: Sedation, hypotension, dry mouth, constipation, urinary retention • May slow the electrical conduction in the heart and cause a prolonged QTc. Check ECG before initiating treatment. • Overdose = lethal **3Cs:** Convulsion (seizure), **Co**ma, **Ca**rdiotoxicity. Treatment: IV sodium bicarb

(Continued)

TABLE 13.3 · Antidepressant Medications (*Continued*)

Class	Drug: Generic (Trade Name)	Mechanism of Action	Use	Side Effects
Monoamine oxidase inhibitors (MAOI)	phenelzine (Nardil) isocarboxazid (Marplan) tranylcypromine (Parnate) selegiline (Emsam)	MAO Inhibitor (↑serotonin, norepinephrine, dopamine)	Depression in patients who had a poor response to at least 2 other antidepressants. Atypical depression (overeating, oversleeping, often in younger patients), phobias	<u>Hypertensive crisis</u>: Can occur within 30 minutes of ingesting tyramine containing foods (aged cheese, aged meats, wine, fava beans). Treatment: Phentolamine, nitroprusside <u>Serotonin syndrome</u>: • Risk factors: Increased risk with >1 serotonergic agent. Often occurs when MAOI is combined with an SSRI, SNRI, linezolid, or antiemetic. • Onset: Acute, typically within 24 hours of ingestion • Symptoms: Autonomic dysfunction (increased HR, increased temperature, sweating, diarrhea), neuromuscular excitation (clonus, hyperreflexia, hypertonicity, rigidity), altered mental status, catatonia. In severe cases, can lead to rhabdomyolysis and renal failure. • Treatment: Stop the offending medication. Provide supportive treatment. Can consider the use of anticonvulsants and benzodiazepines for agitation/muscle rigidity.
Atypical Antidepressants	bupropion (Wellbutrin)	↑norepinephrine, dopamine	Atypical depression	• Overstimulation, insomnia, dry mouth • Lowers seizure threshold: Avoid in epilepsy, eating disorders
	mirtazapine (Remeron)	Blocks multiple receptors: serotonin, α receptors, histamine	Depression, anxiety	• Sedation, weight gain (good for elderly and cancer patients where weight gain is desired)
	trazodone (Desyrl)	Blocks serotonin reuptake	Most often used as non-addictive sleep aids, although sometimes also for depression	• Priapism, sexual dysfunction • Orthostatic hypotension
	vilazodone (Viibryd)	Inhibits serotonin reuptake + has partial 5-HT1A agonism		• Dizziness
	vortioxetine (Trintellix)	Inhibits serotonin reuptake + has full 5-HT1A agonism, partial 5-HT1B agonism + 5-HT3 antagonism		• Nausea, vomiting, constipation

TABLE 13.4 · Antipsychotic Medications

Class	Drug : Generic (Trade Name)	Mechanism of Action	Use	Side Effects
Typical/ 1st Generation	chlorpromazine (Thorazine) fluphenazine (Prolixin) haloperidol (Haldol) perphenazine (Trilafon)	Block D2 dopamine receptor	Schizophrenia (+ symptoms), delirium, Tourette's	• Sedation, orthostatic hypotension, anticholinergic side effects • Metabolic side effects (weight gain, hyperlipidemia, ↑HgA1c) • QTc prolongation, heart block • Hyperprolactinemia <u>Extrapyramidal symptoms (EPS):</u> Abnormal movements and/or tone – Acute dystonia (min–hrs: spasm, twist). Tx: Benztropine (anticholinergic), diphenhydramine (antihistamine) – Akathisia (days–wks). Tx: Lorazepam, propranolol. – Parkinsonism (wks–months). Tx: Benztropine, amantadine. – Tardive dyskinesia (months–years). Tx: Stop medication, can be irreversible. <u>Neuroleptic malignant syndrome (NMS):</u> • Definition: Rare reaction to antipsychotic drug that causes autonomic instability and rigidity • Onset: Subacute, typically within one week of drug initiation • Symptoms: Severe "lead pipe" rigidity, autonomic dysfunction (elevated HR, BP, RR, temp), nausea/vomiting, altered mental status. Make have leukocytosis, elevated CK • Treatment: Stop the offending medication. Provide supportive treatment. Can consider the use of benzodiazepines and dantrolene if severe
Atypical/ 2nd Generation	clozapine (Clozaril) olanzapine (Zyprexa) quetiapine (Seroquel) risperidone (Risperdal) aripiprazole (Abilify) ziprasidone (Geodon)	Block D2 dopamine + 5HT2A serotonin receptor	Schizophrenia (+/– symptoms), bipolar disorder, OCD, depression	1st and 2nd generation are equally effective at reducing psychotic symptoms. EPS is less common with 2nd generation drugs and thus preferred. Drug-specific side effects by medication: • Clozapine: Agranulocytosis, seizure, weight gain, myocarditis • Olanzapine: Weight gain (monitor lipids, glucose at 3 months) • Quetiapine: Weight gain, sedative • Risperidone: Hyperprolactinemia • Aripiprazole: Weight neutral, less risk of metabolic SEs, partial dopamine agonist • Ziprasidone: QT prolongation (monitor EKG)

Drug: Generic (Trade Name)	Mechanism of action	Use	Side Effects
lithium	Stimulates the NMDA receptor, increasing glutamate availability in the postsynaptic neuron. Renally cleared.	Bipolar disorder Lithium blood levels: Safe level is 0.6–1.2 mEq/L Acute: 1–1.5 mEq/L; Chronic 0.6–1.2 mEq/L	• Movement/tremor • Nephrogenic DI (check Cr) • Hyp**O**thyroidism (check TSH) • Pregnancy (♥Ebstein's anomaly of tricuspid leaflets) • Toxic in deliberate overdose • Side effects by level of lithium elevation: - 1.5–2.5 mEq/L: Tremor, nausea. Tx: IV fluids. - 2.5–3.5 mEq/L: Renal failure. Tx: Dialysis. - 3.5+ mEq/L: Coma, cardiac collapse, death. Tx: Dialysis.
valproate (Depakote)	Precise mechanism of action unclear – may affect GABA levels and/or block Na⁺ channels	Bipolar disorder – Acute mania (Load 20 mg/kg/d) or for chronic bipolar disorder if lithium contraindicated	• Sedation, nausea, diarrhea, weight gain, hair loss • Hepatic toxicity (check LFTs); pancreatitis • Pregnancy: Neural tube defects • Non-toxic in deliberate overdose
carbamazepine	Blocks Na⁺ channel	Bipolar disorder, trigeminal neuralgia	• Agranulocytosis, aplastic anemia • Liver injury (check LFTs) • Teratogenic
lamotrigine (Lamictal)	Blocks Na⁺ channel	Bipolar disorder	• Steven Johnson syndrome (rare, although drug rash is relatively common)

TABLE 13.5 • Mood Stabilizing Medications

TABLE 13.6 · Anxiolytic Medications

Onset of action (indication)	Drugs and select details

Rapid-acting (i.e., for treatment of acute anxiety)	• Benzodiazapines (potentiate GABA)
	  - Long-acting: diazepam (Valium), clonazepam (Klonopin)
	  - Intermediate-acting: alprazolam (Xanax), lorazepam (Ativan), oxazepam (Serax), temazepam (Restoril)
	  - Short acting: triazolam (Halcion), midazolam (Versed) used in medical/surgical settings
	    • Side effects: Less motor coordination (careful in elderly), abuse, dependence
	    • Overdose: Respiratory depression. Treatment: Flumazenil.
	    • Withdrawal: Can cause seizures
	• Antipsychotics (e.g., quetiapine, olanzapine) can also be used to treat anxiety
	• Propranolol (Inderal): Often used for anxiety related to public speaking

Long-acting (i.e., for treatment of chronic anxiety)	• Buspirone (BuSpar) - 5-HT$_{1A}$ and 5-HT$_2$ partial agonist. Does not act on GABA. Most commonly used for generalized anxiety disorder • Serotonergic antidepressants can also help with chronic anxiety in addition to depression • Anticonvulsants: pregabalin (Lyrica), gabapentin (Neurontin) are often used for anxiety in clinical practice, although they are not approved for that use

KEY CLINICAL TRIALS & PUBLICATIONS

Major Depressive Disorder

- **STAR*D Study**. *Cleve Clin J Med* 2008;75(1):57–66.
  - The Sequenced Treatment Alternatives to Relieve Depression study evaluated treatment strategies for depression and produced the sequential treatment algorithm frequently used in clinical practice.
- **Efficacy and safety of ECT in depressive disorders.** *Lancet* 2003;361(9360):799–808.
  - Systematic overview and meta-analysis of randomized clinical trials and observational studies evaluating the efficacy and safety of electroconvulsive therapy (ECT) for patients with depressive illness. Concluded ECT is an effective short-term treatment for depression (bilateral > unilateral, high dose > low dose) and likely more effective than drug therapy.

Bipolar Disorder

- **The STEP-BD Trial.** *N Engl J Med* 2007;356:1711–1722.
  - Double-blind, placebo-controlled, randomized clinical trial assessing the use of a mood stabilizer plus an antidepressant vs. a mood stabilizer alone for reducing bipolar depression symptoms (without increasing the risk of mania). Combined therapy did not demonstrate increased efficacy and demonstrated similar rates of treatment-emergent affective switch.
- **BALANCE Trial.** *Lancet* 2010;375(9712):385–95.
  - Open-label, randomized clinical trial evaluating lithium monotherapy, valproic acid (VPA) monotherapy, and combination therapy in the treatment of bipolar disorder. Lithium monotherapy or lithium + VPA > VPA monotherapy. Results could neither confirm nor refute a benefit of lithium + VPA compared to lithium alone.

Antipsychotic Medications

- **CATIE Study (Phase 1).** *N Engl J Med* 2005;353:1209–1223.
  - Double-blind, randomized clinical trial that compared the use of a first-generation antipsychotic (perphenazine) with several newer drugs ("atypical" or "second-generation" antipsychotics) in patients with schizophrenia. The efficacy of perphenazine was similar to that of quetiapine, risperidone, and ziprasidone; however, the majority of patients in each group discontinued treatment due to inefficacy or side effects.

Panic Disorder

- **CBT, imipramine, or their combination for panic disorder.** *JAMA* 2000;283(19):2529–2536.
  - Randomized, double-blind, placebo-controlled trial, which concluded that combination CBT + imipramine conferred substantial advantage over either treatment alone over the long term.

Delirium

- **A double-blind trial of haloperidol, chlorpromazine, and lorazepam in the treatment of delirium in hospitalized AIDS patients.** *Am J Psychiatry* 1996;153(2):231–237.
  - Double blind clinical trial that demonstrated that low-dose neuroleptics could be used to treat symptoms of delirium in medically hospitalized patients with HIV/AIDS, whereas lorazepam was ineffective. This trial provided foundational evidence for the use of anti-psychotics in patients with delirium.

Dementia

- **Risk of death with atypical anti-psychotic treatment for dementia.** *JAMA* 2005;294(15):1934–1943.
  - Meta-analysis of 15 randomized clinical trials that used atypical antipsychotics to treat patients with Alzheimer's disease or dementia (3353 patients randomized to study drug; 1757 randomized to placebo). Concluded that atypical antipsychotic drugs may be associated with a small increased risk of death compared to placebo.

Substance Use Disorders and Treatments

- **Methadone maintenance vs. 180-day psychosocially enriched detoxification for treatment of opioid dependence: A randomized controlled trial.** *JAMA* 2000;283(10):1303–1310.
  - Randomized clinical trial that demonstrated that methadone maintenance therapy results in greater treatment retention and lower heroin use rates than detoxification.
- **COMBINE Study.** *JAMA* 2006;295(17):2003–2017.
  - Randomized clinical trial that demonstrated that naltrexone and/or therapy/social interventions are effective in the treatment of alcohol use disorder, whereas acamprosate showed no evidence of efficacy in this trial.

NOTES

Practical Skills for Learners

Early in training, writing an H&P can sometimes seem overwhelming. Developing a consistent approach, particularly to the HPI, can help reduce the time required for documentation and be useful for keeping a mental checklist during the patient encounter to make sure you're collecting all the necessary information.

TABLE A1.1 · Aspects of an Admission Note for Internal Medicine ("H&P")

1. Chief complaint (or chief concern)
2. History of present illness (HPI)
3. Past medical history (PMH)
4. Past surgical history (PSH)
5. Medications
6. Allergies
7. Family history (FHx)
8. Social history (SoHx; information about the person as an individual and their unique life story) and health-related behaviors (HRB; behaviors that change risk profiles for pathology)
9. Physical exam (PE)
10. Labs/data
11. Problem representation (a description of the patient's presentation that highlights the defining features of a case, helping the clinician to summarize their thoughts and create a differential diagnosis).
12. Assessment & Plan (A&P; a plan by problem for the patient's diagnostic and therapeutic work-up)

Now, let's break down each section and provide some specific guidance:

Chief Complaint and History of Present Illness (HPI)

TABLE A1.2 · Chief Complaint and History of Present Illness (HPI)

→ The **chief complaint (or chief concern)** is traditionally described using the patient's own words	**CC:** "I'm short of breath"
→ The **one-liner** should include pertinent prior diagnoses, and can include key information to characterize disease severity (e.g., stage of cancer, most recent echo result, key medications for a disease)	**HPI:** The patient is a 76-year-old man with a history of HTN, HLD, HFrEF (LVEF 30% in 02/2018), who presents with dyspnea for one week.
→ The **1st paragraph** of the HPI can be scaffolded as: **At baseline,** [baseline function]. **He was in usual state of health until** [number of days prior to admission] **at which time he noted onset of** [acuity] [symptom], **with associated** [other symptoms]. [Course over following days]. **On the day of admission,** [reason for coming to hospital].	**At baseline,** the patient can walk 6–8 blocks before developing dyspnea and sleeps with a single pillow. **He was in his usual state of health until** 8 days prior to presentation, **at which time he noted onset of** slow, progressive swelling in his lower extremities **with associated** 4 lbs increase in his weight. In the following 2–3 days, the patient developed onset of a cough productive of frothy sputum, worsening lower extremity swelling, dyspnea on exertion, and a two pillow orthopnea. He attempted to double his home dose of furosemide without improvement in his symptoms. **On the day of admission,** the patient noted his dyspnea occurring after walking 15–20 feet, prompting him to activate EMS.

(Continued)

TABLE A1.2 · Chief Complaint and History of Present Illness (HPI) (*Continued*)	
→ The 2nd paragraph of the HPI includes pertinent negatives from the ROS, as well as historical information about etiology if the condition has a trigger (such as an episode of acute decompensated heart failure).	The patient denies chest pain or diaphoresis. He denies fevers, chills, or sputum production. He denies recent sick contacts. He endorses having access to all his medications. He has attempted to eat as recommended by his cardiologist but notes that a neighbor had recently brought him a casserole which "tasted salty" and that he has been eating it intermittently throughout the week.
→ The 3rd paragraph of the HPI includes the ED course. Common elements are triage vital signs, key initial findings, and what the ED has already done. This is one style of many; at some institutions, this information goes immediately before the assessment and plan.	In the ED, triage VS were T 37.2, HR 90, BP 90/60, RR 22, SpO2 90% on room air. Initial work-up revealed Cr 1.4, BNP 1600. Troponin and ECG were unremarkable, and CXR was consistent with pulmonary edema. The patient was given furosemide 40 mg IV and admitted to cardiology for management of suspected ADHF.
→ The 4th paragraph of the HPI provides a deep dive into the past medical history, and can be started with, "In regards to his [organ system or pathology] history . . . "	In regards to his cardiac history, the patient was diagnosed with HFrEF in 2018, at which time he was admitted to this hospital for dyspnea on exertion. At that time, TTE revealed LVEF 30% with wall motion abnormalities, and LHC performed that admission revealed stenosis of LAD (90%), LCx (80%).

Additional History

TABLE A1.3 · PMH, PSH, Meds, Allergies, FHx, SoHx	
→ Past Medical History: List all of the patient's medical conditions. Note that here you typically list all conditions, whereas in the one liner you can list the ones that are most pertinent to the presentation. For certain conditions, you can list additional info here as well.	PMH: • HFrEF (LVEF 30% in 02/2018) • Hypertension • Hyperlipidemia • GERD • Depression
→ Past Surgical History: List all prior surgeries. Careful documentations of prior abdominal surgeries is particularly important when the patient is presenting with abdominal pain.	PSH: • S/p cholecystectomy (1994) • S/p tonsillectomy (1965)
→ Medications: List all medications, including herbs and supplements if applicable. List doses and frequency of each medication. Can group medications by organ system to help organize the list (e.g., here, cardiac medications are listed first).	Medications: • Furosemide 40 mg PO daily • Metoprolol succinate 25 mg PO daily • Lisinopril 5 mg PO daily • Atorvastatin 40 mg PO daily • Omeprazole 40 mg PO daily • Fluoxetine 10 mg PO daily
→ Allergies: List the patient's allergies. Ask the patient what reaction occurred with each case and indicate if possible, as some allergies are more severe than others.	Allergies: • Penicillins (rash as a child, no recent rechallenge)
→ Family History: Document the patient's family history. Start by asking about what is most relevant to the case (e.g., does anyone in your family have a history of heart disease?). Then document the medical history of first degree relatives as well, at minimum. If possible, indicate the age at diagnosis for certain medical conditions (e.g., heart disease, cancer).	FHx: • Father with CAD (diagnosed in his 50s) • Mother with HTN, DM2 • Paternal grandfather with CAD, heart failure • Son with colon cancer (diagnosed in 40s)

(Continued)

TABLE A1.3 • PMH, PSH, Meds, Allergies, FHx, SoHx *(Continued)*

→ Social History: For the social history, include information about the patient as an individual, their unique life story, and relevant health-related behaviors (HRB; behaviors that change risk profiles for pathology). → For elderly patients, indicate whether they are independent in activities of daily living (ADLs: Feeding, continence, transferring, toileting, dressing, bathing) and/or instrumental activities of daily living (iADLs: Using the telephone, shopping, preparing food, housekeeping, doing laundry, using transportation, handling medications, handling finances). It is important to know their baseline functional status to provide the best care for them in the hospital and also to assist with discharge planning.	SoHx: • Born in San Francisco, has lived here his whole life • Lives in the Sunset District with his husband • Previously worked as a math teacher, retired for 15 years • Never smoker • 1–2 alcoholic drinks/week • No other drug use • Enjoys hiking, sailing, and reading • At baseline, completely ambulatory and independent in ADLs/iADLs

Physical Exam, Labs, and Other Data

TABLE A1.4 • Physical Exam, Labs, and Other Data

→ Physical Exam: List vital signs, can indicate vital sign trends if relevant. → Perform and document your physical examination, focusing in particular on organ systems that are relevant to the patient's presentation. General = how the patient looks from the doorway—do they look well or are they ill-appearing? It is helpful to document a baseline neurologic exam for all patients, particularly elderly patients who are at higher risk for hospital-induced delirium.	PE: 37.2°F, HR 90, BP 90/60 → 100/65, RR, 90% RA → 94% 2L General: Elderly man in moderate distress, able to speak in short sentences only HEENT: NCAT, moist mucous membranes CV: RRR, no murmur, rubs, gallops Pulm: Crackles at the lung bases bilaterally Abd: Soft, NT, ND. No hepatosplenomegaly Extrem: 2+ pitting edema to the knees Skin: No rashes Neuro: AO×3, alert and conversant, grossly intact
→ Labs/Data: Present the labs, imaging, and microbiology. For abnormal labs, include the trends (e.g,. for hemoglobin, platelets, Cr). Present imaging from admission, or recent imaging or data if relevant.	Labs/Data: WBC 9.0, Hg 12, Plt 250 Na 134, K 3.9, Cl 105, HCO3 25, BUN 34, Cr 1.4 from a baseline 1.0 BUN 1600 (previous admissions in 800 range) Trop <0.02 ECG normal sinus rhythm CXR bilateral small pleural effusions and patchy opacities consistent with pulmonary edema

The Assessment and Plan (A&P)

The assessment and plan (A&P) is the most important part of the H&P (and the oral presentation). It shows that you can put the pieces of your history and physical exam together and form a problem representation, discuss a differential diagnosis, and come up with a plan for how to care for the patient.

TABLE A1.5 · The Assessment and Plan	
→ The **problem representation** is a description of the patient's presentation that highlights the defining features of a case, helping the clinician to summarize their thoughts and create a differential diagnosis. → The first problem listed should always be the most important/critical issue (i.e., the indication for admission). One way to organize the paragraph is as follows: • Sentence 1 (if needed): Summarize presenting symptom and severity • Sentence 2: His hypoxia is most likely due to X because... In this case, also identify a suspected trigger for his heart failure exacerbation • Sentence 3: Discuss other conditions on the differential diagnosis and why they seem less likely → Organize the "to do's" into diagnostic vs. therapeutic groups, as it is easier for the reader to follow	**Assessment & Plan:** 76M with a history of HTN, HLD, HFrEF (LVEF 30% in 02/2018) who presents with one week of dyspnea, found to have evidence of volume overload concerning for a heart failure exacerbation. **# Dyspnea** **# HFrEF, acute on chronic with exacerbation** The patient presented with 1 week of dyspnea requiring 2 L O2 on admission. His hypoxia is most likely due to an exacerbation of his heart failure given PND, orthopnea, pitting edema, pulmonary edema on CXR, and elevated BNP; suspect his heart failure was triggered by dietary changes. Hypoxia less likely due to ACS given normal ECG and negative troponin, and there is also no evidence of infection given he is afebrile without leukocytosis. *Diagnostics:* • F/u final read of CXR (prelim: Pulmonary edema) • F/u respiratory viral panel *Treatment:* • Admit to floor • S/p 40 mg IV furosemide in the ED; given an additional 40 mg IV this morning • Neurohormonal blockade: Continue home metoprolol succinate 25 mg PO daily, lisinopril 5 mg daily • Strict ins/outs and daily weights
→ Add other problems based on other symptoms the patient is reporting, vital sign abnormalities, physical exam findings, lab/imaging abnormalities, and chronic medication conditions. If it is a more complex problem, can organize as described above for the first problem, including the diagnostic and treatment steps. If the problem is more straightforward, can just list the necessary information. To be complete, every medication you prescribe should be associated with a problem on the list.	**# Acute kidney injury** On admission, patient with Cr 1.4 up from a baseline 1.0. Suspect pre-renal due to heart failure with poor forward flow. Reassuring that Cr improving s/p diuresis to 1.2 today. • Continue diuresis as above • Continue to monitor Cr • Avoid nephrotoxins **# HTN** • Continue home metoprolol succinate 25 mg PO daily, lisinopril 5 mg PO daily **# HLD** • Continue home atorvastatin 40 mg PO daily **# GERD** • Continue home omeprazole 40mg PO daily **# Depression** • Continue home fluoxetine 10mg PO daily
→ **The inpatient bundle:** At the end of the note indicate whether the patient requires DVT prophylaxis, their diet, their IV access, and their code status. Indicate who you discussed code status with and when if possible.	**# Inpatient bundle** • Telemetry: Yes, during IV diuresis • Continuous pulse oximetry: Yes • Diet: Cardiac diet • Access: PIVs • Contact: Name, number, and relationship to patient • Code status: Full code (confirmed with patient on admission) *Signature of healthcare provider* *Role on team and/or year of training* Date

HOW TO CALL A CONSULT

- Consult question: In general, consults should be structured around a *specific question* in regard to a patient's care (e.g., Should this patient with melena undergo inpatient endoscopic evaluation? Should this patient with suspected DAH in the presence of rheumatologic disease receive high dose steroids?")
- Consult timing: Practice patterns differ across institutions, however when possible non-urgent consults should generally be made early in the day to allow consulting teams to plan their day's workflow.
- Consult template: A template for paging a consultant is provided in Table A1.6.

TABLE A1.6 · How to Write a Page to a Consultant

Example:
CONSULT: 55M h/o osteoarthritis (on home NSAIDS, no PPI) p/w melena for 4 days- VSS, Hg 6 from baseline 10. Should this patient undergo inpatient colonoscopy? -Name, Medicine intern, *x: 33333
*t: 999-999-9999 *p: 444-4444

Elements:
- Label as a new consult
- Abbreviated one-liner
- Specific consult question (indicate urgency if needed)
- Your name and role on the team
- Multiple ways to call back (especially important if your consultants rotate at multiple hospitals), such as your extension (*x), telephone number (*t), and pager number (*p)

HOW TO PRE-ROUND

- Purpose of pre-rounding: Pre-rounding refers to the activity of gathering data prior to rounds, typically including 24 hour and overnight events, nursing updates/concerns, the patient's subjective report, vital signs, physical exam, labs, and other test results. Gathering this data allows you to formulate a plan for each patient that you can present on rounds.
- Pre-rounding template: An example template for pre-rounding is provided in Table A1.7.

TABLE A1.7 · Pre-rounding Template

PATIENT:	A&P:	☐
24 hour events/subjective:		☐
		☐
		☐
		☐
		☐
Tm HR BP RR O$_2$		☐
In /Out		☐
Physical exam:		☐
✕ +++ ✕		☐
Micro:		
Imaging:		
PATIENT:	**A&P:**	☐
24 hour events/subjective:		☐
		☐
		☐
		☐
		☐
Tm HR BP RR O$_2$		☐
In /Out		☐
Physical exam:		☐
✕ +++ ✕		☐
Micro:		
Imaging:		

DAILY PRESENTATIONS AND NOTES

How to Do Daily Presentations and Notes

- Format: Typically, daily presentations about each patient are presented in a **"SOAP"** note format.
  - Typically mention 24-hour events first
  - **S**: **S**ubjective – What are the patient's symptoms today?
  - **O**: **O**bjective – Vitals, physical exam, ins/outs (if relevant), labs, new micro & imaging
  - **A/P**: **A**ssessment and **P**lan – Ensure that the patient one-liner is up to date! Then present by problem, e.g., problem 1: Sepsis, likely from a pulmonary source; problem 2: Diabetes

PREPARING A PATIENT FOR DISCHARGE

Discharge Checklist

- Approach to discharging a patient: Discharges from the hospital are a transition that creates a risk for breakdown in a patient's care. Table A1.8 provides a list of some important considerations to ensure a patient is ready for discharge. It is important to develop an approach to discharges that reflects the system at your institution, but we offer a possible template in Table A1.9.

TABLE A1.8 · Is the Patient Ready for Discharge?

1. Are all medications being administered PO (or is there a plan in place for ongoing IV medications, which often requires special access)?
2. Is the patient able to nourish themselves (typically by tolerating an oral diet, although in other cases may be by G-tube feeding, etc.)?
3. Has the patient passed stool in the last 24 hours (if needed, depending on the admission indication)?
4. Is the patient ambulating and/or at their physical baseline (if not, they likely require a physical therapy assessment)?
5. Does the patient have a ride home from the hospital (or has a plan been made to transport them home)?
6. Is the patient or family member comfortable with the management of any new devices or equipment they need to manage at home?

TABLE A1.9 · Discharge Checklist

☐ Follow-up appointment(s) booked or requested
☐ Discharge services ordered (e.g., home health services)
☐ Medication reconciliation (if possible, confirm that the patient's pharmacy has received the prescriptions and that the patient has the ability to access the new medications; for example, that they can get a ride to the pharmacy and can afford the co-pay associated with any new medications)
☐ Communication with multidisciplinary team
☐ Communication with primary care provider
☐ Discharge summary
☐ Huddle with bedside nurse (e.g., follow-up plans, plan for RN teaching on new devices or equipment, medication changes to highlight with patient, etc.)

Biostatistics

Types of Clinical Studies & Trials

- Case control study: Compares a group of patients with a disease ("cases") to a group of patients who do not have the disease ("controls"). Looks backward in time (i.e., a retrospective study) to determine if there is a difference in exposure to a potential risk factor between cases and controls. Generates an odds ratio (OR). If an outcome is rare, the OR will be close to the risk ratio (RR) ("the rare disease assumption").
- Cohort study: Compares a cohort of patients who were exposed to a potential risk factor with a cohort of patients who were not exposed. May be prospective (follow the two cohorts and compare disease incidence) or retrospective (review records of disease incidence for each cohort).
- Cross-sectional study: "Prevalence study": A snapshot in time with both exposure and outcome measured simultaneously; may establish association but not causation.
- Clinical trial types: Sample and control group
  - <u>Parallel design</u>: Randomizes one treatment to one group and a different treatment to another group (e.g., treatment vs. placebo)
  - <u>Factorial design</u>: Randomizes to different interventions with additional study of two or more variables (e.g., treatment vs. placebo, and in each group also studying one heart rate goal vs. another)
  - <u>Cross-over design</u>: One group randomized to treatment A and another group randomized to treatment B, the treatment received are reversed in the second half of the study
- Clinical trial phases:
  - <u>Phase I</u>: A small number of healthy volunteer participants (or sometimes volunteer participants with the disease of interest, depending on the context), aiming to determine the highest dose of the drug humans can take without serious side effects
  - <u>Phase II</u>: A new drug is given to a small number of volunteer participants with the disease of interest, aiming to determine the preliminary safety and efficacy of the new drug
  - <u>Phase III</u>: A new drug is given to a larger number of volunteer participants with the disease of interest. Participants are typically randomized to receive the new drug/treatment vs. the standard or care or a placebo. The US FDA typically requires a phase III trial before approving a new medication
  - <u>Phase IV</u>: Post-marketing surveillance

Biases

Recruitment

- Selection bias: Bias in selecting the study group. Subtypes: Attrition bias (participants lost to follow-up), non-response bias (can occur with surveys when low response rate), selection bias

Study execution

- Recall bias: Inaccurate recall of past events by patients; common in case-control studies
- Observer bias: Observer may be influenced by prior knowledge or details of the study that affect the results; mitigated by blinding
- Measurement bias: Poor data collection, inaccurate results

Data/result interpretation

- Confounding bias: At least part of the exposure-disease relationship can be explained by another variable
- Susceptibility bias: Treatment regimen is selected for a patient based on the severity of their condition without considering confounders
- Lead time bias: One intervention may diagnose a disease earlier than another intervention, but there is no change in mortality; however, the earlier detection makes it seem like the intervention prolongs survival

- Pygmalion effect: The researcher's expectation of an outcome influences the study; well-established, particularly in psychological or education studies
- Hawthorne effect: The impact on study participants of knowing that they are being monitored or "watched," i.e., the knowledge of being studied affects compliance to a medication and other aspects of a study

STATISTICAL CONCEPTS AND TEST CHARACTERISTICS

Odds Ratio, Risk Ratio, and Related Statistics

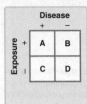

FIGURE A2.1: A 2 × 2 table that compares the presence of disease vs. a given exposure (e.g., disease- lung cancer, exposure- smoking). The columns indicate whether the disease is present (+) or absent (−). The rows indicate whether the exposure is present (+) or absent (−). This table can be used to calculate the odds ratio, risk ratio, and attributable risk – See Table A2.1.

TABLE A2.1 · Common Biostatistics Terms and Formulas		
Term	**Formula***	**Description**
Odds ratio (OR)	$\dfrac{AD}{BC}$	Ratio of odds of an event in one group (e.g., exposed group) versus the odds of the event in the other group (e.g., nonexposed group)
Risk ratio (RR)	$\dfrac{\dfrac{A}{A+B}}{\dfrac{C}{C+D}}$	Ratio of risk of an event in one group (e.g., exposed group) versus the risk of the event in the other group (e.g., nonexposed group)
Attributable risk (AR)	$\dfrac{A}{A+B} - \dfrac{C}{A+D}$	The difference between the risk of an outcome in one group (e.g., exposed group) and another group (e.g., non-exposed group); the portion of an outcome (e.g., disease) attributable to an exposure
Attributable risk percent	$\dfrac{RR-1}{RR}$	Attributable risk, expressed as a percentage
Number needed to harm (NNH)	$\dfrac{1}{ARR}$	How many people need to be exposed to a medication or risk factor in order for one person to have a particular adverse effect
Absolute risk reduction (ARR)	*%risk placebo − %risk treatment*	The difference between the risk of an outcome in a placebo group and a treatment group; the proportion of patients who are spared a particular adverse outcome as a result of a therapy
Number needed to treat (NNT)	$\dfrac{1}{ARR}$	How many people need to be exposed to a medication or therapy in order to have a particular beneficial impact on one person

* A, B, C, and D refer to the positions in the Risk/Disease 2 x 2 contingency table in Figure A2.1

Sensitivity, Specificity, Positive Predictive Value, and Negative Predictive Value

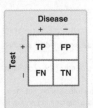

FIGURE A2.2: A 2 × 2 table that compares the presence of disease vs. the results of testing for the disease (e.g., disease- prostate cancer, test- PSA). The columns indicate whether the disease is present (+) or absent (−). The rows indicate whether the test result is positive (+) or negative (−). TP = True positive, FP = False positive, FN = False negative, TN = True negative. This table can be used to calculate sensitivity, specificity, positive predictive value, and negative predictive value. See formulas on the next page.

- Sensitivity = TP/(TP+FN)
  - The probability that when a disease is present, a diagnostic test will have a positive result
  - In other words, what proportion of all positive patients (i.e., TP + FN) will have a positive result?
  - Highly sensitive tests are less likely to miss cases (i.e., unlikely to have false negative results)
  - Therefore, ↑Sensitivity then ↑NPV
- Specificity = TN/(TN+FP)
  - The probability that when a disease is absent, a diagnostic test will have a negative result
  - In other words, what proportion of all negative patients (i.e., TN + FP) will have a negative result?
  - Highly specific tests are less likely to have false positive results
  - Therefore, ↓Specificity then ↓PPV
- Positive predictive value (PPV) = TP/(TP+FP)
  - The probability that a person who has a positive test result actually has a disease
  - In other words, what proportion of positive results are true positives?
- Negative predictive value (NPV) = TN/(TN+FN)
  - The probability that a person who has a negative test result actually does <u>not</u> have a disease
  - In other words, what proportion of negative results and true negatives?
  - If a disease is more prevalent, there is a higher PPV and lower NPV. Sensitivity and specificity are not affected by disease prevalence
- Likelihood ratio (+) = Sensitivity / (1-Specificity)
- Likelihood ratio (−) = (1-Sensitivity) / Specificity

Prevalence vs. Incidence

- Prevalence: Total cases in a population at a given time/total population (↓Prevalance can be due to more prevention or more treatment; ↑Prevalance if those living with the disease have a longer lifespan)
- Incidence: New cases/total in population at risk. Only prevention (not treatment) decreases incidence, since the total population *at-risk* excludes anyone who is already sick

Precision vs. Accuracy

- Precision/reliability: Does a test generate similar results on repeat measurements? Tests that have less random error are more precise/reliable. However, a test can yield consistent results (i.e., be highly precise), but generate results that are inaccurate
- Accuracy/validity: Does a test generate a result that is true or right (imagine: hitting a bullseye)?

Other Statistical Concepts and Formulas

- Standard deviation (SD): For normal distribution, 68% of results within one SD, 95% of results within two SDs, 99% of results within three SDs
- Standard error of the sample mean (SEM): $SD/\sqrt{n}$, where $n =$ sample size
- p-values: Probability that result achieved by chance, e.g., $p = 0.01$ means 1% probability that the result occurred by chance
- Confidence interval (CI): Mean $+/-$ Z(SEM); when $Z = 1.96$, calculates 95% CI
  - When comparing means, if the 95% CI includes 0, then there is no difference (assuming significance is a p-value <0.05)
  - When comparing OR or RR, if the 95% confidence interval includes 1, then there is no difference (assuming significance is a p-value <0.05)
- Comparing means:
  - **T**-test: Compares **T**wo means
  - <u>ANOVA</u>: Compares three or more means
- Comparing categorical variables:
  - **Ch**i²: Compares 2+ proportions (**C**ategorical variables)
- Error:
  - <u>Type I error (α)</u>: Stating that there is an effect when none exists ($\alpha <0.05$)
    - False positive rate = FP/(FP+TN)
  - <u>Type II error (β)</u>: Stating that there is not an effect when there really is one
    - False negative rate = FN/(FN+TP)
  - <u>Power (1-β)</u>: Probability of rejecting the null when it is false

NOTES

Abbreviations/ Acronyms

AAA	Abdominal aortic aneurysm		AVP	Arginine vasopressin
ABPA	Allergic bronchopulmonary aspergillosis		ABG	Arterial blood gas
			AAION	Arteritic anterior ischemic optic neuropathy
ACC	American College of Cardiology		AST	Aspartate aminotransferase
ACS	Acute coronary syndrome		ASA	Aspirin
ACTH	Adrenocorticotrophic hormone		A&P	Assessment and plan
ACEi	Angiotensin-converting enzyme inhibitor		Afib	Atrial fibrillation
ADEM	Acute disseminated encephalomyelitis		ASD	Atrial septal defect
ADPKD	Autosomal dominant polycystic kidney disease		AT	Atrial tachycardia
			AR	Attributable risk
ADH	Antidiuretic hormone		AIHA	Autoimmune hemolytic anemia
AEP	Acute eosinophilic pneumonia		AIP	Autoimmune pancreatitis
AFLP	Acute fatty liver of pregnancy		AVNRT	AV nodal reentrant tachycardia
AFP	Alpha-fetoprotein		AVRT	AV reentrant tachycardia
AGEP	Acute generalized exanthematous pustulosis		ANC	Absolute neutrophil count
			ARR	Absolute risk reduction
AIN	Acute interstitial nephritis		AK	Actinic keratosis
AIP	Acute interstitial pneumonia			
AKI	Acute kidney injury		BV	Bacterial vaginitis
ALF	Acute liver failure		BCC	Basal cell carcinoma
ALL	Acute lymphocytic leukemia		BMP	Basic metabolic panel
AML	Acute myeloid leukemia		BPPV	Benign paroxysmal positional vertigo
APML	Acute promyelocytic leukemia		BB	Beta blocker
ARDS	Acute respiratory distress syndrome		BDG	Beta-D-glucan test
ATN	Acute tubular necrosis		BiPAP	Bilevel positive airway pressure
AI	Adrenal insufficiency		BNP	B-type natriuretic peptide
AOSD	Adult-onset Still's disease			
ARMD	Age-related macular degeneration		CCB	Calcium channel blocker
ALT	Alanine transaminase		CPPD	Calcium pyrophosphate deposition arthropathies
AlkP	Alkaline phosphatase			
tPA	Alteplase		CEA	Carcinoembryonic antigen
AMS	Altered mental status		CRT	Cardiac resynchronization therapy
ALS	Amyotrophic lateral sclerosis		CAUTI	Catheter-associated UTI
AAV	ANCA-associated vasculitides		CCR5	C-C chemokine receptor type 5
ARB	Angiotensin receptor blocker		CLABSI	Central line–associated bloodstream infections
ARNI	Angiotensin receptor neprilysin inhibitor			
			CNS	Central nervous system
AS	Ankylosing spondylitis		CRAO	Central retinal artery occlusion
ANA	Antinuclear antibodies-associated connective tissue disorders		CRVO	Central retinal vein occlusion
			CVP	Central venous pressure
APLS	Antiphospholipid syndrome		CSF	Cerebrospinal fluid
ART	Antiretroviral therapy		CXR	Chest x-ray
AT	Anti-thrombin deficiency		CAR	Chimeric-antigen receptor-T cell therapy
AR	Aortic regurgitation			
AS	Aortic stenosis		CCK	Cholecystokinin

CEP	Chronic eosinophilic pneumonia
CKD	Chronic kidney disease
CLL	Chronic lymphocytic leukemia
CML	Chronic myeloid leukemia
COPD	Chronic obstructive pulmonary disease
CoA	Coarctation of the aorta
CRC	Colorectal cancer
CAP	Community-acquired pneumonia
CBC	Complete blood count
CT	Computed tomography
CI	Confidence interval
CAH	Congenital adrenal hyperplasia
CPAP	Continuous positive airway pressure
CRRT	Continuous renal replacement therapy
CABG	Coronary artery bypass graft
CAD	Coronary artery disease
CCTA	Coronary CT angiography
CBS	Corticobasal syndrome
CJD	Creutzfeldt-Jakob disease
CIM	Critical illness myopathy
CIP	Critical illness polyneuropathy
CrAg	Cryptococcal antigen
COP	Cryptogenic organizing pneumonia
CF	Cystic fibrosis
CRS	Cytokine release syndrome
CMV	Cytomegalovirus
DVT	Deep venous thrombosis
DM	Dermatomyositis
DIP	Desquamative interstitial pneumonia
DI	Diabetes insipidus
DM	Diabetes mellitus
DKA	Diabetic ketoacidosis
DISH	Diffuse idiopathic skeletal hyperostosis
DLBCL	Diffuse large B-cell lymphoma
DPP-4i	Dipeptidyl peptidase 4 inhibitors
DAT	Direct antiglobulin test
DLE	Discoid lupus erythematosus
DMARDs	Disease-modifying antirheumatic drugs
DGI	Disseminated gonococcal infection
DIC	Disseminated intravascular coagulation
DES	Drug-eluting stents
DIHS	Drug-induced hypersensitivity syndrome
ECG	Electrocardiography
EEG	Electroencephalogram
EFWC	Electrolyte-free water clearance
EMG	Electromyography
ETCO$_2$	End tidal CO$_2$
ERCP	Endoscopic retrograde cholangiopancreatography
EUS	Endoscopic ultrasound
ESRD	End-stage renal disease
EGPA	Eosinophilic granulomatosis with polyangiitis
EBV	Epstein-Barr virus
EN	Erythema nodosum
ESAs	Erythropoietin-stimulating agents
ET	Essential thrombocytopenia

eGFR	Estimated glomerular filtration rate
ERV	Expiratory reserve volume
ECMO	Extracorporeal membrane oxygenation
FAP	Familial adenomatous polyposis
FHx	Family history
FN	Febrile neutropenia
FUO	Fever of unknown origin
FNH	Focal nodular hyperplasia
FSGS	Focal segmental glomerulosclerosis
FECA	Fractional excretion of calcium
FFP	Fresh frozen plasma
GGT	Gamma-glutamyl transferase
GRP	Gastrin-releasing peptide
GERD	Gastroesophageal reflux disease
GIB	Gastrointestinal bleed
GU	Genitourinary
GDM	Gestational diabetes
GCA	Giant cell arteritis
GBM	Glioblastoma multiforme
GFR	Glomerular filtration rate
GN	Glomerulonephritis
GLP-1 RA	Glucagon-like peptide 1 receptor agonist
GRA	Glucocorticoid-remedial aldosteronism
G6PD	Glucose-6-phosphate dehydrogenase
GIP	Glucose-dependent insulinotropic peptide
GVHD	Graft vs. host disease
GPA	Granulomatosis with polyangiitis
CGOs	Ground glass opacities
GH	Growth hormone
GYN	Gynecologic
HF	Heart failure
HSC	Hematopoietic stem cell transplant
HD	Hemodialysis
HUS	Hemolytic uremic syndrome
HLH	Hemophagocytic lymphohistiocytosis
HSP	Henoch-Schönlein purpura
HIT	Heparin-induced thrombocytopenia
HE	Hepatic encephalopathy
HAV	Hepatitis A virus
HBV	Hepatitis B virus
HCV	Hepatitis C virus
HDV	Hepatitis D virus
HEV	Hepatitis E virus
HCC	Hepatocellular carcinoma
HRS	Hepatorenal syndrome
HNPCC	Hereditary nonpolyposis colorectal cancer
HSV	Herpes simplex virus
HDL	High-density lipoprotein
HFNC	High-flow nasal cannula
H2	Histamine-2 blocker
H&P	History and physical
HPI	History of present illness
HIVAN	HIV-associated nephropathy
HAP	Hospital-acquired pneumonia

HPV	Human papillomavirus		MR	Mitral regurgitation
HCl	Hydrochloric acid		MS	Mitral stenosis
HHS	Hyperosmolar hyperglycemic syndrome		MCTD	Mixed connective tissue disease
			MMR	(measle, mumps, rubella) vaccine
HP	Hypersensitivity pneumonitis		MELD	Model for End-Stage Liver Disease
HCM	Hypertrophic cardiomyopathy		MAOI	Monoamine oxidase inhibitor
			MGUS	Monoclonal gammopathy of undetermined significance
IBS	Irritable bowel syndrome			
IBD	Inflammatory bowel disease		MAT	Multifocal atrial tachycardia
ICD	Implantable cardioverter defibrillator		MEN	Multiple endocrine neoplasia syndromes
ICP	Increased intracranial pressure			
IC	Inspiratory capacity		MM	Multiple myeloma
ICU	Intensive care unit		MS	Multiple sclerosis
ICH	Intracerebral hemorrhage		MSA	Multiple system atrophy
IIPS	Idiopathic interstitial pneumonias		MAC	*Mycobacterium avium-intracellulare*
ILD	Interstitial lung disease		MTB	*Mycobacterium tuberculosis*
IMNM	Immune-mediated necrotizing myositis		MDS	Myelodysplastic syndrome
IMA	Inferior mesenteric artery		MAP	MYH-associated polyposis
INO	Inhaled nitric oxide			
INR	International Normalized Ratio		NAC	N-acetylcysteine
IRV	Inspiratory reserve volume		NK	Natural killer
ITP	Immune thrombocytopenic purpura		NMS	Neuroleptic malignant syndrome
IUD	Intrauterine device		NMBAs	Neuromuscular blocking agents
IVC	Inferior vena cava		NMO	Neuromyelitis optica
			PMNs	Neutrophils
JVP	Jugular venous pressure		NAFLD	Nonalcoholic fatty liver disease
			NASH	Nonalcoholic steatohepatitis
LBD	Lewy body dementia		NCHCT	Non-contrast head computed tomography
LDH	Lactic dehydrogenase			
LEMS	Lambert-Eaton myasthenic syndrome		NIPPV	Noninvasive positive pressure ventilation
LTBI	Latent tuberculosis			
LBBB	Left bundle branch block		NNRTIs	Nonnucleoside reverse transcriptase inhibitors
LVH	Left ventricular hypertrophy			
LCV	Leukocytoclastic vasculitis		NRB	Nonrebreather
LFTs	Liver function tests		NSCLC	Non-small cell lung cancer
LDL	Low-density lipoprotein		NSIP	Nonspecific interstitial pneumonia
LGIB	Lower GI bleed		NSTEMI	Non-ST elevation myocardial infarction
LMN	Lower motor neuron findings			
LMWH	Low-molecular weight heparin		NSAIDs	Nonsteroidal anti-inflammatory drugs
LP	Lumbar puncture		NTM	Non-tuberculous mycobacteria
LH	Luteinizing hormone deficiency		NPH	Normal pressure hydrocephalus
LAM	Lymphangioleiomyomatosis		NRTIs	Nucleoside reverse transcriptase inhibitors
LCMV	Lymphocytic choriomeningitis virus			
LIP	Lymphoid interstitial pneumonia		NHH	Number needed to harm
			NNT	Number needed to treat
MDF	Maddrey's discriminant function			
Mg^{2+}	Magnesium		OCD	Obsessive compulsive disorder
MRCP	Magnetic resonance cholangiopancreatography		OSA	Obstructive sleep apnea
			OR	Odds ratio
MRI	Magnetic resonance imaging		OIs	Opportunistic infections
MDD	Major depressive disorder		OA	Osteoarthritis
MODY	Maturity-onset diabetes of the young			
MAP	Mean arterial pressure		pRBCs	Packed red blood cells
MCV	Mean corpuscular volume		PNET	Pancreatic neuroendocrine tumors
MGN	Membranous glomerulopathy		PTH	Parathyroid hormone
MAHA	Microangiopathic hemolytic anemia		PNH	Paroxysmal nocturnal hemoglobinuria
MPA	Microscopic polyangiitis		PPT	Partial thromboplastin time
MRA	Mineralocorticoid receptor antagonist		PLR	Passive leg raise
MCG	Minimal change glomerulopathy		PMH	Past medial history

PSH	Past surgical history
PDA	Patent ductus arteriosus
PFO	Patent foramen ovale
PUD	Peptic ulcer disease
PCI	Percutaneous coronary intervention
PAD	Peripheral artery disease
PD	Peritoneal dialysis
phos	Phosphate
PPFE	Pleuroparenchymal fibroelastosis
PJP, PCP	*Pneumocystis jirovecii* pneumonia
POCUS	Point-of-care ultrasound
PAN	Polyarteritis nodosa
PCOS	Polycystic ovarian syndrome
PV	Polycythemia vera
PMR	Polymyalgia rheumatic
PM	Polymyositis
PEP	Post-exposure prophylaxis
PTSD	Post-traumatic stress disorder
PrEP	Pre-exposure prophylaxis
PC	Pressure control
PS	Pressure support
PACNS	Primary angiitis of the central nervous system
PBC	Primary biliary cholangitis
PSC	Primary sclerosis cholangitis
PML	Progressive multifocal leukoencephalopathy
PSP	Progressive supranuclear palsy
PRIS	Propofol-related infusion syndrome
PTU	Propylthiouracil
PIs	Protease inhibitors
PT	Prothrombin time
PPI	Proton pump inhibitor
PAP	Pulmonary alveolar proteinosis
PE	Pulmonary embolism
PFTs	Pulmonary function testing
PH	Pulmonary hypertension
PVR	Pulmonary vascular resistance
PPV	Pulse pressure variation
PEA	Pulseless electrical activity
PG	Pyoderma gangrenosum
RAI	Radioactive iodine
RPGN	Rapidly progressive glomerulonephritis
RBCs	Red blood cells
RBF	Renal blood flow
RCC	Renal cell carcinoma
RTA	Renal tubular acidosis
RAAS	Renin–angiotensin–aldosterone system
RV	Residual volume
RB-ILD	Respiratory bronchiolitis-associated ILD
RSV	Respiratory syncytial virus
RLS	Restless leg syndrome
ROSC	Return of spontaneous circulation
RA	Rheumatoid arthritis
RBBB	Right bundle branch block
RVH	Right ventricular hypertrophy
RR	Risk ratio

SANRT	SA node reentrant tachycardia
SRC	Scleroderma renal crisis
SK	Seborrheic keratosis
SSRI	Selective serotonin reuptake inhibitor
SOFA	Sequential organ failure assessment
SNRI	Serotonin norepinephrine reuptake inhibitor
SAAG	Serum ascites albumin gradient
SARS-CoV-2, COVID-19	Severe acute respiratory syndrome coronavirus 2
STIs	Sexually transmitted infections
ST	Sinus tachycardia
SSTIs	Skin and soft tissue infections
SCLC	Small cell lung cancer
SoHx	Social history
SGLT2i	Sodium-glucose cotransporter-2 inhibitor
SpA	Spondyloarthritis
SBP	Spontaneous bacterial peritonitis
SBT	Spontaneous breathing trial
SCC	Squamous cell carcinoma
STEMI	ST elevation myocardial infarction
SD	Standard deviation
SEM	Standard error of the sample mean
SSSS	Staphylococcal scalded skin syndrome
SJS	Stevens-Johnson syndrome
SAH	Subarachnoid hemorrhage
SDH	Subdural hematoma
SU	Sulfonylureas
SMA	Superior mesenteric artery
SVC	Superior vena cava
SVT	Supraventricular tachycardia
SIAD	Syndrome of inappropriate antidiuresis
SIADH	Syndrome of inappropriate antidiuretic hormone
SIRS	Systemic inflammatory response syndrome
SLE	Systemic lupus erythematosus
SSc	Systemic sclerosis
SVR	Systemic vascular resistance
TTM	Targeted temperature management
Tdap	Tetanus/diphtheria/pertussis
TZD	Thiazolidinedione
TMA	Thrombotic microangiopathy
TTP	Thrombotic thrombocytopenic purpura
TSH	Thyroid-stimulating hormone
TV	Tidal volume
tPA	Tissue plasminogen activator
Tbili	Total bilirubin
TLC	Total lung capacity
TEN	Toxic epidermal necrolysis
TEE	Transesophageal echocardiography
TACO	Transfusion-associated circulatory overload
TRALI	Transfusion-related acute lung injury
TIA	Transient ischemic attack

TIPS	Transjugular intrahepatic portosystemic shunt
TTE	Transthoracic echocardiography
TR	Tricuspid regurgitation
TCA	Tricyclic antidepressant
TACs	Trigeminal autonomic cephalgias
TG	Triglyceride
TNBC	Triple negative breast cancer
TLS	Tumor lysis syndrome
DM1	Type 1 diabetes
DM2	Type 2 diabetes
TKIs	Tyrosine kinase inhibitors
UC	Ulcerative colitis
UCTD	Undifferentiated connective tissue disease
UACS	Upper airway cough syndrome
EGD	Upper endoscopy
UGIB	Upper GI bleed

UMN	Upper motor neuron
UA	Urinalysis
UTI	Urinary tract infection
UIP	Usual interstitial pneumonia
VZV	Varicella zoster virus
VIP	Vasoactive intestinal peptide
VDRL	Venereal Disease Research Laboratory
VAP	Ventilator-associated pneumonia
Vfib	Ventricular fibrillation
VSD	Ventricular septal defect
VT	Ventricular tachycardia
VTach	Ventricular tachycardia
VC	Vital capacity
VC	Volume control
vWD	von Willebrand disease
WBCs	White blood cells
WNV	West Nile virus

NOTES

Index

Tables and figures are indicated by an italic *t* and *f*, respectively, following the page number.

NOTES

NOTES